EMERGENCY IMAGING OF THE ACUTELY ILL OR INJURED CHILD

FOURTH EDITION

EMERGENCY IMAGING OF THE ACUTELY ILL OR INJURED CHILD

FOURTH EDITION

LEONARD E. SWISCHUK, M.D.

Professor of Radiology and Pediatrics
Director, Division of Pediatric Radiology
The University of Texas Medical Branch
Galveston, Texas

LIPPINCOTT WILLIAMS & WILKINS
A **Wolters Kluwer** Company

Philadelphia • Baltimore • New York • London
Buenos Aires • Hong Kong • Sydney • Tokyo

Acquisitions Editor: Beth Barry
Developmental Editor: Anjou K. Dargar
Production Editor: Janice G. Stangel
Manufacturing Manager: Colin Warnock
Cover Designer: Mark Lerner
Compositor: Lippincott Williams & Wilkins Desktop Division
Printer: Maple Vail Book Manufacturing Group

© 2000 by LIPPINCOTT WILLIAMS & WILKINS
530 Walnut Street
Philadelphia, PA 19106 USA
LWW.com

Printed in the USA

Library of Congress Cataloging-in-Publication Data

Swischuk, Leonard E., 1937-
  Emergency imaging of the acutely ill or injured child / Leonard E. Swischuk.—4th ed.
    p. ; cm.
  Includes bibliographical references and index.
  ISBN 0-683-30710-X
    1. Pediatric emergency imaging.   2. Pediatric emergencies.   I. Title.
  [DNLM: 1. Diagnostic Imaging—Child.   2. Emergency Medicine—methods—Child. WN
240 S978e 2000]
  RJ51.D5 S89 2000
  618.92′00754—dc21   00-020040

Care has been taken to confirm the accuracy of the information presented and to describe generally accepted practices. However, the author and publisher are not responsible for errors or omissions or for any consequences from application of the information in this book and make no warranty, expressed or implied, with respect to the currency, completeness, or accuracy of the contents of the publication. Application of this information in a particular situation remains the professional responsibility of the practitioner.

The author and publisher have exerted every effort to ensure that drug selection and dosage set forth in this text are in accordance with current recommendations and practice at the time of publication. However, in view of ongoing research, changes in government regulations, and the constant flow of information relating to drug therapy and drug reactions, the reader is urged to check the package insert for each drug for any change in indications and dosage and for added warnings and precautions. This is particularly important when the recommended agent is a new or infrequently employed drug.

Some drugs and medical devices presented in this publication have Food and Drug Administration (FDA) clearance for limited use in restricted research settings. It is the responsibility of the health care provider to ascertain the FDA status of each drug or device planned for use in their clinical practice.

10 9 8 7 6 5 4 3 2 1

To Janie, my wife and very best friend

CONTENTS

PREFACE TO THE FIRST EDITION

I have always enjoyed the challenge of emergency medicine, for the diseases encountered are varied, and the diagnosis usually must be accomplished promptly. While many of these diagnoses can be established with the history and physical examination, in other instances they are made with the aid of roentgenograms. It is this aspect of emergency medicine to which this book is devoted, and I have attempted to present material and concepts, which, over the years, have proven useful to me. In this regard, my aim was to outline general approaches to diagnostic problems, helpful rules of thumb, and specific diagnostic signs. Every so often, I felt it appropriate to delve more deeply into the pathophysiologic-roentgenographic correlations of certain diseases, but overall the main theme remained: how to approach a problem and then how to utilize the roentgenogram so as to have it yield the desired data.

The subject material in this book truly is "bread and butter" radiology, and I have tried to be as practical and clinical as possible. Most of the acute conditions commonly seen in the emergency room, outpatient clinic, or office practice have been covered, and in this regard, the main emphasis is on the evaluation of the initial films obtained. These films, of course, most often are plain films, and truly this is where the radiologist can excel. The radiologist must remain the expert on the plain film, for in spite of all of the new modalities and augmented diagnostic procedures available, the plain film remains the mainstay of the roentgenographic examination. As far as interpreting the roentgenogram, not only must one know all of the abnormal configurations encountered, but one also must be familiar with all of the normal variations which mimic pathology. In the pediatric age group, this is an especially significant problem in the skull, spine, and extremities. Because of this, I have included considerable material on normal variations causing problems, and as much as possible have placed this material next to the pathology which it mimics.

So many individuals have been of assistance to me during the time it took to write this book that it would be impossible to thank them all personally. There are many who have worked with me, many who have offered their material for inclusion, many who have offered constructive criticism, and many who have offered simple encouragement. I thank all of them, and to those who allowed me to use some of their material in this book, I offer special thanks and hope that I have assigned appropriate credit in every instance. I must also thank the various residents who have passed through the Department of Radiology here in Galveston, for all of them have been most helpful in the accumulation of material on a day-to-day basis. I hope that if they recognize a case they will take some satisfaction in seeing it being used to make a teaching point.

Two individuals, however, stand out so much that it is difficult for me to thank them enough. The first is my former secretary, Jonell Hoffman, and the second , our photographer, Milan Autengruber. Extra effort on their part became a routine daily task, and for this I am deeply indebted to both of them. I would also like to express my appreciation to Lester Murray, Mr. Autengruber's assistant; my former secretary, Cynthia Caldwell, who typed some of the early manuscript; and Donna Lofton in our Department of Medical Illustration for her assistance with the various drawings in this book. In addition, I must thank the radiology technicians who currently work for me and those who have worked for me in the past. There are too many of them to list individually, but all of them are exceptionally devoted, and needless to say, if they had not produced the roentgenograms I use, I would have nothing to illustrate with. My sincerest thanks to all of them.

I also would like to thank Dr. Robert N. Cooley, our former Chairman; and Dr. Melvyn H. Schreiber, our current Chairman, for their constant support for my various projects; and Dr. C. Keith Hayden, my very capable and helpful associate, for his daily physical and moral support. He has been of great assistance to me, and I express my sincerest appreciation to him.

Finally, I would like to express my gratitude to the Williams & Wilkins Company for their unfailing confidence and cooperation. More specifically, however, I am indebted to their astute Chief Radiology Editor, Ruby Richardson, for her perception of the tempo of medical publishing, and her overall flexibility and foresight have once again made it exceptionally easy and rewarding to compile a manuscript. She is a most dynamic and devoted individual whom I am fortunate to know and very pleased to call my friend.

Leonard E. Swischuk, M.D.

PREFACE

This edition of *Emergency Imaging of the Acutely Ill or Injured Child* preserves most of the material that has proven to be worthwhile over the years. There is, however, significant expansion regarding pulmonary infections, certain fractures, and areas relating to the cervical spine. I have also expanded ultrasound of the acute abdomen with new sections on mesenteric adenitis and appendicitis.

The overall content of this book focuses on entities and findings that differ from those seen in adults.

As in the previous edition, normal variations, comparative views, and plain films are stressed. I feel that this is very important as more sophisticated imaging modalities continue to take one's attention away from the plain film.

I am indebted to Carmen Floeck, my secretary, who once again was uniquely instrumental in putting this edition together. I would also like to thank her assistant, Thelma Sanchez, my photographer, John Ellis, and our computer graphics person, Victor Luciano. All of these people constitute a team essential to producing a quality edition of this book.

Leonard E. Swischuk, M.D.

LOWER RESPIRATORY TRACT INFECTION (PNEUMONIA, PNEUMONITIS, BRONCHITIS, AND BRONCHIOLITIS)

Most childhood lower respiratory tract infections are of viral etiology (respiratory syncytial virus, parainfluenza and influenza viruses, adenovirus) or caused by the viruslike organism *Mycoplasma pneumoniae* (1,6). Most of these infections show distinct seasonal variation, and most usually come in epidemics (1,3,6). Because of this, it is of some value to be aware of the "local virus going around the community." Knowledge of this type can aid in evaluating subsequent patients.

Bacterial lower respiratory tract infections show less seasonal variation and certainly are not prone to produce epidemics. Generally, bacterial infections result in airspace disease and hence pneumonia; viral lower respiratory tract infections usually produce a bronchitis or bronchiolitis and thus remain in the interstitial space. This also is true of *Chlamydia*, *Mycoplasma*, and pertussis infections. If consolidations are seen with the latter and with viral infections, they probably represent a pseudoconsolidation. In other words, they represent a disease process that produces intense interstitial inflammatory infiltration and edema, which causes compression of the alveoli. As a result, the involved portion of the lung appears to be consolidated, but it may be more appropriately termed a ***pseudoconsolidation*** (see Fig. 1.6).

Bacterial infections most often are caused by the following organisms: *Streptococcus pneumoniae*, *Staphylococcus aureus*, *Haemophilus influenzae*, and hemolytic *Streptococcus*. *S. pneumoniae* (typical lobar pneumonia) infections are generally more common in older children; *H. influenzae* infections tend to occur more commonly in infants and young children, those between the ages of 2 months and 3 years. *S. aureus* infections also are a little more common in infants and young children, but not to the same extent as *H. influenzae* infections. Currently, however, these latter infections are less common because of prophylactic vaccination programs. *M. pneumoniae* consolidative infections (probably interstitial pseudoconsolidations) are more common in older children and adolescents. These age-group categoriza-

tions, of course, are merely generalizations and are not intended to be used with too much specificity or rigidity.

In addition to these features, there has been increasing attention to the problem of persistent airway hyperreactivity after viral infection. This is especially likely to occur with respiratory syncytial virus–induced bronchiolitis in infants (4,5,7,9) but also is common with *M. pneumoniae* infections (8). Most studies seem to suggest that hyperreactivity results from the initial infection, but there is, of course, the question of whether these individuals have hyperreactive airways to begin with and then overrespond to the infection.

Clinically, over the years, I have found that the two most important items of clinical information in interpreting roentgenograms are the presence of high-grade fever (38–40 °C) and wheezing. In terms of fever, a high fever in the range of 39 to 40 °C (103 to 104 °F) should be present if a bacterial consolidative pneumonia is present. It is almost impossible to find a lesser fever, unless the patient has been treated with antipyretics. On the other hand, although low-grade fevers are the rule with lingering viral infections, in the early viremia stages fevers can be high but high fever alone with no respiratory-tract symptoms generally yields no positive radiographic findings (1,2).

With wheezing, discrimination between bacterial and viral or mycoplasma infections is easier. Wheezing is a hallmark of reactive airway disease, and if it is present, bacterial consolidation is not the cause. The cause, in these cases, is primary viral or mycoplasma infection or inherent reactive airway disease aggravated by superimposed viral or mycoplasma infections. This aspect of pulmonary infections is discussed in more detail in the section on asthma.

Finally, it might be of some value to *review terminology used to describe pulmonary infections in children.* Certainly there is no problem with consolidation, for it infers alveolar, airspace disease. A problem arises, however, if "consolidation" also is used generically to describe atelectasis. It is best if one can avoid this, for atelectasis is associated with volume loss but consolidative pneumonia is not. Consolidation usually produces little, if any, volume loss and infers the presence of alveolar or airspace disease (Fig. 1.1A). A less common pattern of no volume loss airspace disease is that of patchy, fluffy alveolar infiltrates

Emergency Imaging of the Acutely Ill or Injured Child

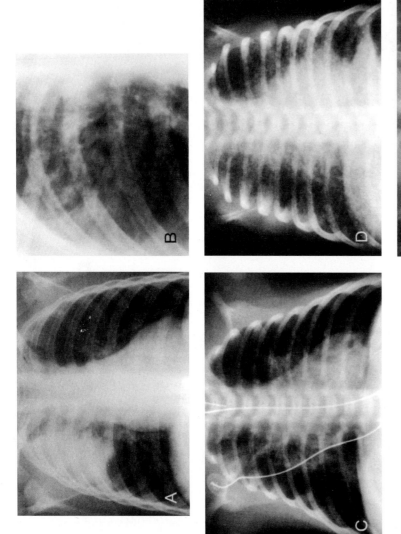

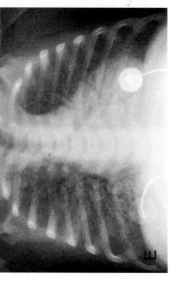

FIGURE 1.1. *Terminology in lower respiratory tract infections.* Pneumonia infers an alveolar process that can manifest in lobar consolidation **(A)** or patchy, fluffy, somewhat nodular infiltrates **(B)**. Bronchitis—peribronchitis infers an interstitial disease process that manifests in thickening of the bronchial walls and peribronchial tissues, resulting in a pattern of perihilar streaky radiations **(C)**. Pneumonitis infers an interstitial disease process, usually viral in origin, that can manifest in diffuse reticulonodularity **(D)** or diffuse haziness of the lungs **(E)**.

(Fig. 1.1B). Perihilar–peribronchial infiltrates (Fig. 1.1C) are synonymous with bronchitis and peribronchitis and infer that the disease process is interstitial (viral or mycoplasma).

If viral infections involve the lung parenchyma beyond the immediate peribronchial space, they still are confined to the interstitium. In such cases, reticulonodular or diffusely hazy lungs can be seen (Fig. 1.1D and E) and *the term "pneumonitis" rather than "pneumonia" is preferred.* Pneumonitis, although a generic term, customarily infers an interstitial, rather than an alveolar inflammatory process.

In summary, then, consolidation is equated with alveolar pneumonia, peribilar–peribronchial infiltration with bronchitis or peribronchitis, and reticulonodular or diffusely hazy infiltrates with an interstitial pneumoni- *tis (Fig. 1.1). It is best not to use the confusing and basically meaningless term "bronchopneumonia."*

REFERENCES

1. Bramson RT, Meyer TL, Silbiger ML, Blickman JG, Halpern E. The futility of the chest radiograph in the febrile infant without respiratory symptoms. *Pediatrics* 1993;92:524–526.
2. Crain EF, Bulas D, Bijur PE, Goldman HS. Is a chest radiograph necessary in the evaluation of every febrile infant less than 8 weeks of age? *Pediatrics* 1991;88:821–824.
3. Glezen WB, Denny FW. Epidemiology of acute lower respiratory disease in children. *N Engl J Med* 1973;288:498–505.
4. Gurwitz D, Mindorff C, Levison H. Increased incidence of bronchial reactivity in children with a history of bronchiolitis. *J Pediatr* 1981;98:551–555.

5. Horn MEC, Reed SE, Taylor P. Role of viruses and bacteria in acute wheezy bronchitis in childhood: A study of sputum. *Arch Dis Child* 1979;54:587–592.
6. Mufson MA, Krause HE, Mocega HE, Dawson FW. Viruses, Mycoplasma pneumoniae and bacteria associated with lower respiratory tract disease among infants. *Am J Epidemiol* 1970;91: 192–202.
7. Rooney JC, Williams HE. Relationship between proved viral bronchiolitis and subsequent wheezing. *J Pediatr* 1971;79:744–747.
8. Sabato AR, Martin AJ, Marmion BP, Kok TW, Cooper DM. Mycoplasma pneumoniae: Acute illness, antibiotics, and subsequent pulmonary function. *Arch Dis Child* 1984;59:1034–1037.
9. Stokes GM, Milner AD, Hodges IGC, Groggins RC. Lung function abnormalities after acute bronchiolitis. *J Pediatr* 1981;98: 871–874.

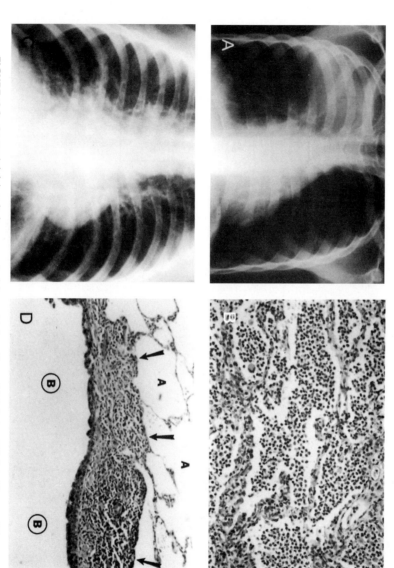

FIGURE 1.2. *Bacterial (alveolar) versus viral bronchial-peribronchial (interstitial) infiltrate.* **(A)** Typical homogeneous bacterial consolidations in the right upper lobes. **(B)** Histologic material in alveolar pneumonia demonstrating the alveoli to be completely full of cells and exudate. **(C)** Typical viral interstitial, bronchitic-peribronchitic pattern of infiltration, with streaky infiltrates radiating along the bronchovascular sheaths out toward the periphery of the lung. **(D)** Histologic material from a patient with viral bronchitis-peribronchitis, demonstrating that the inflammatory reaction, composed primarily of lymphocytes, lies in the immediate peribronchial area (*arrows*). The alveoli (A) are clear. *B, bronchus.*

BASIC ROENTGENOGRAPHIC PATTERNS OF LOWER RESPIRATORY TRACT INFECTION

Introduction

In infants and children it usually is possible to differentiate viral from bacterial infection (3,17,18). This is possible because of the basic underlying differences in pathophysiology between the two types of infection. As noted previously, bacterial infection involves the alveolar airspace (consolidating pneumonia) and viral infection involves the bronchial and peribronchial tissues, resulting in a bronchitis (Fig. 1.2). If no other factors were involved, differentiation between the two types of infection would be relatively simple, but unfortunately atelectasis enters the picture with viral infections. Atelectasis may be segmental or lobar and, if not handled correctly, can lead to erroneous roentgenographic interpretations. On the other hand, if atelectasis is handled correctly, differentiation between the two types of infection is more likely (10,16–18). *Therefore, it is the problem of atelectasis, and how it is managed and interpreted, that becomes the most significant factor in the analysis of chest roentgenograms in infants and children with lower respiratory tract infection.* As the child becomes older and passes into adulthood, all of this becomes less of a problem, because the perihilar-peribronchial pattern fails to materialize and atelectasis is far less common.

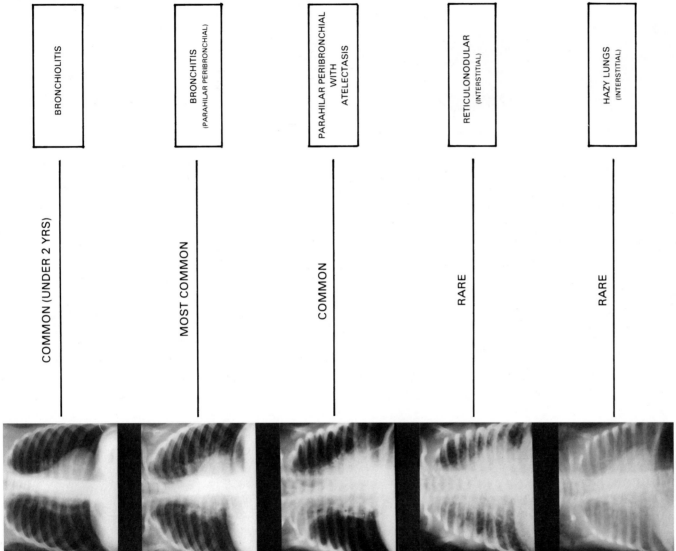

BRONCHIOLITIS

COMMON (UNDER 2 YRS)

BRONCHITIS
(PARAHILAR PERIBRONCHIAL)

MOST COMMON

PARAHILAR PERIBRONCHIAL
WITH
ATELECTASIS

COMMON

RETICULONODULAR
(INTERSTITIAL)

RARE

HAZY LUNGS
(INTERSTITIAL)

RARE

FIGURE 1.3. *Viral lower respiratory tract infection: basic roentgenographic patterns.* Any virus can produce a number of interstitial roentgenographic patterns. The bronchitic spectrum ranges from the often infiltrate-free but overaerated lungs of bronchiolitis through typical perihilar–peribronchial infiltrates. Atelectasis is common and may be segmental or lobar. Less commonly diffuse reticulonodular interstitial infiltrates occur and, equally rarely, one may see diffusely hazy lungs resulting from interstitial parenchymal involvement. The pattern of perihilar–peribronchial infiltration is the most common.

The Viral Spectrum

Any viral infection of the lower respiratory tract can produce roentgenographic patterns ranging from the overinflated, infiltrate-free lungs seen with many cases of bronchiolitis, through perihilar–peribronchial infiltrates with or without atelectasis, to the less commonly seen reticulonodular infiltrates, or hazy lungs (Fig. 1.3). Overall, however, the most common pattern is that of perihilar–peribronchial infiltration, attesting to the fact that these infections are basically airway (i.e., tracheobronchial) infections. Consequently, they result in bronchitis and peribronchitis, rather than an alveolar, consolidative pneumonia.

Roentgenographically, so-called perihilar–peribronchial infiltration results in prominent and "dirty" perihilar regions (Fig. 1.4A). The prominent hilar regions result in part from inflammation of the bronchial walls and peribronchial tissues (2,11) and in part from associated hilar adenopathy. Because of the extreme variability of adenopathy, some children present with well-circumscribed and enlarged lymph nodes (Fig. 1.4), but others show no discrete adenopathy but, rather, a generalized increase in density and raggedness of the perihilar areas (Fig. 1.2C). In addition, in some cases the perihilar–peribronchial infiltrates coalesce to form a more homogeneous perihilar pattern of density (Fig. 1.5). This configuration should not be misinterpreted for airspace consolidative disease: It is another example of pseudoconsolidation seen with intense interstitial disease and viral or *M. pneumoniae* infections. This is important because air bronchograms frequently are seen within these infiltrates. In

all these cases the most important thing to remember is that the infiltrates are bilateral and symmetric and have a central, perihilar predominance.

Air trapping also is a common feature of viral lower respiratory tract infections, because thickening and edema of the bronchial and peribronchial tissues predispose the individual to more than normal narrowing of the airways during expiration. In addition, reactive bronchospasm is present, accentuating the basic problem of air trapping. Such air trapping often is most pronounced in cases of bronchiolitis and also is a greater problem in children with asthma and patients with hyperreactive airway disease.

Clinically, infants and young children with viral infections usually present with a cough, tachypnea, and a generally "miserable" picture of 2 or 3 days' duration. They look sick and feel sick. In addition, upper-airway infection in the form of croup, or at least a croupy cough, nasal congestion, and coryza are common. Most of these children, however, do not require hospitalization, especially if they are older. Actually, what it amounts to is that they have an old-fashioned chest cold with a low-grade fever. Oral temperatures seldom exceed 103 °F in these patients, although children younger than 2 years of age may have higher temperatures. This is especially true in the early viremic stage of these infections, in which fevers may be as high as 104 °F or 39 to 40 °C. *Therefore, fever alone cannot be used as a discriminator in differentiating bacterial from viral infections.*

On auscultation, the lungs in these patients frequently are very noisy and "juicy." Although many of these noises are transmitted upper-airway sounds, true rales, rhonchi, and

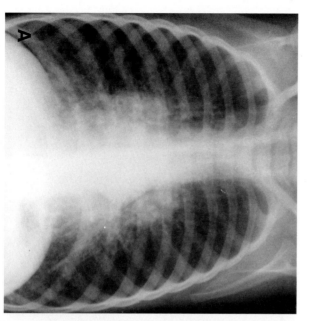
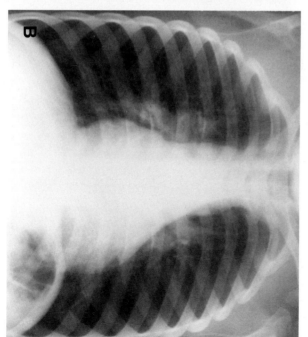

FIGURE 1.4. *Viral perihilar–peribronchial infiltrates with adenopathy.* **(A)** Note the prominent hilar regions and extensive bilateral perihilar–peribronchial infiltrates radiating outward into the periphery. **(B)** In this patient, hilar adenopathy is more easily seen and perihilar infiltrates are minimal.

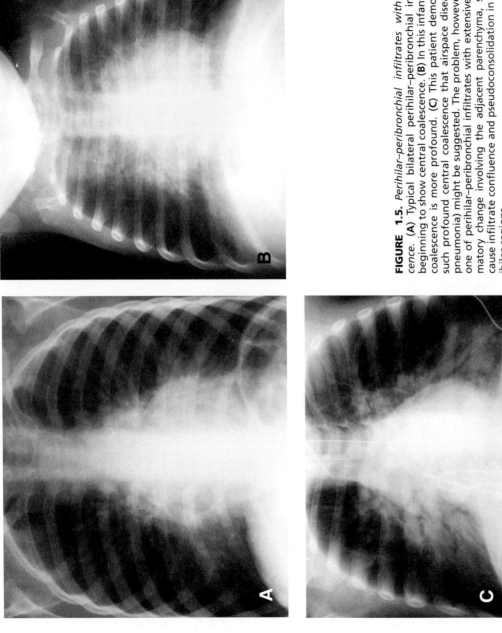

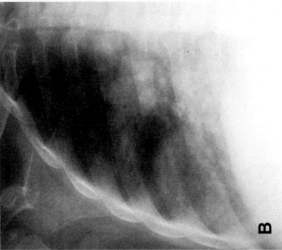

FIGURE 1.5. *Perihilar–peribronchial infiltrates with coalescence.* **(A)** Typical bilateral perihilar–peribronchial infiltrates beginning to show central coalescence. **(B)** In this infant central coalescence is more profound. **(C)** This patient demonstrates such profound central coalescence that airspace disease (i.e., pneumonia) might be suggested. The problem, however, still is one of perihilar–peribronchial infiltrates with extensive inflammatory change involving the adjacent parenchyma, so as to cause infiltrate confluence and pseudoconsolidation in the perihilar regions.

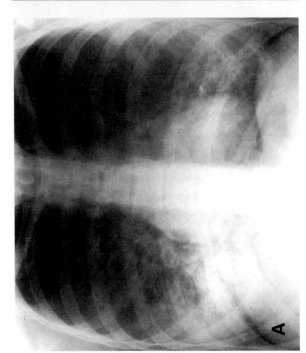

FIGURE 1.6. *Viral pneumonitis: pseudoconsolidation.* **(A)** In this patient there is basal distribution of diffuse hazy, almost opaque infiltrates. **(B)** Older infant with influenza pneumonitis producing a pseudoconsolidation pattern in the right lower and middle lobes.

wheezes also can be heard. These sounds are variable from moment to moment and generally correlate poorly with any attempts to match them, lobe for lobe, with positive roentgenographic findings. The reason for this is that most of the sounds result from incomplete and fleeting obstructions of the airways caused by mucous plugs and bronchospasm, but most of the densities on the chest film represent areas of atelectasis with no airflow, and hence no noise.

If parenchymal involvement occurs with viral lower respiratory tract infection, it usually is widespread and interstitial. Indeed, true alveolar airspace consolidations proba-

bly do not exist. On the other hand, atelectasis is a common problem and frequently is misinterpreted as consolidative pneumonia. If consolidations are seen, they probably are "pseudoconsolidations," resulting from intense interstitial infiltration and edema (8) causing compression of the alveoli (Fig. 1.6). The same phenomenon can occur on a diffuse basis throughout both lungs (Fig. 1.7). Adenoviral infections (4,12,13) have a propensity to produce these pseudoconsolidations, but any virus can be the cause. In addition, *M. pneumoniae* infections can produce this type of infiltrate. Adenoviral infection often is complicated by necrotiz-

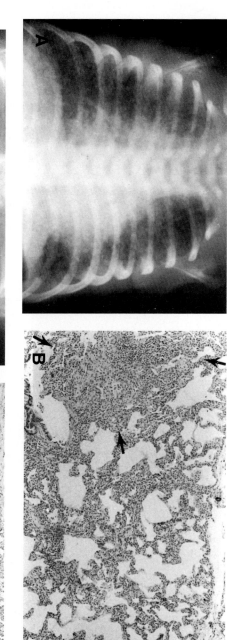

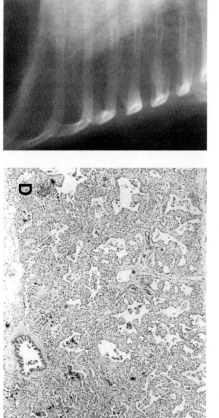

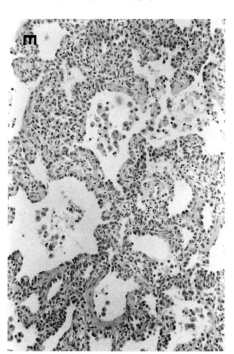

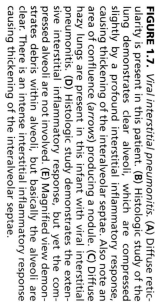

FIGURE 1.7. *Viral interstitial pneumonitis.* (A) Diffuse reticularity is present in this patient. (B) Histologic study of the lung demonstrates clear alveoli, which are compressed slightly by a profound interstitial inflammatory response, causing thickening of the interalveolar septae. Also note an area of confluence (*arrows*) producing a nodule. (C) Diffuse hazy lungs are present in this infant with viral interstitial pneumonitis. (D) Histologic study demonstrates the extensive interstitial inflammatory response, but yet the compressed alveoli are not involved. (E) Magnified view demonstrates debris within alveoli, but basically the alveoli are clear. There is an intense interstitial inflammatory response causing thickening of the interalveolar septae.

ing bronchiolitis and pulmonary hemorrhage; in that case the apparent consolidations become more dense. Hantavirus infection (9) also has a propensity to do this.

The most common pattern of pulmonary infiltration with viral disease is that of streaky or reticular infiltrates, radiating outward from the hilar regions. This pattern leads to the typical perihilar–peribronchial configuration of bronchitis and peribronchitis and, if pronounced, to the "shaggy" heart. This latter phenomenon was described first with pertussis infection but actually is much more common with viral or *M. pneumoniae* infections. With pertussis infection, the reason the shaggy heart is seen is that, just as with viruses, the infection is a bronchitis and not a peripheral alveolar infection. A similar phenomenon occurs with *Chlamydia*

infections, which also are bronchial or peribronchial infiltrative patterns. Typical perihilar–peribronchial infiltrative patterns seen with viral lower respiratory tract infection are presented in Figs. 1.2–1.5.

In other cases of viral lower respiratory tract infection, less commonly, widespread reticulonodularity or diffuse haziness of the lungs is seen (Fig. 1.7). In some of these cases, the pattern of haziness involves both lungs in their entirety; in others, the findings tend to be more pronounced in the lung bases (Fig. 1.6). The latter tends to occur with entities such as desquamative interstitial pneumonitis and similar pneumonitides.

At the other end of the spectrum of viral lower respiratory tract infection is the young infant with bronchiolitis.

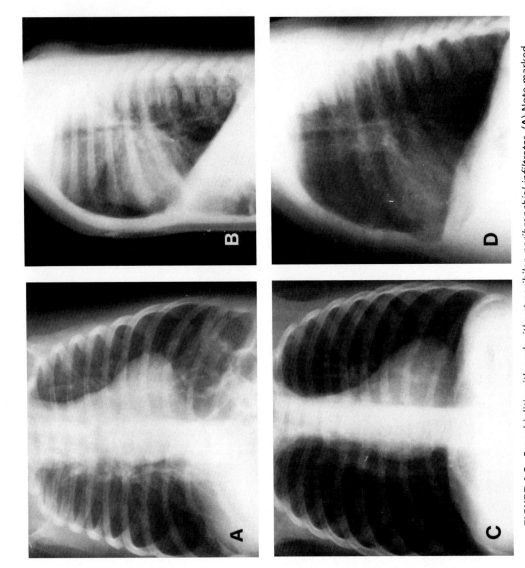

FIGURE 1.8. *Bronchiolitis with and without perihilar–peribronchial infiltrates.* **(A)** Note marked overaeration of both lungs and some perihilar–peribronchial infiltration. **(B)** Lateral view showing marked depression and flattening of the diaphragmatic leaflets secondary to overaeration. In the upper retrosternal area, note how the marked degree of overaeration has caused the thymus gland to separate from the heart. **(C)** In this infant, note that even though there is considerable overaeration, there is minimal, if any, perihilar infiltration. **(D)** Lateral view shows marked overaeration, with a characteristically bell-shaped chest and markedly depressed and flattened diaphragmatic leaflets.

Bronchiolitis is a distinct clinicoroentgenographic entity that usually, but not exclusively, is caused by respiratory syncytial virus. Its incidence peaks at around 6 months of age, but it is common in infants up to 2 years of age. As with all viral infections, perihilar–peribronchial infiltrates and areas of lobar and segmental atelectasis may be seen in these infants (14,15), but many show surprisingly clear chests (Fig. 1.8). Pronounced overaeration as a result of air trapping always is present in bronchiolitis and to be sure is the hallmark of this disease. It leads to severe respiratory distress, and clinically these infants show marked dyspnea, tachypnea, air hunger, paroxysmal coughing, and cyanosis. Fine rales may be heard at the end of inspiration and in early expiration, and in most infants expiratory wheezes are present. Unlike the wheezes in asthma, however, they do not dissipate significantly if epinephrine is administered. Bronchiolar inflammation and expiratory constriction play havoc with the already normally narrow bronchioles in these young infants, and peripheral air trapping becomes pronounced. *Simply speaking, the chests in these infants are "frozen" in deep inspiration, and they do not move air. They are sick, but not toxic.*

Some infants may have multiple bouts of bronchiolitis, and if this occurs, it is important to consider the possibility of underlying asthma or cystic fibrosis, for *it is not unusual for infants with these diseases to first present with what appear to be repeated or especially severe and refractory bouts of bronchiolitis.* Finally, it should be noted that the roentgenographic picture of severe overaeration in bronchiolitis also can be mimicked by centrally obstructing lesions such as vascular rings and mediastinal masses and cysts, and by severe dehydration and acidosis. Acidosis leads to an increase in respiratory rate and diaphragmatic excursion (to blow off excess carbon dioxide), and the low blood volume resulting from the dehydration leads to a diminution in caliber of the pulmonary blood vessels and pulmonary oligemia. Together these findings result in lungs that appear overaerated and underperfused (see Fig. 1.150), a picture virtually indistinguishable from that seen with bronchiolitis, where the lungs are infiltrate-free. Clinical correlation, however, usually quickly deciphers the situation and correctly identifies the problem.

Atelectasis abounds with viral lower respiratory tract infection. It can be segmental or lobar and is much more common than focal obstructive emphysema. Unfortunately, it frequently is misinterpreted as a consolidating pneumonia. It is in such cases that *it should be remembered that roentgenograms are for interpreting and patients for treating.* In other words, if the patient appears to have a relatively mild infection, and the radiographs erroneously suggest that consolidation is present, one should reassess the situation. *The findings should not be discarded but merely reassessed.* If this is done, it becomes apparent that what first was thought to be a consolidation most likely is just atelectasis.

Atelectasis and focal emphysema result from bronchial obstruction secondary to mucosal inflammation, endobronchial secretions, and underlying mucous plugs (15). In any given case, the radiographic picture can be most misleading Figs. 1.9 and 1.10). Areas of segmental atelectasis, in particular, have a propensity to mimic pneumonia and distract one's attention from the real problem. This hardly can be avoided, for often it is truly difficult to be sure that only atelectasis is the problem (Fig. 1.11). If the suspected infiltrates are streaky, linear, or wedgelike, however, the problem is segmental atelectasis (Fig. 1.12). In such cases, if one still is not confident enough to withhold antibiotics, it should be realized that if they are prescribed and the infiltrates clear in just a day or two, it is not because of unusually rapid clearing of the presumed pneumonia but rather because of the dislodging of atelectasis-producing mucous plugs (Fig. 1.13). **Once this phenomenon is appreciated, it becomes easier to understand why some children with viral lower respiratory tract infections seem to show most abnormal and disturbing roentgenographic findings in the face of surprisingly mild symptoms.** The reason for this is that they do not really have pneumonia, as the roentgenograms might at first erroneously suggest. Their basic problem is bronchitis with perihilar–peribronchial infiltrates; it just happens that the multiple areas of lobar and segmental atelectasis confuse the issue by mimicking alveolar consolidation. Such atelectasis is common in infants and children with viral lower respiratory tract infections, including bronchiolitis (16), and occurs because of inefficiency of the collateral air-drift phenomenon occurring through the ducts of Lambert and the pores of Kohn (5). In infants, this mechanism is not as well developed as in adults, and so areas of atelectasis tend to persist. If a major bronchus is plugged by mucus, and the entire lobe collapses, the findings often are easier to assess (Fig. 1.14). On the other hand, in some of these cases, the findings still may be puzzling, for obstructive emphysema rather than atelectasis occurs (Fig. 1.15).

Volume loss is not a prominent feature of acute consolidating pneumonia, for it is only when the pneumonia is healing and contracting (10 days or so later) that significant volume loss occurs. In the acute stages, volume loss usually is minimal (Fig. 1.16). With acute consolidating pneumonia, there is no reason for volume loss to occur, for there is no proximal airway obstruction. Consolidations begin in the periphery of a lobe and work inward. Air in the alveoli slowly is replaced by purulent exudate, the alveoli do not collapse, and volume loss is negligible. This is not so true of the right middle lobe and lingula, in which some volume loss might be suggested (Fig. 1.16E and F). These lobes are smaller than the other lobes of the lungs, and thus the minor degree of volume loss that occurs appears more pronounced than it does in the larger upper and lower lobes. Overall, however, if vol-

Emergency Imaging of the Acutely Ill or Injured Child

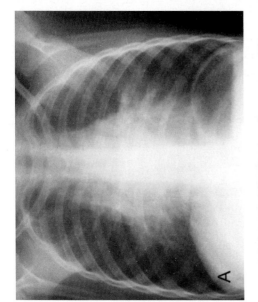

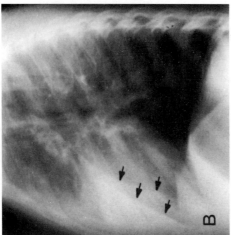

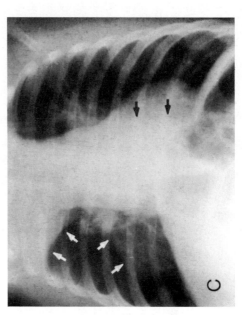

FIGURE 1.10. *Viral bronchitis–peribronchitis with multilobar atelectasis.* **(A)** Note bilateral perihilar–peribronchial infiltrates and haziness along the right and left cardiac borders. **(B)** Lateral view demonstrates that this results from atelectasis of the right middle lobe and lingula (*arrows*). **(C)** Another patient with bilateral perihilar–peribronchial infiltrates and atelectasis of the right upper and lower lobes (*arrows on the right*). In addition, note increased density behind the left side of the heart (*arrows*), resulting from partial atelectasis of the left lower lobe.

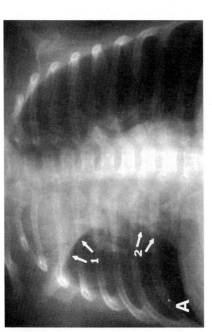

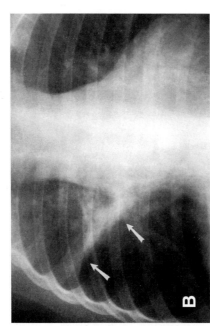

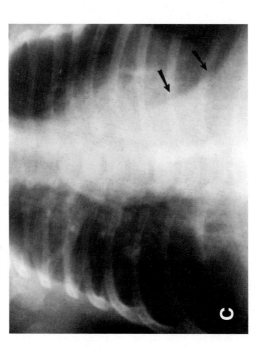

FIGURE 1.9. *Viral bronchitis with lobar atelectasis.* **(A)** Typical configuration of right upper-lobe atelectasis with elevation of the minor fissure (*1*). Medial displacement of the major fissure (*2*) signifies the presence of right lower-lobe atelectasis. Note that the right hemithorax shows considerable volume loss. **(B)** Partial right upper-lobe atelectasis leading to elevation of the minor fissure (*arrows*). **(C)** Classic left lower-lobe atelectasis producing a triangular density behind the heart (*arrows*). Partial atelectasis is present in the right upper and right lower lobes.

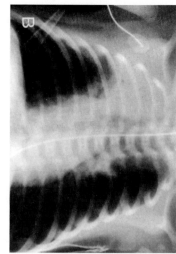

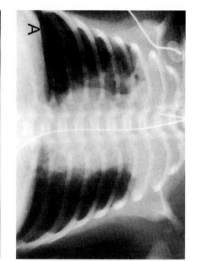

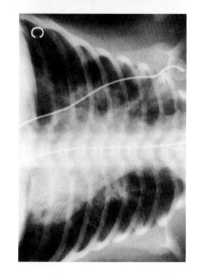

FIGURE 1.11. *Shifting atelectasis masquerading as lobar consolidation.* **(A)** This patient had respiratory syncytial virus infection with typical bilateral perihilar–peribronchial infiltrates. The densities in both upper lobes easily could be misinterpreted as consolidating pneumonias. **(B)** On the next day, however, the left upper-lobe density has disappeared. Clearly this was because of atelectasis. Note that there is a shift of the mediastinum to the right, emphasizing that the problem in the right upper lobe is one of volume loss and, hence, atelectasis. The next day the marked degree of right upper-lobe atelectasis has resolved. Only a minimal degree remains, and typical bilateral perihilar–peribronchial infiltrates, with scattered wedges of segmental atelectasis consistent with a viral bronchitis–peribronchitis, are seen. One must be careful not to misinterpret such lobar atelectasis, which is quite common, for consolidating pneumonia.

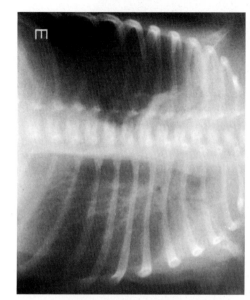

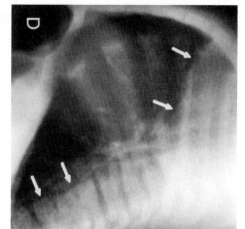

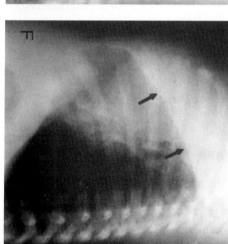

FIGURE 1.10. *(continued)* **(D)** Lateral view demonstrates the right upper-lobe atelectasis (*upper arrows*) and increased density (*arrows*) over the lower thoracic vertebrae, resulting from the bilateral lower-lobe atelectasis. Normally the vertebrae become blacker as one progresses downward along the thoracic spine. **(E)** Another patient with a bizarre chest configuration consisting of marked overaeration of the lungs and densities in both upper lobes (*arrows*). **(F)** Lateral view demonstrates these to be due to atelectasis of the right upper and middle lobes and lingula (*arrows*).

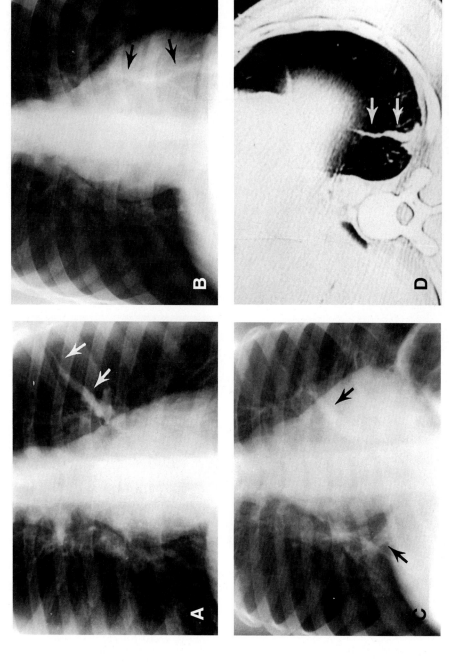

FIGURE 1.12. *Segmental atelectasis: varying configurations.* **(A)** Linear streak of atelectasis *(arrows)* in the left upper lobe. **(B)** Another patient with vertical segmental (discoid) atelectasis *(arrows)*. **(C)** In this patient bilateral areas of segmental atelectasis are seen *(arrows)*. Underlying is a baseline perihilar–peribronchial infiltrate pattern. **(D)** Computed tomographic study demonstrating classic segmental atelectasis *(arrows)*.

ume loss is significant, atelectasis should be favored, and if multilobar involvement is present, atelectasis is more likely. To be sure, multilobar consolidation is far less common than multilobar atelectasis. Finally, it should be noted that pleural effusions are rare with viral infections and usually occur in infants younger than 30 days of age or patients with HIV infection or another immunodeficient state.

Lobar Consolidation– Bacterial Disease

Lobar consolidations most commonly are the result of *S. pneumonia* or *H. influenzae* infections, the latter being more common in infants younger than 2 or 3 years old. *H. influenzae* infections, however, now are less common because of prophylactic vaccination programs. *M. pneumoniae* and *S. aureus* are less common causes and consolida-

tions secondary to infections with *Klebsiella, Pseudomonas,* and other such species generally are rare. *M. pneumoniae* consolidations tend to occur in older children (6). Viral consolidations, if they exist at all, are uncommon, except perhaps in the perinatal period and in immunologically compromised patients. Actually these probably are interstitial pseudoconsolidations, and the same probably occurs with *M. pneumoniae* infections. Fungal infections also can produce consolidations, with or without effusions or empyemas, and of course are more common in endemic areas.

Clinically, patients with bacterial *S. pneumonia* or other lobar consolidations present with abrupt onset of fever (usually 103 °F or greater measured orally), lassitude, malaise, and cough. Auscultatory–roentgenographic correlation, as opposed to that with viral bronchitis, is good, and roentgenograms usually confirm the location of the clinically suspected pneumonia (Fig. 1.16). The appearance of the pneumonia can range from a small peripheral

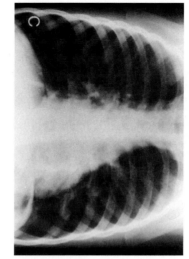
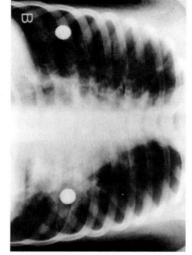
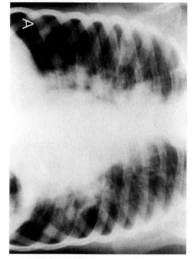

FIGURE 1.13. *Bronchitis with perihilar–peribronchial infiltrates and patchy atelectasis.* (**A**) Note extensive bilateral perihilar–peribronchial infiltrates with a predominantly central distribution. Centrally, the peribronchial inflammatory process has become a little more confluent because of peribronchial edema. Also note scattered densities in almost every lobe, resulting from areas of segmental atelectasis. (**B**) Eighteen hours later, after the patient was treated in a humidifying tent and given antibiotics (unnecessarily given because of misinterpretation of the findings as bacterial disease), considerable improvement has occurred and a more typical pattern of perihilar–peribronchial infiltration is evolving. Areas of segmental atelectasis remain in both lower lobes. (**C**) Thirty-six hours after the first roentgenogram, the original changes have resolved almost totally. A residual pattern of perihilar–peribronchial infiltration with a few typical linear or wedge-like areas of segmental atelectasis in the lower lobes is all that remains. The original pattern of profound perihilar–peribronchial infiltration with numerous superimposed areas of scattered segmental atelectasis most often is misinterpreted as widespread bacterial pneumonia. The central predominance, however, as seen in **A**, is the key to proper diagnosis. Furthermore, no bacterial infection would clear this quickly, and even though antibiotics are frequently administered in these cases, they should not be credited for the rapid clearance of what initially was misinterpreted as widespread bacterial pneumonia. Widespread bacterial pneumonia has a different appearance and is demonstrated in Fig. 1.20D.

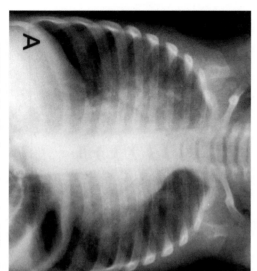
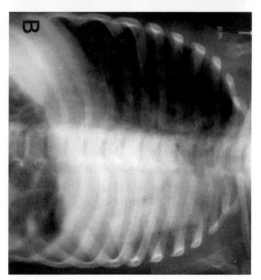

FIGURE 1.14. *Massive atelectasis, shifting from side to side with viral lower respiratory tract infection.* (**A**) Note perihilar–peribronchial infiltrates and what would appear to be a consolidation in the right upper lobe. (**B**) The next day, the apparent consolidation is gone and the entire right lung is clear, attesting to the fact that the problem was atelectasis. Now, however, the left lung has collapsed. The problem in cases such as this is the presence of obstructive and shifting mucous plugs.

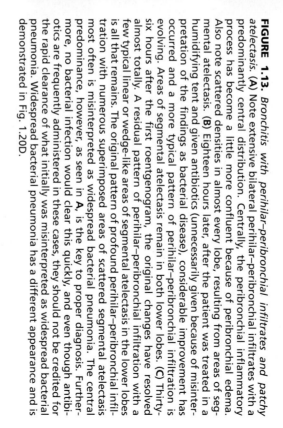

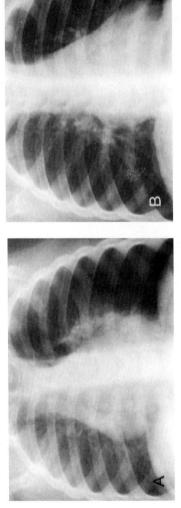

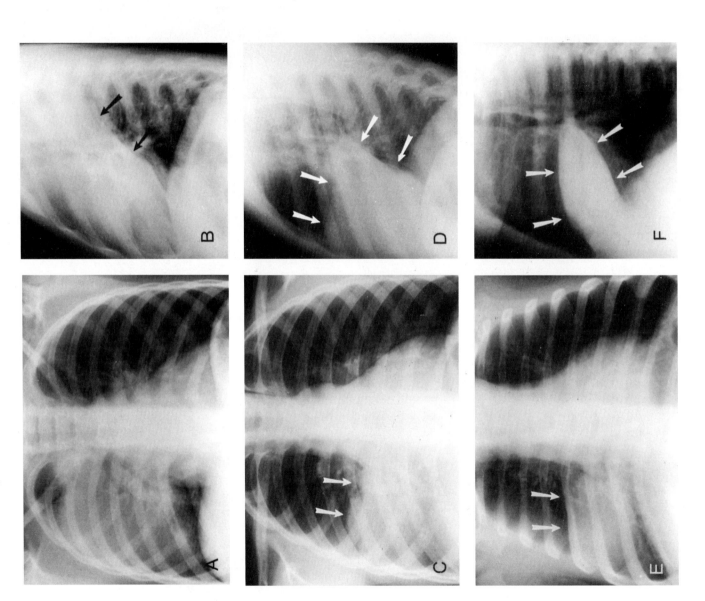

FIGURE 1.15. *Viral bronchitis–peribronchitis with lobar emphysema.* **(A)** In this patient with perihilar–peribronchial infiltrates, note that the left lung is overdistended, hyperlucent, and, in fact, large. This was because of an obstructing mucous plug. **(B)** The next day, with the plug coughed up, only bilateral perihilar–peribronchial infiltrates remain, but there is still some hyperlucency of the left lung.

14

infiltrate to a completely consolidated lobe, and its size depends on the age of the pneumonia (Fig. 1.17). The peripheral origin is important to note, for lobar atelectasis does not begin peripherally, and thus it would be most unusual for atelectasis to present as a peripheral density, as seen in Fig. 1.17A.

Multilobar consolidations also can occur (Fig. 1.18). They can be seen in otherwise completely normal children but also have a definite propensity to occur in infants with prior viral bronchitis and children with underlying sickle cell disease. In the latter patients, it is not clear whether pulmonary venoocclusive disease predisposes to the infection, but multilobar pneumonia is quite common in these patients and in fact may go on to rapidly involve almost all of the parenchyma of both lungs. Consolidations of an entire lung (i.e., totally opaque hemithorax) are rare (Fig. 1.18), and although they do occur, most often if a unilateral hemithorax is totally opacified, the problem is empyema (see Fig. 1.57). A less common pattern of alveolar consolidation is the one in which the infiltrates are soft and patchy or nodular. These may be localized to one lobe or they may be diffuse (Fig. 1.19). They also are seen with fungal disease.

Finally, one or two pitfalls in the interpretation of roentgenograms in patients suspected of having consolidating pneumonia should be borne in mind. The most important of these deals with the patient in whom a chest roentgenogram is obtained early in the course of the disease. *In such cases, because of the usual delay of up to 12 hours from the onset of symptoms to the appearance of a roentgenographically demonstrable infiltrate, the roentgenogram can be normal.* Clinically, however, fever, cough, and decreased air entry in the involved lobe usually are clearly apparent, but because the roentgenogram appears normal, one may be taken aback by the situation. At the other end of the spectrum, it is equally important to note that it is not uncommon for auscultation to fail to detect a well-developed lobar pneumonia that turns out to be present roentgenographically. These cases represent instances of advanced consolidation, and most likely breath sounds from the adjacent normal lung are so well transmitted through the consolidated lobe that they sound normal on cursory auscultation.

FIGURE 1.16. *Consolidating pneumonia (bacterial infection): various lobes.* **(A)** Note extensive consolidation, with clear-cut air bronchograms in the right upper and middle lobes. There is no significant volume loss, and the right lung is of normal size. **(B)** Lateral view demonstrating the same consolidations. Again, note that there is no volume loss and that the major fissure (arrows) is in its normal position. **(C)** Classic right middle-lobe consolidation in another patient. Note again that there is no volume loss and that the minor fissure (arrows) is in its normal place. **(D)** Lateral view also demonstrates that the minor and major fissures (arrows) are in their normal place and, hence, that there is no volume loss. **(E)** Another patient with a right middle-lobe consolidation with the minor fissure (arrows) in its normal place. **(F)** On lateral view, however, there is some volume loss of the right middle lobe (arrows). This occurs primarily with the right middle lobe and lingula, for both are smaller than the upper and lower lobes, and thus even mild degrees of volume loss tend to be exaggerated. Obviously, clinical correlation is important in these latter cases, but in all of the cases, note that even though one or two lobes are completely consolidated, the remainder of the ipsilateral and the entire contralateral lung remain completely clear. In addition, note that there are no perihilar-peribronchial infiltrates.

Mixed Viral and Bacterial Infections

With the approach outlined and with practice, one usually can determine whether an infection is of viral or bacterial origin from the roentgenograms alone (16,17). Problems in interpretation usually do not arise unless the typical perihilar-peribronchial infiltrates are associated with peripheral alveolar infiltrates. The problem, then, is to decide whether these infiltrates result from atelectasis or consolidation, and no matter how experienced one becomes, certain cases remain indeterminate (17). A greater number remains indeterminate if one deals poorly or in a negative fashion with atelectasis and, of course, if one deals infrequently with pediatric roentgenograms.

If mixed infections occur, seldom if ever is there a viral infection the aftermath of a previous bacterial infection. It is the reverse that occurs: a viral infection first and then a bacterial infection. Clinically these patients, for the better part of a week, usually have signs and symptoms of a viral infection and then rather abruptly become quite sick and toxic. This is an important clinical clue and should signal the need for clinical reassessment and another chest roentgenogram.

There is good reason for this sequence of events to occur, for it has been shown that with viral infections bronchial mucosal inflammation and edema, along with increased mucus secretion and bronchospasm, lead to poor tracheobronchial toilet (7). This is further aggravated by impaired ciliary cleansing action (1,12) and overall stagnation and impaired ventilation result. Under such circumstances, chances of pathogenic bacterial growth becoming established are increased, and pneumonia is more likely to develop. If white blood cell counts are obtained in these patients, the original lymphocytosis seen with viral infections changes to an increase in neutrophils, with a concomitant left shift and increase in bands.

If one is dealing with a viral infection and a superimposed bacterial infection, the roentgenograms may be quite confusing. One of the reasons for this is that there is a background of typical viral, perihilar-peribronchial infiltration with or without areas of segmental or lobar atelectasis, and yet a consolidation also is present. In such cases, if the infiltrate in

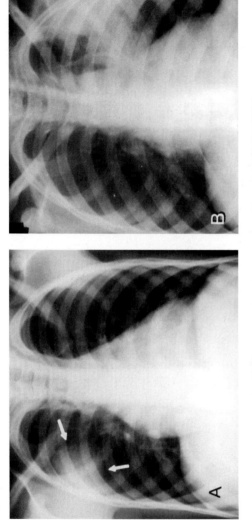

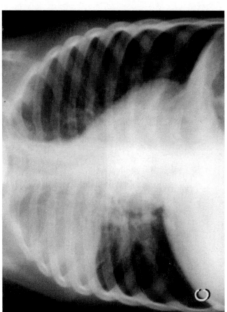

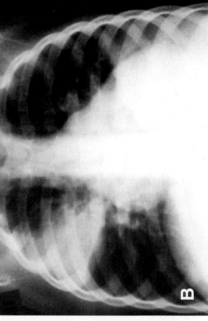

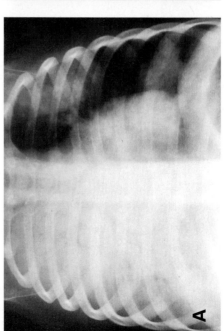

FIGURE 1.17. *Consolidating pneumonia: different stages of development.* **(A)** Note characteristic peripheral location of an early consolidating pneumonia in the right upper lobe (*arrows*). **(B)** Another patient demonstrating a more advanced consolidation in the left upper lobe. The consolidation, however, still is more dense in the periphery, where it originated. **(C)** Well-developed consolidation of the right upper lobe demonstrates total homogeneous opacification with central air bronchograms. Note that the minor fissure is not significantly elevated. Early consolidation also is developing in the right middle lobe.

FIGURE 1.18. *Multilobar consolidations.* **(A)** Note the rather uncommon phenomenon of total consolidation of the right lung and early consolidations developing in the left upper and lower lobes. **(B)** Both right upper-lobe and left lower-lobe consolidations are present. Minimal elevation of the minor fissure is present on the right. The left lower-lobe consolidation causes increased density of the left side of the heart.

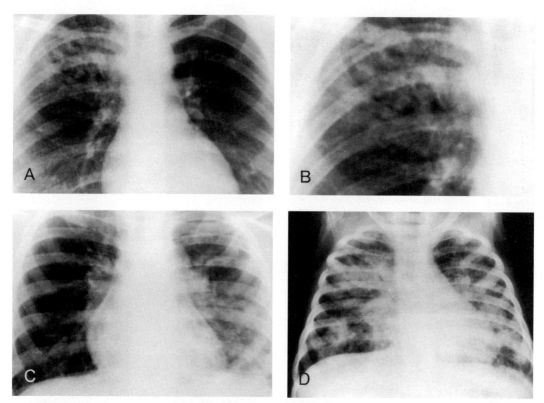

FIGURE 1.19. *Bacterial consolidation: less common patterns.* **(A)** Note the fluffy-to-nodular infiltrate in the right upper lobe. **(B)** Magnified view of the right upper lobe demonstrates the soft fluffy nodules. This pattern also can be seen with *Mycoplasma pneumoniae* infection. **(C)** Another patient with diffuse, fluffy infiltrates, just short of total consolidation of the left lower lobe. **(D)** Infant with diffuse, fluffy infiltrates extending far into the periphery of both lungs. This patient had widespread staphylococcal pneumonia. Note how this pattern differs from the widespread viral pattern of radiating bronchitis–peribronchitis with scattered atelectasis seen in Figure 1.13A. There is no central predominance, and the patchy infiltrates extend far into the periphery of the lung.

question has a smooth, homogeneous appearance rather than a streaky, linear, or wedgelike appearance, one should consider it a superimposed bacterial pneumonia (Fig. 1.20). This is especially true if the involved lobe shows no volume loss and infiltrate is located far in the periphery of the lung, for it

should be remembered that consolidations begin in the periphery of a lobe. Usually such superimposed consolidations involve one lobe only, but multilobar involvement has a propensity to occur in infants suffering from underlying respiratory syncytial viral infections (Fig. 1.21).

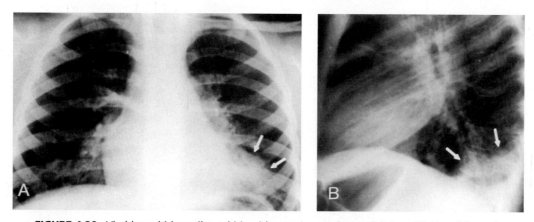

FIGURE 1.20. *Viral bronchitis–peribronchitis with superimposed consolidation.* **(A)** Note bilateral perihilar–peribronchial infiltrates and an area of segmental atelectasis in the right upper lobe. In addition, however, note a homogeneous density, with air bronchograms just adjacent to the left cardiac border (*arrows*). **(B)** Lateral view demonstrates this latter density to be located far in the basal periphery of the left lower lobe (*arrows*). This is a superimposed consolidating pneumonia. *Continued on next page.*

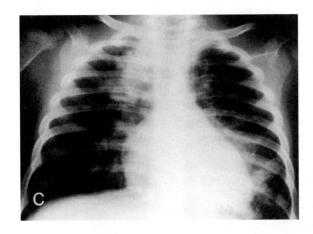

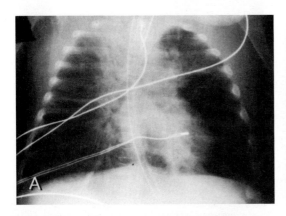

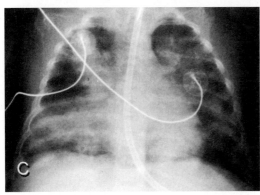

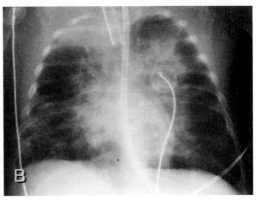

FIGURE 1.20. *(continued)* (C) Another patient with perihilar–peribronchial infiltrates, but with two homogeneous densities, one in the right upper lobe and one in the left lower lobe behind the heart. Neither one of these areas is associated with volume loss, and thus consolidating pneumonia should be favored.

FIGURE 1.21. *Viral bronchitis–peribronchitis, with subsequent superimposed widespread bacterial consolidation.* **(A)** Note the bilateral perihilar–peribronchial infiltrates with perihilar edema and scattered segmental atelectasis in this patient with respiratory syncytial viral infection. **(B)** Five days later the basic perihilar–peribronchial pattern persisted, but the patient was becoming more toxic, and a previously present lymphocytosis had changed to a white blood cell count that now showed a marked increase in segmental neutrophils and bands. These changing clinical and laboratory findings characteristically precede the development of superimposed bacterial consolidations. **(C)** Just 18 hours later, note the development of massive bilateral consolidations involving virtually every lobe on both sides, but best seen in the right lung. This patient developed superimposed bacterial infection.

REFERENCES

1. Carson JL, Collier AM, Hu SS. Acquired ciliary defects in nasal epithelium of children with acute viral upper respiratory infections. *N Engl J Med* 1985;312:463–468.
2. Conte P, Heitzman ER, Markarian B. Viral pneumonia, roentgen pathological correlations. *Radiology* 1970;95:267–272.
3. Donnelly LF. Maximizing the usefulness of imaging in children with community-acquired pneumonia. *AJR* 1999;172:505–512.
4. Gold R, Wilt JC, Adhikari PK, MacPherson RI. Adenoviral pneumonia and its complications in infancy and childhood. *Can J Assoc Radiol* 1969;20:4.
5. Griscom NT, Wohl MEB, Kirkpatrick JA Jr.: Lower respiratory

infections: How infants differ from adults. *Radiol Clin North Am* 1978;16:367–387.
6. Guckel C, Benz-Bohm G, Widemann B. Mycoplasma pneumonias in childhood: Roentgen features, differential diagnosis, and review of literature. *Pediatr Radiol* 1989;19:499–503.
7. Hall CB, Powell KR, Schnabel KC, Gala CL, Pincus PH. Risk of secondary bacterial infection in infants hospitalized with respiratory syncytial viral infection. *Pediatrics* 1988;113:266–271.
8. Ichikado K, Johkoh T, Ikezoe J, Takeuchi N, Kohno N, Arisawa J, Nakamura H, Nagareda T, Itoh H, Ando M. Acute interstitial pneumonia: High-resolution CT findings correlated with pathology. *AJR* 1997;168:333.
9. Ketai LH, Williamson MR, Talepak RJ, Levy H, Koster FT, Nolte KB, Allen SE. Hantavirus pulmonary syndrome: Radiographic findings in 16 patients. *Radiology* 1994;191:665–668.

10. Khamapirad T, Glezen WP. Clinical and radiographic assessment of acute lower respiratory tract disease in infants and children. *Semin Respir Infect* 1977;2:130–144.

11. Muller NL, Miller RR. Diseases of the bronchioles: CT and histopathologic findings. *Radiology* 1995;196:3–12.

12. Murphy S, Florman AL. Lung defenses against infection: A clinical correlation. *Pediatrics* 1983;72:1.

13. Putto A, Ruuskenan O, Meurman O. Fever in respiratory virus infections. *Am J Dis Child* 1986;140:1159–1163.

14. Scanlon GA, Unger JD. The radiology of bacterial and viral pneumonias. *Radiol Clin North Am* 1973;11:317–338.

15. Shopfner CE. Aeration disturbances secondary to pulmonary infection. *AJR* 1974;120:261–273.

16. Swischuk LE. Nontraumatic pediatric thoracic emergencies. *Emergency Radiol* 1995;2:221–233.

17. Swischuk LE, Hayden CK. Viral vs. bacterial pulmonary infections in children (Is roentgenographic differentiation possible?). *Pediatr Radiol* 1986;16:278–284.

18. Wildin SR, Chonmaitree T, Swischuk LE. Roentgenographic features of common pediatric viral respiratory tract infections. *Am J Dis Child* 1988;142:43–46.

Round Pneumonias

If one has never seen a round pneumonia (1–3), one will never guess what it is. Most often these so-called round, spherical, or oval pneumonias represent pneumococcal infections in an early consolidative phase. Some of them appear so round that they defy distinction from a pulmonary nodule or oval mass (Fig. 1.22). In other instances, a mediastinal mass might be suggested (Fig. 1.23), but the fact that one sees these pneumonias in such a configuration is purely fortuitous. If one could examine these patients a few hours later, a more typical picture of consolidation would be present (Fig. 1.24).

The clue to proper diagnosis, of course, is clinical. These children almost always come to the attention of a physician because of abrupt onset of fever, cough, and malaise. Usually they have fevers between 103° F and 105 °F, and auscultative findings that suggest pneumonia. Under these cir-

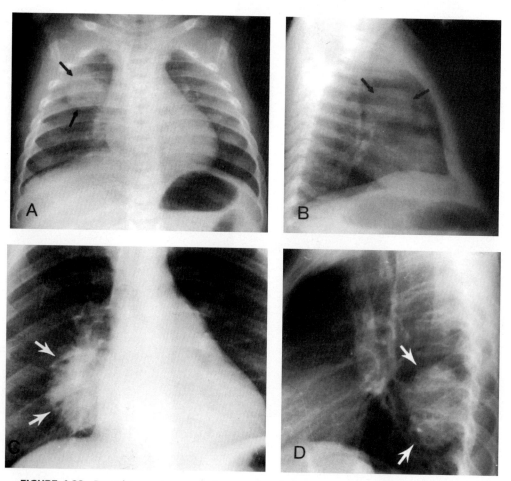

FIGURE 1.22. *Round or oval pneumonias: pseudopulmonary nodules or masses.* **(A)** Note the perfectly round pneumonia in the right upper lobe (*arrows*). This easily could be mistaken for a pulmonary nodule. **(B)** Lateral view demonstrates the same nodulelike appearance of the pneumonia (*arrows*). **(C)** Oval configuration of a lobar pneumonia in the right lower lobe (*arrows*). The configuration might suggest a mass. **(D)** Lateral view confirms the right lower lobe location of this round pneumonia (*arrows*).

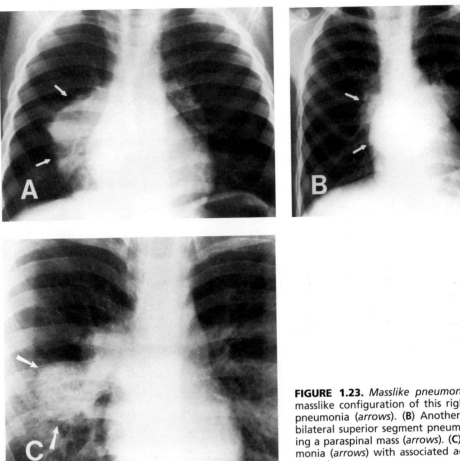

FIGURE 1.23. *Masslike pneumonias.* **(A)** Note masslike configuration of this right lower lobe pneumonia (*arrows*). **(B)** Another patient with bilateral superior segment pneumonias mimicking a paraspinal mass (*arrows*). **(C)** Round pneumonia (*arrows*) with associated adenopathy on the right.

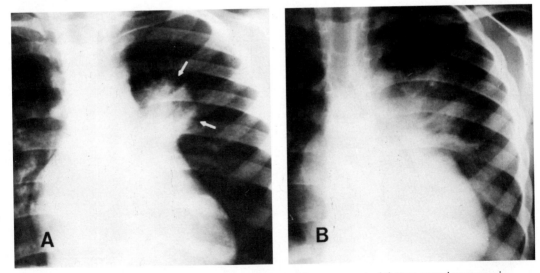

FIGURE 1.24. *Round pneumonia progressing to regular pneumonia.* **(A)** Note round pneumonia mimicking hilar adenopathy on the left (*arrows*). **(B)** On the next day, a more typical consolidation has evolved.

circumstances, one should not think of tumor or pulmonary nodule but rather of a consolidating lobar pneumonia, usually pneumococcal in origin.

REFERENCES

1. Greenfield H, Gyepes MT. Oval-shaped consolidations simulating new growth of the lung. *AJR* 1964;91:125–131.
2. Rose RW, Ward BH. Spherical pneumonias in children simulating pulmonary and mediastinal masses. *Radiology* 1973;106: 179–182.
3. Talner LB. Pulmonary pseudotumors in childhood. *AJR* 1967; 100:208–213.

LOOKING FOR THE PNEUMONIA

Know the Normal Chest First

It is most important that one be thoroughly familiar with the normal chest before one attempts to identify pneumonias; this is a matter of studying the normal shapes and densities of the various structures visualized (Fig. 1.25). For example, both hilar regions should be of relatively equal density, and the cardiac silhouettes to either side of the spine should be about the same density. Indeed, analysis of the chest roentgenogram is a matter of comparing one side with the other, in terms not only of anatomic boundaries but also of comparative densities. To be sure, it is the latter

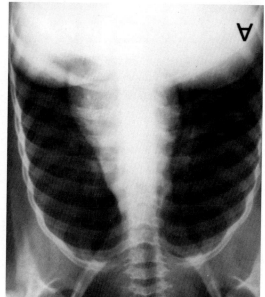

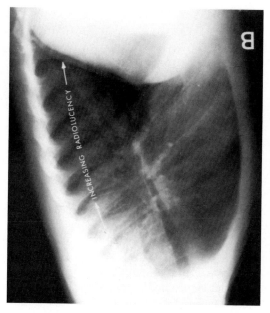

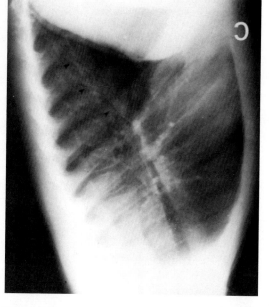

FIGURE 1.25. *Normal chest: pertinent roentgenographic features.* **(A)** On this frontal view, note that both lungs are of equal density and that the mediastinal, cardiac, and diaphragmatic edges are clearly demarcated. In addition, note that both sides of the heart are of equal density and that both hilar regions also appear equal in density and size. **(B)** Lateral view demonstrating increasing radiolucency from top to bottom of the retrocardiac space. Also note how sharp both diaphragmatic leaflets appear. **(C)** Same lateral view as in **B**, demonstrating normal lower-lobe pulmonary vessels *(arrows)*, which often are misinterpreted as pulmonary infiltrates. The characteristic sloping configuration of these vessels aids one in proper interpretation.

comparison that often turns out to be the more useful in detecting early or hidden infiltrates.

One should also note that the margins of the heart and diaphragmatic leaflets, as they lie in juxtaposition to normally aerated lungs, are crisp and distinct. This observation is useful for utilizing and understanding Felson's silhouette sign. This sign is discussed in detail in the next section, but as a preliminary consideration it should be noted that if any of the cardiac or diaphragmatic edges becomes hazy or fuzzy, one should suspect an adjacent abnormality such as a pulmonary infiltrate or atelectasis.

On lateral view, an important normal finding is that the space behind the heart is characteristically radiolucent (Fig. 1.25B); it represents the superimposed, normally aerated, lower lobes. Above this area, the soft tissues of the upper chest wall, axillae, and shoulder cause the lung fields to become progressively more opaque. Characteristically, then, the posterior half of the chest should become more radiolucent as one passes from top to bottom and, if it does not (i.e., the lower retrocardiac space is of equal or greater density than the superior retrocardiac space), one should suspect a pneumonia in one or the other of the lower lobes (compare Fig. 1.25C with Fig. 1.31B). In this area, however, a pitfall to be avoided is misinterpreting normal retro-

cardiac lower-lobe pulmonary vascular markings as being representative of an infiltrate (Fig. 1.25C). The characteristic angle and linear configuration of these pulmonary vessels are the clues to proper diagnosis. The upper retrosternal space should also be radiolucent, except in young infants, in whom the normal thymus gland causes the radiolucency to be replaced by radiodensity or whiteness. If this occurs in older children, one should look for an anterior segment, upper-lobe pneumonia, or a superior mediastinal mass.

The right diaphragmatic leaflet is a little higher than the left, and because of this it is often projected at a higher level on lateral view. Occasionally the leaflets are superimposed, but most often they appear at separate levels. The right diaphragmatic leaflet can also be identified by the fact that it is usually seen in its entirety (Fig. 1.26). In other words, it can be seen as a distinct structure right up to its insertion into the anterior chest wall. The left leaflet, on the other hand, usually is seen only as far as the posterior cardiac wall, for at this point it blends with the cardiac silhouette (Fig. 1.26). Occasionally, however, the left leaflet also can be seen in its entirety, and in such cases the usually visible gastric air bubble or inferior vena cava can be used as differentiating aids. The gastric bubble, of course, lies under the left diaphragmatic leaflet; the inferior vena cava, being under

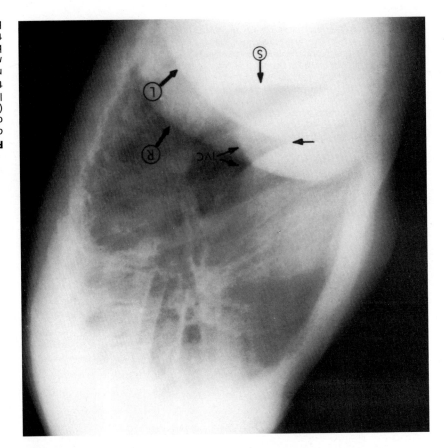

FIGURE 1.26. *Localizing and lateralizing the diaphragmatic leaflets.* Note that the right diaphragmatic leaflet (R) is higher than the left (L). Also note that the right diaphragmatic leaflet is seen in its entirety, but the anterior third of the left leaflet blends with the posterior aspect of the cardiac silhouette (anterior-most arrow). The inferior vena cava (IVC) blends with the right diaphragmatic leaflet; the stomach bubble (S) is located immediately below the left diaphragmatic leaflet.

right-sided, blends with the right diaphragmatic leaflet (Fig. 1.26). All of these findings and relationships may not be present on every lateral chest film, but enough of them usually are present to enable one to determine right- or left-sidedness of a diaphragmatic leaflet, and thus right- or left-sidedness of an adjacent lower-lobe pneumonia.

Picking up Early or Minimal Infiltrates

Early infiltrates often are so subtle that they are totally overlooked or simply misinterpreted as fortuitous conglomerations of rib and bronchovascular densities. The only way to diagnose such pneumonias is to be suspicious of, and then methodically evaluate, any focal area of increased density, no matter how equivocal (Fig. 1.27). In addition to the foregoing, one must remember to always obtain two views of the chest. One may be surprised how well a pneumonia is visible on one view and yet how poorly demarcated it is on the other. The reason for this is that on one view the early pneumonia is seen *en face* and is "too thin" to register on the chest film, but on the other view it is visualized at 90° to the first view and is thick enough to be seen (Fig. 1.28). One should never neglect to get two views of the chest.

Using Felson's Silhouette Sign

Felson's silhouette sign (2) is a most useful sign for detecting an early or subtle infiltrate. It stems from the fact that if two structures of equal roentgenographic density are juxtaposed, the interface between them becomes obliterated. In other words, if an organ such as the heart (water density) is juxta-

posed against a pulmonary infiltrate (also water density), then the interface between them becomes indistinct or frankly obliterated. Normally the heart, mediastinum, and diaphragm (water density) are in juxtaposition to aerated lung (air density), and because they are of such different densities, a sharp line clearly demarcates their interfaces. Once the density of the lung is changed from air to water (i.e., by pneumonia, hemorrhage, edema, or atelectasis), however, the roentgenographic interface between that portion of the lung and the adjacent mediastinum or diaphragm is obliterated and a positive silhouette sign results.

Most often the silhouette sign is applied to pneumonias in the right middle lobe and lingula. In the right middle lobe, the pneumonias that produce a silhouette sign occur in the medial segment. Those in the lateral segment are not juxtaposed with the heart and thus do not produce a positive silhouette sign. In those cases in which a medial-segment pneumonia is present, the adjacent edge of the heart becomes blurred or obliterated (Fig. 1.29). If the pneumonia is in the lingula, it is the left side of the heart that becomes obliterated. Once such blurring of the cardiac silhouette is noted on frontal projection, a lateral view should be obtained for confirmation (Fig. 1.29B). The silhouette sign, utilized in this fashion, also is useful in pneumonias located adjacent to the superior mediastinal structures or the diaphragmatic leaflets (Fig. 1.30). In reverse, the silhouette sign also is helpful in localizing lower-lobe pulmonary infiltrates. For example, if an infiltrate is present in the lower lobes, it lies behind the heart (not in juxtaposition to the lateral edge), and consequently, the heart–lung inter-

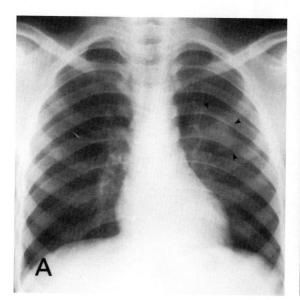
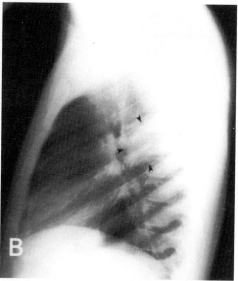

FIGURE 1.27. *Subtle early infiltrate.* **(A)** There is a vague area of focal infiltration in the left upper-lung field, just lateral to the left hilar region (*arrows*). **(B)** Lateral view substantiates the presence of this early pneumonia, as there is a corresponding area of focally increased density in the left lower lobe, superimposed over the spine (*arrows*).

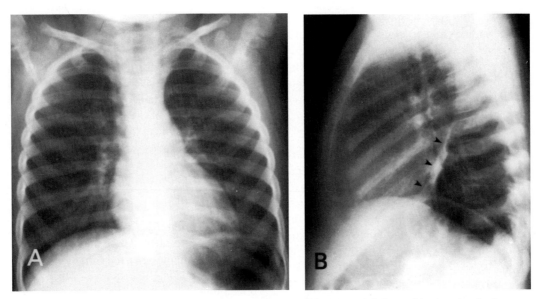

FIGURE 1.28. *Value of obtaining two views.* **(A)** The infiltrate is so subtle on this view that it virtually defies identification. On close inspection, however, one might note that the left diaphragmatic leaflet is a little indistinct and that it is a little higher than usual (probably secondary to splinting). The left lower-lobe pneumonia is seen *en face* and is too "thin" to be visible. **(B)** Lateral view. The pneumonia is seen at a 90-degree angle to that in **A** and now is "thick" enough to register on the roentgenogram (*arrows*).

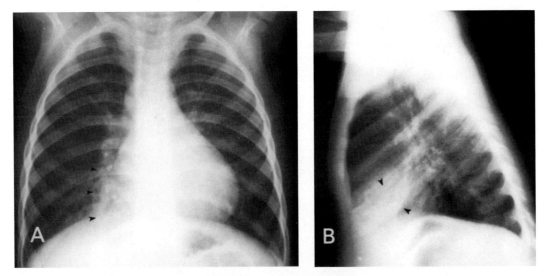

FIGURE 1.29. *Right middle lobe silhouette sign.* **(A)** Note that the right cardiac border is indistinct and, in fact, obliterated over its lower two thirds by an adjacent pneumonia in the medial segment of the right middle lobe (*arrows*). The left cardiac border is sharp. **(B)** Lateral view confirms the presence of a right middle lobe pneumonia seen as an area of increased density anteroinferiorly (*arrows*).

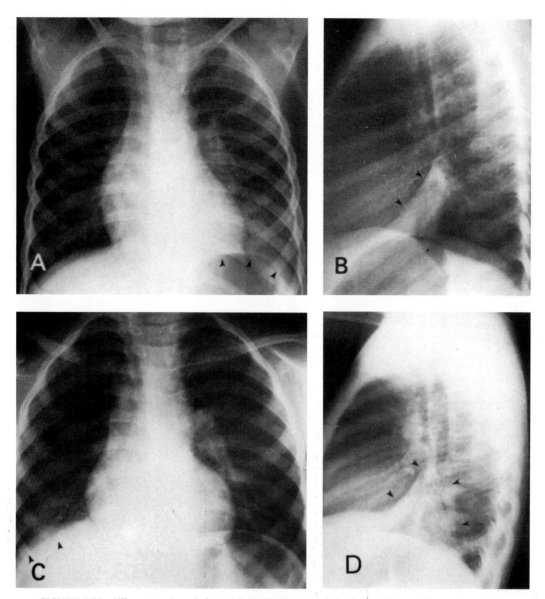

FIGURE 1.30. *Silhouette signs, left and right diaphragmatic leaflets.* **(A)** The infiltrate in the left lower-lung field is difficult to detect on this view, but a strong clue to its presence lies in the fact that the left diaphragmatic leaflet is indistinct *(arrows)*. The gastric bubble is seen below the leaflet, but the leaflet itself is invisible (positive silhouette sign). This finding localizes the pneumonia to the left lower lobe. **(B)** Lateral view substantiates the presence of the left lower-lobe pneumonia lying posterior to the major fissure *(arrows)*. The portion of the diaphragmatic leaflet immediately adjacent to the pneumonia is obliterated, producing another example of a focally positive silhouette sign. **(C)** Positive silhouette sign, right diaphragm *(arrows)*. A lower lobe pneumonia should be suspected. Mediastinal shift to right is caused by rotation. **(D)** Lateral view confirms the right lower-lobe pneumonia *(arrows)*.

face is preserved (Fig. 1.31). This indicates that the infiltrate is far posterior to the heart, that is, in a lower lobe.

Unfortunately, the silhouette sign also occurs in some normal situations. The most frequent site for this is along the right side of the heart. In many children, the bronchovascular markings adjacent to the right side of the heart are so prominent that they blend with the cardiac silhouette and result in a positive silhouette sign. ***If this normal phenomenon is not appreciated, one will continually overcall right***

middle-lobe pneumonia. Most often this occurs if the inspiratory effort is somewhat shallow and the roentgenogram is obtained with the patient in partial lordotic position. The problem is especially common in children with perihilar–peribronchial infiltrates secondary to viral lower respiratory tract infections (Fig. 1.32A) and in some cases may result from a mild degree of atelectasis not pronounced enough to be seen on lateral view (1). The fact that pneumonia is not present can be verified by obtaining a lateral chest roent-

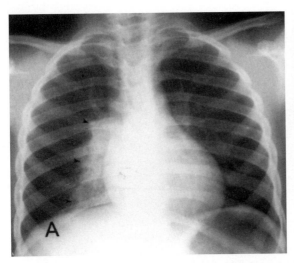
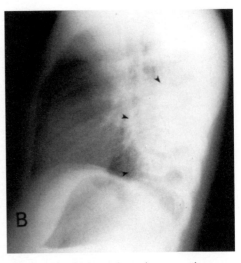

FIGURE 1.31. *Silhouette sign in reverse, right lower-lobe localization.* **(A)** Note the rather extensive pneumonia in the right lower lobe (*arrows*). It is located behind the heart and is causing this portion of the heart to have increased density (i.e., it is more opaque than the left side). Because the pneumonia is behind the heart, however, and not in juxtaposition to its right border, the cardiac border remains distinct. If the pneumonia were in juxtaposition to the right cardiac border, that is, in the medial segment of the right middle lobe, the cardiac border would be obliterated (i.e., as in Fig. 1.29A). **(B)** Lateral view confirms the presence of the extensive right lower-lobe pneumonia, because there is a marked increase in density of the entire posterior retrocardiac space (*arrows*).

genogram, which shows that no middle-lobe infiltrate is present (Fig. 1.32B). It is most unusual to detect a right middle-lobe, medial-segment pneumonia on frontal view and not see even subtle indications of its presence on lateral view.

Another instance in which the silhouette sign can be considered a normal phenomenon is if a pleural fissure blends with the upper aspect of a diaphragmatic leaflet (Fig. 1.33). This can occur with either a normal or an accessory fissure, and it is only if a lateral view is obtained that this positive, but normal, silhouette sign can be deciphered and understood (Fig.1.33). Compare the case illustrated in Figure 1.33 with the one demonstrated in Figure 1.31D, in which a true right

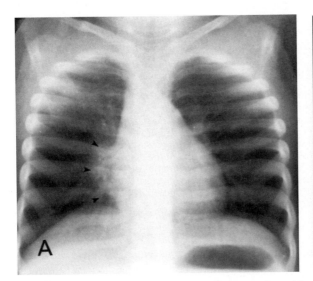
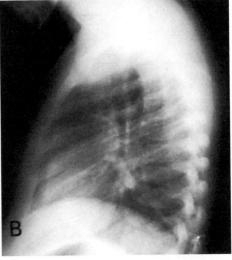

FIGURE 1.32. *Right middle-lobe silhouette sign with perihilar–peribronchial infiltrates: pseudo-focal pneumonia.* **(A)** This infant has widespread perihilar–peribronchial infiltrates. The chest film, however, is quite lordotic (the ribs are horizontal posteriorly and slanted downward anteriorly), and this is causing the bronchovascular markings along the right cardiac silhouette to cluster more than normal (*arrows*). Consequently, the right cardiac border is obliterated, and a right middle-lobe medial-segment pneumonia is suggested. **(B)** On lateral view, however, there is no evidence of a right middle-lobe infiltrate. If an infiltrate were present in the right middle lobe, it would be demonstrable on lateral view. Compare this lateral view with the lateral view in Figure 1.29, in which a true right middle lobe pneumonia is present.

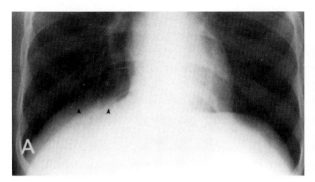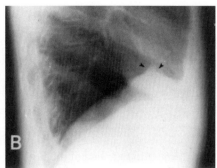

FIGURE 1.33. *Silhouette sign resulting from normal fissure insertion.* **(A)** Note focal obliteration of the right diaphragmatic leaflet (*arrows*). Is this caused by an adjacent pneumonia? **(B)** Lateral view shows that the silhouette sign is produced by blending of the lower aspect of the major fissure with the right diaphragmatic leaflet (*arrows*). On frontal view, this area of blending, caught tangentially by the beam, creates a positive, but normal, silhouette sign. The same phenomenon can occur on the left.

lower-lobe pneumonia and a positive right diaphragmatic-leaflet silhouette sign are present. Felson's silhouette sign is an excellent sign, but one must learn to use it properly. It is always valid in principle but at times may not be abnormal.

REFERENCES

1. Culham JAG. The right heart border in infancy. *Radiology* 1981; 139:381–384.

2. Felson B, Felson H. Localization of intrathoracic lesions by means of the posteroanterior roentgenogram: The silhouette sign. *Radiology* 1950;55:363–374.

Favorite Hiding Places of Pneumonia

There are certain areas that are notorious for hiding early pulmonary infiltrates (1). One should become familiar with all of these sites and give them a second look in inspecting the roentgenogram (Fig. 1.34). Unless one becomes thor-

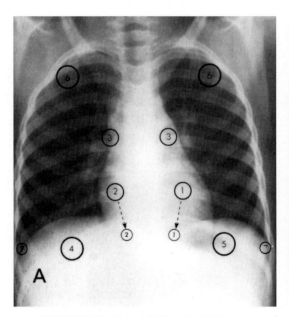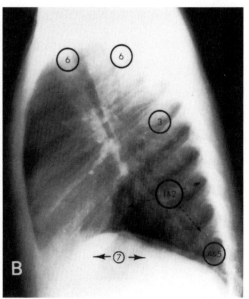

FIGURE 1.34. **(A and B)** *Favorite hiding places of pneumonia.* (*1*) Behind the left side of the heart in the left lower lobe, often extending into the phrenicovertebral angle; (*2*) behind the right side of the heart in the right lower lobe, also often extending into the phrenicovertebral angle; (*3*) behind the hilar regions, in the superior segment of either lower lobe; (*4*) deep in the posterior costophrenic sulcus behind the liver; (*5*) deep in the costophrenic sulcus behind the stomach, spleen, or left lobe of the liver; (*6*) high in the upper lobes; and (*7*) deep in the lateral costophrenic sulci.

oughly familiar with these hiding places, pulmonary infiltrates can be overlooked totally.

The first hiding place the radiology resident is taught is behind the left side of the heart (i.e., in the left lower lobe). In most individuals the bulk of the cardiac silhouette extends to the left of the spine and thus can hide a sizable infiltrate. This is especially true if the film is too light (underpenetrated). In looking for a pneumonia in this location, one should look first for an area of focally increased density projected through the left side of the heart. A good

way to check for this is to quickly compare the densities of both sides of the heart; in normal individuals they are equal, but with left lower-lobe pneumonias they are not. The increase in density in cases in which a pneumonia is present results from the fact that the pneumonia is roentgenographically more dense than normal lung, and thus, if superimposed over the heart, it produces an area of increased density (Fig. 1.35).

Such focal pneumonias are relatively easy to detect, but if the pneumonia is so large that it produces a generalized,

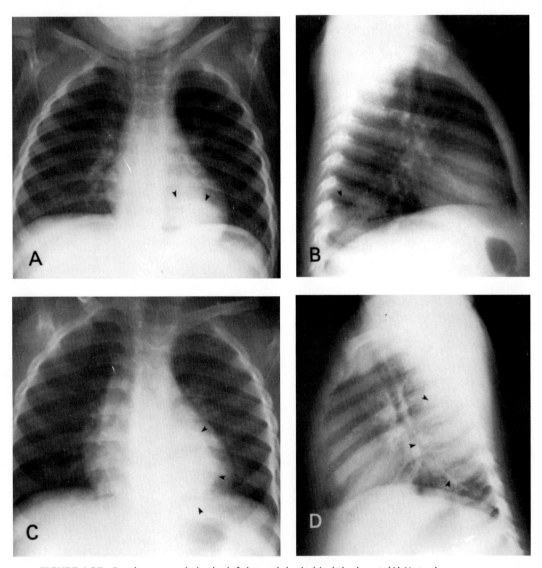

FIGURE 1.35. *Focal pneumonia in the left lower lobe behind the heart.* **(A)** Note the vague area of increased density projected through the left side of the heart (*arrows*). **(B)** Lateral view clearly localizes the pneumonia to the left lower lobe (*arrows*); the left diaphragmatic leaflet is obliterated, producing a positive silhouette sign. The intact leaflet visualized below this area is the right diaphragmatic leaflet. The left leaflet is higher because of splinting. **(C)** Note the large area of increased density behind the left side of the heart (*arrows*). **(D)** The lateral view demonstrates the pneumonia in the left lower lobe, manifesting in somewhat subtle, but still present, diffuse increase in density of the normally radiolucent retrocardiac space (*arrows*).

rather than focal, increase in density of the entire left side of the heart, it can be missed (Fig. 1.36). In still other cases, the infiltrate may be buried deep in the phrenicovertebral sulci. If the sulci are compared one with another, however, it becomes obvious that the abnormal one is whiter or denser than normal (Fig. 1.37). In this regard, the only pitfall to avoid is a normal increase in density in this area produced by overlapping of the cardiac silhouette and the diaphragmatic leaflet on the left (Fig. 1.37C). This usually occurs on supine films, and no such pitfall exists on the right.

So well is it ingrained in us to look behind the left side of the heart for hidden pneumonias that we forget to *look behind the right side of the heart.* Indeed, pneumonias in this area are almost always missed. The best way to recognize a pneumonia in this area again is to follow the rule that both sides of the heart should be of equal density. As on the left, right-side pneumonias may produce focal (Fig. 1.38A) or more generalized (Fig. 1.39A) infiltrates, resulting in a more diffuse increase in density of the entire right side of the cardiac silhouette. Extension into the ipsilateral phrenicovertebral sulcus also is common (Fig. 1.39B) and should be kept in mind in perusing roentgenograms in such cases. Confirmation of all these pneumonias once again is acquired readily with lateral chest roentgenograms (Fig. 1.38B).

Pneumonias in the superior segment of either lower lobe are notorious for hiding behind one or another of the hilar regions. In this location they cause an increase in density, and at times size, of the ipsilateral hilar region (Figs. 1.40 and 1.41). Indeed, the hilus can be so dense and prominent that lymphadenopathy is suggested (as in primary pul-

monary tuberculosis). Once again, however, the lateral view clearly elucidates the problem and confirms the presence of a pneumonia in the superior segment of the involved lower lobe (Figs. 1.40 and 1.41).

Lower-lobe pneumonias deep in the posterior costophrenic sulci also are missed frequently on the frontal projection. On the right side these pneumonias are projected through the liver silhouette, and unless one becomes accustomed to their appearance they are most difficult to recognize (Fig. 1.42). In some cases, one may be surprised at the size of a pneumonia so hidden (Fig. 1.43). On the left side, such pneumonias can be projected through the left lobe of the liver, the stomach bubble, or the spleen (Fig. 1.44). On lateral view, these pneumonias usually lie deep in the posterior costophrenic sulcus and frequently obliterate the adjacent portion of the diaphragmatic leaflet (i.e., positive silhouette sign).

Two other places in which pneumonias can hide are high in the upper lobe and deep in the lateral costophrenic sulcus. In the former instance, the pneumonia often is confused with normal overlying soft tissues (Fig. 1.45). In such cases, one should compare the densities of both apices (actually one should do this for all areas of the chest) and check the lateral view for confirmation. In checking the apices for subtle infiltrates, it is worthwhile to "black out" the remainder of the chest with an opaque piece of cardboard. If this maneuver is performed, comparison of the apices is easier, and subtle infiltrates stand out with more clarity. Pneumonias deep in the lateral costophrenic sulci usually are missed because one simply does not look in this region. These pneumonias are truly subtle and often are seen on frontal projection only (Fig. 1.46).

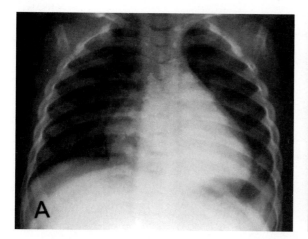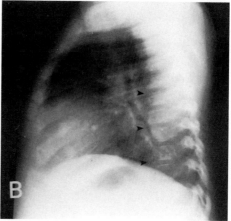

FIGURE 1.36. *Large left lower-lobe consolidation hiding behind the heart.* **(A)** The extensive left lower-lobe consolidation causes an increase in density of the entire left side of the cardiac silhouette. In spite of the size of this consolidation, it can be missed, because the entire left side of the heart rather than a focal area shows increased density. A little of the consolidation projects beyond the left cardiac border, but this is a subtle finding. **(B)** Lateral view clearly defines the presence of the left lower-lobe consolidating pneumonia (*arrows*).

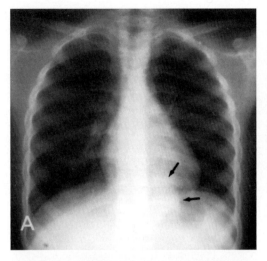
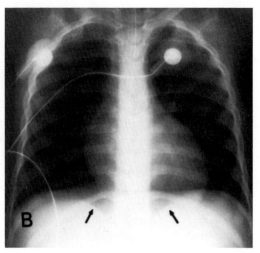
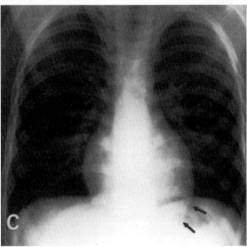

FIGURE 1.37. *Left lower-lobe pneumonia deep in the phrenicovertebral angle.* **(A)** Note how the pneumonia in the left lower lobe extends into the phrenicovertebral angle (*arrows*). Compare this with the normal density of this angle on the other side. Also note that the diaphragmatic leaflet is obliterated in this area. **(B)** Normal chest, somewhat overaerated, showing that both phrenicovertebral angles should be of about equal radiolucency (*arrows*). **(C)** Normal pitfall wherein the left inferior cardiac border and medial left diaphragmatic leaflet overlap to produce an increase in density in the area (*arrows*).

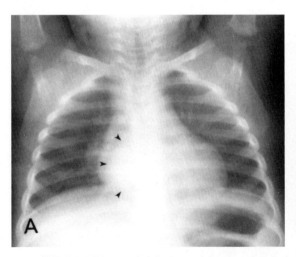
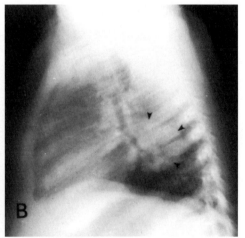

FIGURE 1.38. *Focal right lower-lobe pneumonia behind the right side of the heart.* **(A)** Note focal area of increased density projected through the right side of the cardiac silhouette (*arrows*). **(B)** Lateral view confirms the presence of a right lower-lobe pneumonia (*arrows*) behind the heart.

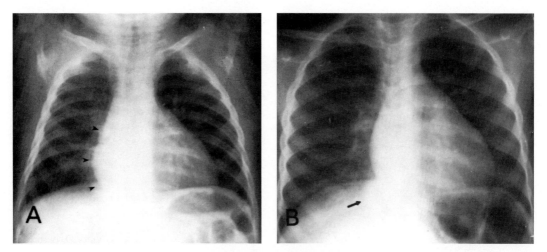

FIGURE 1.39. *Extensive right lower-lobe pneumonia behind the right side of the heart.* **(A)** Note diffuse increase in density of that portion of the cardiac silhouette that lies to the right of the spine. This represents a pneumonia behind the right side of the heart, in the right lower lobe. **(B)** Similar finding in another patient, but in this patient there is extension of the pneumonia into the phrenicovertebral sulcus (*arrow*).

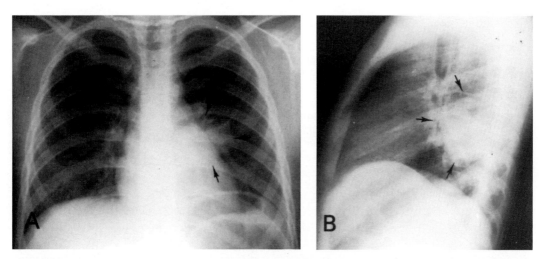

FIGURE 1.40. *Pneumonia behind the left hilus.* **(A)** Note that the left hilus is denser and larger than the right (*arrows*). **(B)** Lateral view shows that the pneumonia is located in the superior segment of the left lower lobe (*arrows*). If one recalls the normal position of the major fissure, it becomes apparent that the pneumonia must be in the superior segment of the lower lobe and not in the upper lobe.

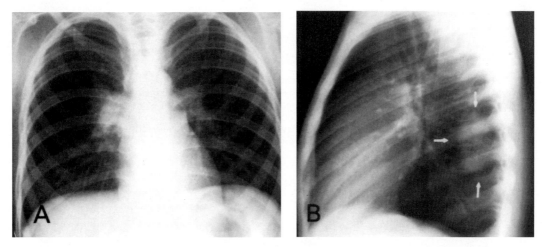

FIGURE 1.41. *Subtle pneumonia behind the right hilus.* **(A)** Note that the right hilus is much whiter (increased density), and slightly larger than the left hilus. At first, this might suggest unilateral hilar adenopathy. **(B)** Lateral view, however, clearly demonstrates the presence of a focal pneumonia in the superior segment of the right lower lobe (*arrows*).

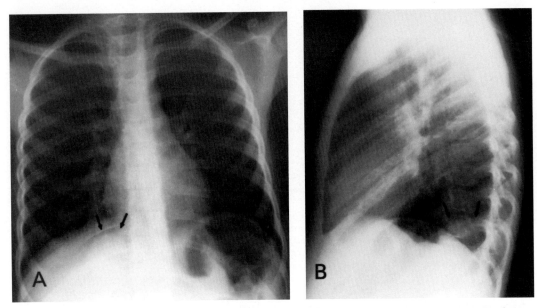

FIGURE 1.42. *Focal pneumonia, right lower lobe behind the liver.* **(A)** Note focal area of increased density (pneumonia) projected through the medial aspect of the liver (*arrows*). **(B)** Lateral view showing how deep this pneumonia lies in the posterior costophrenic sulcus (*arrows*). The right diaphragmatic leaflet is partially obliterated (silhouette sign) by the adjacent infiltrate; the left diaphragmatic leaflet is visualized clearly through the infiltrate.

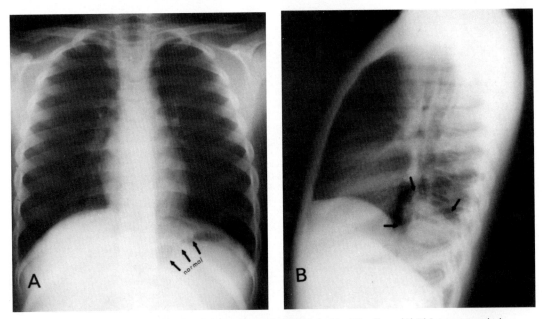

FIGURE 1.43. *Large right lower-lobe pneumonia hiding behind the liver.* **(A)** This pneumonia is so large that it could be missed. Note, however, that there is a general increase in density of the entire area below the right diaphragmatic leaflet but, more importantly, there is increased density of the phrenicovertebral sulcus. It should be radiolucent, just as is the normal one on the left (*arrows*). **(B)** Lateral view shows that the increase in density of the liver results from a large consolidating right lower-lobe pneumonia (*arrows*).

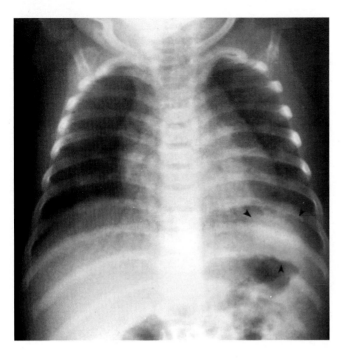

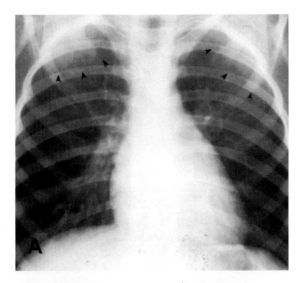

FIGURE 1.44. *Subtle focal pneumonia behind left diaphragmatic leaflet.* Note vague area of increased density projected through the left diaphragmatic leaflet (*arrows*). This was an early consolidating pneumonia of the left lower lobe, deep in the posterior costophrenic sulcus.

FIGURE 1.45. *High apical upper lobe pneumonia versus normal soft tissues.* (**A**) Normal patient with vague increased density high in the apices resulting from normal overlying soft tissues (*arrows*). (**B**) Patient with unilateral increase in density in the same area (*arrows*) representing a pneumonia. This pneumonia easily could be overlooked or mistaken for normal soft-tissue density. (**C**) On lateral view, however, the pneumonia is clearly visualized in the posterior segment of the right upper lobe (*arrows*).

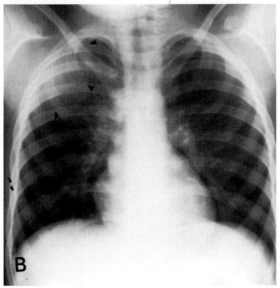

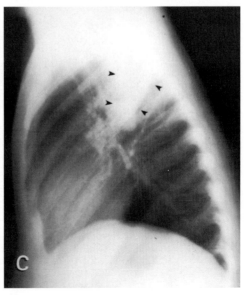

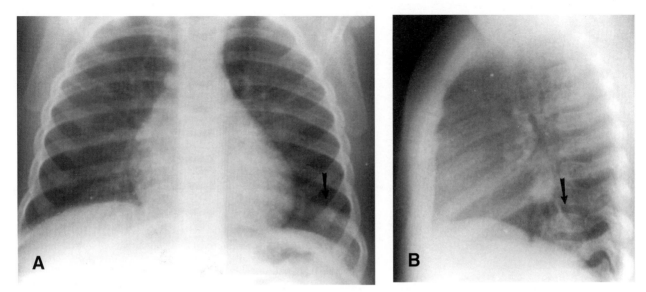

FIGURE 1.46. *Costophrenic sulcus pneumonia.* **(A)** Note the early infiltrate deep in the left costophrenic sulcus (*arrow*). **(B)** Lateral view demonstrates the lower lobe location (*arrow*) of this early consolidation.

REFERENCE

1. Burko H. Considerations in the roentgen diagnosis of pneumonia in children. *AJR* 1962;88:555–565.

Other Pulmonary Infections

The preceding sections deal mainly with the usual bacterial and viral infections presenting in the acute care setting, but a few points regarding other pulmonary infections that can be encountered are in order. First, one might consider pertussis infection, which is still relatively common. For the most part, patients with pertussis present with viral-like perihilar–peribronchial infiltrates (Fig. 1.47A). This should not be a surprise, *because pertussis infection is a bronchitis and peribronchitis, which, in the past, led to the so-called shaggy heart appearance (1).* Interestingly enough, however, although perihilar–peribronchial infiltrates are common, it is also common to see completely clear, but overaerated, lungs (2). *Indeed, over the years we have found this pattern to be more common.* The shaggy heart appearance results from perihilar–peribronchial infiltratives blurring the usually sharp cardiac and mediastinal edges. Currently, of course, the shaggy heart most commonly is seen with

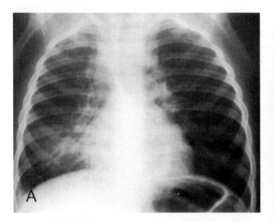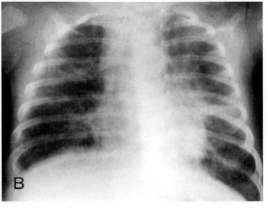

FIGURE 1.47. (A) *Pertussis infection.* Note typical perihilar–peribronchial infiltrates similar to those seen with viral disease. The lungs are overaerated. **(B)** *Chlamydia infection.* The findings are very similar to those seen with pertussis and viral infection. Note an area of segmental atelectasis in the left midlung field.

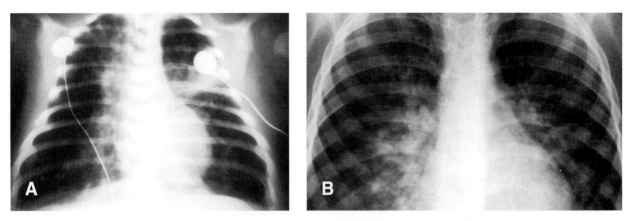

FIGURE 1.48. *Mycoplasma pneumoniae infection: perihilar–peribronchial infiltrates.* **(A)** Note bilateral perihilar–peribronchial infiltrates and segmental atelectasis in the left upper lobe. **(B)** More extensive perihilar–peribronchial infiltrates with some confluence of the infiltrates centrally.

viral or mycoplasmal infections, but it also is seen with chlamydial infections.

With pertussis, it should be remembered that because the basic problem is a bronchitis–peribronchitis, consolidations occur only in those few cases in which superimposed bacterial infection is seen. Therefore, in the usual case of pertussis, the lungs are overaerated and either completely clear or demonstrative of perihilar–peribronchial infiltrates (Fig. 1.47A). Segmental and lobar atelectases also are common and, interestingly enough, a similar appearance usually is seen with chlamydial infections (Fig. 1.47B). This infection also is a bronchial–peribronchial

infection and in the past was referred to as "pertussoid" pneumonia.

Mycoplasma pneumoniae infections are extremely variable in their clinical and roentgenographic presentation (5,6,9), but still the most common presentation is that of a widespread viral-like bronchitis–peribronchitis, with or without associated segmental or lobar atelectasis (Fig. 1.48). On the other hand, *M. pneumoniae* infections also can present with consolidations (Fig. 1.49) and, as noted previously in this chapter, the clinical picture then is not unlike that seen with bacterial pneumonia. The findings probably represent an interstitial pseudoconsolidation,

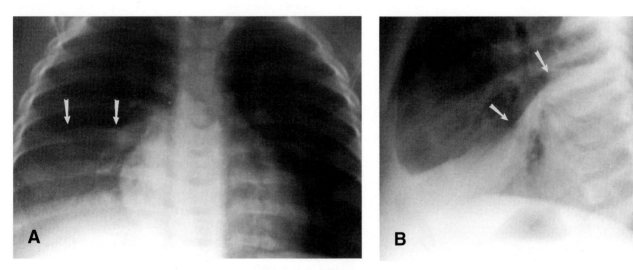

FIGURE 1.49. *Mycoplasma pneumoniae infection: Pseudoconsolidation.* **(A)** Note increased density in the right lower lobe (*arrows*). **(B)** Lateral view demonstrates the same finding (*arrows*). I do not believe that most, if any, of these represent airspace disease. Rather they probably represent extensive disease producing a so-called pseudoconsolidation.

much as with viral disease. If diffuse perihilar–peribronchial infiltrates such as those demonstrated in Fig. 1.48 are seen, the clinical picture more closely resembles that of a viral infection.

Another interesting pattern of infiltration in patients with *M. pneumoniae* infection, especially in older children or adolescents, is that of unilateral, or basically unilobar, distribution of reticulonodular or reticular infiltrates (Figs. 1.50 and 1.51). Associated atelectasis is common in these patients (Fig. 1.50), and in the purest sense they represent patients with *so-called walking pneumonia.* They usually have symptoms for 1 to 2 weeks before they finally come to the physician's attention.

Primary pulmonary tuberculosis also still is common and can present with a wide variety of roentgenographic findings (3,9). Most often, however, one is confronted with unilateral hilar or paratracheal adenopathy and some other finding in the lung (Fig. 1.52), the most common of which is lobar or segmental atelectasis (3,4,9) (Fig. 1.52). Occa-

sionally, a consolidation is encountered (Fig. 1.52F), and rarely a focal, nodular, fluffy parenchymal infiltrate may be seen. Cavitation is not a common problem in primary pulmonary tuberculosis (8) and, if seen, probably is a problem more of pneumatocele formation (4) than actual abscess formation. Obstructive emphysema of a lobe also occasionally can be seen with tuberculosis (Fig. 1.52C), but unilateral hilar or paratracheal adenopathy and associated ipsilateral atelectasis remain the hallmarks of this infection. Bilateral hilar adenopathy is relatively uncommon (see Fig. 1.78B).

Both atelectasis and emphysema usually result from endobronchial granuloma formation rather than external bronchial compression by enlarged nodes, no matter how prominent the nodes appear. Indeed, atelectasis can be seen with little in the way of adenopathy (Fig. 1.52B). Pleural effusions are not as common as in adults but still at times can be massive. In summary, then, *a good rule of thumb for suspecting primary pulmonary tuberculosis in infancy and*

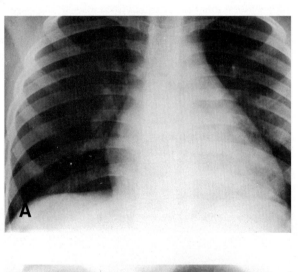

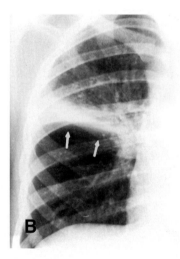

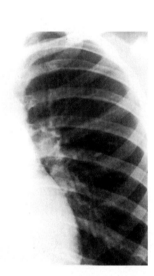

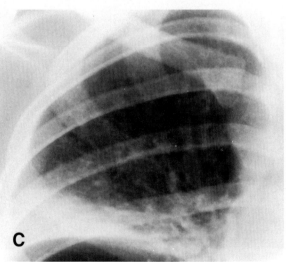

FIGURE 1.50. *Mycoplasma pneumoniae infiltrates with early atelectasis.* **(A)** Note hazy reticular infiltrate in the left upper lobe with scattered areas of streaky segmental atelectasis. **(B)** In this patient reticulonodular infiltrates are present in the right upper lobe and there is early atelectasis, causing increased density in the right upper lobe along the minor fissure (*arrows*). **(C)** Magnified view demonstrates the reticulonodular infiltrates to better advantage.

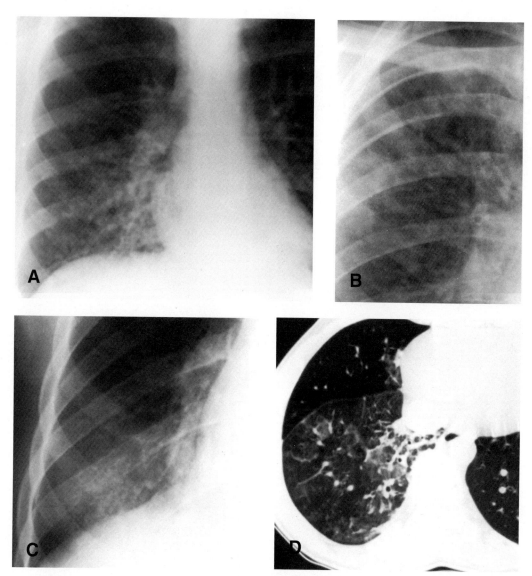

FIGURE 1.51. *Mycoplasma pneumoniae infections: lobar reticulonodular infiltrates.* **(A)** Note extensive reticulonodular infiltrate, basically confined to the right lower lobe. Ipsilateral hilar adenopathy also is present. **(B)** Reticulonodular infiltrates, in this patient, occupy the right upper lobe. **(C)** Reticulonodular infiltrates with some haziness of the lung parenchyma of the right lower lobe. **(D)** High-resolution computed tomography demonstrates patchy ground-glass appearance (interstitial disease) of the involved lung. In addition, note the thickened bronchial walls throughout the pulmonary interstitium.

childhood is the following: Unilateral hilar or paratracheal adenopathy, with or without parenchymal change (almost any type), should be presumed tuberculous in origin until proven otherwise. Even though these findings can be mimicked by atypical tuberculous, fungal, and some cases of *M. pneumoniae* infection, tuberculosis most often is the cause and should be the primary diagnosis until proven otherwise.

Miliary tuberculosis occasionally also can be seen, and although in older children the infiltrates are truly miliary (Fig. 1.52E), in infants the individual nodules are larger and not as miliary. They appear more reticulonodular (Fig. 1.52F). In many of these latter cases, it is difficult to detect underlying hilar adenopathy or associated pulmonary changes, but in others one may see associated adenopathy, atelectasis, and even the peripheral Ghon's lesion.

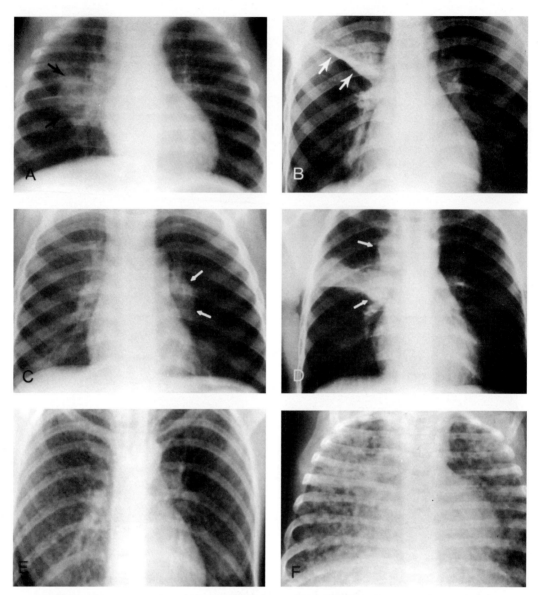

FIGURE 1.52. *Primary tuberculosis.* (**A**) Note characteristic right hilar and paratracheal adenopathy (*arrows*). (**B**) Another patient with atelectasis of the right upper lobe (*arrows*) and little in the way of hilar or paratracheal adenopathy. (**C**) Left hilar adenopathy (*arrows*) with obstructive emphysema of the left lung. A minimal reticular infiltrate is present throughout the right lung, and hilar adenopathy also is present on the right. (**D**) Right hilar and paratracheal adenopathy (*arrows*) with early atelectasis of the right upper lobe. (**E**) Diffuse miliary infiltrates throughout both lungs. There is no hilar adenopathy. (**F**) Infant with more coarse-appearing reticulonodular infiltrates. Right upper lobe consolidation is also suggested.

Fungal infections are not particularly common in childhood, except in the so-called fungus belts. If one resides in such an area, it soon becomes apparent that the roentgenographic findings are very variable (9), ranging from acute disseminated reticulonodular or fluffy infiltrates through lobar consolidations (Fig. 1.53). In still other cases, findings not unlike those seen with primary pulmonary tuberculosis are encountered. This being the case, one soon elevates fungal infections from the bottom of the list of diagnostic possibilities to a higher, more realistic, position. So-called fungus balls (Fig. 1.53B) are seen most often with aspergillosis.

Immunocompromised patients respond differently to infections, and HIV-infected patients are in this category. Basically, however, these patients are chronically ill and tend to have chronic, smoldering infections. For the most part, they do not present with "clean" consolidations or typical perihilar–peribronchial infiltrates. Most often they present with chronic, reticulonodular interstitial infiltrates or patchy alveolar infiltrates (Fig. 1.54), which usually are caused by infection by an opportunistic organism such as cytomegalic inclusion virus or *Pneumocystis carinii* pneumonia. Infections resulting from almost any virus, fungus, tuberculosis, atypical tuberculosis, or other indolent infectious agent, however, can be seen. In advanced cases, extensive consolidations, pleural effusions, and empyemas occur. Finally, it should be noted that patients with sickle cell disease are especially prone to developing pneumococcal and *M. pneumoniae* infections (6,7), and in many cases these can be rather profound and rampant infections. There is, of course, always the added problem of venoocclusive disease resulting from sludging in these patients, and this may prove to be important (i.e., infarction may precede infection).

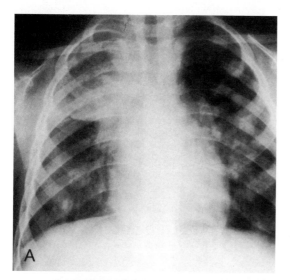

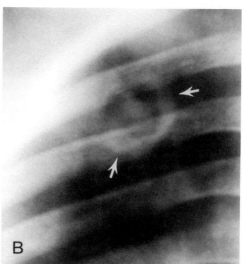

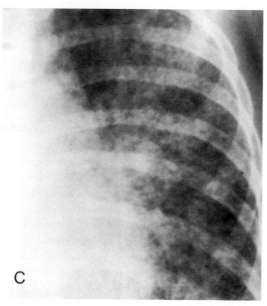

FIGURE 1.53. *Fungal disease.* **(A)** Actinomycosis presenting with consolidation of the right upper lobe and nodules scattered throughout both lungs. **(B)** Aspergillosis with characteristic fungal ball (*arrows*). Note the nidus in the center. **(C)** Acute disseminated histoplasmosis presenting with a diffuse reticulonodular pattern. (From John, S.D., and Swischuk, L.E.: Fungus infections of the chest in infants and children. J. Thorac. Imaging 7: 91–98, 1992, with permission.)

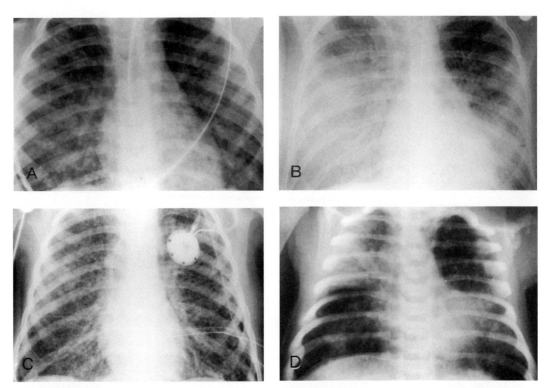

FIGURE 1.54. *Infection in immunocompromised patients.* **(A)** Typical reticulonodular infiltrate throughout both lungs. This can be seen with viral disease, *Pneumoystis carinii* infection, tuberculosis, and nonspecific, reactive lymphoid tissue proliferation. **(B)** Diffuse, interstitial haziness of both lungs, characteristic of *Pneumocystic carinii* infection but also seen with viral infections. **(C)** Diffuse, reticular interstitial infiltrates resulting from herpes pneumonitis. **(D)** Another patient, a very young infant with herpes pneumonitis, showing parenchymal involvement resulting in interstitial pseudoconsolidation of the right upper lobe and lingula.

REFERENCES

1. Barnhard HJ, Kniker WT. Roentgenologic findings in pertussis with particular emphasis on the "shaggy heart" sign. *AJR* 1960;84: 445–450.
2. Bellamy EA, Johnston IDA, Wilson AG. The chest radiograph in whooping cough. *Clin Radiol* 1987;38:39–43.
3. Leung AN, Müller NL, Pineda PR, FitzGerald JM. Primary tuberculosis in childhood: Radiographic manifestations. *Radiology* 1992; 152: 87–91.
4. Matsaniotis N, et al. Bullous emphysema in childhood tuberculosis. *J Pediatr* 1967;71:703.
5. Putman CE, Curtis A, Simeone JF, Jensen P. Mycoplasma pneumonia: Clinical and roentgenographic patterns. *AJR* 1975;124: 417–422.
6. Sabato AR, Martin AJ, Marmion BP, Kok TW, Cooper DM. *Mycoplasma pneumoniae*: Acute illness, antibiotics, and subsequent pulmonary infection. *Arch Dis Child* 1984;59:1034–1037.
7. Seeler RA, Metzger W, Mufson MA. Diplococcus pneumoniae infections in children with sickle cell anemia. *Am J Dis Child* 1972; 123:8–10.
8. Solomon A, Rabinowitz L. Primary cavitating tuberculosis in childhood. *Clin Radiol* 1972;23:483–485.
9. Stansberry SD. Tuberculosis in infants and children. *J Thorac Imaging* 1990;5:17–27.

PLEURAL FLUID COLLECTIONS AND EMPYEMA

The types of fluid that can collect in the pleural space include (a) pus (empyema, pyothorax), (b) serous fluid (hydrothorax), (c) blood (hemothorax), and (d) chyle (chylothorax). Empyema is usually a complication of an underlying pneumonia, and in this regard in the past was seen most commonly with *S. aureus* infections, but this infection is not as common now. Similarly, in patients younger than 3 years of age, *H. influenzae* most often was the causative organism, but with current vaccination programs it is much less common. In the older child, *S. pneumonia* (pneumococcus) is more common. Empyema also can be seen with hemolytic streptococcal pulmonary infections and secondary to osteomyelitis of the spine or subdiaphragmatic infections such as hepatic or subphrenic abscess. Most, however, occur secondary to pneumonias caused by *S. pneumonia*. *Finally, it should be noted that resistant strains of S. pneumonia are becoming more prevalent. As a result, empyemas and protracted clinical courses are much more common.*

Empyemas can develop rapidly. and progression from a subtle collection of fluid to a full-blown empyema in less than 24 hours is not uncommon. Most of these patients, of course, are quite ill, but it is surprising how relatively asymptomatic some of them appear. The roentgenographic changes depend on the size of the pyogenic fluid collection and may range from complete opacification of a hemithorax with massive mediastinal shift (Fig. 1.55A) to less striking and perhaps more puzzling changes. In this regard, it should be remembered that the empyema first must compress the lung and then shift the mediastinum. Consequently, at certain stages

of the development of an empyema, shift may be minimal or absent (Fig. 1.55B), and the incompletely compressed lung can be identified by its air bronchogram (Fig. 1.55C and D). The air bronchogram, however, does not extend far into the periphery, for the peripheral portion of the lung is compressed and surrounded by exudate. Currently, ultrasound is very useful in delineating the empyema in such cases. Indeed, ultrasound is most useful in detecting empyemas in general, whether the fluid collection is free-flowing or loculated. If loculated, the fluid collections may be unilocular or multilocular with many septae (Figs. 1.56 and 1.57). The latter

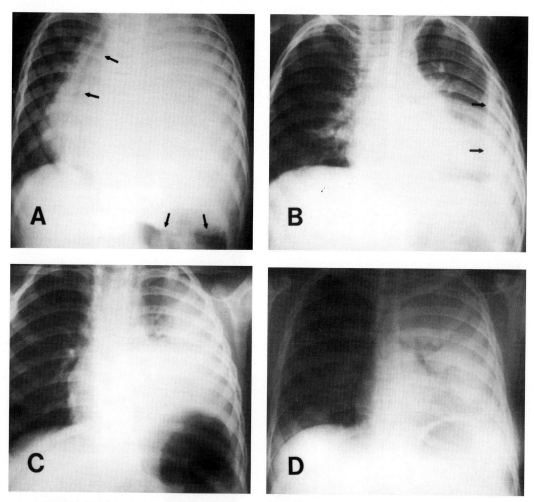

FIGURE 1.55. *Empyema: classic configuration and atypical patterns.* **(A)** Classic massive empyema with contralateral mediastinal displacement and ipsilateral diaphragmatic leaflet depression (*arrows*). **(B)** Another typical case, but with a smaller empyema (*arrows*). **(C)** Empyema with no shift. The developing empyema is not large enough to produce mediastinal shift. **(D)** Pneumonia or empyema? The air bronchogram would at first suggest consolidating pneumonia. One should, however, ask the question, "How many times have I seen a consolidating pneumonia involving the entire lung?" This would be unusual, and furthermore, the air bronchogram does not extend to the periphery. The problem here is a developing empyema, partially compressing the ipsilateral lung.

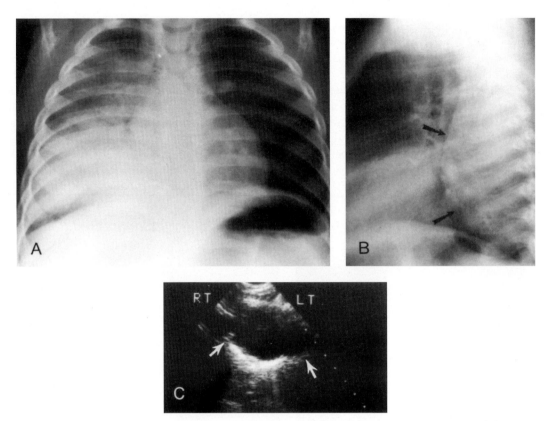

FIGURE 1.56. *Empyema: ultrasonographic detection.* **(A)** Patient with a consolidation of the right middle lobe and a density projected over the lower portion of the upper lobe. **(B)** Lateral view demonstrating increased density in the region of the right middle lobe and a mass located posteriorly (*arrows*). **(C)** Sonogram demonstrates the density to be a hypoechoic, loculated empyema (*arrows*).

collections, of course, are difficult to drain. Pulmonary infiltrates are variable, and in many cases once the purulent fluid is removed, the lungs turn out to be surprisingly clear. This is a common paradox and difficult to explain, for one would presume that a consolidating pneumonia would be seen in all these cases.

If empyema is accompanied by pneumothorax so that pyopneumothorax results, one can be almost completely certain that *S. aureus* is the offending organism. The thick, tenacious secretions characteristic of this infection lead to air trapping secondary to endobronchial obstruction, and as a result complicating pneumothorax is common. In many

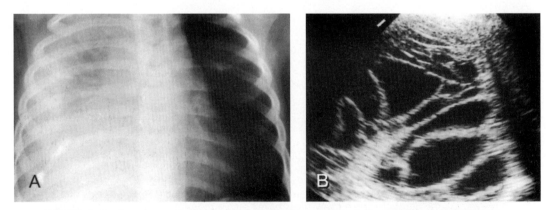

FIGURE 1.57. *Empyema: ultrasonographic confirmation.* **(A)** Note the totally opacified hemithorax and a little aeration of the right upper lobe. There is contralateral mediastinal shift, and a space-occupying process is present on the right. Pleural fluid or a frank empyema compressing the lung circumferentially should be suspected. **(B)** Ultrasonogram demonstrates the presence of a multiloculated empyema.

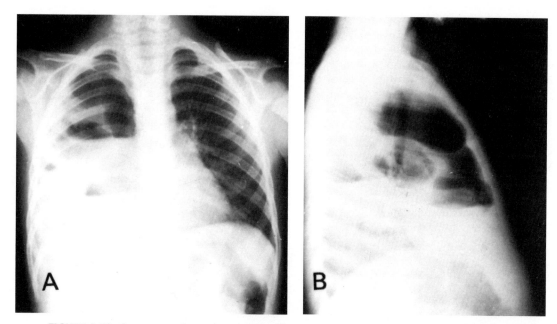

FIGURE 1.58. *Pyopneumothorax (empyema with pneumothorax in staphylococcal infection).* **(A)** Note numerous air–fluid levels on the right. This finding is characteristic of staphylococcal infections. Some of the air collections also could be pneumatoceles. **(B)** Lateral view showing similar findings.

cases, the free air is loculated in numerous compartments, and a multitude of air–fluid levels is seen on the upright film (Fig. 1.58).

Simple pleural effusions, of course, can be seen with pneumonias produced by the same organisms producing empyemas (Fig. 1.59), including *M. pneumoniae*. Pleural effusions also can be seen with primary tuberculous and fungal infections but are rare with viral infections (2). Some modification might be made for newborn infants and patients with HIV and other immunologic problems.

Simple pleural effusions also are commonly seen with kidney disease such as the nephrotic syndrome and acute glomerulonephritis, chest and abdominal tumors such as neuroblastoma and lymphoma, subphrenic or hepatic inflammatory processes, chest-wall or spine lesions, pancreatitis, congestive heart failure, and the collagen vascular diseases. All pleural effusions are readily demonstrable with computed tomographic (CT) and ultrasound imaging, but the latter is more expedient (Fig. 1.60). With CT axial views, pleural fluid is best seen along the posterior and lateral walls of the chest (Fig. 1.61). If such fluid is deep in the

FIGURE 1.59. *Pneumonia with pleural effusion.* This patient has a right lower-lobe consolidating pneumococcal pneumonia, but in addition there is a pleural effusion present (*arrows*).

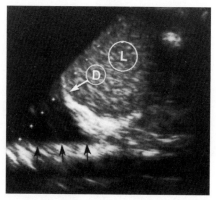

FIGURE 1.60. *Value of ultrasound in detection of pleural fluid.* Note typical sonolucent fluid in the posterior sulcus (*arrows*). *D,* diaphragm; *L,* liver.

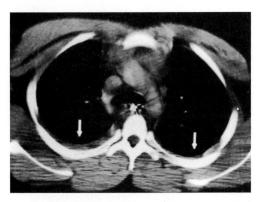

FIGURE 1.61. *Pleural fluid: CT demonstration.* Note small bilateral posterior pleural effusions (*arrows*).

costophrenic sulcus, however, it may be difficult to differentiate it from abdominal fluid. It is here that ultrasound is most useful, because it clearly identifies the diaphragm (Fig. 1.60).

Most often the first roentgenographic sign of a pleural effusion consists of blunting of the costophrenic angles so as to produce wedgelike menisci, which extend upward along the lateral chest wall (Fig.1.62A). Similar collections with characteristically curved or sloping menisci are seen in the posterior costophrenic angles on lateral view (Fig. 1.62B); larger volumes of pleural fluid can be seen to extend up the entire lateral chest wall and eventually over the apex of the lung (Fig. 1.62C). A similar layering phenomenon can

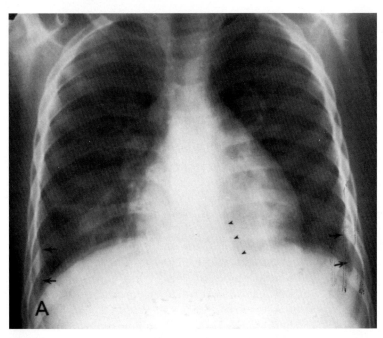

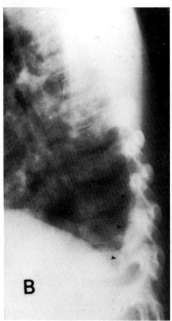

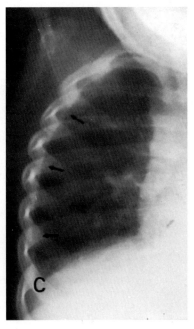

FIGURE 1.62. *Pleural effusions: common presenting configurations.* **(A)** Note characteristic early accumulations of pleural fluid in both costophrenic angles (*large arrows*). In addition, there is accumulation of fluid in the left paraspinal gutter, just barely visible through the cardiac silhouette (*arrowheads*). **(B)** Lateral view demonstrating characteristic sloping or curving configuration of fluid in the posterior costophrenic angles (*arrows*). **(C)** Larger-volume pleural effusion layered along the entire right lateral chest wall and extending over the apex (*arrows*).

occur retrosternally (Fig. 1.63B). In other instances, early pleural effusions may present with what at first appears to be unusual prominence or thickening of the interlobar fissures or with wedgelike tapering accumulations of the fluid at either end of these fissures (Fig. 1.63). Fluid accumulations in the right or left major fissures characteristically appear as thick, sloping lines (Fig. 1.64), the so-called vertical fissure (4).

Pleural effusions in the supine position frequently are overlooked. Most often, one encounters such effusions in a critically ill or severely injured child in whom a supine, instead of an upright, chest film is obtained. In such cases, fluid collects and layers beneath the lung (6), and rather than conforming to one of its more typical configurations, it simply produces a generalized increase in density of the involved hemithorax (Fig. 1.65). If this is the only sign present, one can see why the pleural effusion can be missed. If, on the other hand, other more classic signs of pleural effusion are present, the diagnosis is easier to establish.

Subpulmonic pleural effusions also are often difficult to detect and, in fact, may completely elude the unwary observer. These effusions are free-flowing (6,8) and in the upright position collect between the lung and the diaphragmatic leaflet. In some cases, the fluid so conforms to the normal curvature of the diaphragm that one is led to believe that the diaphragmatic leaflet is elevated (Fig. 1.66). If telltale subtle signs are sought, however, these effusions can be detected with greater certainty. Specifically, these signs consist of (a) unusual flatness of the apparently high diaphragmatic leaflet, (b) a sharp dropoff of the diaphragmatic leaflet laterally, (c) obliteration of the adjacent portion of the cardiac silhouette, (d) increased density of the posterior phrenicovertebral sulcus, (e) paraspinal collections of fluid, especially on the left, (f) peculiar bumps and humps of the apparently high diaphragmatic leaflet, (g) an increase in the space between the top of the apparently elevated diaphragmatic leaflet and stomach bubble, (h) loss of visualization of the normal blood vessels of the lung through the uppermost part of the apparent diaphragmatic leaflet, and (i) evidence

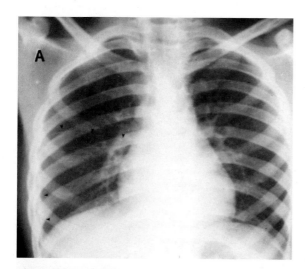

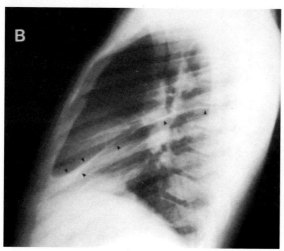

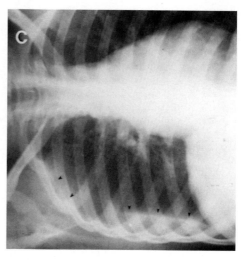

FIGURE 1.63. *Early, subtle pleural effusions.* **(A)** The pleural effusion on the right might be overlooked in this child, who eventually was determined to have a collagen vascular disease. Note however, that there is fluid along the right lateral chest wall (*lateral arrows*) and some fluid in the right minor fissure (*upper arrows*). **(B)** Lateral view showing thin layers of fluid in all the interlobar fissures, but note specifically the typical tapering wedgelike configuration of fluid in the anteriormost portion of the right major fissure (*arrows*). A layer of fluid is also present retrosternally. **(C)** Decubitus film with the right side down demonstrates how much fluid actually is present on the right (*arrows*). Decubitus views are invaluable in demonstrating actual volumes of known pleural effusions and confirming the presence of subtle ones.

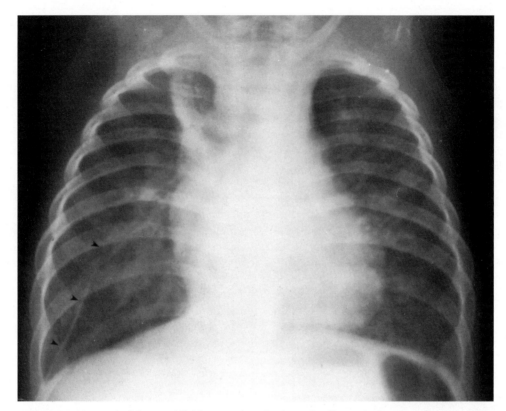

FIGURE 1.64. *Vertical fissure.* If fluid accumulates in the major fissure, its lowermost portion can be seen as a sloping, but basically vertical, line on frontal view (*arrows*). In this case, it is on the right but also can be seen on the left. This patient has congestive heart failure, secondary to congenital heart disease (endocardial cushion defect with left-to-right shunt). Atelectasis of the right upper lobe also is present.

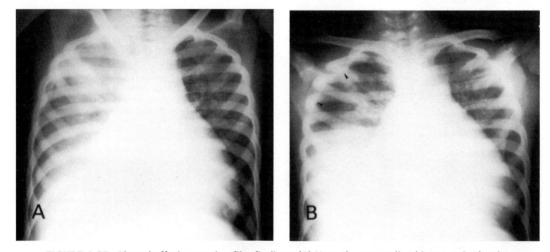

FIGURE 1.65. *Pleural effusion: supine film findings.* **(A)** Note the generalized increase in density of the right hemithorax. Cardiomegaly and pulmonary edema also are present in this patient, who suffered a severe fluid overload. The fact that a large volume of fluid is layered behind the right lung might be overlooked if this were the only film obtained. **(B)** An upright view, however, shows clearing of the right upper lung field secondary to the fluid shifting downward. It now totally opacifies the lower-lung field and mimics a consolidation. Some fluid remains in the apex (*arrows*).

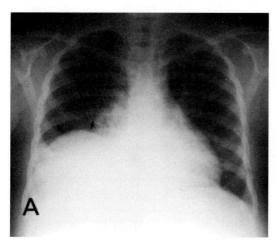 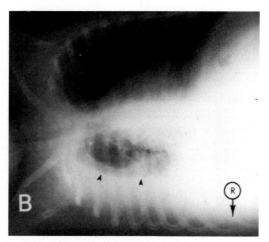

FIGURE 1.66. *Subpulmonic effusion presenting as an apparently elevated diaphragmatic leaflet.* **(A)** The right diaphragmatic leaflet appears elevated (*arrows*). The finding, however, actually represents a subpulmonic effusion. **(B)** Decubitus view with right side down confirms the presence of the large pleural effusion. This patient had nephrotic syndrome.

of pleural fluid collecting in more familiar sites with more familiar configurations. All of these aspects of subpulmonic effusions are illustrated in Fig. 1.67.

In terms of apparent elevation of the diaphragmatic leaflet with subpulmonic effusions and the sharp dropoff laterally, an explanation involving the pulmonary ligament has been offered (1). Evidently the pulmonary ligament more or less tethers the lung medially and does not allow it to be elevated to the same degree as its lateral counterpart. Consequently, if fluid collects between the lung and the diaphragm, the lateral portion of the lung is elevated to a greater degree, and the stepoff occurs.

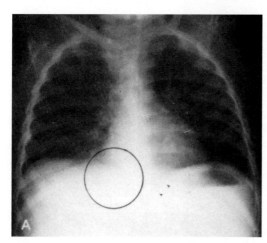 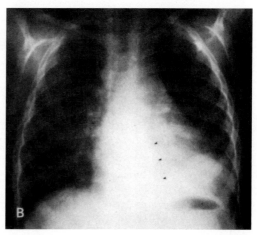

FIGURE 1.67. *Subpulmonic effusion: some subtle telltale signs.* **(A)** There is a subpulmonic effusion on the right. Telltale signs include: slight elevation and flattening of the right diaphragmatic leaflet; a sharp dropoff of the lateral aspect of the diaphragmatic leaflet; minimal fluid along the lateral chest wall extending into the minor fissure (*arrows on the right*); obliteration of the right cardiac border (positive silhouette sign); and opacification of the right phrenicovertebral angle (*circle*). The normal, radiolucent left phrenicovertebral angle is defined by the *arrows* just to the left of the lower thoracic spine. **(B)** Subpulmonic effusion on the left causes apparent elevation of the diaphragmatic leaflet. Note, however, the increased distance between the top of the apparent diaphragmatic leaflet and the stomach bubble and the triangular collection of fluid in the paraspinal gutter (*arrows*). Both of these findings should alert one to the presence of a subpulmonic effusion, but in addition it should be noted that although the pulmonary vascular markings can be seen through the top of the right diaphragmatic leaflet, they are not as easily visible through the top of the apparently high left diaphragmatic leaflet. Such obliteration of the vascular markings by the presence of subpulmonic fluid is another subtle telltale finding of such effusions. In other cases, peculiar bumps along the diaphragmatic leaflets serve to alert one to the presence of a subpulmonic effusion (Fig. 1.68).

In addition to the foregoing considerations regarding subpulmonic effusions, it should be remembered that right-sided subpulmonic effusions can depress the liver downward so as to render it palpable clinically; those on the left can depress the diaphragm and gastric bubble to such an extent that a masslike configuration results (Fig. 1.68). Indeed, one may be surprised at how much fluid can accumulate in the subpulmonic space.

Subpulmonic effusions often are easier to detect on the lateral view, because they fill the posterior costophrenic sulcus in the characteristic meniscoid or sloping fashion of any pleural effusion (Fig. 1.69), but of course if one still is uncertain a decubitus view almost always clarifies the situation (Fig. 1.69). Indeed, with the decubitus view and with the patient in the Trendelenburg position, effusions as small as 5 to 25 mL can be demonstrated (3,7).

Mediastinal and paraspinal gutter effusions also often elude detection. Posteriorly, in the paraspinal gutter, these effusions usually assume a variably long, tapering, triangular, or wedgelike paraspinal configuration (Figs. 1.62A and 1.67B); anteriorly or in the middle mediastinum, these effusions may appear masslike (9) or triangular (Fig. 1.70). Large pleural effusions occasionally can mimic a lobar con-

solidation (Fig. 1.71), and, unquestionably, decubitus views are the answer in these cases. In still other cases, pleural effusions, or empyemas, may become loculated in the various interlobar fissures (Fig. 1.72). Characteristically, these accumulations are round, oval, or spindle-shaped, but some may appear as large pulmonary masses (Fig. 1.73) and others as irregular infiltrates (Fig. 1.74). Many are more typical, however, and show characteristically tapering ends as they lie along the axis of the involved fissure (Fig. 1.75). In this regard, it also should be noted that although on one projection these effusions may appear characteristic, on the other they usually appear atypical. Pleural effusions or empyemas that loculate laterally or posteriorly are less of a problem (Fig. 1.76). Those effusions or empyemas that loculate along the lung base and thus become difficult to differentiate from a subphrenic abscess can be identified with confidence using ultrasonography.

Finally, before leaving the discussion of pleural effusions, it should be noted that many normal children have minimal collections of pleural fluid in their costophrenic angles (5). This is entirely normal and common (Fig. 1.77), and such findings should not be misinterpreted as a pathologic pleural effusion.

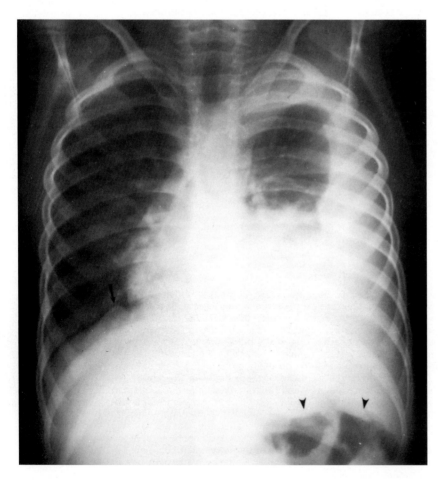

FIGURE 1.68. *Massive pleural effusion with large subpulmonic component.* Note the large effusion on the left. It virtually encircles the aerated lung. There also, however, is a large subpulmonic component that depresses the stomach and splenic flexure to such a degree that a mass might be suggested (*arrows on left*). The *arrow* on the right points to the telltale bump of a subpulmonic effusion, simultaneously present on the right.

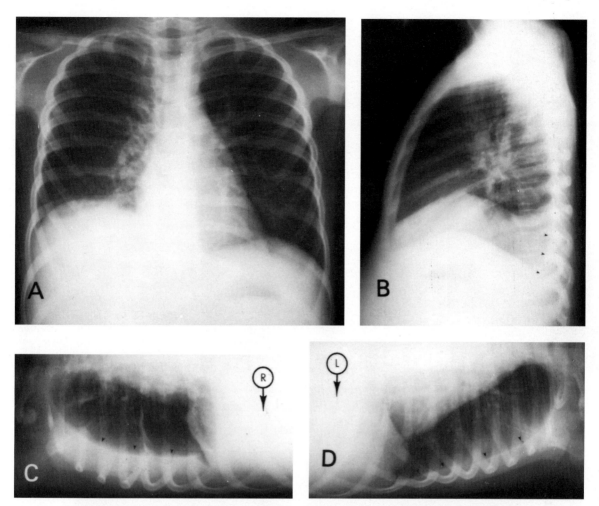

FIGURE 1.69. *Bilateral subpulmonic effusions: value of lateral and decubitus films.* **(A)** Both diaphragmatic leaflets appear elevated in this patient with nephrotic syndrome. Bilateral sub-pulmonic pleural effusions are present. **(B)** Lateral view demonstrates characteristic blunting and obliteration of both posterior costophrenic angles, and a typical sloping edge of one of the posterior collections of pleural fluid (*arrows*). **(C)** Right lateral decubitus film shows how the fluid collects and layers along the right lateral wall. **(D)** Left lateral decubitus view shows similar findings on the left (*arrows*).

Chylothorax is not a common problem in childhood but occasionally can be seen with rupture of the thoracic duct secondary to blunt chest trauma. Otherwise, chylothorax is a problem of newborn and young infants, and of the postthoracotomy patient. Occasionally, the thoracic duct can be obstructed by a hidden mediastinal tumor or cyst and chylothorax can be the presenting problem, but this is a rare situation.

Other pleural fluid collections can be seen with spontaneous or traumatic esophageal rupture, bronchial tears following blunt chest trauma, or bleeding secondary to rib fractures or posttraumatic great vessel rupture. With esophageal perforations and bronchial tears, both air and fluid are seen in the pleural space (i.e., hemopneumothorax or hydropneu-

mothorax). With esophageal perforations, these changes usually occur on the left side in older children and adults but on the right in neonates. These perforations are believed to result from acute increases in intraesophageal pressure secondary to traumatic compression of the abdomen and lower chest, or in some cases from profound vomiting.

Finally, it should be noted that a picture suggesting a large pleural effusion can result in those cases in which there are massive unilateral atelectasis and pronounced contralateral compensatory emphysema (see Fig. 1.87B). It is most important that this pitfall be appreciated so as to avoid needless thoracentesis. The same precaution should be observed in those cases of atypical upper-lobe atelectasis mimicking apical pleural effusions (see Fig. 1.91).

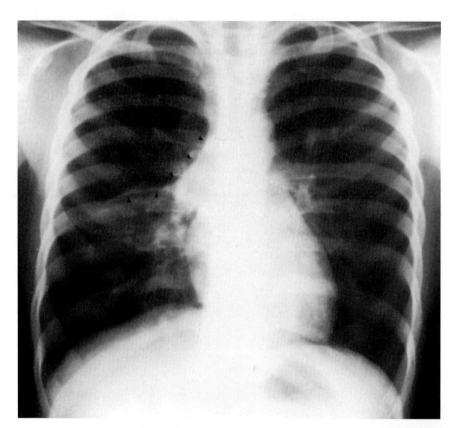

FIGURE 1.70. *Mediastinal effusion.* Note triangular mediastinal effusion (*upper three arrows*). The triangular configuration could be confused with the sail sign of the normal thymus gland in a younger infant, or an area of segmental atelectasis. If the fluid also extends into the minor fissure (*lower two arrows*), however, the diagnosis of an effusion should be favored.

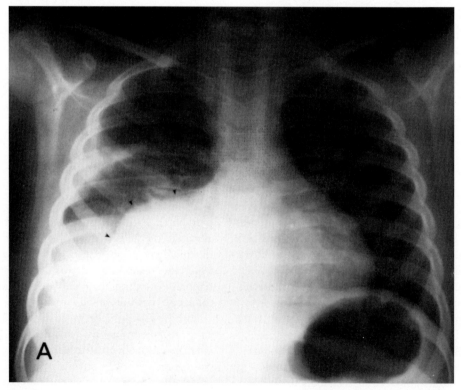

FIGURE 1.71. *Pleural effusion mimicking lobar pneumonia.* **(A)** The pleural effusion on the right could be misinterpreted as a consolidating pneumonia (*arrows*). Note fluid along the right lateral chest wall and some fluid extending into the minor fissure.

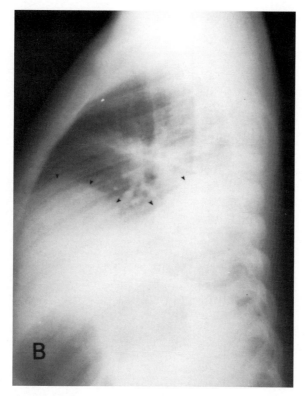

FIGURE 1.71. (continued) **(B)** On lateral view, subpulmonic fluid collections are outlined by the *arrows*. Either one of these configurations could be misinterpreted as a consolidating lobar pneumonia.

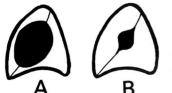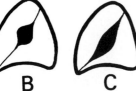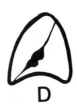

FIGURE 1.72. *Loculated interlobar fissure effusions: diagrammatic representations.* **(A)** Large loculated effusion. The characteristic tapering, spindle-shaped ends often are not present with effusions this large. **(B)** Classic appearance of loculated interlobar effusion presenting as a rounded or oval mass with characteristic tapering, spindle-shaped ends trailing into the fissure. **(C)** Similar configuration but with a longer, more oval effusion. **(D)** Less characteristic, irregular collection of loculated pleural fluid.

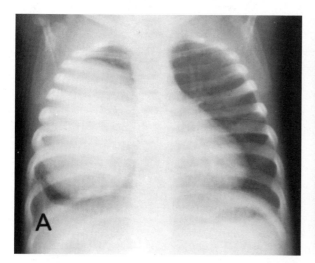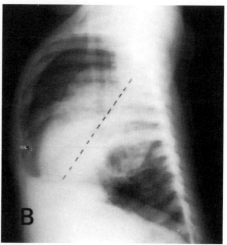

FIGURE 1.73. *Large loculated empyema.* **(A)** This patient originally had a staphylococcal pneumonia with empyema. This roentgenogram was obtained 3 weeks after treatment and shows how the empyema has loculated into a large, perfectly oval, mass-like lesion. The findings defy distinction from a cyst or tumor. **(B)** Lateral view shows the location of the apparent mass. Although the characteristic tapering ends of a loculated pleural effusion are not present, the main axis of the lesion still conforms to the axis of the greater fissure (*dotted line*) and is the clue to the correct diagnosis.

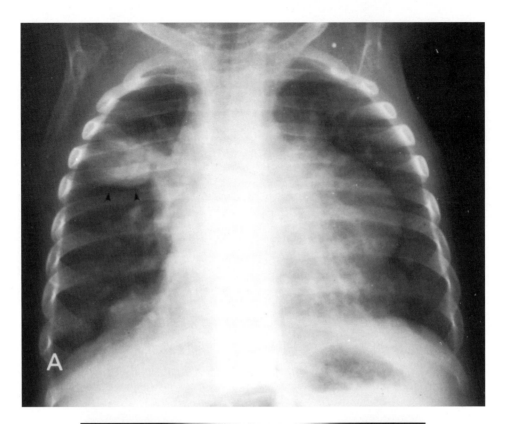

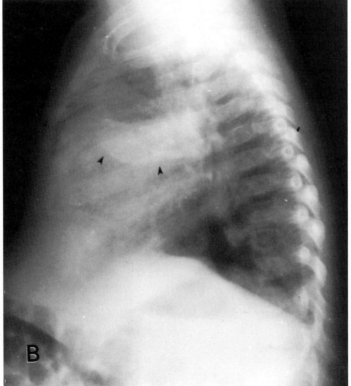

FIGURE 1.74. *Loculated pleural effusion: irregular configuration.* **(A)** On frontal view, this loculated effusion could be misinterpreted as an early consolidating pneumonia (*arrows*). This patient also has an underlying left-to-right shunt, some congestion, and bilateral eventrations. **(B)** Lateral view delineates the somewhat irregular-appearing loculated pleural effusion in the right minor fissure (*arrows*).

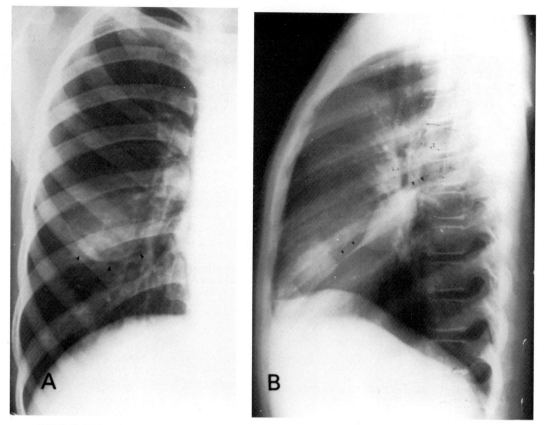

FIGURE 1.75. *Classic loculated pleural effusion.* (**A**) Note the area of increased density in the right midlung field and especially note the sharp rounded lower edge (*arrows*). (**B**) Lateral view clearly establishes that a loculated effusion is present in the right major fissure. Notice the characteristic tapering, spindle-shaped ends of this pseudomass (*arrows*). It lies along the fissure and its tapering ends trail into the fissure. Because these effusions tend to disappear rapidly and unexpectedly, they have been termed vanishing tumors.

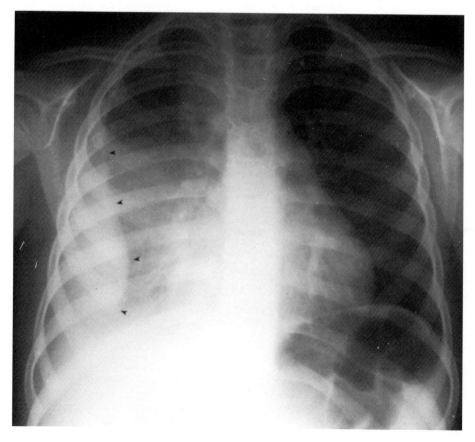

FIGURE 1.76. *Loculated fluid (empyema): lateral chest wall.* This patient had a pneumococcal pneumonia and eventually developed an empyema, which finally loculated laterally (*arrows*). Such loculations are common in the resolving stage of any type of empyema.

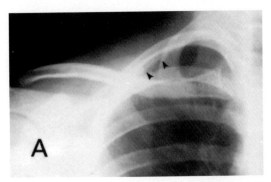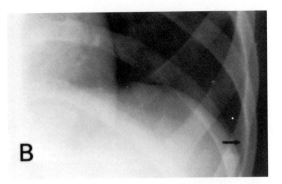

FIGURE 1.77. *Normal pleural reflections mimicking pleural effusions.* **(A)** Apparent fluid over the apex of the right lung (*arrows*). This finding commonly is seen in children and results from normal soft tissues between the lung and ribs. **(B)** Pleural reflection in the left costophrenic angle of a normal child (*arrows*). There is some debate as to whether this finding represents the pleural reflection alone, or a minimal amount of normal pleural fluid. Whichever explanation is correct, the finding is normal, but probably it reflects the presence of a small amount of normal fluid (5).

REFERENCES

1. Budikoff JC. The pulmonary ligament and subpulmonic effusion. *Chest* 1981;80:505-507.
2. Cho CT, Hiatt WO, Behbehani AM. Pneumonia and massive pleural effusion associated with adenovirus type 7. *Am J Dis Child* 1973;126:92–94.
3. Collins JD, Burwell D, Furmanski S, Lorber P, Steckel RJ. Minimal detectable pleural effusions: A roentgenopathology model. *Radiology* 1972;105:51–53.
4. Davis LA. Vertical fissure line. *AJR* 1960;84:451–453.
5. Ecklof O, Torngren A. Pleural fluid in healthy children. *Acta Radiol* 1971;11:346–349.
6. Fleischner FG. Atypical arrangement of free pleural effusion. *Radiol Clin North Am* 1963;1:347–361.
7. Moskowitz H, Platt RT, Schachar R, Mellins H. Roentgen visualization of minute pleural effusion: Experimental study to determine the minimal amount of pleural fluid visible on a radiograph. *Radiology* 1973;109:33–35.
8. Peterson JA. Recognition of infrapulmonary pleural effusion. *Radiology* 1960;74:34–41.
9. Pines A, Kaplinsky N, Rubinstein Z, Bregman J, Meytes D, Frankl O. Massive loculated pleural effusion simulating mediastinal masses. *Br J Radiol* 1982;55:240–242.

HILAR AND PARATRACHEAL ADENOPATHY

Enlarged lymph nodes in the hilar or paratracheal regions are most often inflammatory in nature, and bilateral hilar adenopathy most often is seen with viral lower respiratory tract infections. Of course, bilateral hilar or paratracheal adenopathy also can be seen with conditions such as sarcoidosis (Fig. 1.78A), histoplasmosis and other fungal disease, histiocytosis X, and even tuberculosis (Fig. 1.78B). Most often, however, hilar or paratracheal adenopathy in tuberculosis is unilateral. Discrete hilar adenopathy secondary to lymphoma or leukemia is not as common a presenting feature in children as coalescent mediastinal adenopathy.

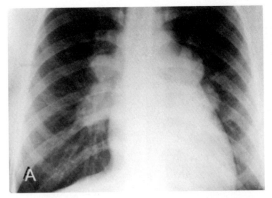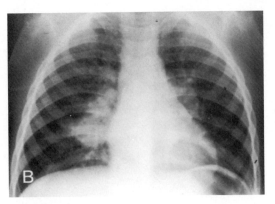

FIGURE 1.78. *Bilateral hilar adenopathy.* **(A)** Typical lumpy bilateral hilar adenopathy in patient with sarcoid. **(B)** Tuberculosis with bilateral hilar adenopathy. Most often in tuberculosis, hilar adenopathy is unilateral.

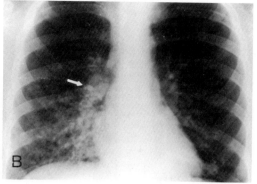
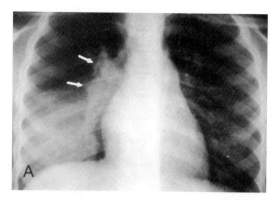

FIGURE 1.79. *Unilateral adenopathy with pulmonary infection.* **(A)** Note classic consolidation caused by bacterial pneumonia in the right lower lobe. There is ipsilateral hilar adenopathy (*arrows*). **(B)** Reticulonodular pattern characteristic of *Mycoplasma pneumoniae* infection in the right lower lobe and associated ipsilateral hilar adenopathy (*arrow*).

Unilateral hilar or paratracheal adenopathy also occurs with bacterial and mycoplasmal infections (Fig. 1.79), but more often such adenopathy is the hallmark of primary pulmonary tuberculosis in childhood. There is good reason for this to occur, for if one considers the basic pathology in tuberculosis, one recalls that adenopathy is secondary to the peripheral Ghon's lesion, and that this lesion usually is single. Because of this, hilar or paratracheal lymph-node involvement usually is unilateral. Indeed, a good rule to follow is that unilateral hilar or paratracheal adenopathy, with or without associated change in the lungs, should be considered tuberculous in origin until proven otherwise. Occasionally, *M. pneumoniae* infections can produce similar findings, but primary pulmonary tuberculosis should be the first consideration in any patient presenting with such a picture. Adenopathy in these cases may be discrete and smooth-edged or fuzzy because of associated, adjacent edema (Fig. 1.80).

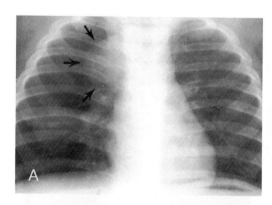
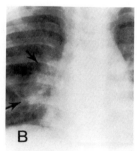
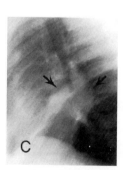
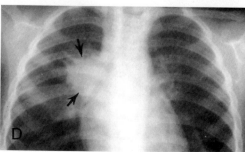

FIGURE 1.80. *Hilar and paratracheal adenopathy.* **(A)** Note smooth-edged right paratracheal adenopathy (*arrows*) in patient with tuberculosis. **(B)** Less distinct but nonetheless clearly evident and prominent right hilar adenopathy (*arrows*) in another patient with tuberculosis. **(C)** Note the typical paracarinal location on lateral view. **(D)** Another patient with right hilar adenopathy but with fuzzy edges (*arrows*) because of adjacent inflammatory edema. Also note that there is an early consolidation developing in the right middle lobe.

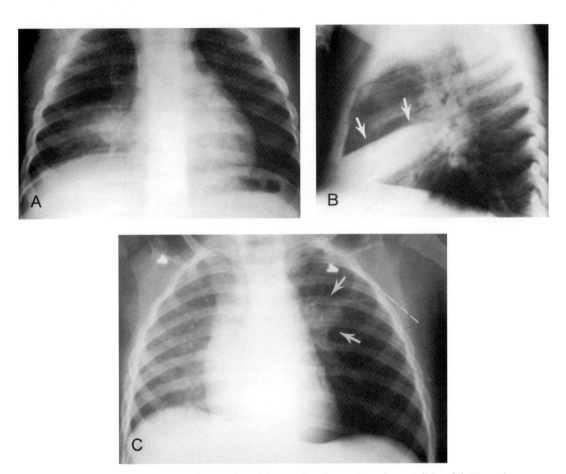

FIGURE 1.81. *Tuberculous adenopathy with associated aeration abnormalities.* **(A)** Note the density in the region of the right middle lobe. Hilar adenopathy is not easy to detect. **(B)** Lateral view demonstrates that the density is caused by classic right middle lobe atelectasis (*arrows*). Also note the prominent hilar region, attesting to the presence of hilar adenopathy. **(C)** Another patient with left hilar adenopathy (*arrows*) associated with obstructive emphysema of the left lung. Both of these patients had primary pulmonary tuberculosis.

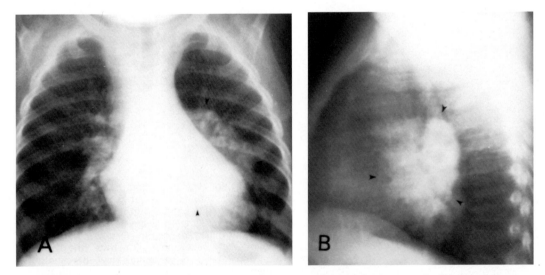

FIGURE 1.82. *Hilar adenopathy versus superior segment lower-lobe pneumonia.* **(A)** Note massive unilateral left hilar adenopathy in this patient with primary pulmonary tuberculosis (*arrows*). **(B)** Lateral view shows typical central, paracarinal location of hilar adenopathy (*arrows*).

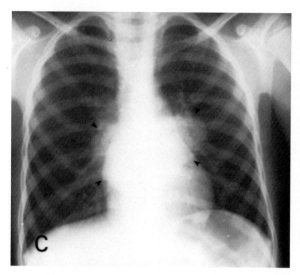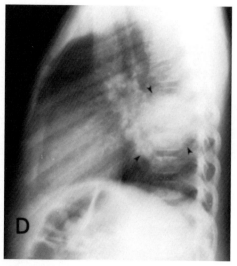

FIGURE 1.82. *(continued)* **(C)** Patient in whom findings might at first suggest bilateral hilar adenopathy or a posterior mediastinal mass *(arrows)*. **(D)** Lateral view shows that the findings represent bilateral superior segment lower-lobe pneumonias *(arrows)*. Characteristically, these pneumonias lie high in the lower lobes, behind the major fissure, and, unlike enlarged hilar lymph nodes, far behind the carina. In most cases, they overlie the spine. This patient had pneumococcal "double" pneumonia with consolidations in the superior segments of both lower lobes.

Atelectasis is a common associated finding in tuberculosis and usually is secondary to endobronchial disease and not the adenopathy. The associated atelectasis, however, may obscure the fact that hilar adenopathy is present (Fig. 1.81A and B). This is less of a problem if obstructive emphysema is present (Fig. 1.81C), but emphysema is far less common than atelectasis.

Before leaving the subject of hilar adenopathy, one should recall that its presence can be mimicked, on frontal view, by superior segment lower-lobe pneumonias. No such problem, however, should last for long, for on lateral view it clearly is seen that hilar adenopathy is central (paracarinal), and superior-segment lower-lobe pneumonias lie posterior to the carina (Fig. 1.82). Large pulmonary arteries, such as might be seen with pulmonary hypertension mimicking hilar adenopathy, are not as great a problem in childhood as in the adult.

ATELECTASIS AND EMPHYSEMA

Which Side Is Abnormal?

Among the most troublesome problems with unilateral, total-lung atelectasis or emphysema is trying to decide which side of the chest is abnormal. In this regard, there is no question that an inspiratory–expiratory sequence of chest roentgenograms is the ultimate answer, but there are *certain rules that can be utilized in determining which side is abnormal* before this is obtained: (a) In obstructive emphysema, the large, hyperlucent lung usually shows diminished pulmonary vascularity; (b) in compensatory emphysema, the large emphysematous, radiolucent (nonobstructed) lung usually shows normal or engorged pulmonary vascularity; and (c) an obstructed, emphysematous lung, no matter how large, cannot compress the other lung to the point of total atelectasis or opacity (Fig. 1.83).

Of course, not every initial film reveals the foregoing findings with clarity, and thus an inspiratory–expiratory film sequence should be obtained. The most important point to note on this study is that usually *the abnormal lung, no matter what its initial appearance, does not significantly change size from inspiration to expiration.* In other words, the lung that changes size most is the normal lung (Fig. 1.83C and D). For the most part, these rules suffice for almost any aeration disturbance encountered except, perhaps, that seen with a congenitally hypoplastic lung. A hypoplastic lung is small and hyperlucent (because of decreased vascularity) but shows change in volume on inspiratory-expiratory film studies.

Atelectasis is a common roentgenographic finding and can involve an entire lung, a lobe, or just a portion of a lung. Indeed, sublobar or segmental atelectasis is quite common in children and, for the most part, occurs with viral lower respiratory tract infections and asthma. To be sure, these areas of atelectasis often are confused with true pulmonary infiltrates (Fig. 1.84). The reason that such atelectasis is common in children is that the collateral airdrift phenomenon, through the pores of Kohn and ducts of Lambert, is not as efficient in children as in adults (5). Consequently, whereas in the adult atelectasis, especially

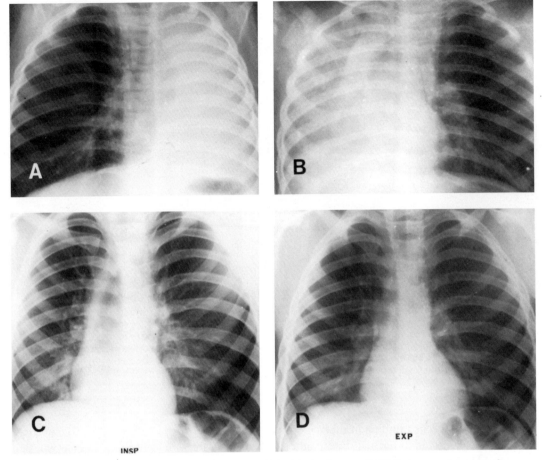

FIGURE 1.83. *Atelectasis and emphysema: Which side is abnormal?* (**A**) Note complete opacification of the left lung. The right lung shows compensatory emphysema and relatively normal vascularity. The fact that the left lung is totally opacified suggests that the problem is atelectasis on the left. An enlarged lung, resulting from obstructed emphysema, no matter how large it gets, seldom, if ever, totally compresses the other lung. (**B**) The right lung is small in this case, but not totally opacified and airless. The problem here is obstructive emphysema on the left. The vascularity may be slightly decreased, but an expiratory view would be necessary for final diagnosis. (**C**) Large left lung. Note that vascularity is normal or even slightly engorged in the left lung, suggesting compensatory emphysema. (**D**) Expiratory film shows the left lung to empty well, but the right lung to change little in size. It is the right lung that is abnormal and, indeed, was obstructed by an endobronchial mucous plug in an asthmatic.

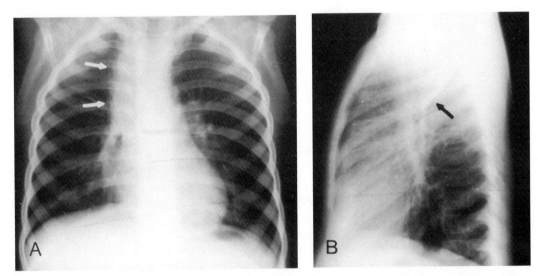

FIGURE 1.84. *Sublobar and segmental atelectasis.* (**A**) Child with acute asthma. Note area of apparent consolidation in the right paratracheal region (*arrows*). This represents collapse of a portion of the right upper lobe. A more subtle finding, assisting in interpretation, is the fact that there is a slight right mediastinal shift. (**B**) Lateral view demonstrates early atelectasis (*arrows*). With such minimal degrees of atelectasis, the fissures may not be markedly displaced, and differentiation from pneumonia is more difficult.

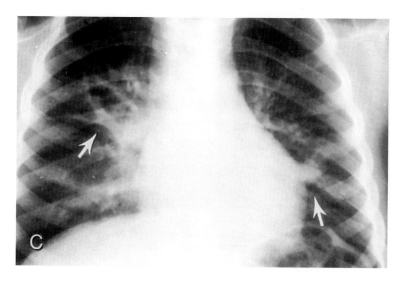

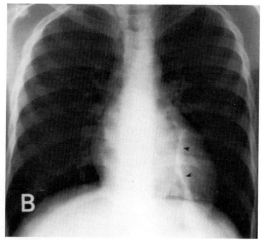

FIGURE 1.84. *(continued)* **(C)** Widespread perihilar–peribronchial infiltrates resulting from viral bronchitis, with scattered linear, wedgelike, and patchy areas of segmental atelectasis *(arrows)*.

segmental, does not last very long, it does tend to linger in children. If such atelectasis is widespread and patchy, it is indeed difficult to differentiate from pulmonary infiltration (Fig. 1.84C). It should be remembered, however, that it is still basically central in distribution. On the other hand, if such atelectasis produces vertical, horizontal, or oblique streaks or wedges, it is easier to appreciate these densities for what they are (Fig. 1.85). Such atelectasis often is referred to as ***discoid, plate-like,*** or ***vertical*** atelectasis.

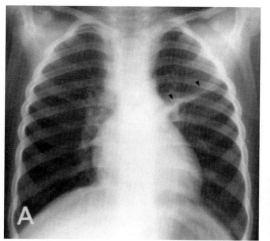

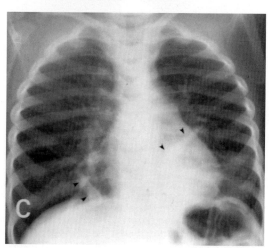

FIGURE 1.85. *Discoid "platelike" or vertical atelectasis.* **(A)** Segmental discoid atelectasis in the left upper lobe *(arrows)*. **(B)** Another patient demonstrating so-called vertical discoid atelectasis *(arrows)*. **(C)** Multiple oblique densities are seen throughout both lung fields, representing multiple areas of segmental, wedgelike atelectasis *(arrows)*.

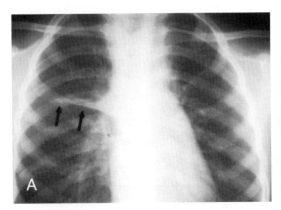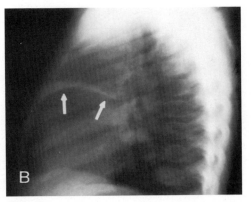

FIGURE 1.86. *Early lobar atelectasis.* **(A)** Note slight elevation of the minor fissure (*arrows*), and that its inferior edge is sharp but its superior edge is fuzzy. **(B)** Lateral view showing similar findings (*arrows*). Without close inspection, these findings often are misinterpreted as small interlobar effusions, but pleural effusions demonstrate sharp edges on both sides.

Atelectasis also can produce a confusing picture when a lobe is just beginning to collapse. The problem arises if the lobe collapses along a major fissure (Fig. 1.86). In such cases, the outer edge of the slightly elevated or inwardly displaced fissure remains sharp, while the inner edge is somewhat indistinct. Indistinctness results from the fact that aeration of the lung still is present. Most likely bronchial obstruction is incomplete in these cases. Overall, therefore, aeration of the collapsing lobe still is present, and thus although the outer edge of the lung abutting the fissure is sharp, the inner aspect is indistinct.

Atelectasis of an entire lung, or a lobe thereof, is most often seen with asthma, viral lower respiratory tract infection, primary pulmonary tuberculosis, and foreign bodies. In the classic case of total lung atelectasis, the findings are clearly apparent, for the entire hemithorax becomes opacified, the mediastinum shifts to the ipsilateral side, and the heart virtually disappears into the atelectatic lung (Fig. 1.87). However, because the other lung becomes overaerated (compensatory emphysema), one very often misinterprets the findings as being abnormal on the wrong side (i.e., obstructive emphysema with mediastinal shift). Expiratory films are the answer

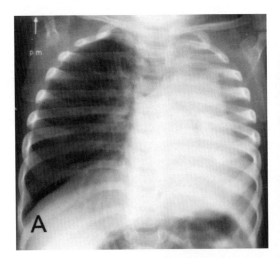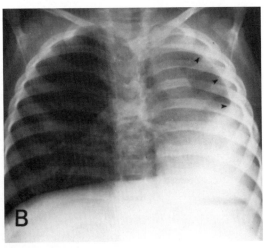

FIGURE 1.87. *Total atelectasis of a lung.* **(A)** In this infant, atelectasis was caused by an obstructing mucous plug. Note the marked loss of volume on the left, pronounced shift of the mediastinum to the left, and compensatory overexpansion of the right lung. The pulmonary vascularity in the right lung is normal or, in fact, a little increased, and this is against obstructive emphysema. With obstructive emphysema the vascularity is diminished. **(B)** Another patient with complete atelectasis of the left lung and pronounced compensatory emphysema of the right lung. The right lung has herniated across the mediastinum to produce a configuration erroneously suggesting a left pleural effusion (*arrows*). This is not pleural fluid; it merely represents the interface between the overaerated, herniated right lung as it is superimposed on the collapsed left lung. The pulmonary vascularity in the right lung is not markedly diminished, and this identifies the problem as one of compensatory, rather than obstructive, emphysema. In other words, blood from the atelectatic left lung is shunted to the right lung. If the right lung were this distended because of obstructive emphysema, the vascularity would be diminished.

here, but before they are obtained one also should evaluate the pulmonary vascularity. In compensatory emphysema, the vascularity in the overaerated lung usually is normal or accentuated; in obstructive emphysema usually it is decreased. Furthermore, it should be noted that in total-lung atelectasis the collapsed lung is totally opaque, even down into the costophrenic angle. This can happen only with atelectasis or agenesis, for an overaerated lung alone, no matter how large, cannot compress the other lung to the point of complete opacity. Some aeration remains and is most evident in the costophrenic angle.

Classic atelectatic patterns for collapse of the various lobes are diagrammatically demonstrated in Fig. 1.88, but from the onset it should be stressed that although on one view an atelectatic lobe may be clearly visualized, on the other it may be difficult to perceive. This occurs because on one view the lobe is seen on edge (easier to see), but on the other, it is seen *en face* (more difficult to see). Indeed,

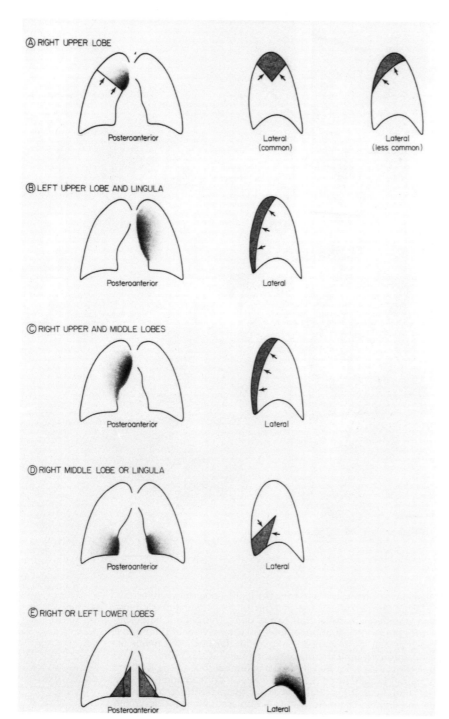

FIGURE 1.88. *Lobar atelectasis: diagrammatic representation of classic patterns.* **(A)** Right upper-lobe atelectasis. **(B)** Left upper-lobe and lingular atelectasis. **(C)** Right upper- and middle-lobe atelectasis. **(D)** Right middle-lobe or lingular atelectasis. **(E)** Right or left lower-lobe atelectasis. *Arrows* indicate direction of collapse and displacement of the involved major fissures. Roentgenographic examples of these patterns are presented in Figures 1.89 through 1.95.

atelectatic lobes visualized *en face* often are so poorly defined that they are misinterpreted as pulmonary infiltrates. It is only if one notes that there is associated volume loss on the other view that one comes to the conclusion that atelectasis only is present.

The pattern of collapse of the upper lobes is different from side to side. This is explained by the fact that on the right the minor fissure separates the right and middle lobes, but on the left the lingula functions as part of the left upper lobe. On the right, on frontal projection, the elevated minor fissure is char-

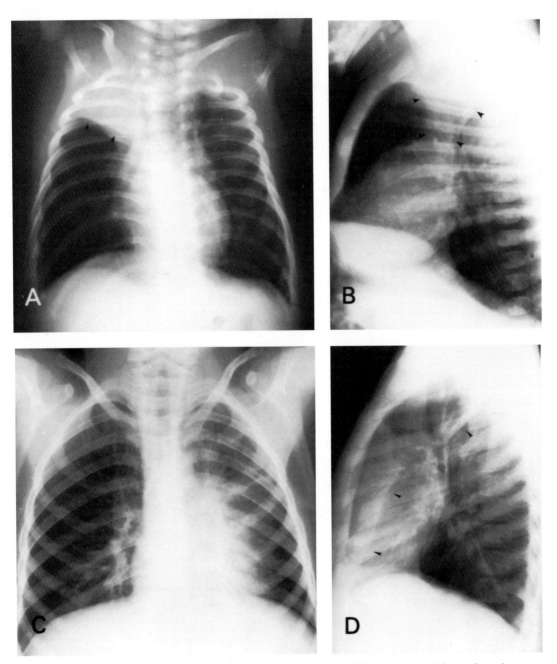

FIGURE 1.89. *Right and left upper-lobe atelectatic patterns.* **(A)** Right upper-lobe atelectasis, classic configuration. The minor fissure (*arrows*) is elevated, and the collapsed upper lobe is dense and triangular. In addition, there is some mediastinal shift to the right. This patient had bronchiolitis with a complicating mucous plug in the right upper lobe. **(B)** Lateral view of right upper lobe atelectasis demonstrating a characteristic V-shaped configuration (*arrows*). The minor fissure delineates the collapsed lobe anteriorly, and the major fissure delineates it posteriorly. **(C)** Left upper-lobe and lingular atelectasis. First note that there is mediastinal shift to the left, and then that the entire left cardiac border is obliterated (positive silhouette sign). In addition, note diffuse central haziness in the left lung field. **(D)** Lateral view shows characteristic configuration of the collapsed left upper lobe and lingula. The major fissure is displaced anteriorly and more or less parallels the anterior chest wall (*arrows*).

acteristic (Fig. 1.89A). On lateral view, the minor and major fissures often outline the collapsed right upper lobe in the shape of a V (Fig. 1.89B), but it is not always easy to see the V in its entirety. On the left side, because no minor fissure is present, one sees only a vague area of increased density over the left upper and midlung fields (Fig. 1.89C). On lateral view, the left upper lobe and lingula collapse anteriorly and are demarcated posteriorly by the forwardly displaced major

fissure (Fig. 1.89D). In most of these cases, the displaced major fissure parallels the anterior chest wall. On the right, a similar configuration results only if the middle and upper lobes are collapsed together (Fig. 1.90).

Finally, it should be noted that either the right or left upper lobe can collapse in atypical fashion (3) and in so doing produce a pleural effusionlike picture (Fig. 1.91). To the unwary, the findings strongly suggest a pleural effusion,

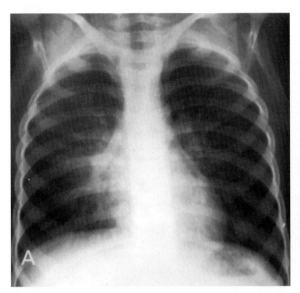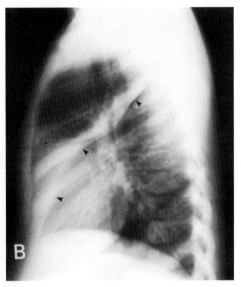

FIGURE 1.90. *Right upper- and middle-lobe atelectasis.* **(A)** Note diffuse haziness over the medial portion of the right lung field. An adjacent positive silhouette sign obliterates the entire right mediastinal edge, and the right hemithorax is slightly smaller than the left. There is some ipsilateral mediastinal shift and slight elevation of the right diaphragmatic leaflet (secondary signs of collapse). **(B)** Lateral view showing characteristic forward displacement of the major fissure as it outlines the collapsed upper and middle lobes (*arrows*).

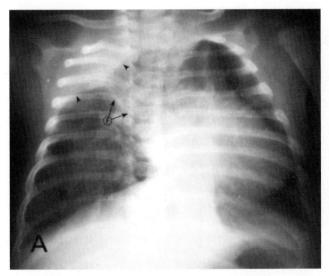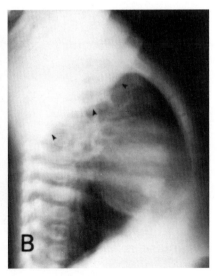

FIGURE 1.91. *Atypical right upper-lobe atelectasis.* **(A)** Note the peculiar configuration of the atelectatic right upper lobe displaced into the apex of the right hemithorax (*arrows*). The minor fissure (*F*) is barely visible but elevated. Because the right upper lobe has collapsed, the right middle lobe has become overaerated and herniated across the anterior mediastinum to the left side. This patient also has left lower-lobe atelectasis as demonstrated by the dense area behind the left side of the heart. **(B)** Lateral view demonstrating the atypically collapsed right upper lobe in the apex of the thorax (*arrows*).

and an unwarranted thoracentesis may even be performed. This can be avoided, however, by becoming familiar with this type of upper-lobe collapse.

Right middle-lobe and lingular collapse produce focal areas of increased density along the lower right or left cardiac borders (Fig. 1.92). In many cases, these findings may at first suggest pneumonia, but the characteristic V-shaped configuration of the collapsed right middle lobe or lingula on lateral view should enable one to make the proper diagnosis. However, it should be mentioned that some variation in the discreteness and density of the V-shaped collapse pattern should be expected, for it is entirely dependent on the degree of atelectasis present.

Lower-lobe collapse is best appreciated on frontal view (Figs. 1.93 and 1.94), for on lateral view it may be totally invisible. At most, the lateral view may reveal a diffuse increase in density over the lower posterior half of the chest and, in some cases, loss of visualization of the adjacent diaphragmatic leaflet (i.e., positive silhouette sign; Fig. 1.94B). Only rarely is the edge of the major fissure seen demarcating the lower lobe anteriorly.

On a frontal view, differentiation of lower-lobe collapse from right middle lobe or lingular collapse is accomplished by noting the presence or absence of an adjacent positive silhouette sign. With right middle-lobe or lingular atelectasis, the ipsilateral cardiac border is obliterated; with lower-lobe

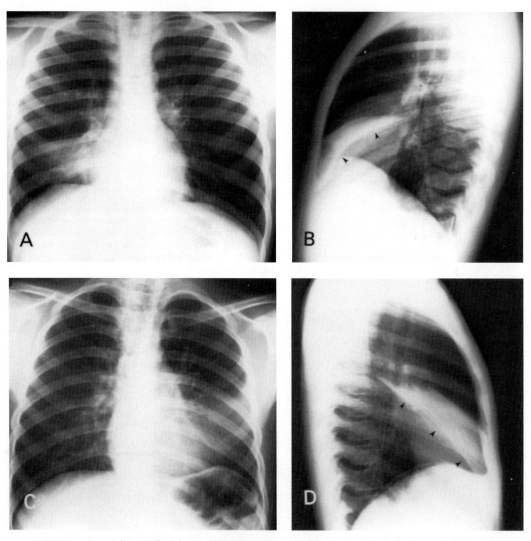

FIGURE 1.92. *Right middle-lobe and lingular atelectasis.* **(A)** Characteristic findings of right middle-lobe atelectasis consisting of an area of increased density just to the right of the lower cardiac border, obliteration of the adjacent portion of the cardiac border (positive silhouette sign), elevation of the diaphragmatic leaflet, and depression of the right hilum. The last two findings, plus the slight mediastinal shift to the right, are secondary signs that indicate that a volume-loss problem is present. **(B)** Lateral view shows the typical V-shaped configuration of the collapsed right middle lobe (*arrows*). **(C)** Lingular atelectasis producing findings similar to those of right middle-lobe atelectasis but on the left side. **(D)** *Arrows* delineate the characteristically triangular collapsed lingula.

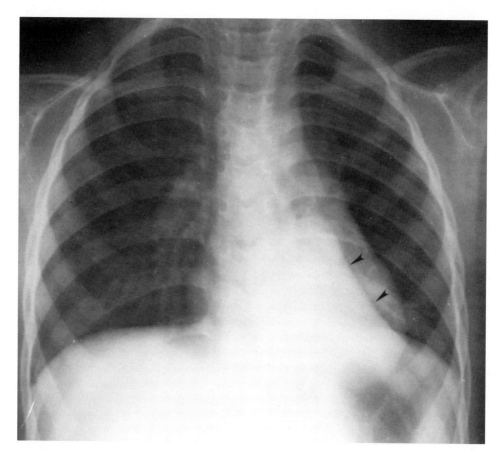

FIGURE 1.93. *Left lower-lobe atelectasis.* Note the characteristic triangular area of increased density behind the left side of the heart adjacent to the spine (*arrows*). The sharp lateral edge reflects the location of the displaced major fissure. In less pronounced cases, the triangular configuration is not as distinct and only a vague area of increased density is seen.

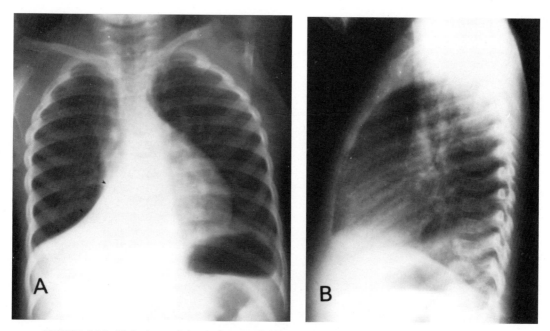

FIGURE 1.94. *Right lower-lobe atelectasis.* (**A**) Note the dense triangular configuration of the collapsed right lower lobe (*arrows*) extending beyond the right cardiac border. The sharp lateral edge delineates the position of the displaced major fissure. In addition, the right diaphragmatic leaflet is obliterated and elevated, and there is slight mediastinal shift to the right. (**B**) Lateral view shows only a vague area of increased density over the spine. The left diaphragmatic leaflet is clearly visualized (note the stomach bubble beneath it), but the right is obliterated because of a positive silhouette sign.

atelectasis it is not (compare Fig. 1.92 with Fig. 1.93). Classically, left lower-lobe collapse produces a triangular area of increased density confined, more or less, to the area behind the left side of the heart (Fig. 1.93). On the right, because there is less cardiac mass, the triangular density of the collapsed right lower lobe often extends beyond the right cardiac border (Fig. 1.94). On the left, if the lower portion of the inferior pulmonary ligament is congenitally defective, anchoring of the left lower lobe is less than normal, and the lobe collapses against the spine in a rounded fashion (4). A paraspinal mass then is suggested, for the characteristic triangular shape of left lower-lobe collapse is absent.

If more than one lobe is collapsed in a patient and the lobes are adjacent, problems in interpretation can arise. Peculiar patterns result and usually reflect a combination of the findings seen if either lobe collapses separately (Figs. 1.89C and D and 1.95).

All of the foregoing patterns of lobar atelectasis are understandably somewhat variable from patient to patient, for they depend to a large extent on the degree of atelectasis present. Because of this, it is of value to be familiar with certain accessory signs that become useful in subtle cases. For example, elevation or depression of a hilus from its usual location (remember that the left hilus is normally a little higher than the right) suggests that there is atelectasis of the upper (elevated hilus) or lower (depressed hilus) lobe. By the same token, elevation of the ipsilateral diaphragmatic leaflet usually is present with lower-lobe atelectasis, and with all types

of lobar collapse there is the inevitable ipsilateral shift of the mediastinum. This latter finding, however, may not always be striking and often becomes more convincing with inspiratory–expiratory film sequences. So-called round atelectasis in adults (2,7) is not commonly seen in children. Atelectasis may appear so round in these patients that a pulmonary nodule or mass is erroneously suggested.

Before leaving the subject of atelectasis, a comment regarding the so-called right middle-lobe syndrome (1,3) is worthwhile. This is a poorly defined "syndrome" that simply reflects the fact that the right middle lobe is chronically or recurrently atelectatic. Because this phenomenon occurs more commonly in the right middle lobe, the term "right middle-lobe syndrome" has been coined.

There is no specificity with regard to the cause of the right middle-lobe syndrome. It can be seen as the aftermath of viral or tuberculous infections and in some cases is a feature of asthma. The presence of the right middle-lobe syndrome suggests a chronic aeration disturbance, and eventually further investigation is required. Most often, this consists of bronchoscopy, whereupon proximal, inflammatory narrowing of the right middle lobe bronchus may be delineated. If repeated pulmonary infections are a problem, the right middle lobe may well require surgical removal. In most cases, however, only expectant treatment is necessary.

Emphysema can be generalized or lobar. Generalized emphysema is seen with central obstructing lesions such as

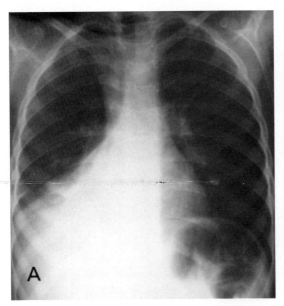
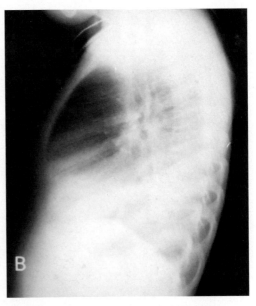

FIGURE 1.95. *Right lower- and middle-lobe atelectasis.* **(A)** Frontal view showing characteristic configuration of the collapsed right lower and middle lobes. The triangular configuration suggests lower-lobe collapse, and the fact that the cardiac border is obliterated indicates that, in addition, the right middle lobe is collapsed. **(B)** Lateral view showing a large area of increased density behind and over the heart, resulting from the atelectatic right lower and middle lobes.

foreign bodies in the trachea, multiple peripheral foreign bodies, paratracheal masses, vascular rings, diffuse peripheral small-airway disease with air trapping (i.e., viral- or thermal injury–induced bronchitis or bronchiolitis), and bronchospasm secondary to asthma and cystic fibrosis (Fig. 1.96). A similar problem can be seen with α_1-antitrypsin deficiency.

Emphysema caused by tracheal obstruction often is accompanied by expiratory wheezing and stridor. The roentgenographic findings may not be striking, for the only feature may be what initially would be considered an apparently "overexuberant" normal inspiration. If it is remembered that it is difficult to obtain a film in deep inspiration in young infants, however, this finding alone should alert one to the fact that generalized air trapping is present.

Thereafter, one should look for more specific findings such as (a) abnormal tracheal deviation, (b) a right-side aortic arch (indicating a vascular ring problem), (c) a mediastinal mass, or (d) opaque airway foreign bodies.

Lobar emphysema is best known in its congenital form and, in this regard, most often involves the left upper lobe (Fig. 1.97A). The right upper lobe and right middle lobe (Fig. 1.97B) also frequently are involved, but lower-lobe involvement is rare. Many of these patients present as newborns; others are asymptomatic into adulthood. Still others can come to the attention of the physician when a superimposed lower respiratory tract infection aggravates the air-trapping problem and renders the patient symptomatic. The whole problem can wax and wane (6) and frequently is dependent on whether or

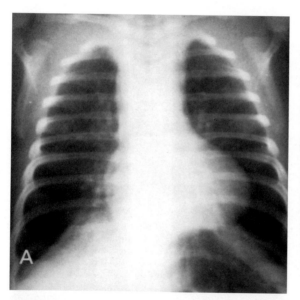
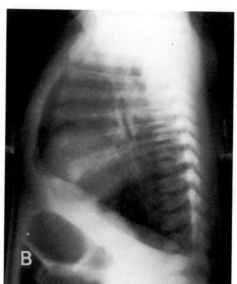
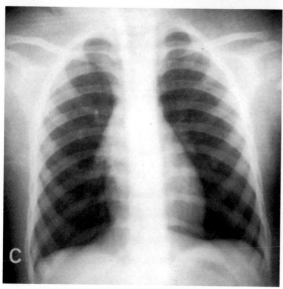

FIGURE 1.96. *Obstructive emphysema: generalized.* **(A)** Note the overdistended lungs in this patient, with a vascular ring producing expiratory air trapping. **(B)** Lateral view showing marked overdistension of the chest with a typical bell-shaped configuration and flat diaphragmatic leaflets. **(C)** Marked overaeration secondary to thermal injury–induced bronchiolitis. This patient suffered from smoke inhalation and died shortly thereafter. Note how depressed the diaphragmatic leaflets are. The soft tissues of the chest wall show extensive edema secondary to widespread skin burns.

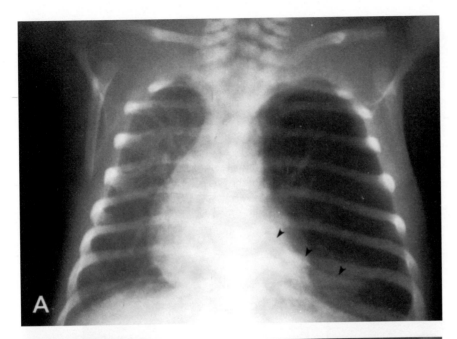

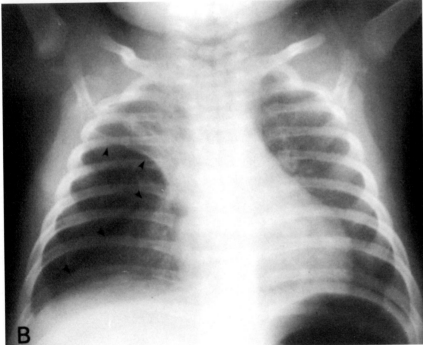

FIGURE 1.97. *Lobar emphysema.* **(A)** Classic findings in congenital left upper-lobe emphysema. The left upper lobe is hyperlucent, the left lower lobe collapsed in a small triangle (*arrows*), and the mediastinum shifted to the right. **(B)** Right middle-lobe emphysema producing an overaerated right middle lobe defined by the upwardly displaced minor fissure (*upper arrows*), and the downwardly and medially displaced major fissure (*lower arrows*). The right upper and lower lobes show slight increase in density because they are partially compressed (i.e., secondary atelectasis).

not an associated viral bronchitis is present. Transient lobar emphysema secondary to endobronchial mucous plugging as seen in asthma and viral lower respiratory tract infections also is frequently encountered. In addition, lobar emphysema can be seen with other obstructing lesions such as the pulmonary sling (aberrant left pulmonary artery) syndrome, mediastinal masses or cysts, and foreign bodies.

Most instances of well-developed lobar emphysema pose no real problem as far as roentgenographic interpretation is concerned, but a modification might be made in those cases in which the right middle lobe alone is involved. In such cases, the unwary observer may be fooled and pick the right middle lobe as being normal (i.e., compensatorily overinflated) and the right upper and right lower lobes as showing primary collapse. ***In these cases, it is only if one realizes that the combination of right upper-lobe and lower-lobe atelectasis is rather uncommon that one begins to focus attention on the right middle lobe as the one abnormally overaerated*** (Fig. 1.97B). Of course, if the interpretation is still in doubt and as part of a general policy of confirming a suspected abnormality of aeration, inspiratory–expiratory film sequences should be obtained.

In the odd case, congenital lobar emphysema is mimicked by cystic disease of the lung (i.e., congenital adenomatoid malformation). In these cases, air trapping in the multiple cysts becomes so profound that the septa between the cysts are almost obliterated, and a picture of lobar emphysema or even pneumothorax is suggested.

Before leaving the topic of emphysema, a note might be made regarding those times when bilateral obstructive emphysema is mimicked by overaeration of the lungs because of some other nonpulmonary problem. In this regard, the most common situation is that of overaeration of the lungs secondary to dehydration and acidosis, as seen with viral gastroenteritis (see Fig. 1.151). The clinical picture in these infants, of course, usually quickly clarifies the situation. The other time when lungs appear overdistended and suggest obstructive emphysema is if a child takes an overexuberant inspiration for the roentgenographic examination. All that is required here is that one be aware of this pitfall and remember not to interpret the roentgenograms in the absence of clinical history.

REFERENCES

1. Billig DM, Darling DB. Middle lobe atelectasis in children: Clinical and bronchographic criteria in the selection of patients for surgery. *Am J Dis Child* 1972;123:96–98.
2. Cho SR, Henry DA, Beachley MC, Brooks JW. Round (helical) atelectasis. *Br J Radiol* 1981;54:643–650.
3. Fanken EA Jr, Klatte BC. Atypical (peripheral) upper lobe collapse. *Ann Radiol* 1977;20:87–93.
4. Glay J, Palayew MJ. Unusual pattern of left lower lobe atelectasis. *Radiology* 1981;141:331–333.
5. Griscom NT, Wohl MEB, Kirkpatrick JA Jr. Lower respiratory infections: How infants differ from adults. *Radiol Clin North Am* 1978;16:367–387.
6. Morgan WJ, Lemen RJ, Rojas R. Acute worsening of congenital lobar emphysema with subsequent spontaneous improvement. *Pediatrics* 1983;71:844–848.
7. Schneider HJ, Felson B, Gonzalez LL. Rounded atelectasis. *AJR* 1980;134:225–232.

PNEUMATOCELES AND PULMONARY ABSCESS

A ***pneumatocele*** is an air-filled cyst, variable in size, usually thin-walled and fluid-free and most frequently seen as a complication of a staphylococcal pulmonary infection. Pneumatoceles may be single or multiple, and some are subject to rapid changes in size (Fig. 1.98). Others may rupture to produce complicating pneumothoraces, but most remain relatively static for extended periods of time. Eventually, they disappear and overall the vast majority are asymptomatic.

In addition to being seen with *S. aureus* infection, pneumatoceles can be seen with other bacterial pneumonias and occasionally with tuberculosis. They also have been documented with hydrocarbon pneumonia (4) and hyperimmunoglobulinemia E syndrome (2,3) and are a common feature of closed or blunt chest trauma. For the most part, little needs to be done about a pneumatocele, for regardless of the cause, it is only if complications such as pneumothorax or infection arise that definitive therapy is required.

Various causes have been considered for the development of pneumatoceles, and it has been suggested that pneumatoceles represent subpleural blebs rather than intra-

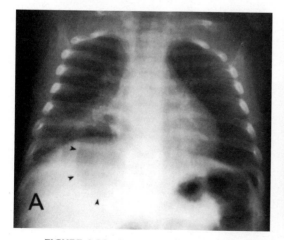 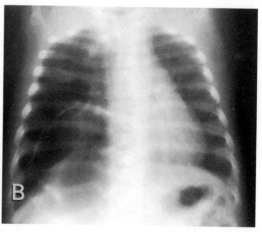

FIGURE 1.98. *Pneumatocele.* **(A)** Note a large pneumatocele developing in the right lower lung of an infant with staphylococcal pneumonia (*arrows*). A smaller pneumatocele is seen just lateral to the large one. **(B)** Seven days later, note how large the pneumatoceles have become. Indeed, there is a tension phenomenon present, with the mediastinum being shifted to the left. Eventually, some 30 days later, the chest film in this infant was completely normal.

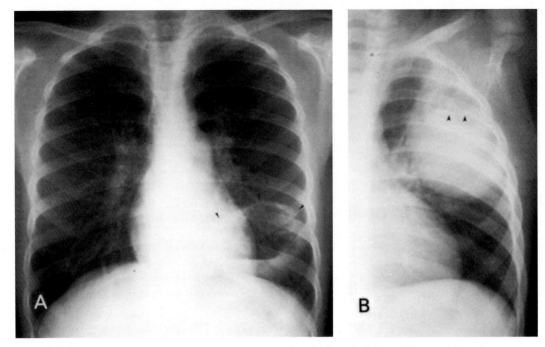

FIGURE 1.99. *Pulmonary abscess.* **(A)** Note the rather thick-walled, irregular-appearing abscess cavity in the left lower lobe (*arrows*). There is an air–fluid level at the bottom of the abscess. **(B)** Another patient with an abscess in the left upper lung. Its hazy margin reflects adjacent inflammatory change. The abscess is nearly full of fluid with only a small air–fluid level noted at the top (*arrows*).

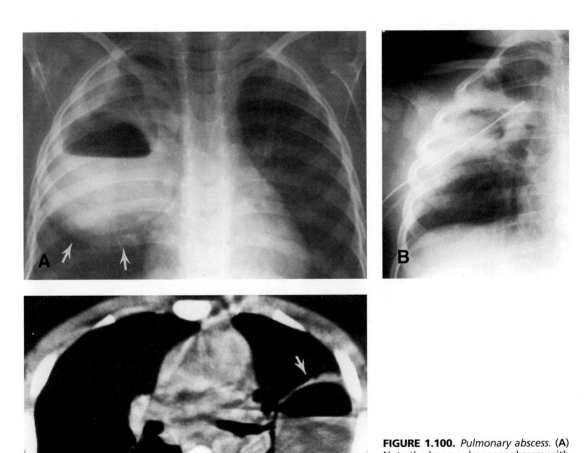

FIGURE 1.100. *Pulmonary abscess.* **(A)** Note the large pulmonary abscess with an air–fluid level (*arrows*) in the right upper lobe. **(B)** After percutaneous catheter drainage the abscess has markedly decreased in size. **(C)** Another patient with a classic appearance of an abscess with an air fluid level on computed tomography (*arrows*).

parenchymal blebs (1). Whatever the exact cause, most agree that pneumatoceles result from alveolar or broncheolar rupture secondary to air-trapping distal to areas of small-airway obstruction.

Pulmonary abscesses are a complication of lobar pneumonia or chronic bronchial obstructions. They are recognized easily by their round or oval configuration, air–fluid levels, and relatively thick walls (Fig. 1.99). Overall, most pulmonary abscesses tend to appear different from pneumatoceles primarily in that they contain fluid and that their walls are thicker and more irregular. Of course, if infection supervenes in a pneumatocele, differentiation may be more difficult, but this is not a particularly common occurrence. CT study is excellent in providing final anatomic data in all of these lesions but is no better than the chest film in differentiating one from the other (Fig. 1.100). Currently pulmonary abscesses are treatable by percutaneous drainage.

REFERENCES

1. Boissett GF. Subpleural emphysema complicating staphylococcal and other pneumonias. *J Pediatr* 1972;8:259–266.
2. Hill HR. The syndrome of hyperimmunoglobulinemia E and recurrent infections. *Am J Dis Child* 1982;136:767–771.
3. Merten DF, Buckley RH, Pratt PC, Effmann EL, Grossman H. Hyperimmunoglobulinemia E syndrome: Radiographic observations. *Radiology* 1979;132:71–78.
4. Stones DK, van Niekerk CH, Cilliers C. Computerized tomography in pneumatoceles after paraffin ingestion. *Pediatr Radiol* 1987;17:443–446.

PNEUMOMEDIASTINUM, PNEUMOTHORAX, AND PNEUMOPERICARDIUM

Pneumomediastinum in childhood can be seen with closed or penetrating chest or neck trauma (3,8), asthma, pulmonary infections with air trapping, airway foreign bodies (2,14), and occasionally with other obstructing airway lesions. On a nontraumatic basis, however, pneumomediastinum in childhood occurs most commonly in patients with asthma. A rather rare cause of pneumomediastinum or pneumothorax is diabetic ketoacidosis (20). In these cases it is the "overbreathing" associated with acidosis that leads to airway rupture. Finally, pneumomediastinal air can be seen after abruptly increased intrathoracic pressures, as can occur with violent coughing episodes and after vomiting (11) (Fig. 1.101). Pneumomediastinum also can occur after esophageal rupture (13).

Pneumothorax is seen with chest trauma, asthma, or foreign bodies and spontaneously. The latter, however, is uncommon in children, and if it occurs, it tends to be seen in thin, adolescent boys. In these cases apical subpleural blebs (18) are believed to be the predisposing cause. The problem tends to be recurrent.

Pneumopericardium usually is traumatic in origin and not particularly difficult to recognize. It can be seen with penetrating or blunt chest trauma. The latter, of course, is less common. In addition, it has been noted with airway foreign bodies (16), and it has been suggested that air enters the pericardium through tears between it and the adjacent connective tissue attachments to the pleura. *Pneumocardium* is

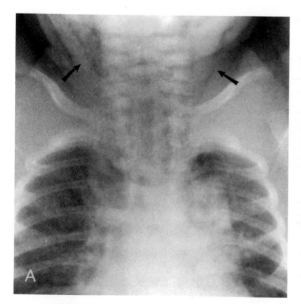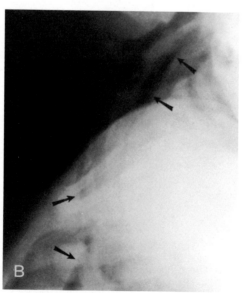

FIGURE 1.101. *Mediastinal emphysema resulting from spasmodic coughing.* **(A)** In this patient with perihilar–peribronchial infiltrates and a viral bronchitis, note considerable free air in the soft tissues of the neck (*arrows*). This was induced by spasmodic coughing. **(B)** Lateral view demonstrates free air in the mediastinum anterior to the trachea (*lower arrows*) and in the retropharyngeal space (*upper arrows*).

relatively uncommon but again can be seen with chest trauma. In small amounts it is innocuous, but if large volumes of air are present cardiac tamponade can result, and on the roentgenogram a small cardiac silhouette is seen (9).

Pneumomediastinal air collections are central in location (4) and of an endless assortment of shapes and sizes. They tend to outline, and surround, the various mediastinal structures such as the thymus, the aorta, and the pulmonary artery. In some cases, the free air extends upward to outline the great vessels and soft tissues of the superior

mediastinum and neck, and in other cases the air may outline the heart (Fig. 1.102). In the latter case, the findings should not be confused with a medial pneumothorax (see Fig. 1.104), or pneumopericardium (see Fig. 1.108). In addition, one should be aware of the fact that pneumomediastinal air can collect subpleurally along the diaphragm (7) and may even extend across the mediastinum to result in the "continuous diaphragm sign" of Levin (6). In the latter cases, the heart virtually is lifted off the diaphragm so that the diaphragm is seen in its entirety (Fig. 1.102B). So gross

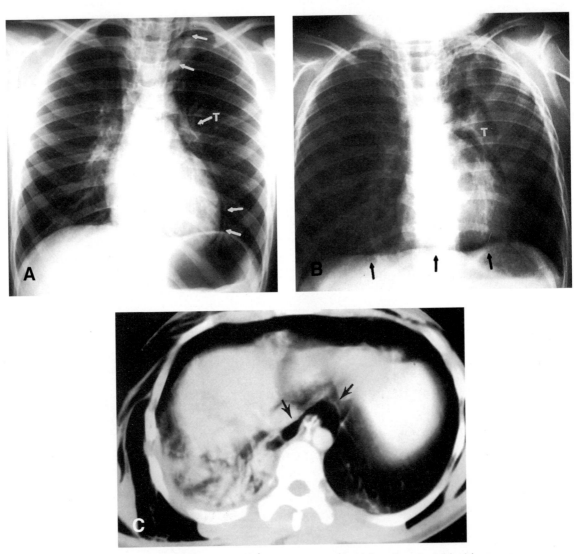

FIGURE 1.102. *Pneumomediastinum: varying configurations.* **(A)** Asthmatic child with pneumomediastinum showing air (a) surrounding the small triangular thymus gland (*T*), (b) extending as linear sheaths into the neck and superior mediastinum (*upper arrows*), and (c) extending along the lower left cardiac edge (*lower arrows*). **(B)** Another asthmatic child with pneumomediastinal air outlining the thymic gland (*T*) on the left and the bottom of the heart. This produces the continuous diaphragm sign: The diaphragm is seen in its entirety from side to side, including that portion just beneath the cardiac silhouette (*arrows*). Smallness of the left hemithorax and increased density over the left upper lobe are caused by partial atelectasis of the left upper lobe and lingula. **(C)** Posttraumatic pneumomediastinum (*arrows*) demonstrated with computed tomography. Also note the pulmonary contusion.

is the finding that it may be missed for this reason alone. In those cases in which air collects subpleurally, that is, beneath the visceral pleura of the diaphragm, a variably thick strip of air is seen along the diaphragmatic leaflet. Clinically, mediastinal air often produces so-called crunching or crackling noises, but seldom is simple pneumomediastinum a cause for alarm, for even extensive air collections are relatively, if not entirely, asymptomatic. Only occasionally does one encounter such severe pneumomediastinum that surgical intervention might be required.

Pneumothorax, on the other hand, usually is accompanied by pain on inspiration and, if large enough and under tension, by respiratory distress. Auscultatory findings include decreased air entry or muffled breath sounds on the involved side, contralateral shift of the cardiac apical impulse, and, in some cases of left-side pneumothorax, a

"click" that might be confused with the crunch of a pneumomediastinum (19).

The job of the radiologist, in cases of pneumothorax, is not so much to detect the large one, for this is relatively easy, but rather to detect the one under tension or the one so subtle that it would otherwise be missed. In the patient in the supine position, because air collects anterior to the lung, a free lung edge may not be visualized. Certain telltale signs, however, are usually present (15,17) and should be sought for. They include (a) increased lucency, and size, of the involved hemithorax (air under tension over the anterior surface of the lung); (b) contralateral shift of the mediastinum (tension phenomenon); and (c) increased sharpness or crispness of the ipsilateral mediastinal edge (Fig. 1.103). The last finding results from the fact that free air rather than aerated lung abuts the heart, and because of this

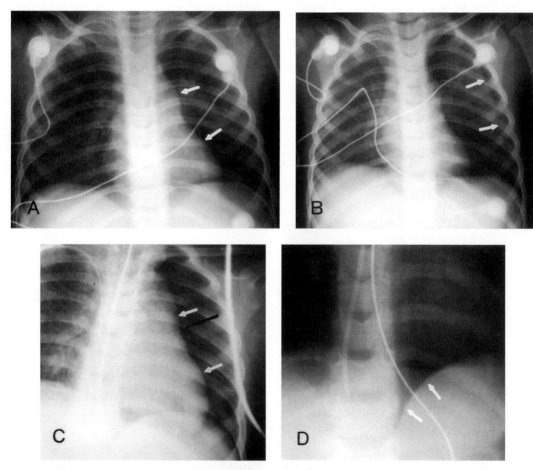

FIGURE 1.103. *Pneumothorax: supine film findings.* **(A)** The fact that a pneumothorax is present on the left might be missed. Note, however, that the left mediastinal edge is "sharper" or "crisper" than the one on the right (*arrows*). This sign indicates that free air is present, lying anterior to the lung and against the heart. **(B)** Moments later, an expiratory film more clearly demonstrates the pneumothorax. The free lung edge on the left is visualized clearly (*arrows*), and the compressed left lung, virtually bathed in an envelope of free air, is easy to detect. Note that the trapped air on the left causes the left hemithorax to remain large and hyperlucent, and that the left cardiomediastinal edge is still sharper than the right edge. **(C)** Another patient with similar findings resulting from an anterior pneumothorax on the left (*arrows*). **(D)** Deep sulcus sign (5) in the same patient, consisting of increased radiolucency of the left paravertebral sulcus (*arrows*).

the edges of the heart and other mediastinal structures become more clearly demarcated, that is, they appear "sharper" or "crisper." The same phenomenon occurs over the diaphragmatic leaflets if air happens to accumulate solely along the bottom of the lung. In addition, the diaphragmatic leaflet may be depressed or show a double contour (21). In still other cases, air may accumulate deep in the costophrenic angle or paravertebral sulci (5) and produce increased radiolucency in this area (Fig. 1.103D).

For the most part, the foregoing findings are quite dependable in allowing one to detect an anterior pneumothorax on supine films; it should be remembered, however, that increased "sharpness" or "crispness" of the mediastinal edge of the diaphragmatic leaflet also can be seen if a lung becomes overdistended, either because of obstruction or because of compensatory emphysema. Consequently, if one suspects an anterior or basal pneumothorax on a supine film, some other film should be obtained for confirmation. For the most part this can be a cross-table lateral, regular lateral, decubitus, or expiratory-phase roentgenogram. During expiration, the lungs empty and become smaller, but the free air of the pneumothorax does not (Fig. 1.103B). One can use any or all of these views to aid in detecting a subtle pneumothorax, and one should not limit oneself to a single additional view. Another misleading configuration of pneumothorax occurs if air collects along the medial aspect of the lung so as to mimic a pneumomediastinum or pneumopericardium (Fig. 1.104). In such cases, an expiratory,

regular or cross-table lateral, or decubitus view once again becomes useful for differentiation (10,15).

On upright view, large pneumothoraces are not difficult to detect; the free lung edge usually is readily discernable, and the area lateral to it appears blacker than usual and free of vascular markings (Fig. 1.105). Smaller pneumothoraces, however, require astute inspection and careful scrutiny of the lung over the apex and lateral aspect, and in the costophrenic angle (Fig. 1.105B and C). In the costophrenic angle, one should look for the typical, laterally pointing, V-shaped air–fluid level. If this finding is seen, one should look harder for a pneumothorax, because it is there (Fig. 1.106). The V-shaped configuration results from the fact that fluid lies both in the anterior and posterior pleural spaces, and as the beam travels through the chest, the two fluid levels are traversed at two different angles and appear as the two limbs of the V. Over the apex of the lung, free air is seen as a slender, radiolucent apical cap; finally, if a localized pneumothorax is seen next to a collapsed lobe (1), bronchial obstruction should be considered (Fig. 1.107). Ordinarily, pneumothorax does not compress a single lobe.

Pneumopericardium is identified by noting free air around the heart (Fig. 1.108). More often than not, however, it is some other roentgenographic finding that usually is misinterpreted as being representative of pneumopericardium, that is, medial pneumothorax, pneumomediastinum, and the artifactual Mach effect (4,15). This causes enhancement of the normal pericardial radiolucency occur-

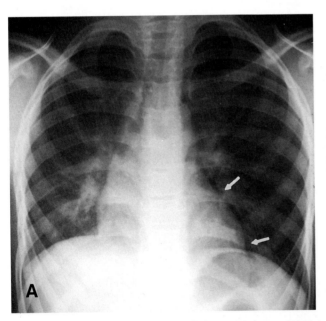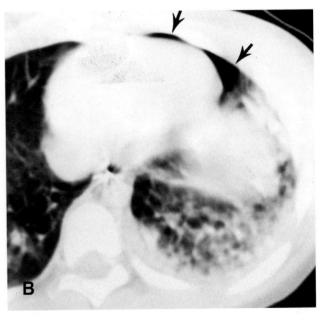

FIGURE 1.104. *Medial pneumothorax.* **(A)** Note the thin strip of free air along the left cardiac border (*arrows*). The finding represents a medial pneumothorax and should not be confused with pneumomediastinum or pneumopericardium. **(B)** Another patient with an antero-medial pneumothorax (*arrows*) demonstrated on computed tomography. Also note the underlying pulmonary contusion.

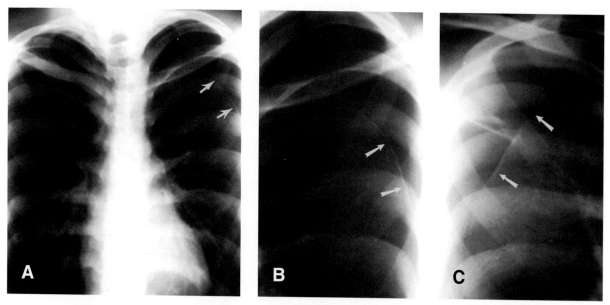

FIGURE 1.105. *Typical pneumothorax.* **(A)** This patient was tall and thin. Note the pneumothorax on the left (*arrows*). **(B)** Magnified view demonstrates the pneumothorax on the left (*arrows*). **(C)** Another pneumothorax is present on the right (*arrows*). These were spontaneous pneumothoraces in a tall, thin individual.

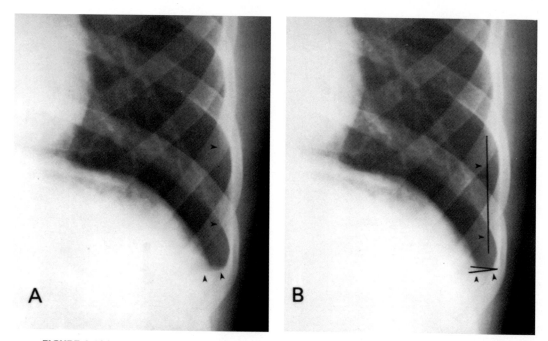

FIGURE 1.106. *Horizontal "V" sign in pneumothorax.* **(A)** At first the V-shaped collection of fluid in the left costophrenic angle (*lower two arrows*) might be overlooked. The free lung edge is barely discernable (*upper two arrows*). **(B)** Diagrammatic representation of the horizontal V sign and the free lung edge.

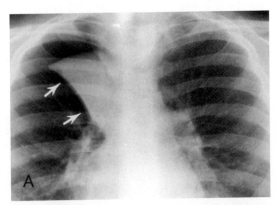
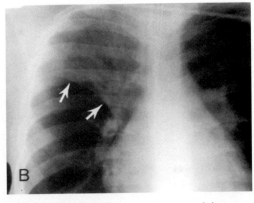

FIGURE 1.107. *Pneumothorax with atelectasis.* **(A)** Note atelectasis of the right upper lobe (*arrows*) and increased lucency in the area. This is caused by an associated pneumothorax. **(B)** After the pneumothorax clears, residual atelectasis of the right upper lobe (*arrows*) is seen.

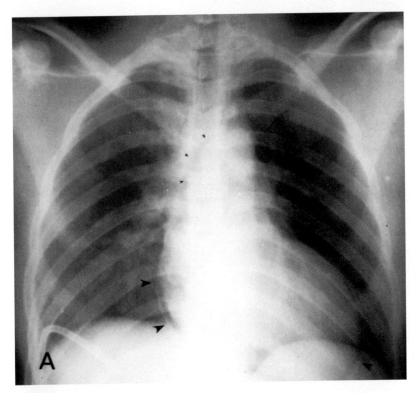

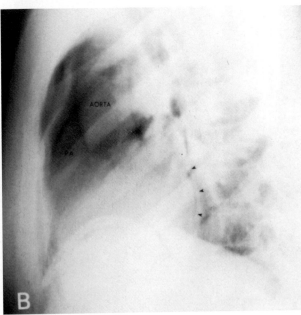

FIGURE 1.108. *Pneumopericardium.* **(A)** Traumatic pneumopericardium. Note the halo of free air around the heart and the clearly visualized pericardial sac (*large arrows*). Air also extends along the aorta (*small arrows*). **(B)** Note air in the pericardial sac posteriorly (*arrows*), but also note that air clearly outlines both the pulmonary artery (*PA*) and aorta. The pericardium attaches to the base of the great vessels, and with larger volume pericardial air collections, the aorta and pulmonary artery are outlined by the air.

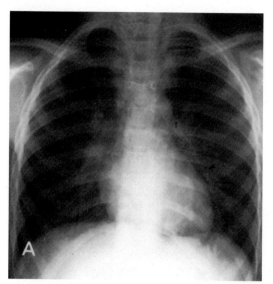 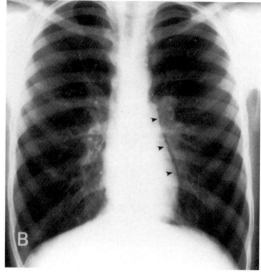

FIGURE 1.109. *Pseudopneumopericardium.* **(A)** Pneumomediastinum mimicking pneumopericardium. Note what appears to be the pericardial sac on the left (*arrows*). If this truly were the pericardial sac, however, enough air is present that it should surround the entire cardiac silhouette. The thymus gland (*T*) is elevated and visualized as a separate structure. This finding is of no particular help, because it occurs both with pneumopericardium and pneumomediastinum. **(B)** Mach effect. Note what would appear to be free air along the left cardiac border (*arrows*). This artifact is produced by a thin strip of normally aerated lung being projected between the cardiac border and the descending left lower-lobe pulmonary artery. Radiolucency of this strip of apparent air is enhanced by the Mach effect.

ring between the cardiac edge and the adjacent lower-lobe pulmonary artery branches (Fig. 1.109B).

The key to distinguishing pneumopericardium from these other entities is to actually note the fine white line of the pericardium as it is separated from the heart by air (Fig. 1.108). Unfortunately, this configuration also can be seen with pneumomediastinum. Pneumomediastinal air, however, usually outlines one side of the heart only (see Fig. 1.109A), but with pneumopericardium, air usually outlines the entire heart (Fig. 1.108). Nonetheless, in cases in which air collections are minimal, if no other signs of pneumomediastinum are present, it may be difficult to make the distinction.

Finally, a note regarding air in the inferior pulmonary ligament is in order. Most often seen with blunt chest trauma (see Fig. 1.138), this also can occur with mediastinal air from other causes. Its characteristic location and usually somewhat oval configuration just along the spine on frontal view are the keys to proper diagnosis.

REFERENCES

1. Berdon WE, Dee GJ, Abramson SJ, Altman RP, Wung J.-T. Localized pneumothorax adjacent to a collapsed lobe: A sign of bronchial obstruction. *Radiology* 1984;150:691–694.
2. Burton EM, Riggs W Jr, Kaufman RA, Houston CS. Pneumomediastinum caused by foreign body aspiration in children. *Pediatr Radiol* 1989;20:45–47.
3. Eklof O, Thomasson B. Subcutaneous emphysema, pneumomediastinum and pneumothorax secondary to blunt injury to the throat. *Ann Radiol* 1980;23:169–173.
4. Friedman AC, Lautin EM, Rothenberg L. Mach bands and pneumomediastinum. *Can J Assoc Radiol* 1981;32:232–235.
5. Gordon R. The deep sulcus sign of pneumothorax. *Radiology* 1980;136:25–27.
6. Levin B. Continuous diaphragm sign: Newly recognized sign of pneumomediastinum. *Clin Radiol* 1973;24:337–338.
7. Lillard RL, Allen RP. The extrapleural air sign in pneumomediastinum. *Radiology* 1965;85:1093–1098.
8. McHugh TP. Pneumomediastinum following penetrating oral trauma. *Pediatr Emergency Care* 1997;13:211-213.
9. Mirvis SE, Indeck M, Schorr RM, Diaconis JN. Posttraumatic tension pneumopericardium: The "small heart" sign, *Radiology* 1986;158:663.
10. Moskowitz PS, Griscom NT. The medial pneumothorax. *Radiology* 1976;120:143–147.
11. Overby KJ, Litt IF. Mediastinal emphysema in an adolescent with anorexia nervosa and self-induced emesis. *Pediatrics* 81:134–136.
12. Poenaru D, Yazbeck S, Murphy S. Primary spontaneous pneumothorax in children. *J Pediatr Surg* 1994;29:1183–1185.
13. Reino AJ, Jahn AF, Parsons J, Lubin A. Traumatic pneumomediastinum in a child secondary to corn chip perforation of the esophagus. *Pediatric Emergency Care* 1993;9:211–216.
14. Saoji R, Ramchandra C, D'Cruz AJ. Subcutaneous emphysema: an unusual presentation of foreign body in the airway. *J Pediatr Surg* 1995;30:860–862.
15. Swischuk LE. Two lesser known but useful signs of neonatal pneumothorax. *AJR* 1976;127:623–627.
16. Tjen KY, Schmaltz AA, Ibrahim A, Nolte K. Pneumopericardium as a complication of foreign body aspiration. *Pediatr Radiol* 1978;7:121–123.

17. Tocino IM, Miller MH, Fairfax WF. Distribution of pneumothorax in the supine and semi-recumbent critically ill adult. *AJR* 1985;144:901–905.

18. Wilcox DT, Glick PL, Karamanoukian H, Allen JE, Azizkhan RG. Spontaneous pneumothorax: A single institution, 12-year experience in patients under 16 years of age. *J Pediatr Surg* 1995; 30:1452–1454.

19. Wright JT. The radiological sign of "clicking" pneumothorax. *Clin Radiol* 1965;16:292–294.

20. Zahller MC, Skoglund RR, Larson JM. Pneumomediastinum associated with diabetic ketoacidosis. *J Pediatr* 1978;93:529–530.

21. Ziter FMH Jr., Westcott JL. Supine subpulmonary pneumothorax. *AJR* 1981;137:699–701.

PULMONARY CONGESTION AND EDEMA

Pulmonary congestion, and eventually frank pulmonary edema, can arise from a number of cardiac and extracardiac causes. Before discussing the roentgenographic features of pulmonary congestion and edema, however, it is wise to first address the problem of "pneumonia" versus congestion. I suspect that this is the question most frequently asked by the clinician of the roentgenologist. Unfortunately, there is no simple answer to the problem, for the solution comes only through experience, but there are one or two points that might be utilized to differentiate the two conditions.

First, one should be aware that problems arising in the differentiation of pulmonary congestion from pneumonia are most frequently encountered in young infants. Almost always the problem is one of differentiating the findings of a viral lower respiratory tract infection with a perihilar–peribronchial pattern of infiltration from true congestion. Indeed, in some of these cases the roentgenographic patterns virtually defy distinction from one another, and if one were to limit the examination to the lung fields alone, it certainly would be nearly impossible to differentiate the two.

One also should look at the heart, however, for if cardiomegaly is present, cardiac disease is most likely, and if it is not, viral pulmonary infection should be the determination (Fig. 1.110). It should be remembered that these patients have a viral bronchitis and not a true pneumonia, and that their disease process is in the interstitial compartment, just like early pulmonary edema.

Pulmonary vascular congestion can be divided into two broad groups, active and passive (Fig. 1.111). Active congestion is seen most often with underlying left-to-right shunts and admixture lesions, and thus its presence virtually assures that a congenital heart lesion is present. In such cases, more blood flows through the lungs than normal, and because of this the pulmonary vessels enlarge, become more tortuous, and, as opposed to normal vessels, are visualized far into the periphery (outer third) of the lung (Fig. 1.111A). Once this pattern of pulmonary congestion is appreciated, one can go on to differentiate one lesion from another, but a discussion of this finding is beyond the scope of this book.

Passive congestion, on a purely cardiac basis, infers the presence of an obstructing lesion on the left or a failing left heart. This can occur with obstructing lesions such as aortic stenosis and coarctation of the aorta, but more often it occurs with myocardial dysfunction such as is present with left side–overload heart lesions, acute myocarditis, or some form of cardiomyopathy. The roentgenographic pattern of passive congestion differs completely from that of active congestion, for in the former, the volume of blood flowing through the lungs is not increased. Rather, because pulmonary venous pressures are elevated, bloodflow through the lungs is impeded, the pulmonary veins distend, fluid oozes out into the perivascular interstitium (transudate), and an overall fuzzy appearance of the vessels results (Fig. 1.111B). Actually, what one is witnessing is the development of interstitial pulmonary edema.

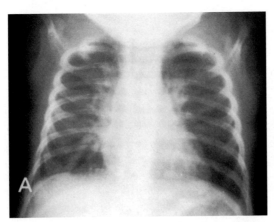 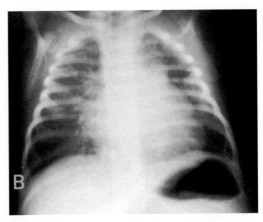

FIGURE 1.110. *Viral perihilar–peribronchial infiltration versus congestion.* **(A)** The perihilar distribution of infiltrates in this infant with a viral lower respiratory tract infection might be mistaken for pulmonary congestion. The heart, however, is not enlarged. **(B)** Contrarily, the perihilar pattern of pulmonary congestion secondary to heart disease in this patient might be misinterpreted as perihilar–peribronchial infiltration except that the heart is enlarged.

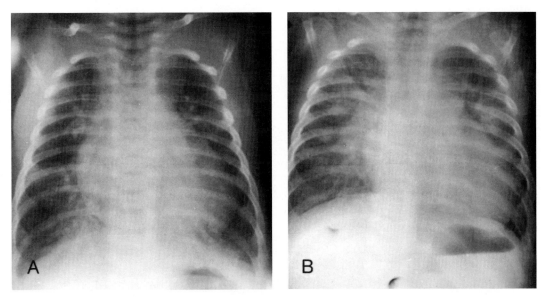

FIGURE 1.111. *Active versus passive congestion.* **(A)** In this patient with a large ventricular septal defect, note cardiomegaly and prominent pulmonary vessels bilaterally. Although the vessels are somewhat indistinct, they still are identifiable as individual structures. **(B)** Same patient, now with myocardial decompensation and passive congestion. Note that the perihilar regions are prominent and hazy because of pulmonary edema. The individual vessels, as identified in **A**, are no longer discretely visible.

Pulmonary edema results from increased permeability of the pulmonary capillaries, because of either increased pulmonary venous pressures secondary to a failing left heart or direct damage to the capillaries. In the latter case, pulmonary vascular pressures usually are normal, but in either instance, when fluid first seeps out of the vessels it accumulates in the pulmonary interstitium. This being the case, one notes first the development of stringy or reticular white lines in the chest and then increasing opacity or haziness of the lungs (Figs. 1.112 and 1.113). The white lines represent fluid in the interstitial septa of the lungs and commonly are referred to as Kerley "A" and "B" lines. The B lines are the

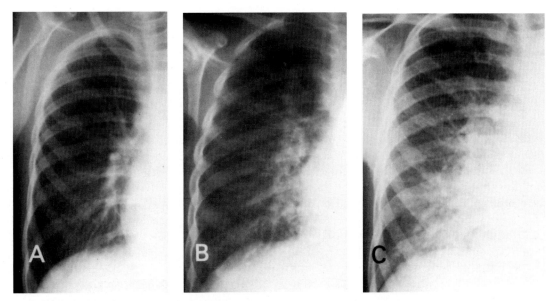

FIGURE 1.112. *Pulmonary edema: interstitial stage.* **(A)** Note the early development of streaky white lines (interstitial septal edema) radiating from the hilar region. In this case, the lines primarily are Kerley A lines. This patient had acute glomerulonephritis. **(B)** More extensive reticular pattern of pulmonary interstitial edema in a patient with cardiac failure secondary to aortic stenosis. **(C)** Very extensive interstitial edema producing pronounced reticulation throughout the lung and some underlying parenchymal haziness. Kerley A and B lines are present. This patient had acute glomerulonephritis.

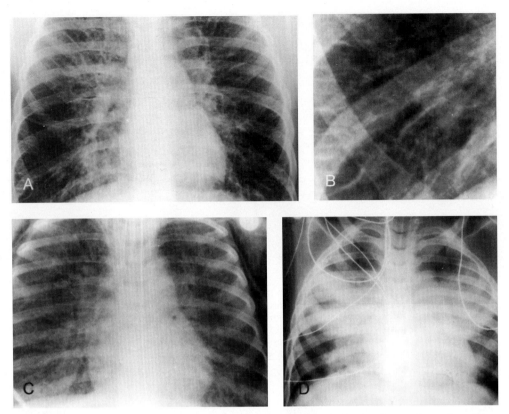

FIGURE 1.113. *Pulmonary edema: various interstitial through fluffy alveolar configurations.* **(A)** Widespread interstitial pulmonary edema leading to a streaky perihilar pattern with Kerley A and B lines in a patient suspected of inhaling a noxious substance. **(B)** Coned view of the right base more clearly demonstrates the Kerley A and B lines characteristic of an interstitial disease process. **(C)** Another patient with extensive pulmonary edema, primarily interstitial, leading to hazy lungs. This patient had adult respiratory distress syndrome. **(D)** Alveolar pulmonary edema in a typical butterfly configuration. Note that the densities resulting from the edema now are very confluent and very opaque. Edema in this case was caused by fluid overload.

small, transverse lines usually best seen in the costophrenic sulci; the A lines are the longer lines, generally running outward from the hilar regions (Figs. 1.112 and 1.113). The hazy appearance that eventually develops may at first suggest alveolar fluid accumulation but actually still probably represents fluid in the interstitial space (Fig. 1.113C). Alveolar fluid is much more dense and usually is patchy, fluffy, or totally confluent (Fig. 1.113D).

Once fluid saturates the interstitium, alveolar pulmonary edema begins to develop. In other words, fluid then oozes out into the alveolar space, and in a few instances edema fluid collects more centrally in the perihilar regions, leaving the periphery of the lungs relatively clear and producing the typical "butterfly" configuration (Fig. 1.113D). In many of these cases, the patchy and asymmetric nature of the infiltrate makes it most difficult to differentiate from widespread pneumonia, but the basically central predominance favors edema. In the past, one of the most common

causes of pulmonary edema in childhood was acute glomerulonephritis (7). These patients often demonstrate a combination of interstitial and alveolar edema, and overall the findings frequently first suggest myocarditis with cardiac failure. Indeed, the pattern of congestion, including the presence of Kerley B lines and pleural effusions, is virtually indistinguishable from that seen with acute myocarditis (Fig. 1.112C). At first, this roentgenographic picture may seem strange for the disease, but it is more common than generally believed and actually quite typical. The most likely cause for pulmonary congestion and cardiomegaly in these patients is circulatory overload (hypervolemia) secondary to sodium and fluid retention (7). No cardiac disease has been demonstrated in these patients, and, indeed, once the fluid overload is corrected, the chest findings return to normal. Some of these patients may demonstrate a little cardiomegaly, but normal heart size is generally the rule. The problem now is less common because of the widespread treatment of streptococcal infections with antibiotics.

Other causes of pulmonary edema include iatrogenic fluid overload, smoke or hot-air inhalation (4,14), noxious-fume inhalation, near drowning (15), neurogenic pulmonary edema secondary to increased intracranial pressure (2,8), collagen vascular disease, massive aspiration (5), fat embolism (1), allergic pneumonitis, and the shocked-lung syndrome (3,6,10). In addition, pulmonary edema can occur secondary to poisoning by drugs such as cocaine, methadone, carbon monoxide, and certain insecticides. Edema in such cases results from damage to the capillaries, with resultant increased capillary permeability and extravasation of fluid into the interstitial space.

Pulmonary edema also has been described as an aftermath of upper-airway obstruction and hypoxia (11). The exact mechanism for the production of pulmonary edema in these cases is not completely understood, but it is believed that it results from capillary damage secondary to hypoxia.

Neurogenic pulmonary edema occurs as an aftermath of an acute rise in intracranial pressure, but its precise cause is incompletely understood. Generally, however, it has been noted that these patients demonstrate bradycardia, peripheral vasoconstriction, lowered cardiac output, and elevated pulmonary venous pressures (2,8). Because of this, hydrostatic pressure across the pulmonary capillaries becomes excessive, and fluid extravasates into the surrounding lung tissue. Hyperactivity of the vagus nerve has been implicated as leading to bradycardia and lowered cardiac output in these patients, but the precise cause is unclear.

Near drowning is not so much a matter of pulmonary edema as one of aspirating water into the lungs. As far as the roentgenographic findings are concerned, it makes little difference as to whether one aspirates salt or fresh water. Only the volume is important, for the more water aspirated, the more striking the roentgenographic findings. The chest film for these patients usually shows patchy alveolar infiltrates and serves as a baseline study (see Fig. 1.146B). It must be stressed, however, that clinical assessment, with serial blood-gas determinations, is more important than judging the patient's condition from the roentgenograms. Fluid aspirated into the lung usually clears quickly, but if asphyxia also occurs, neurogenic pulmonary edema and even shocked lung can develop. In these cases, the patchy pattern of alveolar fluid often gives way to one of diffuse interstitial edema.

Pulmonary edema secondary to smoke inhalation or noxious-fume inhalation is self-explanatory. It should be noted, however, that if smoke or hot-air inhalation has caused bronchiolar damage, the chest film may show pronounced air trapping rather than pulmonary edema. These changes may clear after 1 or 2 days and later be replaced by nonspecific infiltrates caused by edema and microatelectasis

secondary to pulmonary microemboli (4). In severe cases, a necrotizing bronchiolitis with widespread patchy atelectasis and hemorrhage can develop. Very often these patients go on to rapid demise.

Fat embolism with subsequent pulmonary congestion results from the trapping of fat droplets in the pulmonary circulation after they have been dispersed into the bloodstream by the fracturing of a long bone such as the femur. It is not a common complication in childhood, however, and although many patients with fractures have evidence of fat droplets in the bloodstream, only a few develop pulmonary complications.

Shocked-lung or adult respiratory distress syndrome (3,6,10) occurs after profound hypoxia and hypotension, and the latter is seen with any number of conditions leading to these problems: trauma, severe burns, blood loss, septic shock, neurogenic shock, and so forth. The roentgenographic findings (Fig. 1.113C) develop after the state of shock has resolved. The cause of shocked lung is unknown, but a central neurologic origin has been suggested (9). In this regard, it has been suggested that cerebral hypoxia leads to reactive arterial spasm in the lungs and, hence, hypoxia of the lungs. The net result is a loss of surfactant, increased cell-wall permeability, and small-vessel thrombosis (12). Roentgenographically, this results in interstitial and then alveolar pulmonary edema and scattered areas of segmental atelectasis and hemorrhage. The problem, in reality, is similar to that seen in newborns with surfactant deficiency (hyaline-membrane disease), or the respiratory distress syndrome, and hence the term "adult respiratory distress syndrome" is used. The problem in the neonate recently has been termed the "leaky lung syndrome" (13).

REFERENCES

1. Feldman F, Ellis K, Green W. Fat embolism syndrome. *Radiology* 1975;114:535–542.
2. Felman AH. Neurogenic pulmonary edema: Observations in 6 patients. *AJR* 1971;112:393–396.
3. Greene R. Adult respiratory distress syndrome: Acute alveolar damage. *Radiology* 1987;163:57–66.
4. Kangarloo H, Beachley MC, Ghahremani GG. The radiographic spectrum of pulmonary complications in burn victims. *AJR* 1977;128:441–445.
5. Landay MJ, Christensen EE, Bynum LJ. Pulmonary manifestations of acute aspiration of gastric contents. *AJR* 1978;131: 587–592.
6. Lyrene RK, Truog WE. Adult respiratory distress syndrome in a pediatric intensive care unit: Predisposing conditions, clinical course, and outcome. *Pediatrics* 1981;67:790–795.
7. Macpherson RI, Banerjee AJ. Acute glomerulonephritis: A chest film diagnosis? *Can J Assoc Radiol* 1974;25:58–64.
8. Milley JR, Nugent SK, Rogers MC. Neurogenic pulmonary edema in childhood. *J Pediatr* 1979;94:706–709.
9. Moss G. The role of the central nervous system in shock: The centroneurogenic etiology of the respiratory distress syndrome. *Crit Care Med* 1974;4:181–185.

10. Ostendorf P, Birzle H, Vogel W, Mittermayer C. Pulmonary radiographic abnormalities in shock: Roentgen-clinical-pathological correlation. *Radiology* 1975;115:257–263.
11. Oudjhane K, Bowen A, Oh KS, Young LW. Pulmonary edema complicating upper airway obstruction in infants and children. *Can J Assoc Radiol* 1992;43:278-282.
12. Pinet F, Tabib A, Clermont A, Loire R, Motin J, Artru F. Post-traumatic-shock lung: Post-mortem microangiographic and pathologic correlation. *AJR* 1982;139:449–454.
13. Swischuk LE, Shetty BP, John SD. The lungs in immature infants: How important is surfactant therapy in preventing chronic lung problems? *Pediatr Radiol* 1996;26:508–511.
14. Teixidor HS, Rubin E, Novick GS, Alonso DR. Smoke inhalation: Radiologic manifestations. *Radiology* 1983;149:383–387.
15. Wunderlich P, Ruprecht E, Treffz F, Thomsen H, Burhardt J. Chest radiographs of near-drowned children. *Pediatr Radiol* 1985;15:297–299.

PERICARDIAL FLUID AND MYOCARDITIS

Myocarditis and pericardial effusions can occur together, and differentiation of the two may be difficult. In their pure forms, however, the major difference between them is that with myocarditis passive vascular congestion is present, but with pericardial effusion it is not (Fig. 1.114). Of course, if both are present the findings may well overlap. Pericardial fluid accumulations can occur with rheumatic, viral, bacterial, or tuberculous pericarditis, kidney disease (glomerulonephritis and the nephrotic syndrome), or collagen vascular diseases, and as hemopericardium with chest trauma. Chylopericardium is very rare.

The roentgenographic identification of pericardial effusions of enough volume to cause cardiac enlargement entails study of the superior mediastinum. If such effusions are present, the great-vessel silhouettes (aorta and pulmonary artery) become obliterated, for fluid accumulates in that portion of the pericardial sac that extends over their

bases (2). This is, perhaps, the most important roentgenographic finding to detect, for enlargement of the cardiac silhouette is relatively nonspecific. Displacement of the epicardial fat pad also has been described with pericardial effusion (1,3), but in my experience this finding is difficult to utilize in most cases. Actually, ***if one suspects a pericardial effusion, one should turn to ultrasonography for diagnosis*** (Fig. 1.114C).

REFERENCES

1. Lane EJ Jr., Carsky EW. Epicardial fat: Lateral plain film analysis in normals and in pericardial effusion. *Radiology* 1968;91:1–5.
2. Soulen RL, Lapayowker MS, Cortex FM. Distribution of pericardial fluid: Dynamic and static influences. *AJR* 1968;103:583–588.
3. Torrance DJ. Demonstration of subepicardial fat as an aid in diagnosis of pericardial effusion or thickening. *AJR* 1955;74:850–855.

ASTHMATIC CHILD

The child with asthma comes to the emergency room not so much for the diagnosis of asthma but for the diagnosis or exclusion of one of its complications. On a practical basis, the problem often boils down to the following: (a) Is infection present and, if so, what kind? (b) Are there any focal aeration disturbances (i.e., atelectasis or obstructive emphysema)? (c) Is there evidence of pneumomediastinum or pneumothorax? In this regard, the value of chest roentgenograms for patients with their first attack of asthma has been questioned (4,5). On a practical basis it often is difficult to deny a chest roentgenogram for these patients, but at the same time, not every child with an asthmatic attack requires a chest roentgenogram. The chest roentgenogram should be used

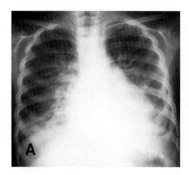 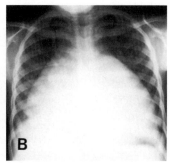 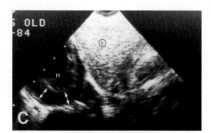

FIGURE 1.114. *Myocarditis* versus *pericardial effusion.* **(A)** Moderate generalized cardiomegaly and marked passive congestion of the pulmonary vasculature are seen in this patient with myocarditis. The superior mediastinum, however, in the region of the aorta and pulmonary artery, is not widened. Bilateral pleural effusions also are present. **(B)** Pericardial effusion producing diffuse globular enlargement of the cardiac silhouette. Note, however, that the superior mediastinum is widened, the aorta and pulmonary artery are completely obscured, and that no pulmonary vasculature congestion is present. **(C)** Ultrasound study demonstrating pericardial effusion (*arrows*). *H*, heart; *D*, diaphragm; *L*, liver.

to determine air-block complications that might be present, and it has been suggested that the presence of subcutaneous emphysema and severe desaturation often herald the presence of such complications (12). In the end, one has to use one's own judgment as to when a roentgenogram should be obtained, but it should not be a standard procedure.

In answer to the question of whether infection is present in a patient with asthma, one should note that, although asthmatic children are more susceptible to lower respiratory tract infections, these more often are viral than bacterial (6,8–10). This is especially true if increased wheezing accompanies the infections (10), for bacterial infections usually do not cause or lead to wheezing in asthmatic children (6). There is good reason for this to be so, for bacterial infections usually are parenchymal (alveolar) infections, with little in the way of associated bronchitis. Viral infections, on the other hand, manifest as a widespread bronchitis–peribronchitis, and it is this aspect of these infections that predisposes to bronchospasm, mucous-plug formation, and aggravation of the basic pathophysiology of asthma. This, of course, is not to say that bacterial infections with

parenchymal consolidations do not occur in asthmatic children, for indeed they do, but only to emphasize that such infections are much less common than generally believed. Bacterial infections generally do not aggravate asthmatic symptoms, for they do not have a significant bronchitic component. For the most part, they present just as they do in nonasthmatics.

In asthmatics, therefore, most of the time what is at first suspected to be a parenchymal infiltrate turns out to be an area of segmental atelectasis (Fig. 1.115). The problem here is much the same as in those patients with viral bronchitis and areas of atelectasis. Segmental and lobar atelectasis are extremely common in asthma, and once this is appreciated one comes to the realization that the single most common cause of pulmonary density on the chest films of asthmatic children is transient atelectasis secondary to endobronchial mucous plugging, and not pneumonia (6).

In many asthmatic children, a characteristic baseline roentgenogram is seen. It consists of widespread overaeration, perihilar–peribronchial infiltration with bronchial cuffing, and an overall picture very similar to that seen with

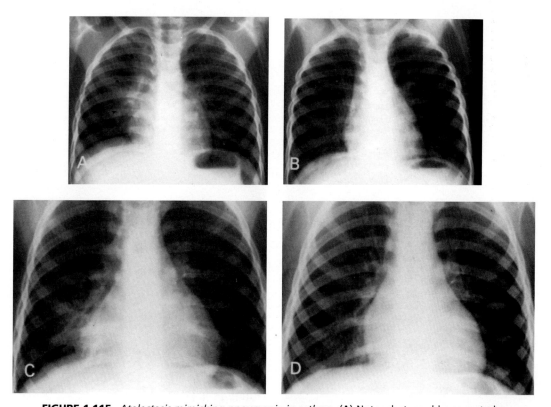

FIGURE 1.115. *Atelectasis mimicking pneumonia in asthma.* **(A)** Note what would appear to be an infiltrate in the right upper lobe (*arrows*). **(B)** Less than 24 hours later the infiltrate has disappeared. It had been caused by partial atelectasis of the right upper and middle lobes. Such areas of atelectasis are common in asthma and frequently are misinterpreted as patchy pneumonia. **(C)** Another patient with an apparent right middle-lobe infiltrate (*arrows*) that suggests a pneumonia. Also note generalized overaeration. **(D)** Twenty-four hours later, the chest film is normal. No pneumonia would clear this rapidly. The findings resulted from transient middle-lobe atelectasis.

viral lower respiratory tract infections (Fig. 1.116). To be sure, so similar are the findings that it is often difficult to determine whether or not an asthmatic child has a superimposed viral lower respiratory tract infection. All of these findings may at first appear relatively nonspecific, but familiarity with them soon leads to a typical template for the so-called asthmatic chest in childhood. As in patients with viral lower respiratory tract infections, asthmatics demonstrate thickening of the bronchi and peribronchial tissues leading to typical perihilar–peribronchial infiltrates. It must be noted, however, that not all asthmatic patients have this typical baseline chest appearance. Indeed, there are those who merely show overaeration and never really develop a pattern of chronic, perihilar–peribronchial infiltration.

The generalized air trapping commonly seen in asthmatics is, of course, secondary to bronchospasm. During acute attacks such air trapping may be profound, and it is at these times that there is a greater tendency for complications such as pneumomediastinum and pneumothorax to occur (1,7, 11). Pneumomediastinum, however, is by far the more common of the two (Fig. 1.117A and B), and in some of these cases the mediastinal air can leak into the interstitial tissues of the neck and chest wall (Fig. 1.117C and D). Most often, pneumomediastinum is treated conservatively, but pneumothorax often requires decompression. A peculiar complication of pneumomediastinum has been documented in the form of retropharyngeal air producing upper-airway obstruction (3).

Endobronchial mucous plugs, as noted previously, are common in asthmatic children and may lead either to atelectasis or obstructive emphysema (5), but atelectasis is much more common. The presence of these plugs may not be appreciated until expiratory films are obtained (Figs. 1.118 and 1.119).

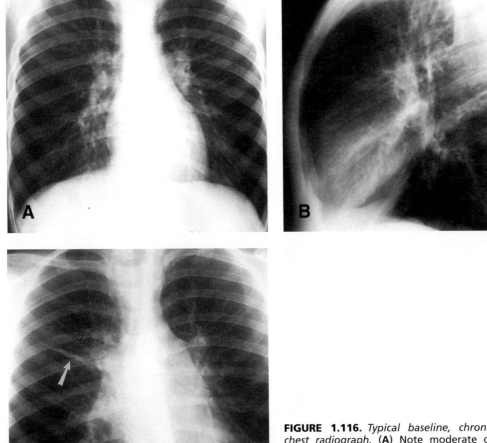

FIGURE 1.116. *Typical baseline, chronic asthmatic chest radiograph.* **(A)** Note moderate overaeration, pronounced perihilar–peribronchial infiltration, some bronchial cuffing, and hilar adenopathy. **(B)** Lateral view showing overdistended chest. Note how the heart is pushed away from the sternum. **(C)** Another patient with overaeration, perihilar–peribronchial infiltrates, and scattered areas of segmental atelectasis (*arrows*).

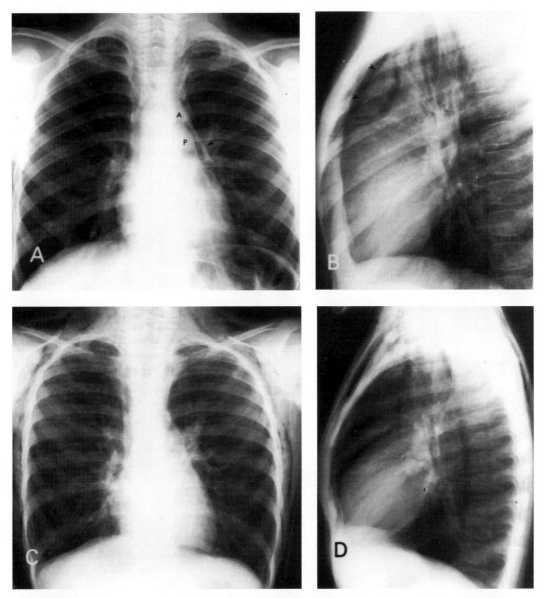

FIGURE 1.117. *Pneumomediastinum and interstitial air complicating asthma.* **(A)** Note pneumo-mediastinal air outlining the aorta (*A*), pulmonary artery (*P*), and a slender left thymic lobe (arrow). **(B)** Lateral view in another patient demonstrating a small thymus gland (*arrows*) surrounded by pneumomediastinal air. **(C)** Note the typically overdistended chest with chronic per-ahilar–peribronchial infiltrates in this child with an acute asthmatic attack. Some air is present in the superior mediastinum, but most has escaped into the soft tissues of the neck and chest wall. **(D)** Lateral view. Note interstitial air in the soft tissues of the chest wall, both anteriorly and posteriorly. Some air is seen in the mediastinum.

Other findings seen in acute asthma include prominence of the pulmonary artery and elongation of the entire cardiac silhouette (Fig. 1.120). The latter finding is explained by the fact that the diaphragm is depressed, and the heart is elongated and squeezed by the overdistended lungs. Prominence of the pulmonary artery usually is explained on the basis of transient pulmonary hypertension secondary to increased pulmonary vascular resistance produced by the profound degree of emphysema and sludging of the blood in the pulmonary arteries.

Chronic mucous plugging with superimposed aspergillosis infection (2,13) is not particularly common in childhood asthma, but it can occur. In these cases, the mucous plugs can be seen as oval, elongated, or sometimes Y-shaped densities in the lung field. Distal to these areas, one usually sees focal air trapping and increased lucency of the involved lobe. Transient mucous plugs without superimposed aspergillosis infection also occur and probably are more common than generally realized (Fig. 1.121).

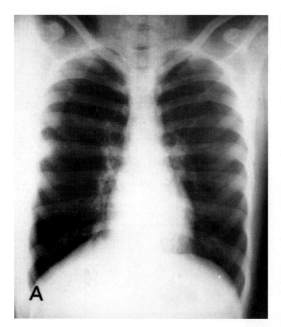 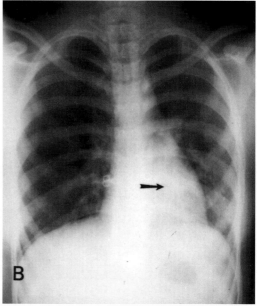

FIGURE 1.118. *Mucous plug causing unsuspected obstructive emphysema.* **(A)** On this inspiratory chest film, the lungs are markedly overdistended, but apart from this, the roentgenogram most likely would be interpreted as normal. One would not suspect that any focal aeration disturbance was present, and yet, as is seen in **B**, an obstructing mucous plug is present on the right. **(B)** On expiration, note that the mediastinum has shifted to the left (arrow), and that although the left lung has emptied partially, the right lung remains large and radiolucent. This attests to the fact that obstructive emphysema of the right lung is present. In such cases, obstruction is of such a degree that enough air escapes during expiration to keep the obstructed lung from getting overly large.

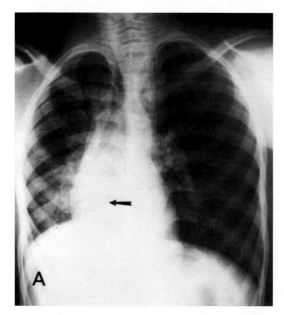 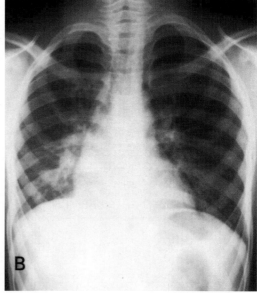

FIGURE 1.119. *Mucous plug with distracting contralateral compensatory emphysema.* **(A)** On this inspiratory view, there is marked mediastinal shift to the right (arrow), and the left lung might be suspected of being abnormal. As shown in **B**, however, it is normal. **(B)** Expiratory film showing that the problem lies on the right. Note that the left lung has emptied but the right lung has not changed in size. The thin radiolucent band outlining the left pericardial border represents a small medial pneumothorax.

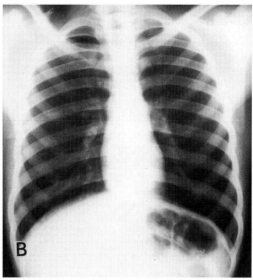
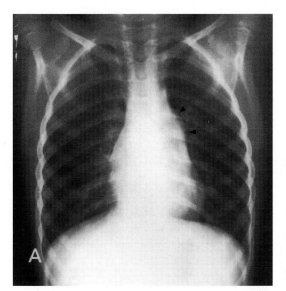

FIGURE 1.120. *Prominent pulmonary artery in asthma.* **(A)** Note the prominent pulmonary artery (*arrows*) in this patient with an acute asthmatic attack. This is a common finding in asthmatic children and is a reflection of acute pulmonary hypertension. **(B)** Elongated, small heart in asthma. Note the long thin cardiac silhouette in this asthmatic child suffering from status asthmaticus. Such stretching of the heart with resultant smallness of the cardiac silhouette (microcardia) is not uncommon in asthma. If dehydration is present in these patients, it further accentuates the findings of microcardia. Note that in this patient, perihilar–peribronchial infiltrates are virtually absent, which demonstrates that not all asthmatic children show the degree of perihilar–peribronchial infiltration seen in Figure 1.116.

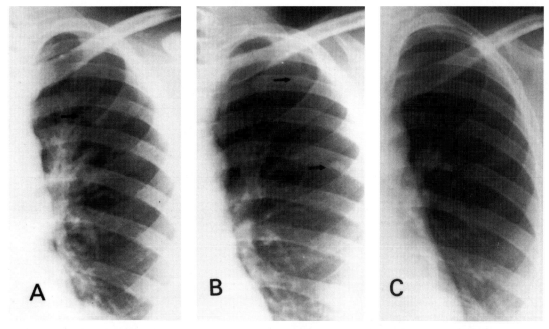

FIGURE 1.121. *Transient peripheral mucous plugs.* **(A)** Adolescent asthmatic with round nodule in left upper lobe (arrow). **(B)** During another admission the previous nodule disappeared but two new ones appeared (*arrows*). **(C)** At a later date, no nodules are present. These nodules represent transient peripheral mucous plugs, with focal, subsegmental atelectasis.

REFERENCES

1. Bierman CW. Pneumomediastinum and pneumothorax complicating asthma in children. *Am J Dis Child* 1967;114:42–50.
2. Carlson V, Martin J, Keegan J, Dailey J. Roentgenographic features of mucoid impaction of the bronchi. *AJR* 1966;96: 947–952.
3. Cohn RC, Steffen ME, Spohn WA. Retropharyngeal air accumulation as a complication of pneumomediastinum and a cause of airway obstruction in asthma. *Pediatr Emerg Care* 1995;11: 298–299.
4. Faiqa Q. Management of children with acute asthma in the emergency department. *Pediatr Emerg Care* 1999;15:206–213.
5. Gershel JC, Goldman HS, Stein REK, Shelov SP, Ziprokowski M. The usefulness of chest radiographs in first asthma attacks. *N Engl J Med* 1983;336–340.
6. McIntosh K, Ellis EF, Hoffman LS, Lybass TG, Eller JJ, Fulginiti VA. The association of viral and bacterial respiratory infections with exacerbations of wheezing in young asthmatic children. *J Pediatr* 1973;82:578–590.
7. McSweeney WJ, Stempel DA. Non-iatrogenic pneumomediastinum in infancy and childhood. *Pediatr Radiol* 1973;1: 139–144.
8. Minor TE, Baker JW, Dick EC, DeMeo AN, Ouellette JJ, Cohen M, Reed CE. Greater frequency of viral respiratory infections in asthmatic children as compared with their non-asthmatic siblings. *J Pediatr* 1974;85:472–477.
9. Minor TE, Dick EC, DeMeo AN, Ouellette JJ, Cohen M, Reed CE. Viruses as precipitants of asthmatic attacks in children. *JAMA* 1974;227:292–298.
10. Mitchell I, Inglis H, Simpson H. Viral infection in wheezy bronchitis and asthma in children. *Arch Dis Child* 1976;51:707–711.
11. Ozonoff M. Pneumomediastinum associated with asthma and pneumonia in children. *AJR* 1965;95:112–117.
12. Stack AM, Caputo GL. Pneumomediastinum in childhood asthma. *Pediatr Emerg Care* 1996;12:98-101.
13. Wang JLF, Patterson R, Mintzer R, Roberts M, Rosenberg M. Allergic bronchopulmonary aspergillosis in pediatric practice. *J Pediatr* 1979;94:376–381.

FOREIGN BODIES IN THE LOWER AIRWAY

Small infants are virtual vacuum cleaners, for anything they see goes into their mouths, and foreign body aspirations into the airway are as common as ever. Clinically, the problem often is clearly apparent, for the aspiration, followed by coughing, gagging, vomiting, varying degrees of respiratory distress, and even cyanosis, is clearly documented. *Interestingly, however, these symptoms often subside quickly, and the patient may appear surprisingly well and even asymptomatic (7) shortly after the acute problem.* The reason for this is that the endobronchial receptors responsible for producing the initial symptoms soon lose their sensitivity and react less to the foreign body (1). However, do not be fooled by this lull in the clinical picture, for the foreign body is still present and, if not detected, may lead to the development of recurrent pneumonias or wheezing suggestive of asthma. Indeed, *wheezing in the absence of known pulmonary disease such as asthma, especially if it is unilateral, should be considered to result from a for-eign body until it is proven otherwise*. Similarly, one should not expect classic findings of diminished air entry (wheezing, coughing, and so forth) in all cases. Indeed, in one study they frequently were noted to be absent (8).

Once foreign-body aspiration is suspected, the roentgenographic workup should be thorough and undertaken immediately. The patterns of aeration disturbance are varied; many are subtle and many are missed. Even the experienced observer cannot let his guard down if a foreign-body problem is being investigated; every possible clue should be sought. Of course, if the foreign body is opaque (e.g., teeth, pebbles, metal tacks), the problem is lessened (8), but most foreign bodies are nonopaque, and thus one must rely on an evaluation of disturbances of aeration. Unfortunately, these may not always be apparent, and in one series, 31% of patients studied had normal initial chest roentgenograms (7). In another study, however, the initial radiographs were abnormal in all 96 cases (8).

Before embarking on a discussion of aeration disturbances, a few general considerations might be in order. First, it should be noted that there is a difference between tracheal (central) and bronchial (peripheral) foreign bodies. The latter, of course, are much more common (1,9), and there is a slight preponderance of right-bronchial foreign bodies (1,9). At first, one might expect that the overwhelming majority of aspirated foreign bodies would settle in the right bronchus, but it has been shown that in infants and young children the right and left bronchial angles are rather symmetric, and it is only in the older child and adult that the right bronchus offers a more direct route for aspirated foreign bodies (5).

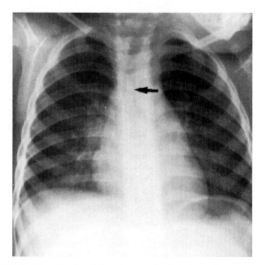

FIGURE 1.122. *Tracheal foreign body.* This is an inspiratory film that easily could be interpreted as normal: One might note that the lungs are not as large as one would expect for a full inspiration, but almost always the film would be read as normal. A peanut (arrow), however, just barely visible, was present in the trachea. The trachea is well distended, confirming that the film is an inspiratory film and not an expiratory film. The trachea normally narrows on expiration.

Central foreign bodies located in the trachea, but below the larynx, can be difficult to diagnose, and plain films can be deceptively normal (Fig. 1.122). The reason for this is that the aeration disturbance is generalized and not lateralized to one or the other of the lungs. Furthermore, the problem more often is one of inspiratory underaeration rather than overaeration. In other words, restricted air entry more than air exit and obstructive emphysema is the pathophysiologic malady. At the same time there may be paradoxic enlargement of the cardiac and mediastinal silhouettes (4,6). Ordinarily, with inspiration, as the lungs enlarge and diaphragmatic leaflets become depressed, heart size diminishes. With central obstruction, however, be it in the trachea or the larynx, intrathoracic pressures become more negative during inspiration, and the heart and mediastinum enlarge. This certainly is a useful sign, but not one easy to detect.

As far as endobronchial foreign bodies are concerned, the plain chest film frequently demonstrates the unilateral aeration abnormality, but if it does not, the mandatory expiratory chest film will. If this fails, fluoroscopy can be performed but usually is not necessary. Indeed, plain films are quite accurate (11), and in terms of abnormalities encountered, the most common is obstructive emphysema. In advanced cases, obstructive emphysema is not difficult to identify (Fig. 1.123). Obstructive emphysema develops because, during inspiration, there is enough physiologic dilatation of the bronchus to allow some air to get around the foreign body and enter the lung. On expiration, however, physiologic narrowing of the bronchus occurs, and in the presence of an occluding foreign body a check-valve phenomenon develops and air is trapped in the lung. Ensuing mucosal edema aggravates the problem, and these events, cycling over and over, eventually lead to progressive air trapping and overdistension of the involved lung or lobe. In these children, such a lobe or lung appears larger and more radiolucent than the other lung (Fig. 1.123). Largeness is explained on the basis of chronic air trapping; hyperlucency occurs because more air than normal is present in the lung, and because pulmonary bloodflow is diminished. Indeed, this latter finding is the hallmark of obstructive, emphysematous overdistension of a lung and as such can be used to differentiate obstructive emphysema from compensatory emphysema. With compensatory emphysema, although the lung may appear large during inspiration, pulmonary bloodflow is not compromised. Decreased bloodflow in an obstructed lung results in part from compression of the vessels, and in part from hypoxia-induced vasospasm.

In other cases of obstructive emphysema, the findings may not be so obvious. In these cases, entry and exit of air are abnormal but neither predominates to the point that frank obstructive emphysema or total atelectasis results. Consequently, the lung may be of normal or nearly normal size, and it is only during expiration that one notes that the

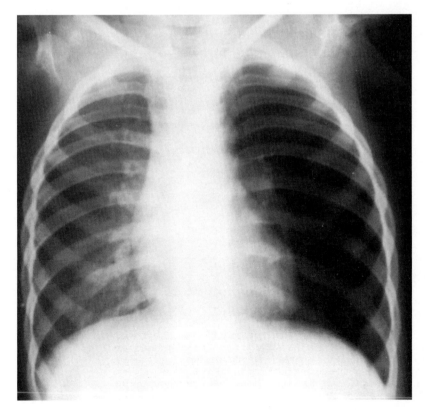

FIGURE 1.123. *Foreign body in the left main stem bronchus with obstructive emphysema.* Note the large hyperlucent, underperfused (oligemic) left lung. Such underperfusion is characteristic of obstructive emphysema and is not seen with compensatory emphysema. The mediastinum is shifted to the right, and the left diaphragmatic leaflet is displaced downward. The findings are classic for a check valve foreign body producing obstructive emphysema on the left.

involved lung does not deflate and is pathologically obstructed. In many of these cases, a clue to the fact that some degree of obstructive emphysema exists is that the pulmonary vascularity in the involved lung or lobe is somewhat diminished (Fig. 1.124). A good rule to follow is that the lung with diminished bloodflow is the abnormal lung whether it is large and hyperlucent or small and hyperlucent. Another good rule to follow is that the lung that changes shape least or not at all between inspiration and expiration is the abnormal lung.

Clearly, inspiratory–expiratory film sequences are the key to identifying obstructed lungs. In some cases, however, one may resort to decubitus films (3), for with lateral decubitus positioning, a normal lung, if it is the dependent lung, empties and becomes smaller (i.e., it is compressed). With an obstructed lung, however, the trapped air prevents it from collapsing and becoming smaller in the dependent, decubitus position (Fig. 1.125). Simply speaking, the obstructed lung acts as an air cushion or inflated balloon and does not deflate on compression. These points notwithstanding, however, with regular inspiratory–expiratory films one can almost always identify the abnormal lung, and although fluoroscopic examination of the chest may

demonstrate more vividly findings such as contralateral mediastinal shift and fixation of the involved diaphragmatic leaflet, it is seldom necessary.

If patchy atelectasis or pneumonic infiltrates are associated with obstructing foreign bodies, they may distract one from the actual problem (10). Indeed, it is not unusual for such children to be treated for a presumed pneumonia for a number of days or even weeks but in the final analysis be determined to have an obstructing foreign body (Fig. 1.126). In other instances, if the foreign body is not recognized, emphysema eventually is replaced by atelectasis. This is especially likely to occur with a foreign body of low irritation such as a piece of plastic, metal, or bone. Peanuts and popcorn, on the other hand, because of their fat content, produce a more pronounced and rapidly ensuing local inflammatory reaction. Because of this, the obstructive problem is accelerated and the patient comes to the attention of the physician sooner. Unrecognized foreign bodies also eventually may present as chronic infections, including pulmonary abscess and bronchiectasis. After emphysema, however, atelectasis is the most common manifestation of a bronchial foreign body (Fig. 1.127).

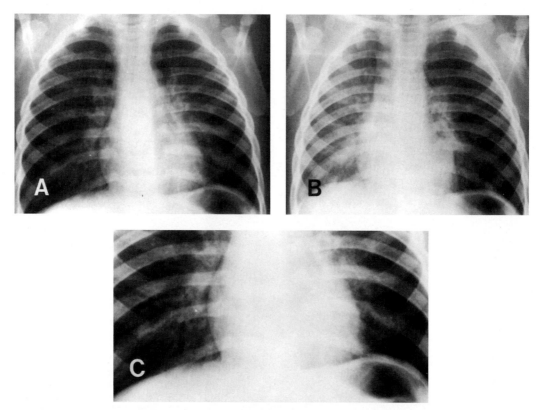

FIGURE 1.124. *Obstructed lung, subtle findings.* **(A)** On this inspiratory film, note that, even though the right lung is a little larger than the left, it is the left lung that shows decreased vascularity. **(B)** Subsequent expiratory film shows that the right lung empties normally (i.e., changes size dramatically); the left lung retains its original size and does not empty. A foreign body was present in the left main bronchus. **(C)** Coned view of the lungs as shown in **A** demonstrates the decrease in vascularity in the left lung base to better advantage.

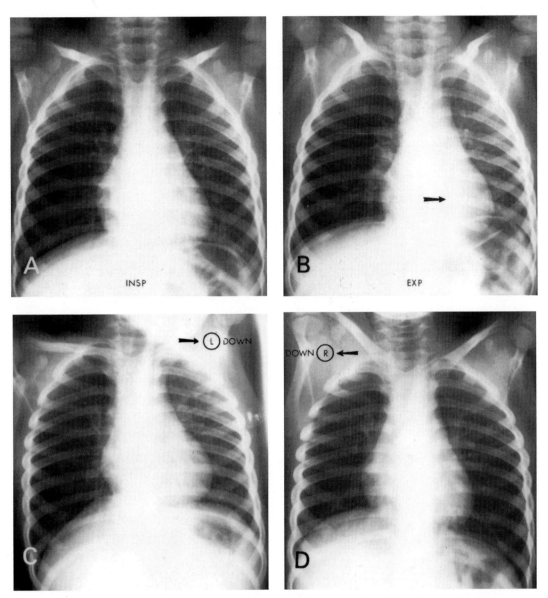

FIGURE 1.125. *Foreign body: value of expiratory and decubitus films.* **(A)** Inspiratory (*INSP*) view shows a large, hyperlucent right lung. An obstructing foreign body in the right main bronchus should be suspected. **(B)** Expiratory (*EXP*) film accentuates the hyperlucent large right lung. Air has emptied from the normal left lung, and the mediastinum is now clearly shifted to the left (arrow). **(C)** Left lateral decubitus film. The left side is down and the left lung is partially deflated (compressed). This is normal. The right lung remains relatively overinflated. **(D)** Right lateral decubitus. This time the right side is down and the right lung should have deflated. Because it is obstructed, however, it remains radiolucent and large (i.e., the presence of obstructive emphysema does not allow it to deflate). The decubitus films in **C** and **D** are illustrated in the upright position for ease of comparison.

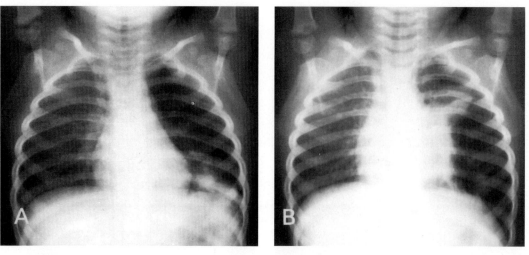

FIGURE 1.126. *Foreign body disguised as pneumonia.* **(A)** Note the infiltrate in the left lower lung field. Clinically, pneumonia was suspected. The overaerated left upper lobe was believed to represent compensatory emphysema. **(B)** On the next day, note that obstructive emphysema has developed in the left lower lobe. There was an underlying foreign body (peanut fragments) in the left lower lobe.

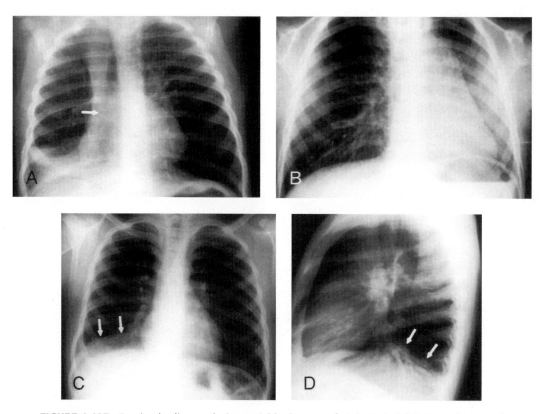

FIGURE 1.127. *Foreign bodies producing variable degrees of atelectasis.* **(A)** Note atelectasis of right lower lobe and compensatory emphysema of the right upper lobe and entire left lung. Also, note tack (arrow) in the right main bronchus. If this tack were not seen, a foreign body might not be suspected. **(B)** Another patient with partial collapse of the left lung caused by carrot particles in the left bronchus for 3 days. There is marked shift of the mediastinum to the left, and the right lung is overdistended. Because the blood vessels in the right lung still are prominent, however, one should consider overdistension of the right lung to result from compensatory, and not obstructive, emphysema. If the problem was one of obstructive emphysema of the right lung, the vessels would be less prominent and, indeed, attenuated. **(C)** Chronic foreign body in the right lower lobe producing basilar atelectasis (*arrows*). **(D)** Lateral view demonstrating the atelectasis (*arrows*) to better advantage.

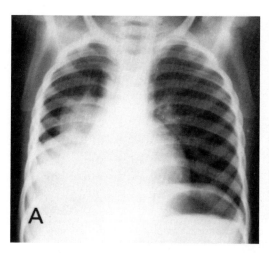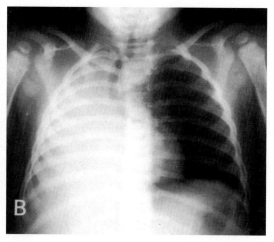

FIGURE 1.128. *Foreign body causing total massive atelectasis.* **(A)** Note right lower-lobe and right middle-lobe atelectasis resulting from a longstanding foreign body of low irritation (plastic bottle cap). The findings, except that there is marked volume loss, could be misinterpreted as a simple pneumonia. **(B)** Massive, total atelectasis of the right lung. This infant inhaled a pinto bean into the right main bronchus. In less than 60 min, total atelectasis of the right lung occurred, with pronounced respiratory distress, cyanosis, and syncope.

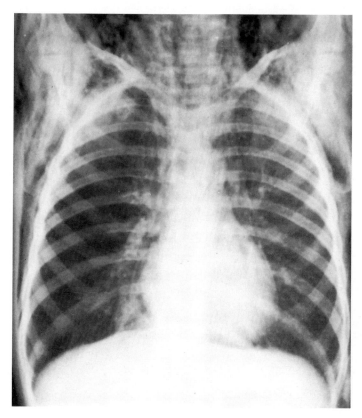

FIGURE 1.129. *Foreign body with mediastinal and interstitial air.* Note extensive free air in the mediastinum and soft tissues of the neck and chest. So striking are the findings that one might miss the fact that the right lung is a little more radiolucent than the left. The reason for this discrepancy in radiolucency is that a foreign body was present in the right bronchus and the right lung was trapping air. (Courtesy of Webster Riggs, M.D.)

Foreign bodies that totally occlude a bronchus can produce lobar or total-lung atelectasis (Fig. 1.128). In some of these cases, occlusion of the bronchus may occur so rapidly that cyanosis and syncope are surprisingly rapid in onset. In these cases, the abrupt mediastinal shift leads to syncope by producing acute kinking and obstruction of the inferior and superior vena cavae, and also by rendering one lung abruptly functionless. Some foreign bodies produce such gross aeration disturbances that complicating pneumomediastinum (2) and pneumothorax can result. In such cases, the roentgenographic findings may be very puzzling, for the presence of the mediastinal air often distracts one's attention from the basic underlying problem (Fig. 1.129). These complications usually result from rupture of the lung that is obstructed.

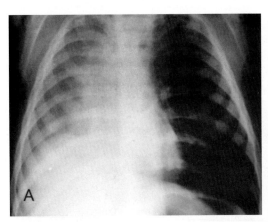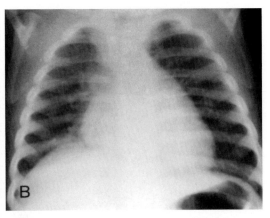

FIGURE 1.130. *Foreign body: coughed up.* **(A)** Note classic obstructive emphysema of the left lung. **(B)** This patient had a coughing spell and coughed up the foreign body; the left lung now is nearly normal. A little emphysema remains, however, probably secondary to some residual mucosal edema. This is not an uncommon finding just after foreign bodies are dislodged or removed.

Finally, it should be noted that not all foreign bodies need to remain lodged in any one position for the entire time they are in the tracheobronchial tree. Indeed, some foreign bodies tend to move back and forth and may even move from one bronchus to another. If this is the case, they produce confusing clinical and roentgenographic findings. By the same token, one should not be surprised to encounter a patient who, on his or her own, coughs up the foreign body and becomes symptom-free, even while awaiting initial or further diagnostic studies (Fig. 1.130). Still another peculiarity of endobronchial foreign bodies deals with multiple foreign bodies. Very often the aspirated material has been chewed or partially chewed and numerous small fragments are aspirated. Such fragments are "sprayed"

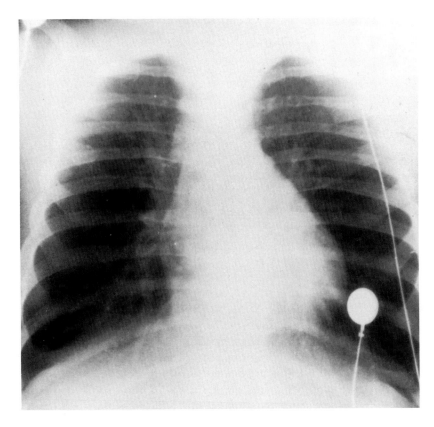

FIGURE 1.131. *Multiple foreign bodies.* This patient had acute onset of marked generalized wheezing and severe respiratory compromise. History of foreign body aspiration was vague, but the patient's condition deteriorated rapidly, and bronchoscopy was performed. Numerous peanut fragments were found scattered throughout the bronchi of both lungs.

throughout the peripheral bronchi, and diffuse, catastrophic air trapping with numerous peripheral obstructions occurs (Fig. 1.131).

REFERENCES

1. Blazer S, Naveh Y, Friedman A. Foreign body in the airway: Review of 200 cases. *Am J Dis Child* 1980;134:68–71.
2. Burton EM, Riggs W Jr. Kaufman RA, Houston CS. Pneumomediastinum caused by foreign body aspiration in children. *Pediatr Radiol* 1989;20:45–47.
3. Capitanio MA, Kirkpatrick JA. The lateral decubitus film, and aid in determining air-trapping in children. *Radiology* 1972;103:460–462.
4. Capitanio MA, Kirkpatrick JA. Obstructions of the upper airway in children as reflected on the chest radiograph. *Radiology* 1973;107:159–161.
5. Cleveland RH. Symmetry of bronchial angles in children. *Radiology* 1979;133:89–93.
6. Grunebaum M, Adler S, Varsano I. The paradoxical movement of the mediastinum: A diagnostic sign of foreign body aspiration during childhood. *Pediatr Radiol* 1979;8:213–218.
7. Laks Y, Barzilay Z. Foreign body aspiration in childhood. *Pediatr Emerg Care* 1988;4:102–106.
8. Linegar AG, van Oppel UO, Hegemann S, et al. Tracheobronchial foreign bodies experience at Red Cross Children's Hospital. *S Afr Med J* 1992;82:164–167.
9. Reed MH. Radiology of airway foreign bodies in children. *Can J Assoc Radiol* 1977;28:111–118.
10. Seibert RW, Seibert JJ, Williamson SL. The opaque chest: When to suspect a bronchial foreign body. *Pediatr Radiol* 1986;16:193–196.
11. Svedstrom E, Puhakka H, Kero P. How accurate is chest radiography in the diagnosis of tracheobronchial foreign bodies in children? *Pediatr Radiol* 1989;19:520–522.

PENETRATING AND NONPENETRATING (BLUNT) CHEST TRAUMA

Blunt chest trauma is more common than penetrating trauma, but assessing either is not an easy task. There are many subtle findings to look for, and the thoracic cage, cardiovascular structures, pleural space, and pulmonary parenchyma must be examined quickly and carefully. Plain films usually identify significant problems, but eventually CT scans usually are required for final analysis (19,28,33,38). In terms of the thoracic cage, although rib fractures are common, unless they are grossly displaced or multiple, they are not particularly easy to detect on initial films. This is not such a great drawback, however, for it is much more important to determine whether complications such as pneumothorax or hemothorax are present (Fig. 1.132A and B). A rib fracture may also be detected by the presence of a local subpleural hematoma (Fig. 1.132C), but most often rib fractures are detected more easily later, when they are healing.

Rib fractures also aid in directing one's attention to more serious intrathoracic or abdominal injuries. For example,

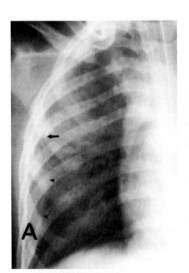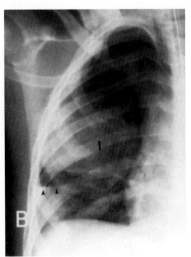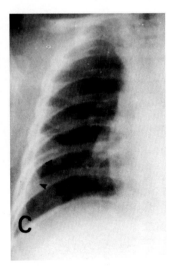

FIGURE 1.132. *Rib fractures.* **(A)** Rib fracture with pneumohemothorax. Note the rib fracture involving the fifth rib on the right (*large arrow*). Diffuse haziness of the right lung results from blood in the pleural space (*lower small arrows*), and an associated pulmonary contusion. **(B)** Upright view showing an air–fluid level (*arrows*) substantiating the presence of a pneumohemothorax. The pulmonary contusion is more clearly visualized on this view, and in addition, fractures of the posterior third, fourth, and fifth ribs are visible. **(C) Rib fracture with subpleural hematoma.** There is a small subpleural hematoma (*arrows*) in this patient, who was sat upon by his older sibling. He had chest pain and point tenderness over the area. Although a rib fracture is not visualized, it should be suspected if a subpleural hematoma is identified.

anterior or lateral rib fractures over the lower thoracic area should cause one to look more earnestly for evidence of splenic or liver trauma. Low posterior rib fractures should alert one to the possibility of underlying renal trauma, and fractures of the first three ribs should obligate one to rule out great-vessel injury (25). By no means, however, does fracturing of these ribs mean that vascular injury is inevitable. Indeed, most often it is not present (37). Nonetheless, the possibility must be kept in mind, and in searching for rib fractures in this area, one should look for collections of fluid (blood) over the apex of the lung (Fig. 1.133).

Fractures of the sternum are best visualized on the lateral view and, of course, on CT scans. They usually result from blunt trauma to the chest such as occurs with steering-wheel injuries or other direct, severe blows to the chest (Fig. 1.134). Retro- and presternal soft-tissue swelling from associated edema and bleeding are noted commonly, but the most important aspect of sternal fractures is that

they frequently are associated with underlying cardiac injury.

Pulmonary parenchymal manifestations of blunt trauma are numerous and include pulmonary contusion, pulmonary hematoma (23), and traumatic pneumatoceles (4,7,10,26). Pulmonary contusions produce pneumonia-like areas of homogeneous or nodular consolidation (Fig. 1.135), which usually become larger and denser during the first 24 to 48 hours after injury. Pulmonary contusions clear slowly and eventually may contract to the point of suggesting a pulmonary mass. Densities that appear round or oval from the onset probably represent pulmonary hematomas. Usually they are slow to resolve, and they may cavitate during the course of their resolution (Fig. 1.136).

Traumatic pneumatoceles or air cysts frequently occur with blunt chest trauma and may be seen either in the pulmonary parenchyma or in the mediastinum (6,7,27). They usually are seen with other manifestations of pulmonary

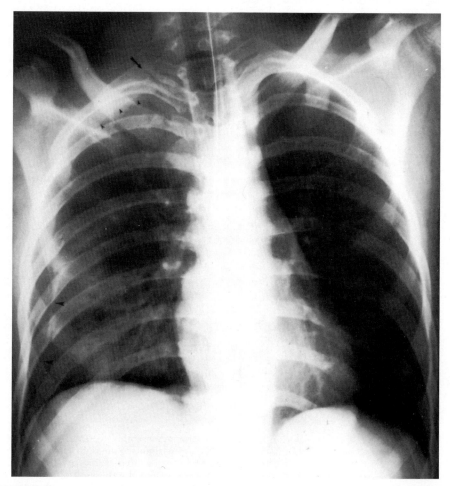

FIGURE 1.133. *Fracture of the first rib with apical blood.* Note the fracture of the first rib on the right (*upper large* arrow). Just beneath it note blood over the apex of the right lung (*upper three small arrows*). A pneumothorax also is delineated (*lower arrows*).

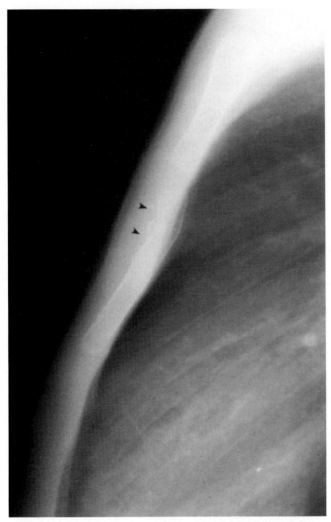

FIGURE 1.134. *Sternal fracture.* This patient was wrestling and suffered blunt chest trauma. The sternum is fractured (*arrows*), and there is some pre- and retrosternal soft tissue swelling.

injury and develop within minutes or hours of the injury. These air cysts or pneumatoceles may be round or oval, single or multiple, and some may contain blood (Fig. 1.137). Generally, they are thin-walled and may increase in size rather rapidly after they first appear. Similar air collections in the mediastinum tend to be more elongated and paraspinal in position (Fig. 1.137D). These air collections are believed to lie in the inferior pulmonary ligament (6,7), although similar collections can occur in the retroesophageal ligament. Overall, traumatic pneumatoceles are relatively innocuous, for seldom do they rupture or become infected. For the most part, they slowly become smaller and disappear over a 2 to 3-week period. To the uninitiated, however, they frequently constitute distractions from other potentially more serious problems that also might be present. In addition, if multiple (2), they can be misinterpreted

as the findings of a traumatic diaphragmatic hernia (Fig. 1.138).

More catastrophic injuries to the respiratory system include bronchial and tracheal fracture or tear (12,21,24, 27,36) and torsion of the lung (8,22). Torsion of the lung, with subsequent infarction, is often difficult to diagnose roentgenographically, but it has been pointed out that because such a lung makes a 180-degree turn around its hilus, the vascular pattern of the upper and lower lobes is inverted (8,22). This finding, however, first requires awareness of its existence and then close scrutiny of the roentgenogram for its presence.

With **bronchial fracture** one may see massive pneumothorax or massive atelectasis (Fig. 1.139A), and indeed with blunt chest trauma, massive atelectasis and refractory pneumothorax or air leak should be presumed secondary to bronchial or tracheal fracture until it is proven otherwise (12,21,24,36). With tracheal lacerations, pneumomediastinum is more common than pneumothorax, and if bleeding into the mediastinum occurs, it appears widened. If a pneumothorax results from a bronchial tear, it usually is massive, and if the lung is completely detached from its bronchus, upright views show it at the bottom of the hemithorax (Fig. 1.139B). In other cases of bronchial fracture, the air column in the proximal portion of the fractured bronchus appears tapered or beveled, and in still other instances, air may be seen tracking along the bronchial or tracheal wall itself (14,27). If bleeding also occurs, fluid is seen in the ipsilateral hemithorax. With tracheal tears, the endotracheal tube may lie outside the trachea, and the balloon, because it is not contained by the ruptured trachea, may be overdistended (28). Unfortunately, however, many cases of fractured bronchi are cases of incomplete fracture, and neither atelectasis nor pneumothorax is present at the onset. It is only later, if a frank tear occurs, that these complications develop.

Cardiovascular manifestations of blunt chest trauma also are varied and include bloody or serous pericardial effusions, myocardial contusions (3,5,15), and traumatic aneurysms of the heart or aorta. In one study (5), 95% of cases resulted in cardiac contusion. In more severe cases, frank tears or ruptures of the heart or vessels can occur (1,20,32,34), and in addition, aortic insufficiency associated with traumatic aneurysms of the ascending aorta and traumatic ventricular septal defects can be encountered (17,29). Minimal myocardial injuries are detected best with electrocardiograms or myocardial scintograms, or perhaps magnetic resonance imaging. Such myocardial injuries are not detectable roentgenographically, but with more extensive contusions nonspecific cardiomegaly is seen. Pericardial effusions, if large enough, produce enlargement of the cardiac silhouette, but with smaller effusions, ultrasonography is the diagnostic procedure of choice.

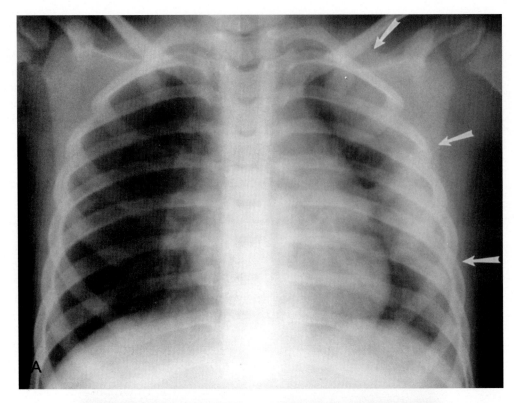

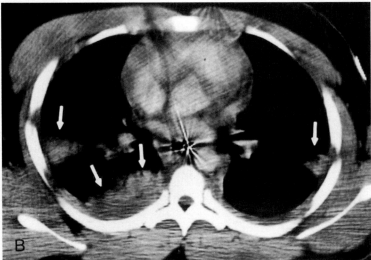

FIGURE 1.135. *Pulmonary contusion.* **(A)** Young patient with an extensive contusion in the left lung (*arrows*). **(B)** Computed tomographic study in another patient demonstrating multiple contusions (*arrows*) and bilateral pleural effusions.

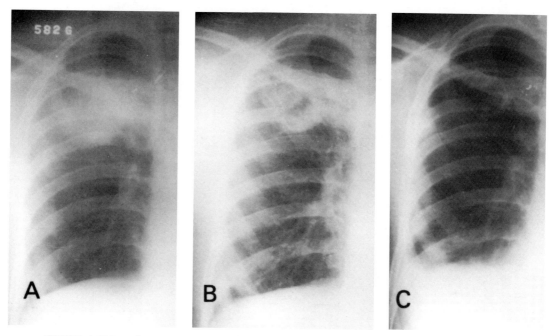

FIGURE 1.136. *Pulmonary hematoma with cavitation.* **(A)** Note a masslike lesion in the right upper lobe. **(B)** A few days later, note that a cavity is developing in this hematoma. **(C)** More than a month later, a thin-walled cavity remains. (From Fagan CJ, and Swischuk LE: Traumatic lung and paramediastinal pneumatoceles. *Radiology* 120:11–18, 1976, with permission.)

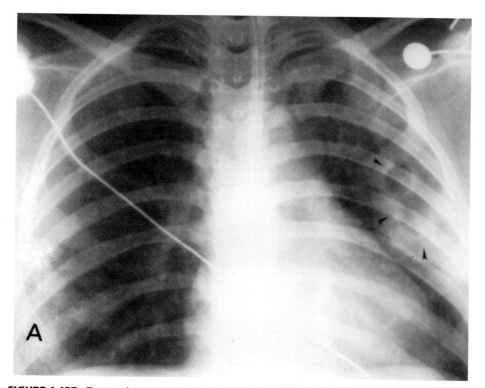

FIGURE 1.137. *Traumatic pneumatoceles.* **(A)** Note the two spherical, thin-walled pneumatoceles (*arrows*) in the contused left lung of this child, who had been run over by a truck. *Continued on next page.*

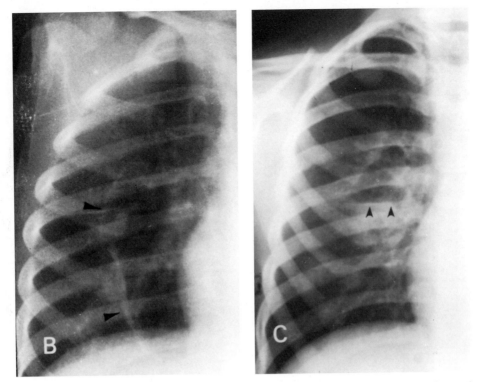

FIGURE 1.137. *(continued)* (B) Large posttraumatic pneumatocele on the right side (*arrows*). (C) Another patient with a traumatic pneumatocele demonstrating an air–fluid level (*arrows*) on upright view. The air–fluid level represents air and blood in the pneumatocele. (From Fagan CJ, and Swischuk LE: Traumatic lung and paramediastinal pneumatoceles. *Radiology* 120:11–18, 1976, with permission)

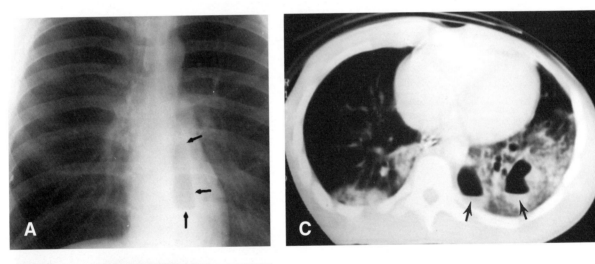

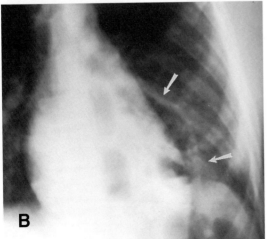

FIGURE 1.138. *Less typical traumatic pneumatoceles.* (A) Traumatic pneumatocele in inferior pulmonary ligament (*upper arrows*). The *lower arrow* points to an air–fluid level. (B) Multiple traumatic pneumatoceles (*arrows*) mimicking a congenital diaphragmatic hernia. (C) Computed tomographic study demonstrates the numerous pneumatoceles present in the left lower lobe (*arrows*). (From Fagan CJ, and Swischuk LE: Traumatic lung and paramediastinal pneumatoceles. *Radiology* 120: 11–18, 1976, with permission.)

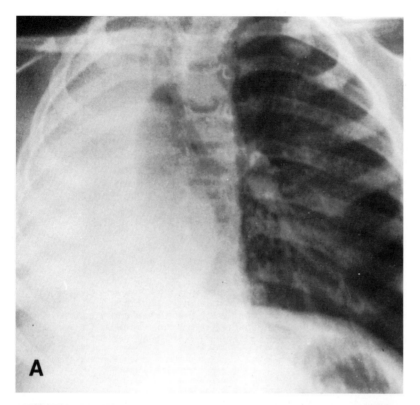

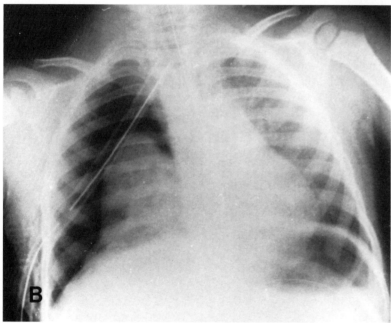

FIGURE 1.139. (A) Bronchial rupture of right lung, manifesting as total atelectasis of the right lung. Rib fractures are present on the other side. (From Mahboubi S, and O'Hara AE: Bronchial rupture in children following blunt chest trauma. *Pediatr Radiol* 10: 133–138, 1981, with permission.) **(B)** Avulsion of a bronchus. Note the massive pneumothorax and collapsed, dropped right lung. (From Grover FL, et al.: Diagnosis and management of major tracheobronchial injuries. *Ann Thorac Surg* 28: 385–391, 1979, with permission.)

Injury to the aorta or great vessels is most important to detect, but unfortunately the roentgenographic findings often tend to elude initial observation. Because of this, one must constantly be on guard for signs of superior mediastinal widening (20,31,34) or the collecting of blood over the apex of the left lung (Fig. 1.140A). This latter finding has been termed the ***left apical extrapleural cap sign*** (33) and

results from leaking of blood from a ruptured aortic arch into the pleural space over the left lung. There is a normal defect in the pleural covering over the aorta in this area (transverse arch), and mediastinal blood can track directly into the left apical pleural space. The finding is subtle but important and should be sought with diligence. Unfortunately, however, it is not always present, and it also can be

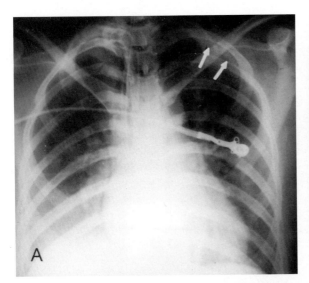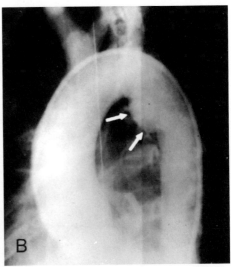

FIGURE 1.140. *Traumatic aortic aneurysm.* **(A)** Note the collection of fluid over the left lung apex (*arrows*). This constitutes the apical cap sign. There is a posterior fracture of the right third rib. The superior mediastinum is widened slightly, but more importantly, the endotracheal and esophageal tubes are shifted to the right. These findings substantiate the fact that a mediastinal hematoma is present. **(B)** Subsequent aortogram demonstrates a traumatic aortic aneurysm (*arrows*).

seen with nonaortic trauma. For this reason it is not specific, but in combination with other signs of aortic rupture, especially mediastinal widening (30,31), it should arouse considerable suspicion. Thereafter, if aortic or great-vessel injury is suspected, immediate CT scanning or preferably aortography (34) is required (Fig. 1.140). However, with spiral, contrast-enhanced CT, arteriography can be avoided in a significant number of cases (13).

Mediastinal widening as seen with aortic rupture must be differentiated from widening secondary to the presence of normal thymus and supine positioning. Most injured patients are examined in the supine position, and the superior mediastinum may appear wide. It has been noted that with widening resulting from aortic rupture, the trachea and esophagus are displaced to the right (11,34,35) (Fig. 1.140). If widening results from thymus gland and

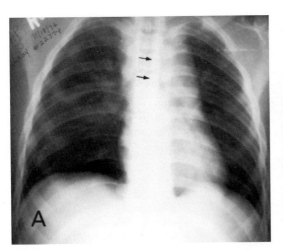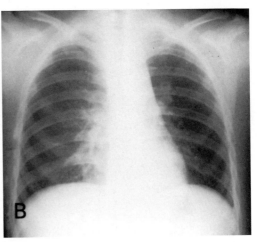

FIGURE 1.141. *Widened superior mediastinum and pleural fluid but no traumatic aortic rupture.* **(A)** Note that there is a pneumothorax on the right and that there is blood layered over the apex of the left lung. The superior mediastinum is widened, but note that the tube in the esophagus is in a normal location (*arrows*). It is not shifted to the right. **(B)** Repeat film the next day with the patient in an upright position shows persistence of the right pneumothorax but a normal-appearing superior mediastinum. Some fluid still is present on the left. The findings in **A** were caused by supine positioning, and not a hematoma resulting from aortic rupture.

supine positioning, these structures are not displaced to the right (Fig. 1.141). This is an important observation to make, and frequently it is facilitated by the fact that these patients have indwelling tubes in either the trachea or esophagus, or in both of these structures. Recently, it has been noted that if these midline structures are not displaced, one can confidently exclude aortic injury (18,34). This is important in confusing cases (Fig. 1.142), in which a simple mediastinal hematoma may mimic aortic rupture (9).

Pneumopericardium is not particularly common with blunt chest trauma but does occur. It is, of course, more common with penetrating wounds to the chest, and roentgenographically it is identified by air surrounding the cardiac silhouette. In these cases, the pericardium itself is usually visible, and it is most important that a pneumopericardium not be confused with a medial pneumo-

thorax or pneumomediastinum (Figs. 1.102 and 1.104). An uncommon injury is rupture of the pericardium. In such cases, the heart is displaced or dislocated to the left (16), and because of this the findings resemble those seen with unilateral congenital absence of the left pericardium, or shifting of the heart to the left by a pronounced pectus excavatum deformity of the chest.

Penetrating injuries to the chest, heart, and great vessels can produce all of the findings seen with closed (blunt) chest trauma, but, in addition, one can see air in the heart and great vessels (Fig. 1.143). Delayed complications such as cardiac or great vessel tears with hemopericardium also can be encountered, and with metallic foreign bodies such as bullets one may see the bullet in one of the chambers of the heart or great vessels. In other instances, the bullet may be lodged in the mediastinum, lung, or spine (Fig. 1.143).

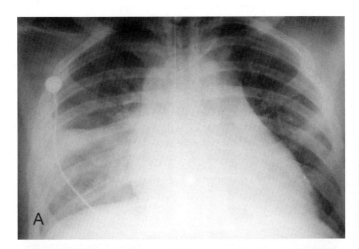

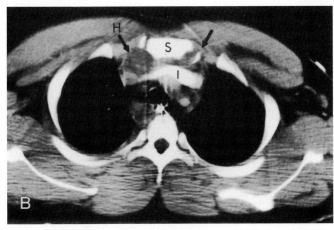

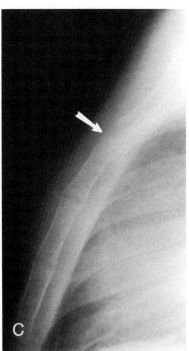

FIGURE 1.142. *Widened mediastinum without traumatic aortic aneurysm.* **(A)** Note the wide mediastinum in this patient. The esophageal tube and trachea, however, are not displaced to the right. There is a contusion on the right. **(B)** Computed tomographic scan with contrast identifies the innominate vein (*I*) and sternum (*S*), and in between these two structures, a hematoma (*H*). Mediastinal widening resulted from this hematoma. Note the displaced sternal fracture fragment (arrow). **(C)** Lateral view of the sternum demonstrates the fracture through the sternomanubrial junction (arrow).

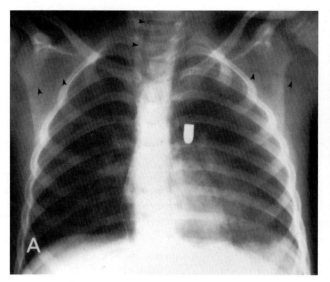
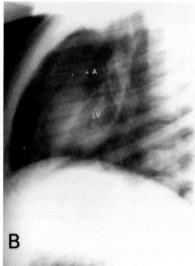

FIGURE 1.143. *Penetrating injury of the heart with free air.* **(A)** Note the bullet lodged in the back of this patient. Also note (a) contusion of the left lung, (b) air in the heart, (c) air in the pericardium (best seen on the right), and (d) air in the subclavian and carotid arteries (*upper arrows*). **(B)** Lateral view demonstrates air in the left ventricle (*LV*) and aorta (*A*). The patient soon died. The bullet is not seen on this view but was lodged in the soft tissues of the back. (Courtesy of Virgil B. Graves, M.D.).

REFERENCES

1. Ali IS, Fitzgerald PG, Gillis DA, Lau HYC. Blunt traumatic disruption of the thoracic aorta: A rare injury in children. *J Pediatr Surg* 1992;27:1281–1284.
2. Allbery AM, Swischuk LE, John SD. Posttraumatic pneumatoceles mimicking diaphragmatic hernia. *Emerg Radiol* 1997;4:94–96.
3. Bromberg BI, Mazziotti MV, Canter CE, Spray TL, Strauss AW, Foglia RP. Recognition and management of nonpenetrating cardiac trauma in children. *J Pediatr* 1996;128:536–541.
4. Cochlin DL, Shaw MRP. Traumatic lung cysts following minor blunt chest trauma. *Clin Radiol* 1978;29:151–158.
5. Dowd MD, Krug S. Pediatric blunt cardiac injury: Epidemiology, clinical features, and diagnosis. *J Trauma* 1996;40:61–67.
6. Elyaderani MK, Gabriele OF. Traumatic paramediastinal air cysts. *Br J Radiol* 1979;52:458–460.
7. Fagan CJ, Swischuk LE. Traumatic lung and paramediastinal pneumatoceles. *Radiology* 1976;120:11–18.
8. Felson B. Lung torsion: Radiographic findings in nine cases. *Radiology* 1987;162:631–638.
9. Fleisher AG, David I, Hilfer C, Mekhjian HA, Stanley-Brown EG. Mediastinal hematoma mimicking aortic rupture. *J Pediatr Surg* 1986;21:445–446.
10. Galea MH, Williams N, Mayell MJ. Traumatic pneumatocele. *J Pediatr Surg* 1992;27:1523–1524.
11. Gerlock AJ Jr. Muhletaler CA, Coulam CM, Hayes PT. Traumatic aortic aneurysm: Validity of esophageal tube displacement sign. *AJR* 1980;135:713–718.
12. Hancock BJ, Wiseman NE. Tracheobronchial injuries in children. *J Pediatr Surg* 1991;26:1316–1319.
13. Haramati LB, Hochsztein JG, Marciano N, Nathanson N. Evaluation of the role of chest computed tomography in the management of trauma patients. *Emerg Radiol* 1996;3:225–230.
14. Harvey-Smith W, Bush W, Northrop C. Traumatic bronchial rupture. *AJR* 1980;134:1189–1193.
15. Ildstad ST, Tollerud DJ, Weiss RG, Cox JA, Martin LW. Cardiac contusion in pediatric patients with blunt thoracic trauma. *J Pediatr Surg* 1990;25:287–289.
16. Kermond AJ. The dislocated heart: An unusual complication of major chest injury. *Radiology* 1976;119:59–60.
17. Knapp JF, Sharma V, Wasserman G, Hoover CJ, Walsh I. Ventricular septal defect following blunt chest trauma in childhood: A case report. *Pediatr Emerg Care* 1986;2:242–243.
18. Mahboubi S, O'Hara AE. Bronchial rupture in children following blunt chest trauma. *Pediatr Radiol* 1981;10:133–138.
19. Manson D, Babyn PS, Palder S, Bergman K. CT of blunt chest trauma in children. *Pediatr Radiol* 1993;23:1–5.
20. Marnocha KE, Maglinte DDT. Plain-film criteria for excluding aortic rupture in blunt chest trauma. *AJR* 1985;144:19–22.
21. Mordehai J, Kurzbart E, Kapuller V, Mares AJ. Tracheal rupture after blunt chest trauma in a child. *J Pediatr Surg* 1997;32:104–105.
22. Moser ES Jr., Proto AV. Lung torsion: Case report and literature review. *Radiology* 1987;162:639–643.
23. Parsai D, Nussle D, Cuendet A. Presentation of two cases of pulmonary hematoma in child after closed chest trauma, and review of literature. *Ann Radiol* 1974;17:831–836.
24. Perchinsky M, Long W, Rosoff J, Campbell TJ. Traumatic rupture of the tracheobronchial tree in a 2-year-old. *J Pediatr Surg* 1994;29:1548-1549.
25. Pierce G, Maxwell J, Boggan M. Special hazards of 1st rib fractures. *J Trauma* 1975;15:264–267.
26. Ravin C, Smith GW, Lester PD, McLoud TC, Putman CE. Posttraumatic pneumatocele in the inferior pulmonary ligament. *Radiology* 1976;121:39–41.
27. Rollins RJ, Tocino I. Early radiographic signs of tracheal rupture. *AJR* 1987;148:695–698.
28. Roux P, Fisher RM. Chest injuries in children: an analysis of 100

cases of blunt chest trauma from motor vehicle accidents. *J Pediatr Surg* 1992;27:551–555.

29. Rowland TW. Traumatic aortic insufficiency in children: Case report and reviews of the literature. *Pediatrics* 1977;60:893–895.
30. Savastano S, Feltrin GP, Miotto D, Chiesura-Corona M. Value of plain chest film predicting traumatic aortic rupture. *Ann Radiol* 1989;32:196–200.
31. Sefczek DM, Sefczek RJ, Deeb ZL. Radiographic signs of acute traumatic rupture of the thoracic aorta. *AJR* 1983;141:1259–1262.
32. Simeone JF, Minagi H, Putman CE. Traumatic disruption of the thoracic aorta: Significance of the left apical extrapleural cap. *Radiology* 1975;117:265–268.
33. Sivit CJ, Taylor GA, Eichelberger MR. Chest injury in children with blunt abdominal trauma: Evaluation with CT. *Radiology* 1989;171: 815–818.
34. Spouge AR, Burrows PE, Armstrong D, Daneman A. Traumatic aortic rupture in the pediatric population: Role of plain film, CT and angiography in the diagnosis. *Pediatr Radiol* 1991;21:324–328.
35. Tisnado J, Tsai FY, Als A, Roach JF. A new radiographic sign of acute traumatic rupture of the thoracic aorta: Displacement of the nasogastric tube to the right. *Radiology* 1977;125:603–608.
36. Wiener Y, Simansky D, Yellin A. Main bronchial rupture from blunt trauma in a 2-year-old child. *J Pediatr Surg* 1994;28:1530–1531.
37. Woodring JH, Fried AM, Hatfield DR, Stevens RK, Todd EP. Fractures of first and second ribs: Predictive value for arterial and bronchial injury. *AJR* 1982;138:211–215.
38. Vyas PK, Sivit CJ. Imaging of blunt pediatric thoracic trauma. *Emerg Radiol* 1997;4:16–25.

MISCELLANEOUS CHEST PROBLEMS

Hydrocarbon Pneumonitis

The most commonly ingested hydrocarbons include furniture polish, gasoline, kerosene, and charcoal lighter fluid, and the most important aspect of these hydrocarbons is that the lower their viscosity and surface tension, the greater the

likelihood that they will be diffusely aspirated into the tracheobronchial tree. In this regard, it is mineral seal oil in certain furniture polishes (i.e., red furniture polish) that causes most of the difficulty, for it is one of the lightest of hydrocarbon distillates (2,3,6). Consequently, an infant does not have to aspirate a large volume of a hydrocarbon-containing mineral seal oil to be in serious difficulty.

There still is some controversy as to whether the pneumonitis resulting from ingestion of hydrocarbons occurs because of aspiration or because of absorption of the hydrocarbon from the stomach, but most now favor aspiration as the major mechanism (5,6). Although a small amount of the hydrocarbon probably is absorbed from the gastrointestinal tract and expelled through the lungs, it is not enough to explain the pulmonary changes. It may explain the cerebral depression that some of these children demonstrate after such ingestion, but in most cases, resulting damage to the lungs from hydrocarbons circulating in the bloodstream is negligible.

Characteristically, with hydrocarbon ingestion and inhalation, roentgenographic pulmonary changes are absent for the first 6 to 12 hours, unless massive aspiration occurs. Consequently, a normal chest film during this lag period can be misleading, and it is much more important to evaluate the patient clinically and to obtain blood-gas values early. Often the values are abnormal, for the local effects of lipid dissolution (i.e., surfactant destruction and the development of microatelectasis) lead to serious gas-exchange problems (3). In addition, cell membrane destruction occurs, and all of this, along with small-vessel thrombosis, soon leads to bronchiolar necrosis and a necrotizing bronchopneumonia (5).

After the usual clear-lung period, infiltrates quickly develop in the lung bases (Fig. 1.144). This characteristic

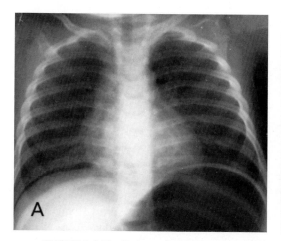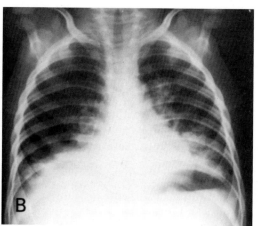

FIGURE 1.144. *Hydrocarbon pneumonitis.* **(A)** This patient aspirated red furniture polish, but 2 hours after ingestion, the lungs are clear. **(B)** By 12 hours, however, note extensive infiltrates in the lung bases.

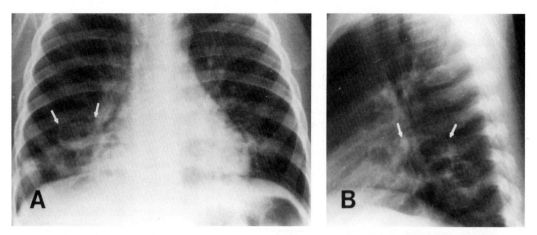

FIGURE 1.145. *Pneumatoceles with hydrocarbon aspiration.* **(A)** Frontal view demonstrating bilateral, basal, and medial infiltrates and pneumatoceles in the right lower lobe (*arrows*). **(B)** Lateral view demonstrates these pneumatoceles (*arrows*) to better advantage.

location basal supports aspiration as the cause of hydrocarbon pneumonitis, and the changes can range from minimal fluffy infiltrates to dense, confluent infiltrates involving a good portion of the lungs bilaterally. In the latter case, focal emphysema and pneumatocele formation are not uncommon (Fig. 1.145) and most likely result from air trapping from the damaged small bronchi and bronchioles (1,4). All of these changes are slow to clear, often taking up to 2 or 3 weeks to completely disappear (3,6). Currently, in addition to regular therapy in these patients, extracorporeal membranous oxygenation has been used in severe cases.

REFERENCES

1. Bergeson PS, Hales SW, Lustgarten MD, Lipow HW. Pneumatoceles following hydrocarbon ingestion. *Am J Dis Child* 1975;129:49–54.
2. Giamonna ST. Effects of furniture polish on pulmonary surfactant. *Am J Dis Child* 1967;113:658–663.
3. Griffin JW, Daeschner CW, Collins VP, Eaton WL. Hydrocarbon pneumonitis following furniture polish ingestion: Report of fifteen cases. *J Pediatr* 1954;45:13–26.
4. Harris VJ, Brown R. Pneumatoceles as a complication of chemical pneumonia after hydrocarbon ingestion. *AJR* 1975;125:531–537.
5. Heinisch HM, Levejohann R. The pathogenesis of radiological changes in the lungs after ingestion of petroleum distillates: An experimental study in rabbits and extrapolation of the results in children. *Ann Radiol* 1973;16:263–266.
6. Jimenez JB, Lester RG. Pulmonary complications following furniture polish ingestion: A report of 21 cases. *AJR* 1966;98:323–333.

Other Pulmonary Aspiration Problems

Aspiration of gastric contents into the tracheobronchial tree with resultant pneumonia can be focal or widespread, and the findings depend on the volume of fluid aspirated and the patient's position during the aspiration episode. In small infants, aspiration often occurs into the right upper lobe and results in right upper-lobe atelectasis. Presumably, aspiration occurs into the right upper lobes of these infants because they are fed in the recumbent position on their right sides. Aspiration in the upright position leads to medial lower-lobe infiltrates, and the roentgenographic findings are not unlike those seen with hydrocarbon pneumonitis. With massive aspiration, the findings may mimic those of pulmonary edema or widespread bacterial pneumonia. Severe cases are referred to as constituting ***Mendelson's syndrome*** (5,7). In these cases, a severe chemical pneumonitis secondary to the aspiration of acid gastric contents occurs, and the roentgenographic findings reflect extensive pulmonary edema.

Chronic aspiration problems lead to pulmonary fibrosis, bronchitis, and even bronchiectasis. Infiltrates secondary to significant aspirations usually take weeks, or even months, to completely clear. This is especially true of lipid aspiration, which often leads to very dense, hazy lungs (Fig. 1.146A). Aspiration of detergents also can lead to serious damage to the lungs (4).

Causes of aspiration are numerous and include swallowing mechanism defects, tracheoesophageal fistulae, aspiration during episodes of seizure activity or unconsciousness, drowning, and, as mentioned previously, incidental aspiration during normal feeding of young infants. In addition, aspiration can occur secondary to gastroesophageal reflux. Massive aspiration of particulate matter such as dirt, sand, or cornstarch (1,3,6) can be severe and often leads to sud-

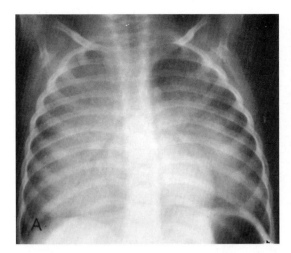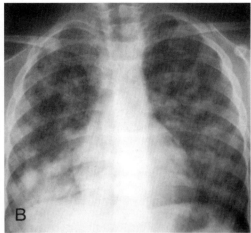

FIGURE 1.146. *Other aspiration problems.* **(A)** Diffuse, widespread hazy infiltrates resulting from lipid aspiration. **(B)** Diffuse fluffy nodular infiltrates resulting from aspiration of water in near drowning.

den death. If the foreign material contains calcium carbonate (2), it can be seen as opaque material filling the bronchi on chest films.

Near drowning presents another common aspiration problem. In this regard, it makes no difference whether salt or fresh water is aspirated; it is the volume of water that makes the difference. Usually the aspirated water clears quickly, although if a patient aspirates a great deal of associated debris, problems may be more prolonged, and certainly infection becomes a common complication. The findings in near drowning are usually nonspecific and consist of a variable degree of patchy, fluffy alveolar pulmonary infiltration (Fig. 1.146B). With near drowning it should be noted that many patients also are asphyxiated. As a result, they develop brain edema and in some cases neurogenic pulmonary edema. In addition, they may develop, as they recover from the initial aspiration, superimposed adult respiratory distress syndrome.

REFERENCES

1. Bergeson PS, Hinchcliffe WA, Crawford RF, Sorenson MJ, Trump DS. Asphyxia secondary to massive dirt aspiration. *J Pediatr* 1978; 92:506–507.
2. Bonilla-Santiago J, Fill WL. Sand aspiration in drowning and near drowning. *Radiology* 1978;128:301–302.
3. Choy IO, Idowu O. Sand aspiration: A case report. *J Pediatr Surg* 1996;31:1448–1450.
4. Einhorn A, Horton L, Altieri M, Ochsenschlager D, Klein B. Serious respiratory consequences of detergent ingestions in children. *Pediatrics* 1989;84:472–474.
5. Richman H, Abramson SF. Mendelson's syndrome. *Am J Surg* 1970;120:531–536.
6. Silver P, Sagy M, Rubin L. Respiratory failure from cornstarch aspiration: A hazard of diaper changing. *Pediatr Emerg Care* 1996; 12:108–110.
7. Wilkins RA, Lacey GJ, Flor R, Taylor S. Radiology in Mendelson's syndrome. *Clin Radiol* 1976;27:81–85.

Delayed Diaphragmatic Hernia

Occasionally, an older child presents with acute respiratory distress secondary to herniation of the abdominal viscera into the thoracic cavity. Indeed, such occurrences in older children are being documented more often (1–11). These patients frequently present with acute respiratory distress, which may or may not be preceded by vomiting. The resulting roentgenographic findings may be startling and puzzling, and unless the possibility of delayed diaphragmatic hernia is kept in mind, the proper diagnosis may elude the initial observer. Misinterpretation as a large pneumothorax, pulmonary cyst, or diaphragmaatic hernia is not unusual (Fig. 1.147). In those cases in which the stomach contains fluid, the findings may be misinterpreted as an intrathoracic mass. Rarely, gastric rupture or small bowel necrosis can occur (3).

An upper gastrointestinal series may be needed for verification that the stomach or other portion of the gastrointestinal tract is in the chest, but, if gastric volvulus also is present, barium may not pass from the esophagus to the stomach. If volvulus is not present, barium is seen to pass from the esophagus upward into the stomach, which, of course, is in the chest cavity. Most of these cases are presumed to be instances of delayed herniation through a congenital diaphragmatic defect, but it also should be noted

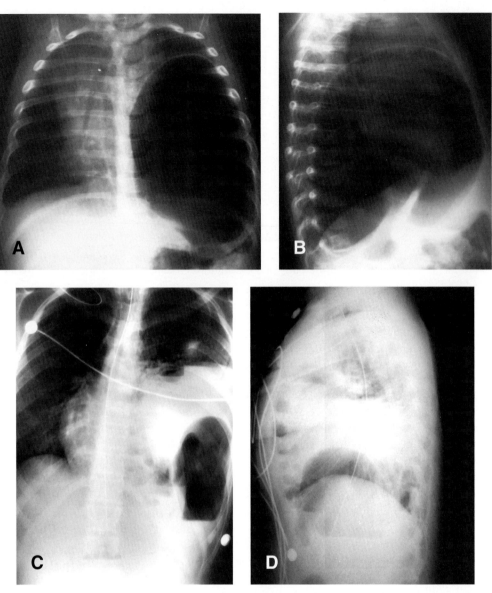

FIGURE 1.147. *Diaphragmatic hernia, delayed presentation in older children.* (**A**) Note a large cyst-like structure in the left hemithorax. It displaces the heart and mediastinum to the right. The findings might be misinterpreted as a large lung cyst or pneumothorax. Note, however, that there is no gastric bubble visualized in the abdomen. (**B**) Lateral view shows the incarcerated, dilated stomach herniated into the chest of this young child, who presented with an acute vomiting episode followed by severe respiratory distress. (Courtesy of Virgil B. Graves, M.D.). (**C**) In this older child, numerous loops of intestine and stomach are present in the left hemithorax. This patient was completely asymptomatic before this occurred. (**D**) Lateral view demonstrates the massive hernia.

that such hernias can occur after blunt abdominal trauma either on an acute or delayed basis. In addition, rupture of the diaphragm has been documented in association with coughing in pertussis (4).

REFERENCES

1. Berman L, Stringer D, Ein SH, Shandling B. The late presenting pediatric Bochdalek hernia: A 20-year review. *J Pediatr Surg* 1988;23:735–739.
2. Booker PD, Meerstadt PWD, Bush GH. Congenital diaphragmatic hernia in the older child. *Arch Dis Child* 1981;56:253–257.
3. Byard RW, Bourne AJ, Cockington RA. Fatal gastric perforation in a 4-year-old child with a late presenting congenital diaphragmatic hernia. *Pediatr Surg Int* 1991;6:44–46.
4. Dutta T. Spontaneous rupture of diaphragm due to pertussis. *J Pediatr Surg* 1975;10:147–148.
5. Gaisie G, Young LW, Oh KS. Late onset Bochdalek's hernia with obstruction: Radiographic spectrum of presentation. *Clin Radiol* 1983;34:267–270.
6. Glasson MJ, Barter W, Cohen DH, Bowdler JD. Congenital left posterolateral diaphragmatic hernia with previously normal chest x-ray. *Pediatr Radiol* 1975;3:201–205.
7. Kirchner SG, Burko H, O'Neill JA, Stahlman M. Delayed radiographic presentation of congenital right diaphragmatic hernia. *Radiology* 1975;115:155–156.
8. Quah BS, Hashim I, Simpson H. Bochdalek diaphragmatic hernia presenting with acute gastric dilatation. *J Pediatr Surg* 1999;34:512–514.
9. Malone PS, Brain AJ, Kiely EM, et al. Congenital diaphragmatic defects that present late. *Arch Dis Child* 1989;64:1542–1544.
10. McCue J, Ball A, Brereton RJ, Wright VM, Shaw D. Congenital diaphragmatic hernia in older children. *J R Coll Surg Edinb* 1985;30:305–310.
11. Swischuk LE. Vomiting blood for three days. *Pediatr Emerg Care* 1994;10:241–243.

Delayed Congenital Lobar Emphysema

Congenital lobar emphysema usually is considered a neonatal problem, but this condition occasionally presents at a later point in childhood (1). Indeed, a superimposed viral infection can convert or aggravate a relatively asymptomatic case into one with full-blown symptoms (Fig. 1.148). The problem most often involves the upper lobes, with the left being more involved than the right. The next most common lobe to be involved is the right middle lobe, and in some series right middle-lobe involvement is a little more common than right upper-lobe involvement. Lower-lobe involvement is virtually unheard of. With upper-lobe emphysema, the key to proper diagnosis is visualization of the compressed, triangular-appearing lower lobe deep in the costovertebral angle (Fig. 1.148). In

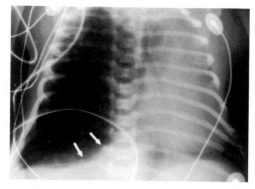

FIGURE 1.148. *Congenital lobar emphysema: delayed presentation.* In this patient with triggering respiratory syncytial viral infection, emphysema in the right upper lobe is very profound. Note the collapsed right lower lobe (*arrows*). The right lung is so overdistended that it is herniating to the left across the upper mediastinum. There is contralateral shift of the heart to the left. Note that there are virtually no lung markings in the emphysematous right upper lobe.

many of these cases, the lung is so overdistended that parenchymal markings, for the most part, are invisible, and the findings are misinterpreted as massive tension pneumothorax. With middle-lobe involvement, the upper and lower lobes become atelectatic, and usually the atelectatic lobes erroneously are believed to be primarily atelectatic rather than compressed by the overdistended middle lobe.

REFERENCE

1. Taber P, Benveniste H, Gans SL. Delayed infantile lobar emphysema. *J Pediatr Surg* 1974;9:245–246.

Allergic Pneumonitis

Allergic manifestations in a lung can occur with toxic substances that are either inhaled or ingested. The resultant infiltrates may be widespread (Fig. 1.149) or focal. If such infiltrates come and go rapidly in different areas of the lung, the terms ***Löffler's pneumonia*** or ***pulmonary infiltrates with eosinophilia*** often are applied. A detailed discussion of all of the causes of allergic pneumonitis is beyond the scope of this book, but it should be stressed that proper questioning of the patient regarding the intake of any medication or drugs is mandatory if unexplained infiltrates are seen on chest roentgenograms. Nonspecific pulmonary infiltrates also are seen in the milk allergy or Heiner's syndrome (1,2). In most instances, the findings are nonspecific.

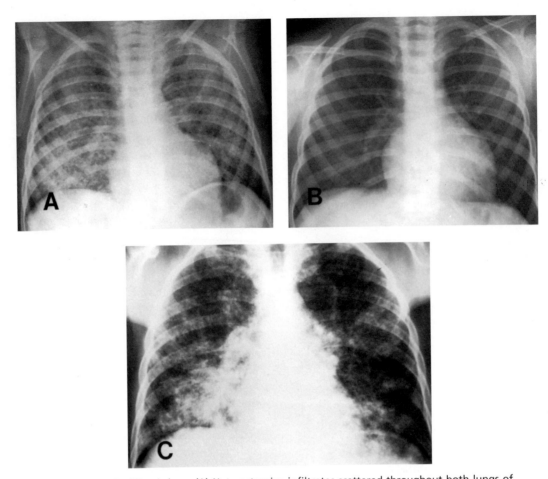

FIGURE 1.149. *Allergic lung.* **(A)** Note extensive infiltrates scattered throughout both lungs of this child, with an allergic lung manifestation caused by cytotoxic drug administration for treatment of leukemia. **(B)** Twenty-four hours later, after steroid administration, the lungs are clear. **(C)** Patchy infiltrates in another patient with an "allergic lung" secondary to inhaled fungal antigens. ***Farmer's lung*** is the term often applied to these cases. (Courtesy of A. Selke, M.D.)

REFERENCES

1. Diner WC, Knicker WT, Heiner DC. Roentgenologic manifestations in the lungs in milk allergy. *Radiology* 1961;77:564–572.
2. Heiner DC, Sears JW, Knicker WT. Multiple precipitins to cow's milk in chronic respiratory disease: A syndrome involving poor growth, gastrointestinal symptoms, evidence of allergy, iron deficiency anemia, and pulmonary hemosiderosis. *Am J Dis Child* 1962;103:634–654.

Acute Chest Syndrome in Sickle Cell Disease

This is a common problem in patients with sickle-cell disease. There is ongoing controversy as to whether the problem is caused by pulmonary infarction or infection, but data are accumulating to suggest that microvascular occlusive disease may be the important predisposing factor (1,2). Indeed, identifiable responsible infectious agents were not found in 87% of cases in one series (4). All of this notwithstanding, these patients present with acute respiratory distress and chest pain. Very often findings include consolidations of both lower lobes. It is interesting that lower-lobe involvement is more common than upper-lobe involvement, and at the same time bilateral lower-lobe involvement is common (Fig. 1.150). The radiographic changes often are rapidly progressive, and in most cases the patient is considered to have a pneumonia and treated. Nonetheless, if changes clear rapidly, support for the hypothesis that venoocclusive disease is the cause of these episodes becomes more evident. Whatever the cause, these patients often can benefit from transfusion (3).

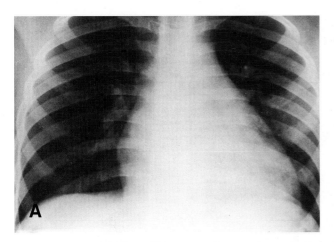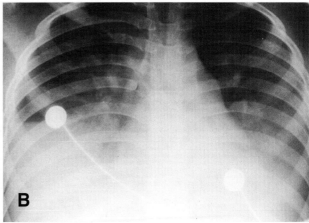

FIGURE 1.150. *Acute chest syndrome: sickle cell disease.* **(A)** Early findings demonstrate slight increased density behind the left side of the heart. The heart is enlarged. **(B)** Within hours bilateral lower-lobe consolidations develop.

REFERENCES

1. Bhala M, Abboud MR, McLoud TC, Shepard J-AO, Munden MM, Jackson SM, Beaty JR, Laver JH. Acute chest syndrome in sickle cell disease: CT evidence of microvascular occlusion. *Radiology* 1993;187:45–49.
2. Castro O, Brambilla DJ, Thorington B, Reindorf CA, Scott RB, Gillette P, Vera JC, Levy PS, et al. The acute chest syndrome in sickle cell disease: Incidence and risk factors. *Blood* 1994;84: 643–649.
3. Emre U, Miller ST, Gutierez M, Steiner P, Rao SP, Rao M. Effect of transfusion in acute chest syndrome of sickle cell disease. *J Pediatr* 1995;127:901–904.
4. Martin L, Buonomo C. Acute chest syndrome of sickle cell disease: radiographic and clinical analysis of 70 cases. *Pediatr Radiol* 1997;27: 637–641.

Dehydration, Acidosis, Overaeration, and Microcardia

Dehydration with acidosis commonly reflects itself on the chest roentgenograms of young infants. In such cases, the findings result from dehydration secondary to vomiting or diarrhea, and the patient's lungs appear overaerated and undervascularized (Fig. 1.151). In addition, the cardiac silhouette often is small, and the findings frequently are confused with those of bronchiolitis. Decreased vascularity and smallness of the cardiac silhouette (microcardia) result from hypovolemia; overaeration results from the metabolic acidosis present. These infants attempt to blow off carbon dioxide and, in so doing, overaerate. Microcardia, with overdistended lungs, also can be seen with acute, large-volume blood loss, and with more severe asthmatic attacks. In the latter instance, the overdistended lungs depress the diaphragmatic leaflets, and this causes the heart to be stretched. In addition, the heart is compressed by the emphysematous lungs.

Other causes of microcardia include Addison's disease, anorexia nervosa, and, of course, a normal long thin heart in an asthenic individual (usually a young female patient). Microcardia secondary to cardiac atrophy, with actual loss of muscle bulk (protein), as a result of longstanding debilitating disease (malignancy, malnutrition, severe burns, chronic infection, and so forth) is a less common cause of a small cardiac silhouette (1).

REFERENCE

1. Swischuk LE. Microcardia: an uncommon diagnostic problem. *J Radiol* 1968;103:115–118.

Pulmonary Hemorrhage

Pulmonary hemorrhage, of course, is common with pulmonary contusions sustained with blunt or penetrating chest trauma. On a nontraumatic basis it can occur with idiopathic pulmonary hemosiderosis and Henoch–Schönlein purpura (2). In either case, the roentgenographic findings consist of diffuse opacification of the lungs. Another cause of focal pulmonary hemorrhage is rupture of a mycotic aneurysm secondary to pulmonary infection (1). This is a rare cause of focal pulmonary hemorrhage, but the aneurysms can be demonstrated with ordinary or digital arteriography (1).

REFERENCES

1. Moorthy C, Walser E, John SD, Angel C, Swischuk LE. Rupture of a solitary, erosive peripheral pulmonary artery aneurysm. *Emerg Radiol* 1996;3:253–257.
2. Olson JC, Kelly KJ, Pan CG, Wortmann DW. Pulmonary disease with hemorrhage in Henoch-Schoenlein Purpura. *Pediatrics* 1992; 89:1177–1181.

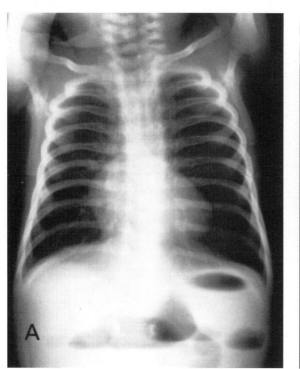
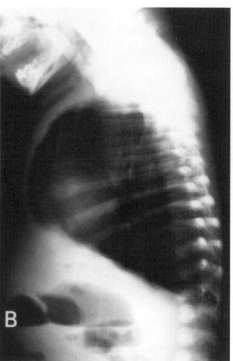

FIGURE 1.151. *Dehydration and overaeration.* **(A)** Note the overdistended hyperlucent appearance of the lungs in this infant with severe gastroenteritis, diarrhea, and dehydration. The vascularity is diminished and the heart somewhat small in size. Air–fluid levels scattered throughout the abdomen indicate the presence of gastroenteritis. In other cases, the cardiac silhouette is even smaller than in this infant. **(B)** Lateral view showing emphysematous appearance of the lungs, not unlike that seen with bronchiolitis.

Hypoplastic–Agenetic Lung

Lung hypoplasia and agenesis of a lung generally are asymptomatic problems (1,2), unless they declare themselves in the neonatal period. Hypoplasia of the lung results in a small, hyperlucent lung with diminished pulmonary blood-flow, for the pulmonary artery also is hypoplastic (Fig. 1.152A). The small, hyperlucent lung ventilates normally;

that is, there is normal decrease in size with expiration, and therefore such lungs are not predisposed to infection. Pulmonary angiography, pulmonary perfusion and ventilation scintigraphy studies, and even CT scans have been utilized in the evaluation of these patients, but all of these studies are superfluous, because they lend nothing more to the information obtained from the plain films. Simply speak-

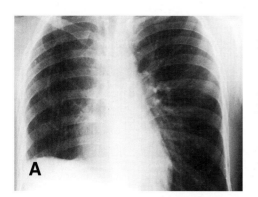
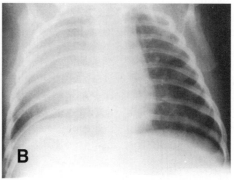
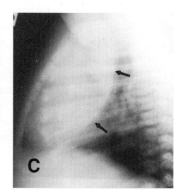

FIGURE 1.152. *Hypoplastic lung.* **(A)** Note that the right lung is smaller than the left. In addition, note that vascularity is diminished on the right and a little increased on the left. **(B)** Infant with agenesis of the right upper and middle lobes. Only the right lower lobe shows aeration. Mediastinal shift is to the right. **(C)** Lateral view demonstrates the typical retrosternal density of the agenetic right upper and middle lobes (*arrows*).

ing, these patients have a small lung that has decreased pulmonary bloodflow, and thus the lung appears small and hyperlucent. Ventilatory excursion is relatively normal, but because of the decreased pulmonary bloodflow the lung is basically less efficient in terms of gas exchange. Only severe cases require workup.

If the entire lung is agenetic, the problem usually declares itself in the neonatal period. In such cases, the involved hemithorax is small and completely opaque, and there is marked shift of the mediastinum to the ipsilateral side. Concomitantly, there is overdistension (compensatory emphysema) of the other lung, and because the agenetic lung cannot receive blood from the right ventricle, all of the blood is diverted to the normal lung and vascularity in the normal lung appears increased. A more difficult problem arises if only one or two lobes are agenetic. Most often, this occurs on the right, which has been termed the "hypogenetic right-lung syndrome" (3). The lobes involved usually are the upper and middle lobes, and they lead to decreased volume of the hemithorax. At the same time, there is increased density of the involved hemithorax and a very confusing picture results, which often is misinterpreted as pneumonia (Fig. 1.152B). The key deterrent to this misinterpretation should be the fact that these patients demonstrate significant volume loss (Fig. 1.152C and D) and, as has been reiterated many times, consolidating pneumonias generally are not associated with any significant volume loss.

REFERENCES

1. Cremin BJ, Bass EM. Retrosternal density: A sign of pulmonary hypoplasia. *Pediatr Radiol* 1975;3:145–147.
2. Currarino G, Williams B. Causes of congenital unilateral pulmonary hypoplasia: A study of 33 cases. *Pediatr Radiol* 1985;15:15–24.
3. Felson B. Pulmonary agenesis and related anomalies. *Semin Roentgenol* 1972;7:17–30.

Hemoptysis in Childhood

Hemoptysis in childhood is not as common as in the adult, but it can occur with hemangiomas in the hypopharynx or upper airway, bacterial pneumonias, other acute and chronic pulmonary infections (5), cystic fibrosis (5), bronchial adenomas (6), and intrathoracic gastroenteric cysts (1,2). Pulmonary infections and foreign bodies, however, have been shown to account for approximately half of the cases (5).

With gastroenteric cysts, pulmonary changes may range from discrete cystic masses to nonspecific, consolidative-like lesions. If ulceration of the cysts leads to perforation, blood and free air also are seen in the thoracic cavity (2). With bronchial adenoma, the findings vary from a solitary pulmonary nodule to focal atelectasis or emphysema caused by airway obstruction by the nodule. In children, however, bronchial adenomas are rare.

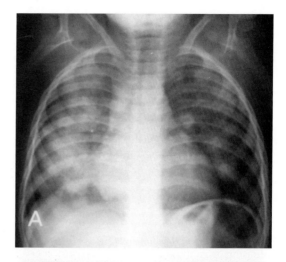

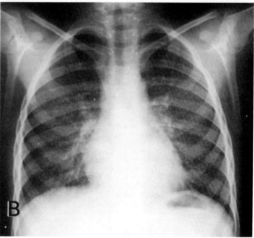

FIGURE 1.153. *Pulmonary hemosiderosis: varying configurations.* **(A)** Fluffy, asymmetric infiltrates, resembling widespread pneumonia or even pulmonary edema. **(B)** Another child showing diffuse miliary infiltrates not unlike those seen with miliary tuberculosis.

Pulmonary hemosiderosis also is a cause of hemoptysis in childhood (3,4), and in that case the condition is associated with iron-deficiency anemia, variable respiratory distress, oxygen-diffusion difficulties, and a wide variety of roentgenographic findings. In acute cases, parenchymal bleeding leads to fluffy, bilateral parenchymal infiltrates (Fig. 1.153A), but with repeated bleeding, chronic fibrosis ensues and pulmonary changes may consist of hazy lungs or lungs with miliary-like reticulonodularity (Fig. 1.153B). In any given patient the findings may be different, but chronic, progressive fibrosis eventually ensues (3,4).

REFERENCES

1. Chang SH, Morrison L, Shaffner L, Crowe JE. Intrathoracic gastrogenic cysts and hemoptysis. *J Pediatr* 1976;88:594–596.
2. Macpherson RI, Reed MH, Ferguson CC. Intrathoracic gastro-

genic cysts: Cause of lethal pulmonary hemorrhage in infants. *Can J Assoc Radiol* 1973;24:362–369.

3. Matsaniotis N, Karpouzas J, Apostolopoulou E, Messaritakis J. Idiopathic pulmonary hemosiderosis in children. *Arch Dis Child* 1968;43:307–309.
4. Repetto G, Lisboa CM, Emparanza E, Ferretti R, Neira N, Etchart M, Maneghello J. Idiopathic pulmonary hemosiderosis. *Pediatrics* 1967;40:24–32.
5. Tom LWC, Weisman RA, Handler SD. Hemoptysis in children. *Ann Otol Rhinol Laryngol* 1980;89:419–424.
6. Wellons HA, Eggleston P, Golden GT, Allen M. Bronchial adenoma in childhood. *Am J Dis Child* 1976;130:301–304.

Anterior Chest Pain

Anterior chest pain is a common complaint of children, but most often it is musculoskeletal and frequently secondary to overexercising or viral infections. In this regard, it can result from Tietze's syndrome, a costochondritis of the upper costochondral junctions of presumed viral origin. In other cases, it may be pleuritic, but anterior chest pain in children seldom is caused by heart disease (1,3). Chest pain also can be seen after exercise in patients with so-called exercised-induced asthma (2).

REFERENCES

1. Driscoll DJ, Glicklich LB, Galen WJ. Chest pain in children: A prospective study. *Pediatrics* 1976;57:648–651.

2. Wiens L, Sabath R, Ewing L, Gowdamarajan R, Portnoy R, Scagliotti J. Chest pain in otherwise healthy children and adolescents is frequently caused by exercise-induced asthma. *Pediatrics* 1992;90:350–353.
3. Zavaras-Angelidou KA, Weinhouse E, Nelson DB. Review of 180 episodes of chest pain in 134 children. *Pediatr Emerg Care* 1992;8:819.

Rapidly Expanding Chest Masses and Cysts

A complete discussion of pulmonary and mediastinal masses is beyond the scope of this book and not particularly relevant to its theme of emergency medicine. Only one or two points need be made regarding a child who might present with a chest mass in the emergency room. Such children can present with chest pain, respiratory distress, wheezing, or asthma-like symptoms (1). The more common masses include mediastinal lymphoma and thymus glands infiltrated with leukemic cells. These have similar appearances, and the roentgenographic findings are quite characteristic (Fig. 1.154A). Other tumors also can be encountered and pulmonary cysts that become infected also can compress the airway and cause respiratory distress (Fig. 1.154B and C). Tumors can expand rapidly because of rampant malignant growth or hemorrhage, while pulmonary cysts usually become larger because of supervening infection, or occasionally, hemorrhage.

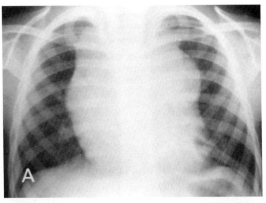

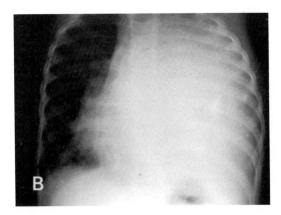

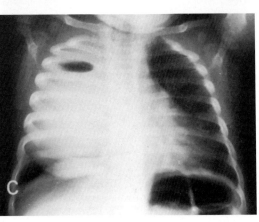

FIGURE 1.154. *Rapidly expanding masses and cysts.* **(A)** Note the large mediastinal mass in this child presenting with a 4-day history of wheezing and respiratory distress, suggesting a pulmonary infection. The mass was a biopsy-proven lymphoma. **(B)** This child also presented with asthma-like symptoms. Note the large mass with calcification in the left chest. It was a teratoma. **(C)** Infant presenting with respiratory distress. Note the large infected bronchogenic cyst in the right chest. It is compressing the trachea and right bronchus.

REFERENCE

1. Swischuk LE. Acute respiratory distress in the infant. *Radiol Clin North Am* 1977;16:77–90.

NORMAL FINDINGS CAUSING PROBLEMS

Technically Poor Examination

The fallacy of assessing a chest roentgenogram obtained during expiration is well known and cannot be overstressed. On the expiratory film, the normal lungs and heart may erroneously appear totally abnormal (Fig. 1.155), and it is only after proper inspiration is accomplished that this is appreciated. Rotation of the chest to one side or the other causes obvious problems, and lordotic position can throw the heart and pulmonary vessel into such projection that abnormality is suggested. Lordotic positioning tends to accentuate the hilar regions and upper-lobe vascularity and cause the heart to assume a right-ventricular hypertrophy configuration.

Normal Thymus Gland

The normal thymus gland is notorious for mimicking pathology. Ordinarily it covers the superior aspect of the heart like an umbrella and blends imperceptibly with the cardiac silhouette (Fig. 1.156A). Subtle notches may delineate its inferior extent, and on lateral view it occupies the

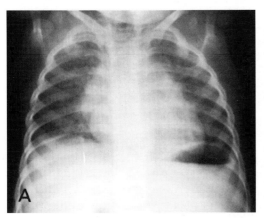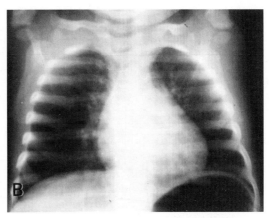

FIGURE 1.155. *Technically poor films.* **(A)** Expiratory view causes the lungs to appear infiltrated and the heart enlarged. The thymus gland drapes the superior cardiac silhouette and on the right might suggest hilar adenopathy or a mediastinal mass. **(B)** Same infant with deeper inspiration but lordotic positioning. Lordotic positioning is manifested by horizontal positioning of the posterior ribs, downward-pointing anterior ribs, and accentuation of the vascular markings in the upper lobes. This infant was normal.

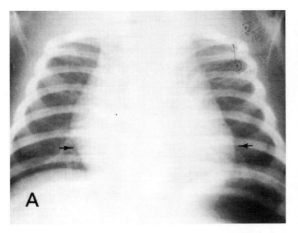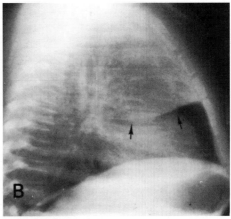

FIGURE 1.156. *Normal thymus.* **(A)** The normal thymic silhouette blends with the cardiac silhouette. Faint notches are seen at the junctions of the thymic lobes and heart (*arrows*). The great vessels are difficult to define. **(B)** Lateral view showing the normal position of the thymus gland, and its undulating lower edge (*arrows*). (From Swischuk LE: *Radiology of the newborn and young infant.* Baltimore: Williams and Wilkins, 1997, with permission.)

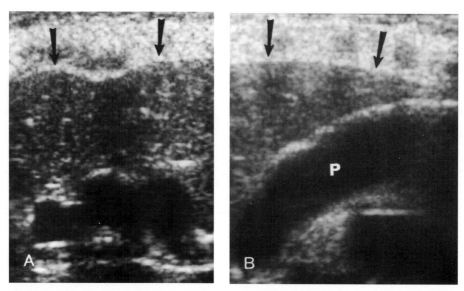

FIGURE 1.157. *Normal thymus: ultrasonographic findings.* **(A)** Axial view demonstrates characteristic thymic texture of this large but normal thymus gland (*arrows*) in an infant with a cardiac murmur. Note the great vessels behind the thymus. **(B)** Midsagittal view demonstrates the characteristic sail-like configuration of the normal thymus gland (*arrows*). It lies just over the pulmonary artery (*P*).

anterior superior mediastinal compartment and is delineated by a straight or undulating line along its inferior border (Fig. 1.156B). In other cases, the thymus (right lobe especially) may be very large and erroneously suggest a mediastinal or cardiac mass (see Fig. 1.158). An important feature of the normal thymus gland is that no matter how large it is, it does not displace the trachea. The normal thymus gland now also is readily studied with ultrasound, CT, or magnetic resonance imaging (Fig. 1.157).

In some cases, the thymus gland is triangular in shape, producing the so-called sail sign (Fig. 1.158A). If rotation is present in these patients, the sail-like lobe of the thymus may be thrown into such projection that a consolidating upper-lobe pneumonia is suggested (Fig. 1.158B). In older children, residual normal thymus also erroneously may suggest a mediastinal mass (Figs. 1.159 and 1.160). In such cases one should remain practical and calm and ask oneself the question, "Why was this child examined?" If the answer

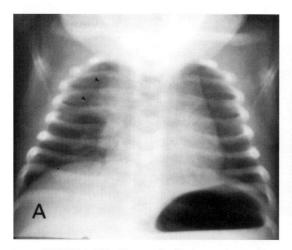
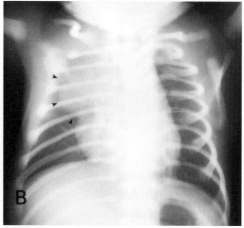

FIGURE 1.158. *Thymus "sail" sign and pseudopneumonia.* **(A)** Typical sail sign of normal thymus (*arrows*). **(B)** Rotation to the right in this infant causes the normal thymus to appear as though it were a consolidating pneumonia of the right upper lobe (*arrows*).

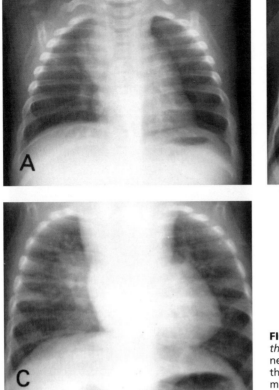

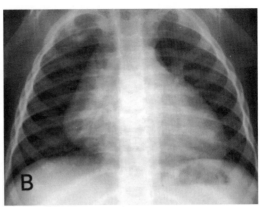

FIGURE 1.159. *Masslike configuration of normal thymus gland.* (**A**) Bilateral superior mediastinal fullness caused by normal thymus gland. (**B**) Large right thymic lobe suggesting a mass. (**C**) Peculiar superior medial widening, secondary to incomplete descent of normal thymus gland and lordotic positioning.

is because of possible pneumonia, chest cold, routine chest, preoperative chest, or so forth, one should ask oneself the next question: "***Could I be dealing with normal thymus?***" Certainly a normal thymus is the most likely possibility, and thereafter a repeat chest film in 30 days would be in order. A mass resulting from a lymphoma would not remain the

same size; normal thymus almost invariably would remain the same in size and configuration. Taking a little time to assess the findings may be more productive than going on to CT or magnetic resonance imaging. The reason for this is that very often even on these studies the thymus gland has a peculiar configuration and the problem is not solved. In

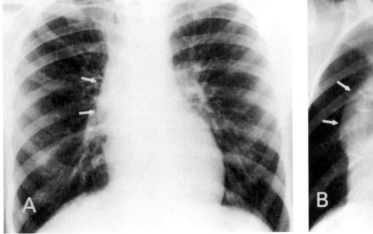

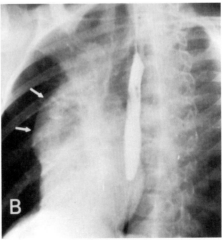

FIGURE 1.160. *Large thymus: older child.* (**A**) This 10-year-old child was examined for a possible pneumonia. Incidentally, note what was at first interpreted to be a superior mediastinal mass (*arrows*). (**B**) Oblique view with barium demonstrates the same mass (*arrows*). It was normal thymus gland.

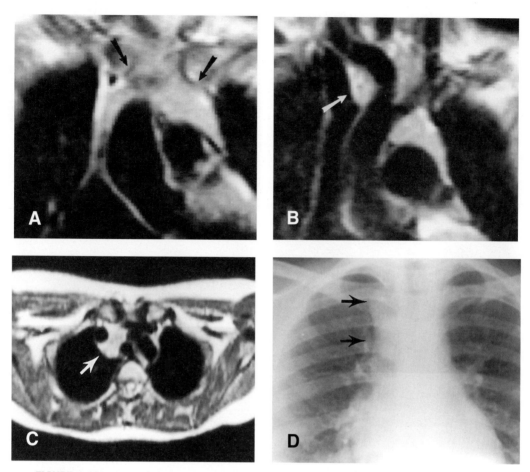

FIGURE 1.161. *Normal thymus extending between innominate artery and superior vena cava.* **(A)** Note normal thymus gland (*arrows*). **(B)** A portion of the thymus gland (*arrow*) is seen to extend between the superior vena cava and innominate artery. **(C)** On axial view, the same extension is seen (*arrow*). **(D)** Plain films demonstrate right side mediastinal widening (*arrows*). (From Swischuk LE, and John SD: Normal thymus extending between the right brachiocephalic vein and the innominate artery. *AJR* 1996;166:1462–1464).

this regard, even CT scanning can lead to difficulties. The reason for this is that CT scanning now commonly demonstrates normal extension of the thymus gland between the right bracheocephalic vein and innominate artery (1). This finding should not be misinterpreted as a mediastinal mass (Fig. 1.161).

Normal thymus most commonly is seen in patients younger than the age of 2 years, but it can be seen in older children. Indeed, one can see normal thymus in children even up to the age of 10 to 14 years, not routinely, but not so uncommonly that the possibility should be discounted completely.

REFERENCE

1. Swischuk LE, John SD. Case report: Normal thymus extending between the right brachiocephalic vein and innominate artery. *AJR* 1996;166:1462–1464.

2

UPPER AIRWAY, NASAL PASSAGES, SINUSES, AND MASTOIDS

NORMAL ANATOMY OF UPPER AIRWAY

One must be thoroughly familiar with the normal anatomy of the upper airway before attempting to identify pathology. Fortunately, this is not too difficult a task, for air in the airway provides one with an ideal contrast agent. However, unless a proper roentgenogram is obtained, pathologic determination is seriously compromised. The upper-airway roentgenogram must be obtained during inspiration, with the patient in true lateral position and, preferably, the neck extended (Fig. 2.1). This, of course, requires some degree of technical expertise, but if the study is obtained during expiration, or with forward flexion of the neck, an endless number of peculiar, misleading, or virtually noninterpretable configurations of the buckled upper airway result (Fig. 2.2). This also results in problems with the retropharyngeal soft tissues, which erroneously may appear pathologically thickened. Frontal views of the upper airway also are helpful, but they do not provide as much information as do lateral views.

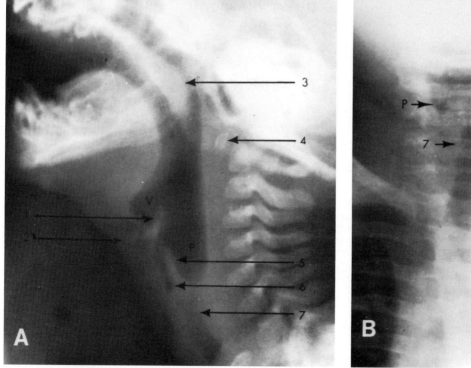
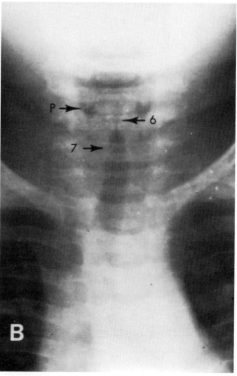

FIGURE 2.1. (A and B) *Normal upper airway.* Note the following structures: epiglottis (*1*), body of the hyoid bone (*2*), uvula (*3*), anterior arch of C1 (*4*), aryepiglottic folds (*5*), ventricle of glottis (*6*), subglottic portion of trachea (*7*), vallecula (*V*), and piriform fossa (*P*).

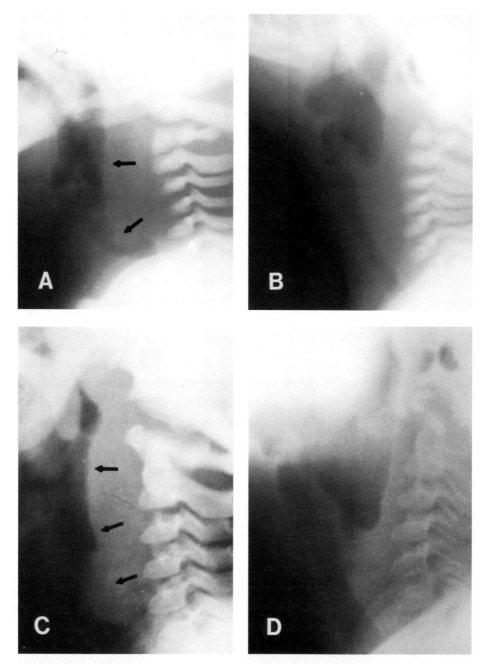

FIGURE 2.2. *Technically poor film with pseudomass configuration.* **(A)** This patient was examined with the neck flexed forward and the airway incompletely distended. A retropharyngeal mass (*arrows*) is suggested. **(B)** With proper positioning, however, note that no mass is present, and the stepoff between the hypopharynx and subglottic trachea is preserved. **(C)** Another patient showing what would appear to be a lumpy retropharyngeal mass (*arrows*). Lumpiness favors normal tissue. **(D)** Properly obtained film with full distension of the airway shows no mass.

In terms of normal retropharyngeal soft tissues, there is a normal increase in thickness at the level of the larynx, producing a stepoff of the posterior wall of the airway. In other words, the fully distended hypopharynx extends further posteriorly than does the subglottic trachea (Fig. 2.2B and D). With true retropharyngeal soft-tissue thickening this stepoff usually is obliterated and the airway displaced anteriorly in a smoothly curving fashion (see Fig. 2.20). This usually does not occur with normal buckling, for even though gross distortions occur (Fig. 2.2A), the stepoff, on full inspiration, is preserved (Fig. 2.2B). In these cases, part of the problem is that normal lymphoid tissue may extend into the retropharynx and cause the normal soft tissues to appear disturbingly thick and lumpy (see Fig. 2.21). In those younger than 3 months of age, however, adenoidal tissue is normally quite sparse (1).

REFERENCE

1. Capitanio MA, Kirkpatrick JA. Nasopharyngeal lymphoid tissue: Roentgen observations in 257 children two years of age or less. *Radiology* 1970;96:389–391.

UPPER-AIRWAY OBSTRUCTION AND ACUTE STRIDOR

Stridor is descriptive of noisy breathing and usually infers the presence of a lesion in the upper airway. However, before one embarks on an imaging workup of patients with stridor, the clinical features should be reviewed to determine whether the stridor is inspiratory or expiratory, associated with wheezing, associated with voice alterations, or associated with dysphagia (Fig. 2.3).

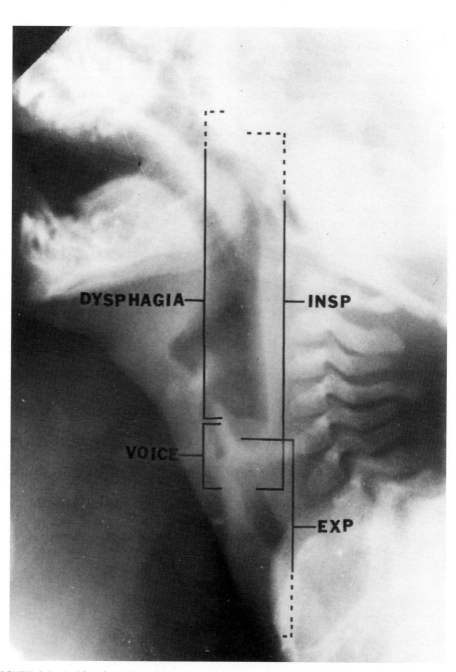

FIGURE 2.3. *Stridor: location of lesion according to symptoms.* Note zones of predominantly inspiratory or expiratory stridor and the area of overlap. Also note the area for dysphagia and voice problems.

If it is inspiratory, or both inspiratory and expiratory, chances are that the lesion is in the glottic or paraglottic region; if it is purely expiratory, however, the lesion probably exists below the glottis, often in the chest. In the latter cases, expiratory wheezing also is present and may predominate. Alterations in voice or cry associated with stridor almost always place the lesion in the glottis; dysphagia with stridor usually is seen with lesions in the hypopharynx (e.g., epiglottitis, retropharyngeal abscess, hypopharyngeal tumors or cysts). Dysphagia also can be seen with problems in the chest (e.g., vascular rings or mediastinal masses or cysts).

After one's clinical assessment of the patient with stridor, the next investigative procedure should be a lateral roentgenogram of the upper airway, and not endoscopy. With a proper lateral neck roentgenogram, hardly a lesion goes undetected, and if a chest film and an occasional barium swallow study also are obtained, virtually nothing should escape detection (10).

Epiglottitis

Epiglottitis usually affects older children, with the peak incidence occurring between 3 and 6 years of age. It usually presents abruptly with variable inspiratory stridor and dysphagia, and most often is caused by *Haemophilus influenzae* infection. However, viral epiglottitis also can occur (7), and at the same time, now that vaccine programs are in effect for *H. influenzae* infection, epiglottitis secondary to this organism is becoming less common. Other causes of epiglottitis include thermal injury resulting from ingestion of hot fluids (8,14), angioneurotic edema (9), and chronic infection with Monilia organisms, especially in HIV patients (1).

Dysphagia in epiglottitis is secondary to the marked degree of supraglottic inflammation and edema present, and clinically the cherry red epiglottis is classic. However, most physicians still are cautious regarding examination of the oropharynx in these patients, because of the possibility of inducing glottic spasm. For this reason, the roentgenogram has become a more popular method of diagnosing epiglottitis, and indeed this relatively innocuous study can clearly demonstrate its presence (6,11). However, it should be stressed that these patients should not be sent to the roentgenographic examination room unattended, for the possibility of acute airway obstruction is always present, and it can be precipitated by neck extension necessary for the roentgenographic study.

In the classic case of epiglottitis, on lateral view, the roentgenographic findings of epiglottitis are typical and consist of thickening and edema of the aryepiglottic folds and epiglottis (Fig. 2.4A). In advanced cases, the swollen epiglottis looks like an upward-pointing thumb, and hence reference is made to the "thumb" sign. With more extensive disease, a supraglottic mass may be suggested (Fig. 2.4C). Mild to moderate hypopharyngeal overdis-

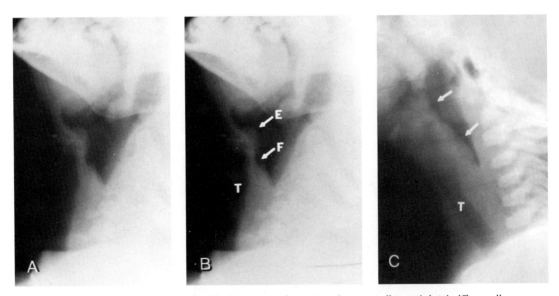

FIGURE 2.4. *Epiglottitis.* **(A and B)** Classic case demonstrating a swollen epiglottis (*E*), swollen aryepiglottic folds (*F*) and no narrowing of the subglottic trachea (*T*). There is moderate hypopharyngeal overdistension. The configuration of the epiglottis constitutes the so-called thumb sign. Evaluation of the aryepiglottic folds should be made at their midpoint, or just behind the epiglottis, and not at their base, where they normally appear thick (11). **(C)** A more pronounced case has resulted in the epiglottis and aryepiglottic folds fusing so as to present as a large supraglottic mass (*arrows*). Note that the subglottic portion of the trachea (*T*) is of normal diameter.

tension also occurs, but seldom is it as marked as in croup. In addition, as opposed to croup, the subglottic portion of the trachea appears normal, on lateral view. On frontal view, however, some cases of epiglottitis demonstrate subglottic edema and a funnel-shaped glottic area indistinguishable from that seen in croup (Fig. 2.5). In these cases, although the primary problem still is supraglottic and glottic edema, enough edema extends into the subglottic portion of the trachea to produce the funnel deformity (17).

It is most important to note that the aryepiglottic folds in epiglottitis are thickened, for with croup and other causes of stridor the aryepiglottic folds are thin and normal (11). However, one must evaluate fold thickening at the proper level. In this regard, it has been noted that the folds should be evaluated at their midpoint, or just behind the epiglottis, and not at their base (11). At the base, as they drape over the arytenoid cartilage, they normally are thick, and the overlap with abnormal thickening is too great to be of value. This does not occur at the other two levels (11).

In addition, in epiglottis, it is important to note whether the posterior wall of the midportion of the epiglottis is still visible. In most cases of epiglottitis, because the epiglottis swells, the posterior wall becomes invisible (Fig. 2.4).

Unfortunately, in mild cases of epiglottitis the posterior wall of the epiglottis still may be visible and the aryepiglottic folds only minimally thickened (Fig. 2.6). This, however, is the exception more than the rule, for in most cases of epiglottitis the posterior wall of the body of the epiglottis is obliterated (11). All of these points are important in the evaluation of these patients, and if one is not certain of the findings, then a repeat examination should be done. Finally, clinical correlation with endoscopy, if deemed necessary, should follow.

It is also important not to misinterpret the normal, so-called omega epiglottis as a thickened epiglottitis. In these patients, stridor may result from croup or some other cause, but the epiglottis may appear a little thickened. This impression is erroneous, for it is merely a floppy epiglottis with prominent downward-curving lateral flaps (10). This results in an inverted U– or omega-shaped epiglottis that appears thickened on lateral view (Fig. 2.7). However, in these cases no thickening of the aryepiglottic folds is seen, and this should strongly rule against epiglottitis (10). *If one is not able to make this distinction on a lateral neck roentgenogram, it usually is because the inspiratory effort is not deep enough, and thus the study should be repeated. One must be absolutely sure about the diagnosis of epiglottitis.*

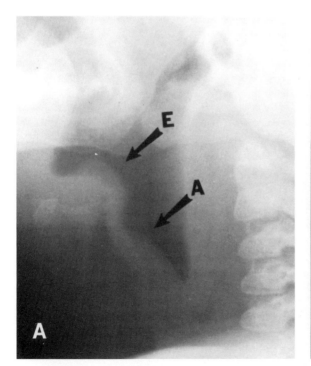
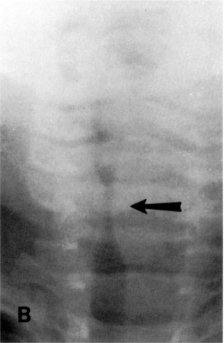

FIGURE 2.5. *Epiglottitis with subglottic edema.* **(A)** Note typical findings of epiglottitis on lateral view. Note, however, that the subglottic portion of the trachea is of normal diameter. The epiglottis (*E*) and aryepiglottic folds (*A*) are thickened. **(B)** Frontal view shows a funnel-shaped glottic and subglottic region (*arrow*) resulting from glottic edema. The findings, on this view, mimic those of croup.

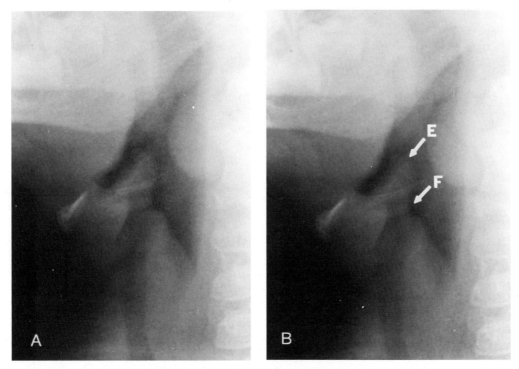

FIGURE 2.6. *Mild epiglottitis; evaluation of aryepiglottic folds.* (**A** and **B**) In this patient note that the epiglottis (*E*) is swollen. The posterior wall of the midportion of the epiglottis is barely visible. The aryepiglottic folds (*F*) themselves are indistinct but mildly thickened.

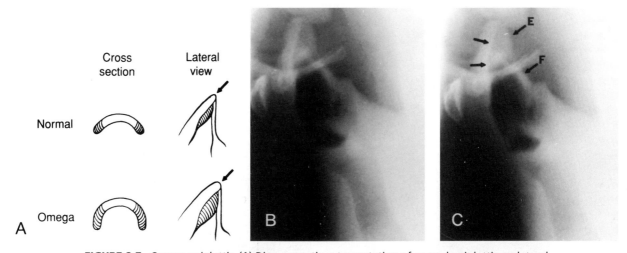

FIGURE 2.7. *Omega epiglottis.* (**A**) Diagrammatic representation of normal epiglottis on lateral view. Note that the normal epiglottis (*arrows*) is thin and the lateral walls (*shaded area*) are not prominent. With an omega epiglottis, the lateral walls (*shaded areas*) are more prominent and on lateral view can cause the epiglottis to appear thickened. (From John SD, Swischuk LE. Stridor and upper airway obstruction in infants and children. *RadioGraphics* 1992;12:625–643, with permission.) (**B** and **C**) Note pseudothickening of the epiglottis (*E*) resulting from an omega epiglottis. The aryepiglottic folds (*F*) are normal. However, also note that the posterior wall (*arrows*) of the body of the epiglottis still is clearly visible. This usually does not occur with epiglotittis.

Croup

Most cases of croup are of viral origin (10), but bacterial croup, often severe and refractory, can occur. It is referred to by terms such as ***membranous croup, pseudomembranous croup, membranous tracheitis, bacterial croup,*** or ***refrac-*** ***tory croup*** (15). In these cases, symptoms often are more severe, subglottic narrowing more pronounced, and response to usual treatment refractory. Indeed, intubation often is required. Organisms responsible include *Staphylococcus aureus, H. influenzae,* and occasionally anaerobic bacteria (2). Croup also has been demonstrated to be more common in allergic children (19), and this also has been our experience. Indeed, in older children, croup can occur on a purely allergic basis. In these cases, it is not associated with any type of infection at all and can be very abrupt and severe in onset.

Classically, in croup, stridor primarily is inspiratory, and the entire picture, including the barking cough, is rather typical. Characteristically, the disease is one of infants and young children, with the peak age incidence being between 6 months and 3 years. Many of these children also have a full-blown viral lower respiratory tract infection, and in the evening croup develops. Overall, the clinical findings are so typical that there is question as to why roentgenograms should be obtained in these children. Nonetheless, the study seems to be quite popular, mostly because it easily can differentiate croup from epiglottitis (5,6,10,16).

Roentgenographically, with croup, there is marked hypopharyngeal overdistension during inspiration, but the epiglottis and aryepiglottic folds are normal. The vocal cords, however, usually appear thickened and fuzzy, and the subglottic portion of the trachea narrowed (Fig. 2.8A). This narrowing is primarily paradoxic and represents tracheal collapse secondary to negative intraluminal pressures that develop in this area during inspiration (16). This is a non-specific response that occurs with any glottic obstruction,

but in childhood it is seen most commonly with croup and is an important feature of this condition (Fig. 2.9). On expiration, it should be noted that such narrowing is not as fixed as it first appears (Fig. 2.8B). Indeed, it usually diminishes or completely disappears, further attesting to the fact that in typical viral, or spasmodic, allergic croup, such narrowing is not caused by fixed edematous, subglottic tracheal narrowing. In more severe cases, however, and these usually are cases of bacterial croup, inflammation may extend into the subglottic trachea and render the narrowing more pronounced and persistent. Indeed, it may not completely disappear on expiration. In addition, actual membranes in the trachea may be seen in some of these cases (Fig. 2.10).

On frontal view, in croup, the vocal cords appear thickened and funnel-like in configuration (Fig. 2.11A). They appear this way because they are edematous and in spasm. Normally, on inspiration, the vocal cords should fall away and reveal a wide open airway (Fig. 2.11B); with crying or forced expiration (e.g., Valsalva's maneuver), the inferior aspect of the vocal cord should appear shoulderlike or squared-off (Fig. 2.11C). With croup, there is little change in the appearance of the cords between inspiration and expiration, and thus the funnel-shaped configuration or "steeple" sign is almost always present and, interestingly enough, often seen on frontal chest roentgenograms.

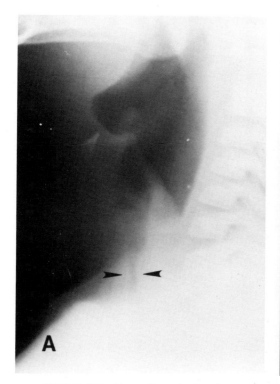
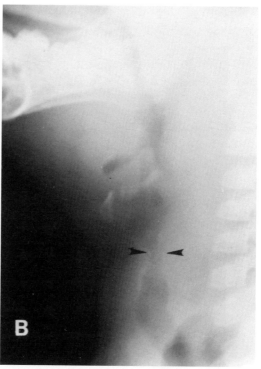

FIGURE 2.8. *Croup: lateral view.* (A) Typical findings include marked overdistension of the hypopharynx and paradoxical narrowing of the subglottic portion of the trachea (*arrows*). The epiglottis and aryepiglottic folds are normal. (B) Expiratory film demonstrating that the subglottic narrowing is not fixed, for on this view the subglottic area appears much wider (*arrows*). In most cases, the narrowing disappears entirely. Also note overdistension of the subglottic trachea.

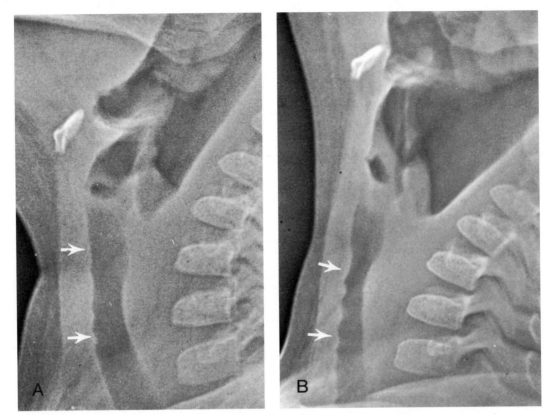

FIGURE 2.9. *Croup: paradoxical subglottic tracheal narrowing.* (**A**) Moderate inspiration. Note that the diameter of the subglottic trachea (*arrows*) is normal. (**B**) With deep inspiration, the hypopharynx shows gross overdistension and the subglottic portion of the trachea (*arrows*) now shows paradoxical narrowing. Also note that with marked overdistension of the hypopharynx the aryepiglottic folds appear thin and normal but with the lesser degree of hypopharyngeal distension noted in A the folds erroneously appear thickened. This study is a xeroradiogram, which is not currently used or advised. However, it does demonstrate the tracheal dynamics to greater advantage. (From John SD, Swischuk LE. Stridor and upper airway obstruction in infants and children. *RadioGraphics* 1992;12:625–643, with permission.)

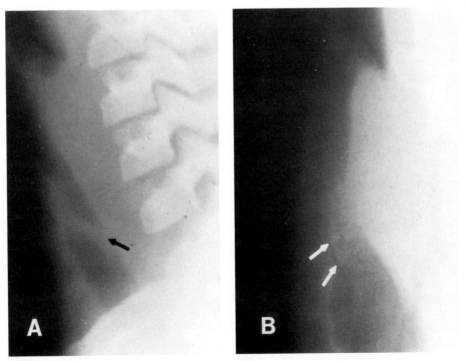

FIGURE 2.10. *Membranous croup or bacterial tracheitis.* (**A**) Note the membrane (*arrow*) in the trachea of this patient with severe respiratory stridor. (Courtesy of Robin Gaup, MD.) (**B**) Another patient with severe stenosis of the trachea (*arrows*) and an indistinct, subglottic membrane.

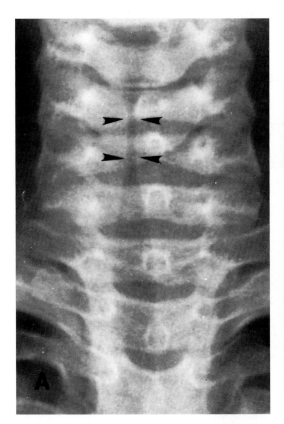

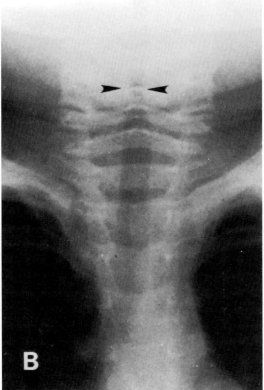

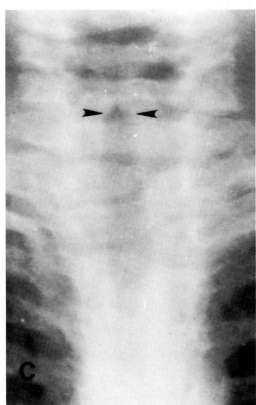

FIGURE 2.11. *Croup: frontal view.* **(A)** Typical funnel-shaped glottic and subglottic narrowing in infant with croup (*arrows*). Edema and spasm of the glottis and, to a lesser extent, edema of the subglottic portion of the trachea lead to this typical funnel-shaped upper-airway narrowing. **(B)** In a normal child, inspiratory film for comparative purposes, showing how normal vocal cords open during inspiration to leave a wide airway (*arrows*). **(C)** In a normal child, expiratory film (forced Valsalva's maneuver) for comparative purposes, showing the normal right-angle configuration of the inferior aspect of the closed vocal cords (*arrows*).

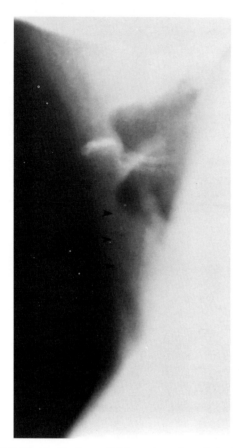

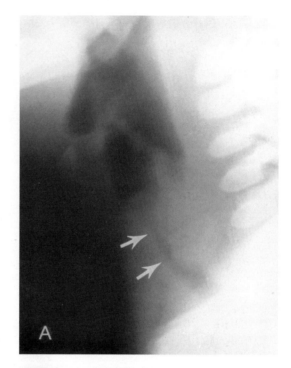

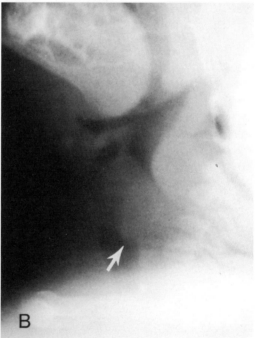

FIGURE 2.12. *Croup: fuzzy, thickened vocal cords.* Lateral view showing moderate hypopharyngeal overdistension and a normal epiglottis and aryepiglottic folds. However, the region of the vocal cords is fuzzy and thickened (*arrows*). This configuration is just as typical for croup as is the one demonstrated in Fig. 2.8, and if the inspiratory effort were deeper, one would be able to see paradoxical collapse of the subglottic trachea.

Unfortunately, not all children display as classic a picture of croup as that outlined here, for if obstruction is less marked, and/or the inspiratory effort not as deep, less hypopharyngeal overdistension and paradoxical subglottic tracheal narrowing occur. In these patients, the only finding may be thickening or fuzziness of the vocal cords (Fig. 2.12). However, this configuration is just as suggestive of croup as is the classic one illustrated in Fig. 2.8. In such instances, with a deeper inspiratory effort the findings become more classic. To be sure, the degree of roentgenographic abnormality in croup is more dependent on the degree of inspiration than on the severity of disease. In severe cases, steroid therapy can be utilized (4).

There are one or two other lesions that might present with crouplike symptoms and initially might be misdiagnosed as croup. These include congenital subglottic stenosis (6) and subglottic hemangioma. In congenital subglottic stenosis, the findings are remarkably similar to those of croup, for there is hypopharyngeal overdistension and narrowing of the subglottic portion of the trachea (Fig. 2.13A).

FIGURE 2.13. *Subglottic stenosis.* **(A)** Note narrowing of the subglottic portion of the trachea (*arrows*). On expiration, such narrowing does not disappear. **(B)** *Subglottic hemangioma.* Note the characteristic posterior location of the subglottic hemangioma (*arrow*). In other cases, the mass may come off the lateral wall of the subglottic portion of the trachea.

However, compared to most cases of croup, the degree of narrowing does not diminish during expiration, for it is truly fixed and stenotic. With subglottic hemangioma, the characteristic finding is an eccentric posterior or lateral mass projecting into the subglottic portion of the trachea (Fig. 2.13B). These tumors most often are posterior or lateral but occasionally can be anterior. Hemangiomas may be present elsewhere in the body or on the skin and, under such circumstances, make the diagnosis even more binding. Both congenital subglottic stenosis and subglottic hemangioma are mentioned at this point because, during episodes of viral respiratory tract infection, they may become more symptomatic and lead to a clinical picture suggestive of acute croup.

Another lesion that may mimic the roentgenographic findings of croup is a laryngeal web; this is the one lesion that is almost impossible to demonstrate roentgenographically. Generally the findings mimic croup, and consequently endoscopy usually is required for diagnosis. Vocal cord paralysis also can produce findings similar to croup on frontal and lateral views, but of course hoarseness, or aphonia, also usually are present. Finally, it might be noted that other infections of the larynx such as candidal and herpes infections can lead to croup or epiglottitis and stridor, and that upper airway obstruction in general has been shown to cause pulmonary edema (12,18) and systemic hypertension. Although its cause is unknown, hypoxia is suspected as the basic trigger for these complications.

Uvulitis

Uvulitis as a part of pharyngitis (13) or in association with epiglottitis also can cause airway obstruction. In such cases, however, the uvula becomes quite large and swollen and may be a cause of inspiratory stridor or even dysphagia. Roentgenographically, the enlarged uvula is readily demonstrable (Fig. 2.14).

REFERENCES

1. Balsam D, Sorrano D, Barax C. Candida epiglottitis presenting as stridor in a child with HIV infection. *Pediatr Radiol* 1992;22: 235–236.
2. Brook I. Aerobic and anaerobic microbiology of bacterial tracheitis in children. *Pediatr Emerg Care* 1997;13:16–18.
3. Brook I. Uvulitis caused by anaerobic bacteria. *Pediatr Emerg Care* 1997;13:221.
4. Connors K, Gavula D, DO, T. The use of corticosteroids in croup: A survey. *Pediatr Emerg Care* 1994;10:197–199.
5. Currarino G, Williams B. Lateral inspiration and expiration radiographs of the neck in children with laryngotracheitis (croup). *Radiology* 1982;145:365–366.
6. Dunbar JS. Upper respiratory tract obstruction in infants and children. *AJR* 1970;109:225–247.
7. Grattan-Smith T, Forer M, Kilham HL, Gillis J. Viral supraglottitis. *J Pediatr* 1987;110:434–435.
8. Harjacek M, Kornberg AE, Yates EW, Montgomery P. Thermal epiglottitis after swallowing hot tea. *Pediatr Emerg Care* 1992;8: 342–344.
9. Herman TE, McAlister WH. Epiglottic enlargement: Two unusual causes. *Pediatr Radiol* 1991;21:139–140.
10. John SD, Swischuk LE. Stridor and upper airway obstruction in infants and children. *RadioGraphics* 1992;12:625–643.
11. John SD, Swischuk LE, Hayden CK Jr. Aryepiglottitis fold width in epiglottitis: Where should measurements be obtained? *Radiology* 1994;190:123–125.
12. Kanter RK, Watchko JF. Pulmonary edema associated with upper airway obstruction. *Am J Dis Child* 1984;138:356–358.
13. Kotloff KR, Wald ER. Uvulitis in children. *Pediatr Infect Dis* 1983;2:392–393.
14. Kulick RM, Selbst SM, Baker MD, Woodward GA. Thermal epiglottitis after swallowing hot beverages. *Pediatrics* 1988;81: 441–444.
15. Liston SL, Gehrz RC, Siegel LG, Tilelli J. Bacterial tracheitis. *Am J Dis Child* 1983;137:764–767.
16. Meine FJ, Lorenzo RL, Lynch PF, Capitanio MA, Kirkpatrick JA. Pharyngeal distension associated with upper airway obstruction: Experimental observations in dogs. *Radiology* 1974;111: 395–398.
17. Shackelford GD, Siegel MJ, McAlister WH. Subglottic edema in acute epiglottitis in children. *AJR* 1978;131:603–605.
18. Travis KW, Todres ID, Shannon DC. Pulmonary edema associated with croup and epiglottitis. *Pediatrics* 1977;59:695–698.
19. Zach M, Erben A, Olinsky A. Croup, recurrent croup, allergy and airways hyper-reactivity. *Arch Dis Child* 1981;56:336–341.

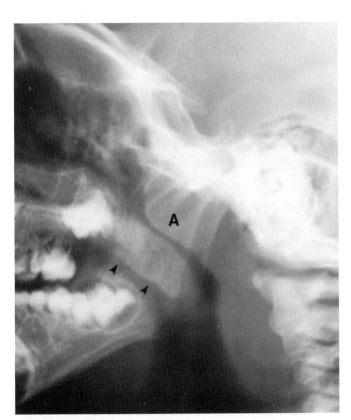

FIGURE 2.14. *Uvulitis.* Note the thickened uvula (*arrows*). Also note prominent, probably inflamed, adenoids (*A*) and retropharyngeal lymphoid tissue.

Chest Film in Airway Obstruction

Obstruction of the airway below the glottis manifests itself primarily as an expiratory problem, and although there may be both inspiratory and expiratory breathing difficulty, it is the expiratory air trapping that predominates roentgenographically. Because of this, the chest tends to be overaerated, and classic examples of lesions leading to such overaeration include obstructing vascular rings and mediastinal masses and cysts. With obstruction in and around the glottis, however, air cannot enter the chest in adequate amounts, and thus the chest often appears underaerated (1). Furthermore, there is a paradoxical increase in heart size during inspiration (1,3). The reason for this is that, with glottic or supraglottic obstruction, inspiratory intrathoracic pressures become negative and, in so doing, cause the cardiac silhouette to become larger and more prominent. Normally, of course, it would become smaller during inspiration.

Pulmonary edema also occurs in some cases of airway obstruction (2,5–7). It can occur during or after the obstruction but occurs most often after the obstruction has been relieved. The exact cause of the pulmonary edema is not known, but most likely it lies in the realm of increased permeability of the capillaries secondary to hypoxia (4). The phenomenon is similar to that seen with postatelectatic pulmonary edema.

REFERENCES

1. Capitanio MA, Kirkpatrick JA. Obstructions of the upper airway in children as reflected on the chest radiograph. *Radiology* 1973;107:159–161.
2. Galvis AG. Pulmonary edema complicating relief of upper airway obstruction. *Am J Emerg Med* 1987;5:294–297.
3. Grunebaum M, Adler S, Varsano I. The paradoxical movement of the mediastinum: A diagnostic sign of foreign-body aspiration during childhood. *Pediatr Radiol* 1979;8:213–218.
4. Izsak E. Pulmonary edema due to acute upper airway obstruction for aspirated foreign body. *Pediatr Emerg Care* 1986;2:235–237.
5. Kanter RK, Watchko JF. Pulmonary edema associated with upper airway obstruction. *Am J Dis Child* 1984;138:356–358.
6. Rivera M, Hadlock FP, O'Meara ME. Pulmonary edema secondary to acute epiglottitis. *AJR* 1979;132:991–992.
7. Travis KW, Todres ID, Shannon DC. Pulmonary edema associated with croup and epiglottitis. *Pediatrics* 1977;59:695–698.

Vocal Cord Dysfunction

Vocal cord dysfunction is a condition defined by abnormal adduction of the vocal cords during inspiration. The clinical findings at first frequently mimic those of asthma, but as the patient is studied it becomes evident that the problem is not so much expiratory wheezing as inspiratory vocal cord closure and dysfunction, which often may be psychogenic (1,2). As a result, roentgenographically the cords are seen to close during inspiration. **Because this is an unexpected finding, it may take a little time to appreciate that this is happening.**

REFERENCES

1. Landwehr LP, Wood RP II, Blager FB, Milgram H. Vocal cord dysfunction mimicking exercise-induced bronchospasm in adolescents. *Pediatrics* 1996;98:971–974.
2. Poirier MP, Pancioli AM, DiGiulio GA. Vocal cord dysfunction presenting as acute asthma in a pediatric patient. *Pediatr Emerg Care* 1996;12:213–214.

Foreign Bodies in the Upper Airway and Hypopharynx

Nasal foreign bodies are common and often detected clinically. However, they can be seen both on plain films and on computed tomographic (CT) studies and often are unexpected findings (Fig. 2.15).

With hypopharyngeal foreign bodies, after the initial coughing episode the foreign body can remain surprisingly silent. Roentgenographically, lateral neck films are invaluable, and if such foreign bodies are opaque, they are identified readily (Fig. 2.16A). If, however, they are radiolucent

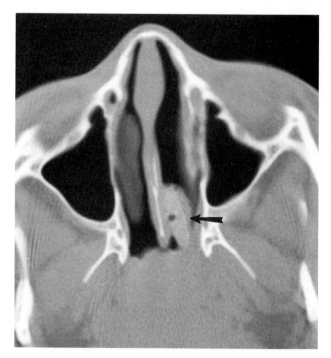

FIGURE 2.15. *Nasal foreign body.* Note the button (*arrow*), incidentally found on this computed tomographic study of the sinuses.

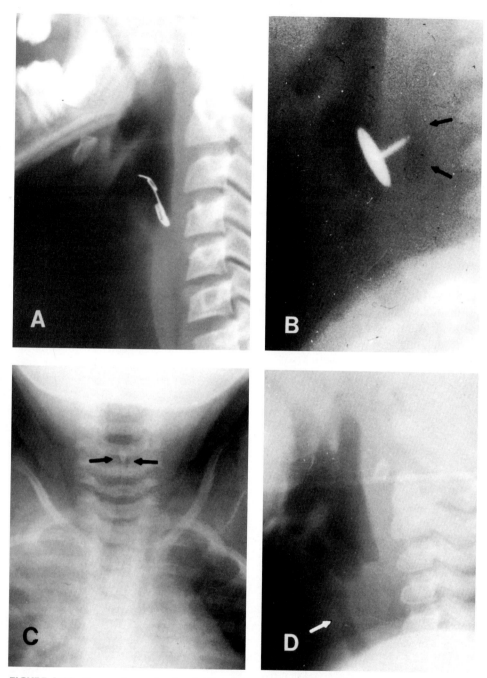

FIGURE 2.16. *Upper-airway foreign bodies.* **(A)** Foreign body (safety pin) in hypopharynx. **(B)** Another infant with a thumbtack in the hypopharynx. Note that the retropharyngeal space is markedly thickened and that air bubbles are present (*arrows*). These findings represent a retropharyngeal abscess secondary to perforation of the posterior pharyngeal wall. **(C)** Opaque laryngeal foreign body. A chicken bone is present in the larynx just at the level of the glottis (*arrows*). **(D)** Radiolucent upper-airway foreign body, indirect findings only. This patient had an acute episode of coughing and hemoptysis, and then persistent stridor for 3 weeks. The only roentgenographic finding was a persistent soft tissue mass bulging from the anterior tracheal wall, just below the glottis (*arrow*). On subsequent endoscopy, a small piece of aluminum foil was found embedded just below the glottic region.

(e.g., aluminum, wood, plastic) they are almost impossible to detect (Fig. 2.16D). If perforation occurs, a retropharyngeal abscess may result (Fig. 2.16B). With other perforations, only free air is seen (Fig. 2.17).

Hypopharyngeal foreign bodies, unless they totally occlude the hypopharynx, seldom result in acute respiratory catastrophes. Laryngeal foreign bodies, on the other hand, commonly present with severe respiratory distress, stridor, and even apnea (Fig. 2.16C). Indeed, the problem often is so acute that there is no time for roentgenograms to be obtained.

Foreign bodies that lodge in the vocal cords usually are slender and either flat or long. The classic such foreign body was an eggshell fragment, but eggshell aspiration is not as common as it was in former days. However, if it should occur, the eggshell fragment may be seen on end, located between the vocal cords. In this position, it appears as a thin, opaque, vertical stripe. Occasionally, other opaque foreign bodies such as chicken and turkey bones can be visualized in the same position (Fig. 2.16C). Fish bones, however, almost always elude detection, for only those that are large and heavily calcified can be detected (1).

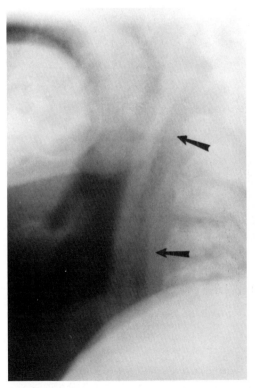

FIGURE 2.17. *Perforation of the hypopharynx.* Note streaks of free air (*arrows*) in the retropharyngeal soft tissues secondary to hypopharyngeal perforation resulting from a swallowed chicken bone.

The problem of confusing a foreign body with normally calcified laryngeal cartilage is not as great in children as it is in adults. These calcifications are discussed with upper esophageal foreign bodies in Chapter 3.

REFERENCE

1. Campbell DR, Brown SJ, Manchester JS. An evaluation of the radio-opacity of various ingested foreign bodies in the pharynx and esophagus. *Can J Assoc Radiol* 1968;19:183–186.

Other Causes of Upper Airway Obstruction

Edema of the larynx and paraglottic structures can be seen with caustic burns secondary to lye ingestion (Fig. 2.18A), laryngeal trauma (Fig. 2.18B), and, in some cases, hot air or smoke inhalation. In such cases, hypopharyngeal overdistension and enlargement or obliteration of the glottic and paraglottic structures is seen. With **trauma to the larynx,** associated fractures of the hyoid bone and laryngeal cartilage also can be seen. In this regard, it is important not to confuse the separate ossification centers of the normal body and wings of the hyoid bone with a fracture (Fig. 2.18B). CT scanning is very valuable in further documenting laryngeal fractures.

Acute stridor occasionally is seen with **angioneurotic (allergic) edema of the epiglottis or uvula** (6). In some of these cases, symptoms may be profound, because nearly total airway occlusion may occur. Roentgenographically, the swollen, enlarged epiglottis (Fig. 2.18C) or uvula is readily demonstrable. In other cases, a chronically lodged foreign body in the upper esophagus may lead to tracheal compression and acute stridor (2–5). These patients often do not present with a history of dysphagia, and roentgenograms may demonstrate compression of the trachea only (see Fig. 3.151).

Vascular rings or other vascular anomalies usually present with chronic airway obstructive problems, but if a superimposed respiratory tract infection is present, acute stridor or wheezing may occur. In such cases, it is most important to identify the presence of a right sided aortic arch, for this is almost always present with a vascular ring (Fig. 2.19). Of course, tracheal compression may be seen on plain films, but generally speaking the workup of stridor secondary to a vascular ring is not an emergency room procedure. A similar statement can be made regarding mediastinal masses and cysts that might present with airway obstruction. An unusual cause of airway obstruction is air dissection into the posterior pharynx secondary to pneumomediastinum in asthmatics (1).

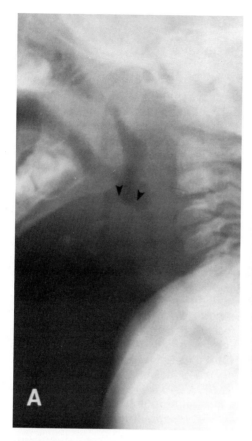

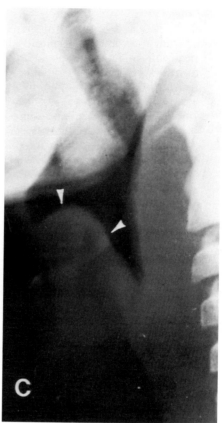

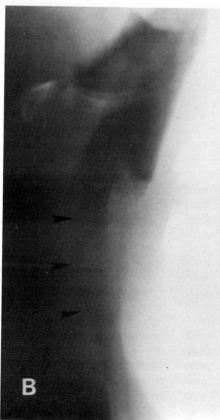

FIGURE 2.18. *Miscellaneous causes of upper-airway obstruction.* (**A**) Lye burns to larynx. Note the edematous cords (*arrows*) in this patient, who sustained lye burns to the esophagus, hypopharynx, and vocal cords. (**B**) Trauma to larynx. This boy was hit in the anterior neck by a fist and became hoarse. Note the edematous, indistinct vocal cords (*arrows*) and the separately ossified body and wings of the hyoid bone. These should not be misinterpreted as a fracture. (**C**) Angioneurotic edema of the epiglottis. Note the markedly thickened epiglottis, aryepiglottic folds (*arrows*), and retropharynx in this patient presenting with acute respiratory distress. (From Watts FB Jr, Slovis TL. The enlarged epiglottis. *Pediatr Radiol* 1977;5:133–316, with permission.)

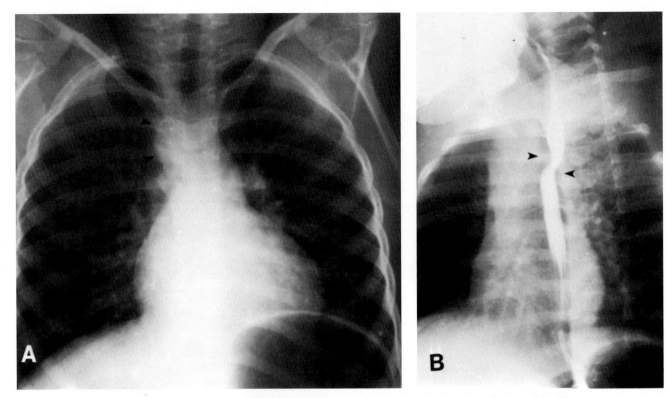

FIGURE 2.19. *Vascular ring causing stridor.* **(A)** Note the right-sided aortic arch (*arrow*) in this patient with a vascular ring (double aortic arch). The trachea is displaced to the left and indented on the right by the right-sided aortic arch. On lateral view in these patients, one occasionally can see anterior displacement of the trachea. **(B)** Barium swallow demonstrating characteristic reverse "S," double indentation of the esophagus (*arrows*).

REFERENCES

1. Cohn RC, Steffen ME, Spohn WA. Retropharyngeal air accumulation as a complication of pneumomediastinum and a cause of airway obstruction in asthma. *Pediatr Emerg Care* 1995;11: 298–299.
2. Lallemand D, Roussel B, Sauvegrain J. Narrowing of the cervical trachea following foreign body aspiration. *Ann Radiol* 1975;18: 413–418.
3. Schidlow DV, Palmer J, Balsara RK, Turtz MG, Williams JL. Chronic stridor and anterior cervical "mass" secondary to an esophageal foreign body. *Am J Dis Child* 1981;135:869–870.
4. Smith PC, Swischuk LE, Fagan CJ. An elusive and often unsuspected cause of stridor or pneumonia (the esophageal foreign body). *Am J Roentgenol Radium The Nucl Med* 1974;122:80–89.
5. Tauscher JW. Esophageal foreign body: An uncommon cause of stridor. *Pediatrics* 1978;61:657–658.
6. Watts FB Jr., Slovis TL. The enlarged epiglottis. *Pediatr Radiol* 1977;5:133–136.

RETROPHARYNGEAL ABSCESS

Retropharyngeal abscess usually presents with fever, neck pain and stiffness, and dysphagia (1). Stridor can be seen in these patients but usually is not a predominant feature. Adenopathy usually is present in the neck and, in some cases, may be striking. In most instances, the retropharyngeal abscess results from suppuration of lymphoid tissue in the retropharyngeal space, but occasionally it can result from perforation of the hypopharynx by a foreign body.

Roentgenographically, the findings consist of thickening of the retropharyngeal soft tissues and forward, displacement of the airway (Fig. 2.20). If gas is present in the abscess, the diagnosis is established more readily (Fig. 2.16B). In those cases in which findings are minimal and one is in doubt, a barium swallow study is helpful. This study shows the abnormal forward position of the esophagus and more clearly demonstrates the presence of soft-tissue swelling in the retropharyngeal space.

The cervical spine usually is straight or flexed in cases of retropharyngeal abscess and often there is some degree of anterior offsetting of C2 on C3. This latter finding results from the intense muscle spasm present and does not represent true dislocation. By the same token, C1 may be displaced forward on C2, and as a result the space between the anterior arch of C1 and the dens becomes widened. It has

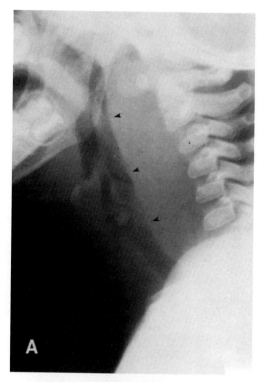

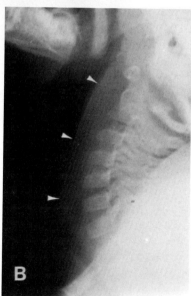

been stated that this finding results from inflammation-induced laxity of the ligaments in the area, and this may be true. However, it should be remembered that normal hypermobility of the upper cervical spine in infants is common.

It is important to differentiate normal tracheal buckling and prominent lymphoid tissue from true thickening of the retropharyngeal soft tissues. In this regard, with true thickening there is loss of the normal stepoff from the posterior pharyngeal wall to the posterior wall of the trachea (Fig. 2.20). With normal retropharyngeal soft tissues, this does not occur and the stepoff generally is preserved (Fig. 2.21). However, if uncertainty persists, a barium swallow can determine whether true thickening is present. Currently in most cases of retropharyngeal inflammation, either ultrasound or CT scan is utilized for defining the abnormality (Figs. 2.22 and 2.23). Ultrasound is very effective at demonstrating parapharyngeal adenopathy, but CT scans better demonstrate disease processes that are truly posterior to the hypopharynx. CT scan also is more rewarding in demonstrating abscess formation and certainly almost always should be utilized before surgical intervention occurs.

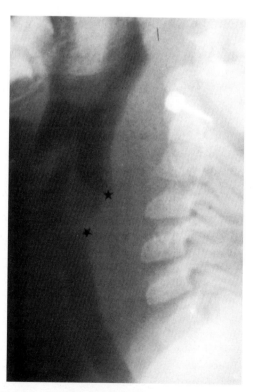

FIGURE 2.20. *Retropharyngeal abscess.* **(A)** Large retropharyngeal abscess causing thickening of the retropharyngeal space and smooth, continuous anterior displacement of the airway (*arrows*). **(B)** Less striking case showing less thickening of the retropharyngeal tissues (*arrows*). Note also that the neck is in its normal extended position. Nonetheless, the prevertebral soft tissues are thickened and the airway displaced anteriorly in a smooth, curving fashion (i.e., the normal stepoff of the airway at the level of the larynx is lost).

FIGURE 2.21. *Normal retropharyngeal soft tissue prominence.* In this patient, normal retropharyngeal lymphoid tissue causes indentation of the posterior wall of the hypopharynx. However, note that the posterior walls of the trachea and hypopharynx (*asterisks*) remain offset. Therefore, even though a retropharyngeal disease process might be suggested, the smooth, curving deformity of the combined posterior hypopharyngeal and tracheal walls as demonstrated in Figure 2.20 is absent.

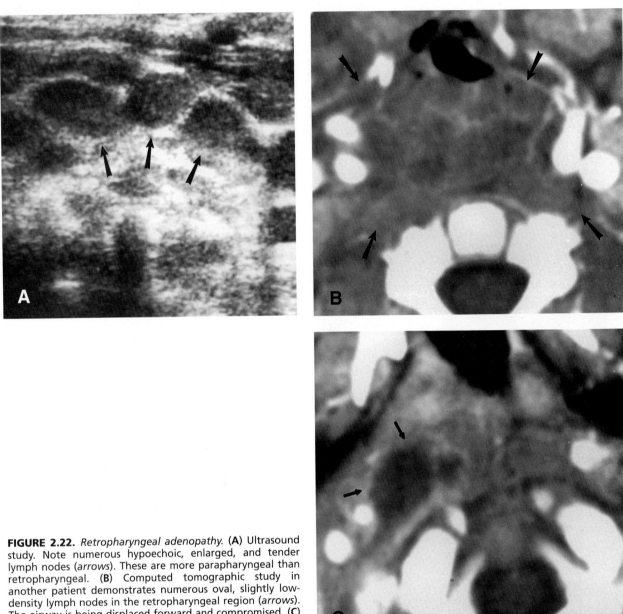

FIGURE 2.22. *Retropharyngeal adenopathy.* **(A)** Ultrasound study. Note numerous hypoechoic, enlarged, and tender lymph nodes (*arrows*). These are more parapharyngeal than retropharyngeal. **(B)** Computed tomographic study in another patient demonstrates numerous oval, slightly low-density lymph nodes in the retropharyngeal region (*arrows*). The airway is being displaced forward and compromised. **(C)** Suppurated lymph node (*arrows*). It has an appearance virtually indistinguishable from an abscess.

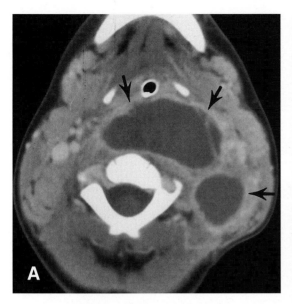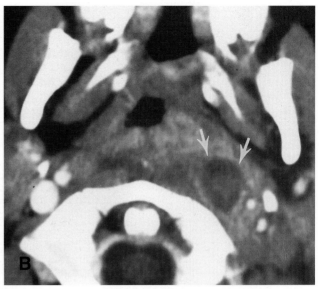

FIGURE 2.23. *Retropharyngeal abscess: findings on computed tomographic scanning.* **(A)** Two large abscesses (*arrows*). One is retropharyngeal and the other parapharyngeal. Note that the airway is markedly anteriorly displaced. **(B)** Another patient with a smaller abscess (*arrow*). This also could represent a suppurated lymph node. Note that the adjacent jugular vein and carotid artery are small secondary to spasm. This is a common phenomenon with retropharyngeal infections.

REFERENCE

1. John SD, Swischuk LE. Stridor and upper airway obstruction in infants and children. *RadioGraphics* 1992;12:625–643.

SINUSITIS, MASTOIDITIS, AND NASAL PASSAGE ABNORMALITIES

Sinusitis

Sinusitis is common in infants and children, and those who suggest that roentgenographic examination of the sinuses in this age group is of limited value do these patients an injustice. This is not to say, however, that dealing with sinusitis in infants and children is easy, but still it must be dealt with. Sinusitis comes in varying degrees of severity, may be allergic or inflammatory, and frequently is subacute (13). In addition, it is variably symptomatic, and if all of these factors are considered it becomes a difficult entity to deal with.

Part of the problem of recognizing sinus disease in children, especially in young infants, arises from the fact that it was, and to a large extent still is, generally held that sinuses are not developed in infants. This is untrue, for the maxillary and ethmoid sinuses often are present at birth and can become infected at ages as young as 3 to 6 months (13). The problem, however, is that roentgenographic examination of the sinuses in infants younger than 1 year of age is difficult to perform, and interpretation of the findings is even more difficult. ***Consequently, it is easier to say that the sinuses have not yet developed than to try to find***

them and interpret the findings. In such cases, it is only if the sinus cavities clear with treatment that one realizes that they were present all the time (Fig. 2.24). Similarly, proof that sinus cavities exist in young infants is present if disease is unilateral (Fig. 2.24C).

In addition, usually the Waters view, the single most important view in evaluating sinusitis in children, is obtained with too steep an angle (Fig. 2.25). Although this most common problem is not always completely circumvented in very young infants, awareness of it can prompt repeat studies and, thus, proper interpretation. This is important, because the Waters view usually suffices in most cases (11). All of this also should be considered in light of the fact that it seems doubtful that, as previously proposed, crying can cause enough mucosal edema and sinus obliteration to mimic disease (2–5,8,13). By the same token, mucosal redundancy, often suggested as a normal phenomenon of young infants causing opacification of sinuses in the very young, also seems a doubtful concept. One only has to ask why, of all the mucosal surfaces in a young infant, would the mucosa in the paranasal sinuses selectively be redundant. ***Consequently, I have come, more and more, to the conclusion that the only normal sinus cavity is the one completely clear.*** However, if a sinus cavity is opacified, one cannot predict the severity of the problem, the exception being the presence of air-fluid levels that signify acute, purulent, bacterial sinusitis. Viral infection seldom produces air-fluid levels. Mucosal thickening is common in allergic sinusitis, a frequently seen problem in children with asthma (2,9,13). It also is seen with viral and bacterial

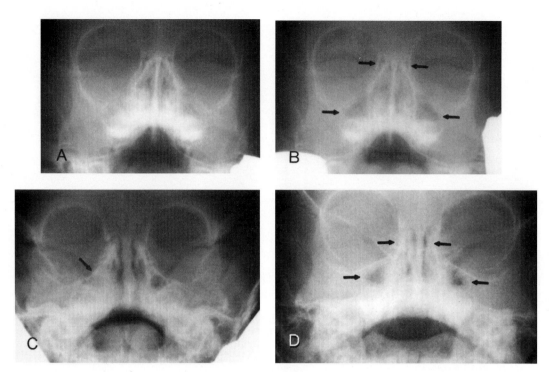

FIGURE 2.24. *Sinusitis in infancy.* **(A)** Note that the maxillary sinuses are difficult to see in this 11-month-old infant. The reason is that they are completely obliterated by inflammatory changes. However, ***one might be tempted to erroneously conclude that the maxillary sinuses are not yet developed***. **(B)** After treatment, just 3 weeks later, one can see the normally aerated maxillary (*lower arrows*) and ethmoid (*upper arrows*) sinuses. **(C)** Another patient with unilateral maxillary sinus opacification on the right (*arrow*). One could see how easy it would be to say that the sinuses were not developed if the left maxillary sinus also were obliterated. ***This patient was 5 months old.*** **(D)** Note bilateral mucosal thickening of the maxillary sinuses (*lower arrows*) and obliteration of the ethmoid sinuses (*upper arrows*). Mucosal thickening in the maxillary sinuses might at first be missed and the maxillary sinuses erroneously believed to be clear, and perhaps a little small.

infection. Complete opacification, of course, also can be seen with all three of the types of "sinusitis."

The fact that the roentgenograms, for the most part, cannot yield data regarding severity of sinusitis explains why some studies have shown that patients with no complaints show opacified sinuses (7). Indeed, most likely, if a random population were examined, a fair number of indi-

viduals would have opacified sinuses and yet not complain overly of them. Sinusitis is a disease with a wide clinical spectrum, and many individuals, including children, can tolerate certain degrees of sinusitis. This does not mean, however, that the sinuses are normal, only that the disease is not very severe. ***Overall, the roentgenogram is quite sensitive in detecting sinus opacification and hence disease,***

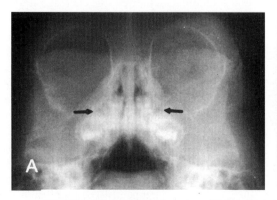
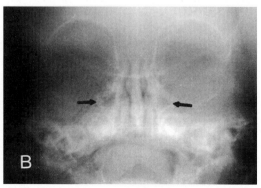

FIGURE 2.25. *Faulty Waters view.* **(A)** This Waters view was obtained too steeply and the maxillary sinuses (*arrows*) appear obliterated. **(B)** With proper angulation (less steep than in adults), the sinuses are seen to be clear (*arrows*).

but it does not define severity. Another useful function of the roentgenographic study of the sinuses is that it often is difficult to differentiate purulent rhinitis from purulent sinusitis on a clinical basis. On the other hand, this usually is easily accomplished if roentgenograms of the sinuses are obtained. With rhinitis, the sinus cavities are clear.

In terms of which views to obtain, it is the Waters view that is most beneficial and indeed has been shown to usually to suffice (11). However, we also obtain the lateral view for evaluation of the sinuses and nasopharynx. The reason the Waters view is so valuable is that it is designed to visualize the maxillary and ethmoid sinus cavities, and, in infants and young children, these are the cavities most often involved. The maxillary sinus cavities, however, are more readily evaluated than the ethmoid and sphenoid sinus cavities. In terms of evaluating these cavities, it might be recalled that although the ethmoid and maxillary sphenoid sinus cavities generally are present by 6 months and the sphenoid sinus cavities by 2 years, the frontal sinuses are usually not present until 7 to 10 years of age. Therefore, frontal sinusitis does not exist in infants and young children.

Before embarking on a discussion of the roentgenographic findings of sinusitis, *it is probably worthwhile to try to understand the pathophysiology of sinusitis.* Nor-mal sinus cavities are well aerated, for drainage is normal, but if drainage becomes impaired, the sinus cavities become occluded, and then superimposed bacterial infection becomes a high risk. There is a question of how the sinus cavities become occluded in the first place—the most common causes are viral upper respiratory tract infections and allergy. In such cases, the mucosa of the sinuses becomes congested, occludes the orifices of the sinus cavities, and leads to impaired drainage. Once this occurs, the possibility of superimposed bacterial infection increases.

In terms of the clinical significance of opacified sinuses, it has been shown that opacified paranasal sinuses in children are bacterially infected in 70% of cases (1). *Of further interest is the fact that the vast majority of these patients did not have symptoms that would have prompted the initial physician to consider sinus disease.* This phenomenon has been correlated by others (5), and certainly this has been our experience. *Once one accepts these aspects of sinus disease in infants and children, one can begin to accept the premise that the only normal sinus cavity is the one that is completely aerated.*

The *roentgenographic manifestations of sinusitis* include total opacification of the sinuses, variable thickness of the mucosa, and air–fluid levels (Figs. 2.24 and 2.26).

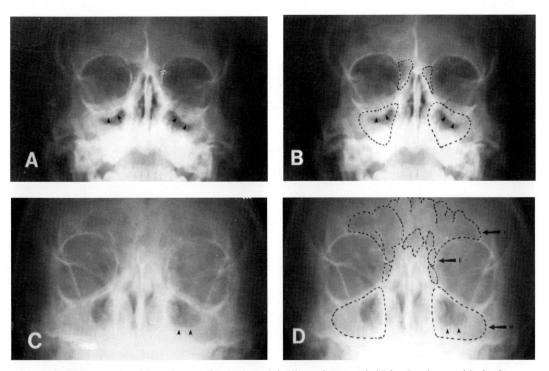

FIGURE 2.26. *Sinusitis: other configurations.* **(A)** Bilateral mucosal thickening is noted in both maxillary sinuses (*arrows*). This configuration frequently is seen in allergic children. In addition, the ethmoid sinuses, located just along the medial aspect of the orbital rims, also are partially obliterated and involved by inflammatory change. **(B)** For comparative purposes, the bony cortex of the maxillary and ethmoid sinuses in this patient have been delineated by dotted lines. **(C)** Another patient with an air–fluid level in the left maxillary sinus (*arrows*). The right maxillary sinus is almost completely obliterated by inflammatory change (exudate and mucosal thickening), and the ethmoid and frontal sinuses also are involved. Air–fluid levels most often are seen with acute sinusitis of bacterial origin. **(D)** Dotted lines once again outline the sinus cavities for comparative purposes. M, maxillary sinus; E, ethmoid sinus; F, frontal sinus.

Mucosal thickening is most common and, as correlated with clinical and magnetic resonance imaging findings in patients examined for reasons other than sinus disease, thickening of the mucosa in the maxillary sinuses of 4 mm or greater proved significant in terms of associated symptomatology consistent with sinusitis (10).

In interpreting mucosal thickening, it is important not to misinterpret the findings as merely being representative of small sinus cavities (Fig. 2.27). This is a common mistake in the assessment of paranasal sinus disease in the pediatric age group, especially in infants and young children, in whom the bony walls of the sinus cavities are thin (Fig. 2.27C). Air–fluid levels in any sinus cavity suggest acute bacterial sinusitis, and for their demonstration upright views are necessary. Totally opacified sinuses, as noted previously, are seen with all types of sinusitis but often escape notice until treatment and clearing of the sinus cavities occur (Fig. 2.24).

Symptoms of sinusitis in childhood often are not like those in adults (2,4,7,9,11,13), and although pain and redness can occur over an acutely infected sinus cavity in a child, more often sinusitis is a chronic problem presenting with a persistent cough (resulting from a postnasal drip and often worse at night) and recurrent bouts of otitis media (4,5,13). Headache is not nearly as common a symptom as it is in adults and, indeed, is a poor heralding finding of sinusitis in children. In other children with maxillary and ethmoid sinusitis, proptosis caused by orbital edema may be the presenting problem and actually is quite common. In such cases, CT studies are invaluable and indeed mandatory. They clearly show whether the pathologic process results from preseptal cellulitis or intraorbital inflammation, even to the point of abscess formation. Preseptal cellulitis manifests in soft-tissue swelling of the tissues anterior to the globe (Fig. 2.28A). If inflammation extends into the retroorbital space, it most often occurs medially and displaces the medial rectus muscle (Fig. 2.28B and C). Abscess formation can occur anywhere (Fig. 2.28D). Computerized tomography studies are invaluable in these patients and should be performed for any patient with inflammatory proptosis. In addition, computerized tomography is essential for preoperative assessment of sinus disease (6), and overall is gaining in popularity in all patients. It is much more informative than plain films, especially for disease in the ethmoid and splenoid sinuses. However, this is not to be misinterpreted as suggesting that CT studies should be obtained in all patients, because they should not.

Finally, in terms of the clinical diagnosis of sinusitis, a problem arises in distinguishing acute viral upper respiratory tract infections with coryza from sinusitis. Our experience has been that in cases of acute viral upper respiratory tract infection, even though the patient may feel congested and look congested, the paranasal sinuses are clear. It is not until later, when enough mucosal thickening and edema have occurred, that the sinuses become abnormal.

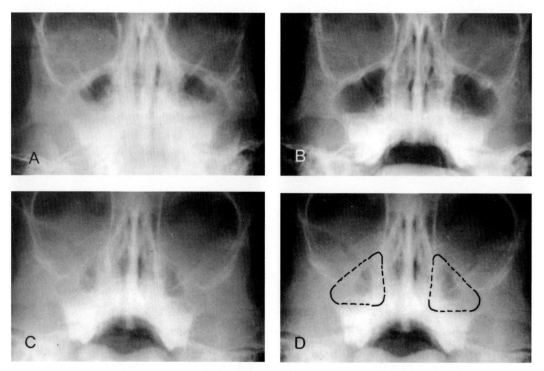

FIGURE 2.27. *Pseudosmall sinus pitfall.* **(A)** Note moderately pronounced mucosal thickening of the maxillary sinuses, which might suggest erroneously that the sinuses are clear but small. **(B)** With treatment the sinuses now are clear and their true size readily apparent. **(C)** Extensive mucosal thickening of the maxillary sinuses in an infant, which, again, at first might suggest erroneously that the maxillary sinuses are clear but small. The bony walls are difficult to see. **(D)** *Dotted lines* outline the true sinus cavities.

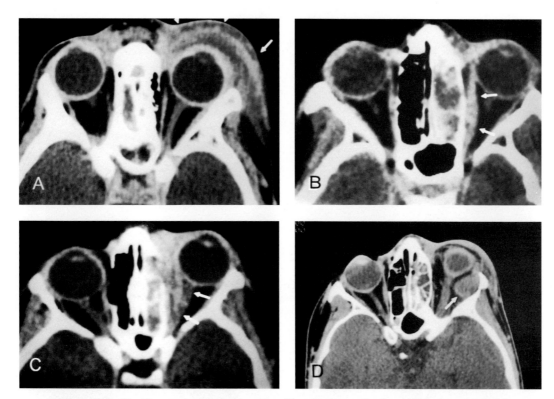

FIGURE 2.28. *Maxillary and ethmoid sinusitis with orbital complications.* **(A)** Preseptal cellulitis. Note extensive swelling of the preseptal soft tissues (*arrows*). There is no edema extending into the retroorbital space, and the medial rectus muscle is normal. **(B)** Another patient with thickening of the medial rectus muscle and adjacent soft tissues (*arrows*). Note adjacent sinusitis in the ethmoid cells. **(C)** Still another patient with more extensive edema along the medial retroorbital space (*arrows*). Adjacent sinusitis is present but a frank abscess is not suggested. **(D)** Another patient with an abscess in the retroorbital region (*arrow*).

Before finally leaving the topic of sinusitis, another pitfall in the interpretation of paranasal sinuses should be discussed in more detail. This pitfall deals with the fact that the maxillary sinuses are not cuboid but rather triangular. As a result, either the superior or lateral orbital walls can be so slanted that pseudothickening of the mucosa erroneously is suggested (Fig. 2.29). Ultrasound also has been utilized to determine the degree of aeration of the sinus cavities, but we have not done so. The procedure is not in widespread use and probably never will become popular.

Rhinitis

Rhinitis is a common problem in the pediatric age group. As with sinusitis, it can be allergic, viral, or bacterial in origin. It is not a roentgenographic diagnosis. ***It becomes important only if it must be differentiated from usually normal paranasal sinuses.***

Acute Mastoiditis

Acute mastoiditis is best demonstrated, in terms of plain films, on Towne's projection of the skull. In these cases, one

has both mastoid areas to compare, and acute mastoiditis is reflected by haziness or obliteration of the mastoid air cells (Fig. 2.30) and, in more acute cases, actual destruction of the bone with abscess formation. Obliteration of the mastoid air cells also occurs with bleeding associated with cal-

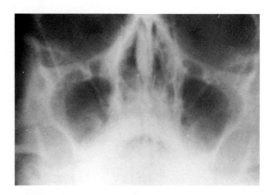

FIGURE 2.29. *Sloping wall artifact.* Note what would appear to be mucosal thickening along the roof and lateral walls of both maxillary sinuses. However, the thickening is not as pronounced laterally and certainly is not present medially or along the floor of the sinus cavities. This would be unusual if mucosal thickening were the problem. The findings result from normal sloping of the roof and lateral wall of the maxillary sinuses, which erroneously suggests mucosal thickening on these slightly steep films.

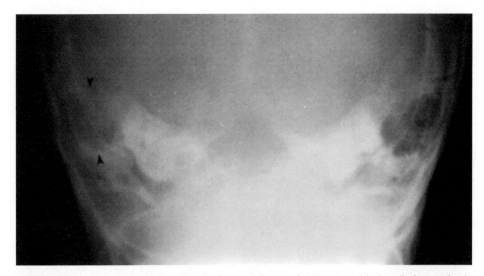

FIGURE 2.30. *Acute mastoiditis.* Note the hazy, obliterated right mastoid air cells (*arrows*). The mastoid air cells on the left are normal and well aerated. In such cases, often it is difficult to determine whether one is dealing with extensive acute inflammatory disease or early destruction secondary to an abscess.

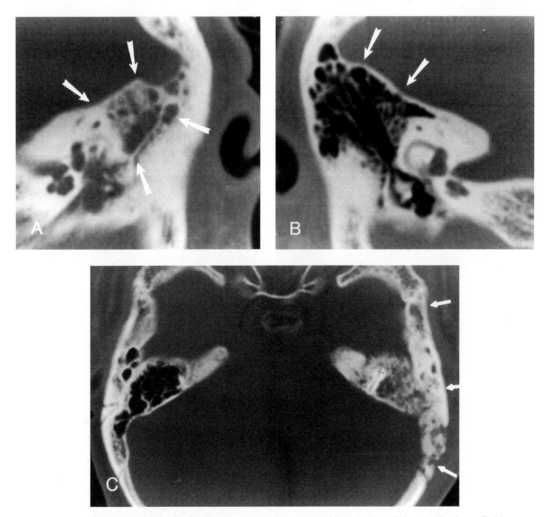

FIGURE 2.31. *Mastoiditis: findings on computed tomographic scanning.* (**A**) Note the hazy fluid-filled, underdeveloped mastoid air cells (*arrows*). (**B**) Normal side for comparison. Note the normal-appearing air-filled mastoid air cells (*arrows*). (**C**) Another patient with chronic mastoiditis and extensive destruction of the adjacent calvarium resulting from osteomyelitis (*arrows*).

varial trauma and bone destruction, as seen with rhabdomyosarcoma, histiocytosis X, leukemia, and lymphoma.

Aeration of the mastoid antra is present at birth, and mastoid air cell development occurs rapidly thereafter. Consequently, mastoid air cell aeration usually is present in infants as young as 3 months of age, and thus the diagnosis of acute mastoiditis with obliteration of the air cells can be made roentgenographically at this age. In those patients who suffer chronic repeated bouts of otitis media, overall air cell development is impaired, and bony sclerosis supervenes (14). Overall, in these patients, there are fewer aerated air cells and dense or white-appearing petrous bones. CT scanning most clearly defines all of these acute and chronic problems (Fig. 2.31).

REFERENCES

1. Arruda LK, Mimica IM, Sole D, et al. Abnormal maxillary sinus radiographs in children: Do they represent bacterial infection? *Pediatrics* 1990;85:553–558.
2. Furukawa CT, Shapiro GG, Rachelefsky GS. Children with sinusitis. *Pediatrics* 1983;71: 133–134.
3. Glasier CM, Mallory GB Jr, Steele RW. Significance of opacification of the maxillary and ethmoid sinuses in infants. *J Pediatr* 1989;114:45–50.
4. Kogutt MS, Swischuk LE. Diagnosis of sinusitis in infants and children. *Pediatrics* 1973;52:121–124.
5. Kovatch AL, Wald ER, Ledesma-Medina J, Chiponis DM, Bedingfield, B. Maxillary sinus radiographs in children with nonrespiratory complaints. *Pediatrics* 1984;73:306–308.
6. McAlister WH, Lusk R, Muntz HR. Comparison of plain radiographs and coronal CT scans in infants and children with recurrent sinusitis. *AJR* 1989;153:1259–1264.
7. McLain DC. Sinusitis in children: Lessons from 25 patients. *Clin Pediatr* 1970;9:342.
8. Odita JC, Akamaguna AI, Ogisi FO, Amu OD, and Ugbodaga CI. Pneumatisation of the maxillary sinus in normal and symptomatic children. *Pediatr Radiol* 1986;16: 365–367.
9. Rachelefsky GS, Shapiro GG. Diseases of the paranasal sinuses in children. In: Bierman C.W., Pearlman, D.S. (eds.): Allergic diseases of infancy, childhood and adolescence. Philadelphia: W.B. Saunders, 1980:526–624.
10. Rak KM, Newell JD II, Yakes WF, Damiano MA, Luethke JM. Paranasal sinuses on MR images of the brain: Significance of mucosal thickening. *AJR* 1991;156:381–384.
11. Ros SP, Herman BE, Azar-Kia B. Acute sinusitis in children: Is the Water's view sufficient? *Pediatr Radiol* 1995;25:306–307.
12. Rulon JT. Sinusitis in children. *Postgrad Med* 1970;48:107.
13. Swischuk LE, Hayden CK Jr, Dillard RA. Sinusitis in children. *RadioGraphics* 1982;2:241–252.
14. Tos M, Strangerup S-E, Hvid G. Mastoid pneumatization: Evidence of the environmental theory. *Arch Otolaryngol* 1984;110: 502–507.

EPISTAXIS

Epistaxis is a common problem in childhood. Most often it results from a simple nosebleed, and no roentgenograms are obtained. However, one should be aware of the fact that juvenile angiofibromas often present with epistaxis and sinusitis (1,2). These angiofibromas occur most commonly in adolescent boys and, on the lateral roentgenogram of the paranasal sinuses, present as masses in the nasopharynx (Fig. 2.32). Such a mass should not be

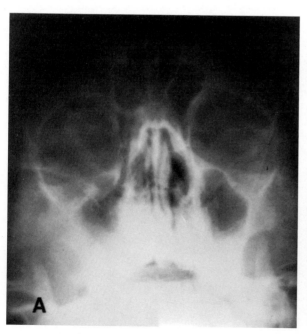

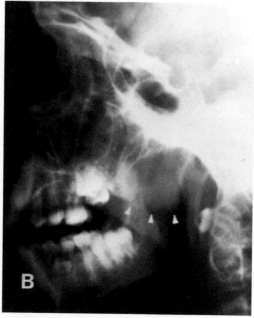

FIGURE 2.32. *Juvenile angiofibroma of nasopharynx presenting with epistaxis.* **(A)** Note the partially obliterated right maxillary sinus in this patient with epistaxis. **(B)** Lateral view showing large nasopharyngeal mass *(arrows)*, which might be mistaken for large adenoids. *Continued on next page.*

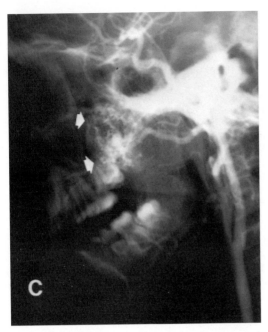

FIGURE 2.32. *(continued)* **C)** Subsequent arteriogram demonstrates extensive tumor vascularity (*arrows*) characteristic of this lesion. It is being supplied by the external maxillary artery.

confused with normal adenoidal tissue, which often is very abundant in normal children. Nasopharyngeal angiofibromas now are best defined with magnetic resonance imaging, on which high signal on second-echo, T2-weighted images is characteristic. Nonetheless, angiogra-

phy still is necessary prior to therapy, which now includes preoperative embolization.

Epistaxis also may result from an acute or chronic foreign body in the nose, and if such a foreign body is radiolucent, it may remain undetected for extended periods of time. In addition, epistaxis also is seen with trauma to the face and nose.

REFERENCES

1. Fitzpatrick PJ. The nasopharyngeal angiofibroma. *Clin Radiol* 1967;18:62–68.
2. Holman CB, Miller WE. Juvenile nasopharyngeal fibroma: Roentgenologic characteristics. *AJR* 1965;94:292–298.

SALIVARY GLANDS

Acute problems involving the salivary glands include, for the most part, infection and stone formation with obstruction. The former is more common. Most infections are viral in origin (e.g., mumps), and suppurative infections usually result from *Staphylococcus aureus* infection. Autoimmune salivary gland inflammation also can occur. Stones can be visualized on plain films or CT scans, but the usual imaging modality first used to study enlarged, tender salivary glands is ultrasound. The findings demonstrate nonspecific echogenicity of the enlarged

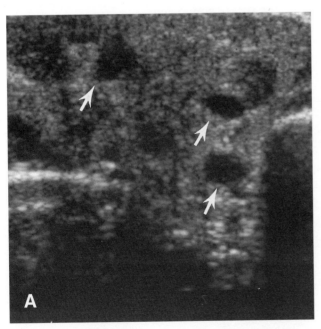
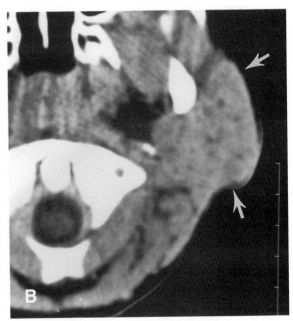

FIGURE 2.33. *Parotid inflammation.* **(A)** Note the enlarged parotid gland with numerous hypoechoic intraglandular lymph tissue collections (*arrows*). **(B)** Computed tomographic study demonstrates the enlarged parotid gland along with adjacent reactive enlarged lymph nodes (*arrows*).

gland. If suppuration occurs, a central hypoechoic collection of pus can be seen. In addition intraglandular lymphoid tissue commonly is seen and should not be misinterpreted as microabscess formation (Fig. 2.33). Such intraglandular lymphoid tissue has a propensity to occur in HIV-positive patients (1,2).

REFERENCES

1. Brilli RG, Benzing G III, Cotcamp DH. Epiglottitis in infants less than two years of age. *Pediatr Emerg Care* 1989;5:16–21.
2. Denny FW, Murphy TF, Clyde WA Jr, Collier AM, Henderson FW. Croup: An 11-year study in a pediatric practice. *Pediatrics* 1983;71:871–876.

3

THE ABDOMEN

Analyzing the abdominal roentgenogram is more difficult and often less rewarding than analyzing the chest roentgenogram, but it is an important study. In the chest, symmetry of structures and densities from side to side is of paramount importance, but in the abdomen symmetry is a minor consideration. In the abdomen, it is a matter of becoming familiar with the appearance of relatively fixed organs seen through changing intestinal gas patterns. *No one normal configuration looks exactly like another, and the overall "normal" picture comes only through examining many roentgenograms over many years.*

In beginning one's assessment of the abdominal roentgenogram, it is worthwhile to locate the stomach, rectum, and both the hepatic and splenic flexures of the colon. These areas of the gastrointestinal tract are relatively fixed, usually contain gas, and look much the same from one patient to another. After this, one should attempt to define the solid abdominal viscera, and of these the easiest to visualize are the liver, spleen, kidneys, psoas muscles, and urinary bladder, if filled (Fig. 3.1). After the abdominal viscera are examined, one should cast an eye over the diaphragmatic leaflets and bony structures such as the vertebrae, ribs, and pelvis. This is especially important in abdominal trauma.

All of these points are most pertinent to plain films, which, of course, continue to be obtained for the evaluation of acute abdominal problems in children. *Ultrasound (4,7,8), even more than computed tomographic (CT) scanning (2,6), however, has come to play a significant if not key role (1,3,5) in the evaluation of the acute abdomen in children.* The reason that ultrasound is superior to CT imaging in infants and children is that CT scans are more rewarding when considerable abodminal fat is present. This occurs in adults but is not the rule in infants and children. In trauma, however, CT scanning is preferred over ultrasound. With the acute abdomen, ultrasound is excellent in identifying appendicitis and other problems such as mesenteric adenitis, enteritis, and adnexal problems in females. In our hands it has proven to be 98% accurate (8).

With ultrasonography, almost invariably the first organs to be imaged are the right kidney and liver (Fig. 3.2). Thereafter, the spleen and left kidney are identified, and then, primarily in cross-section, one can assess the retroperitoneal structures (Fig. 3.2). The lower abdomen and pelvic regions also can be assessed in longitudinal and cross-sectional views, but to do so, the urinary bladder must be full, either with urine or with saline introduced by the examiner. CT scanning yields cross-sectional anatomic data (Fig. 3.3).

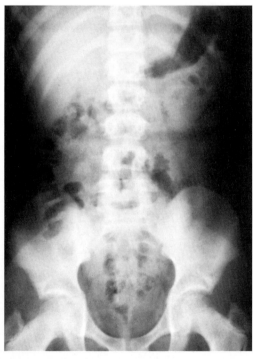

FIGURE 3.1. Normal abdomen. The distribution and volume of gastrointestinal gas are about average. The renal silhouettes are clearly visible, and the psoas shadows are seen as broad triangular structures on either side of the spine. A distended urinary bladder is seen in the pelvis.

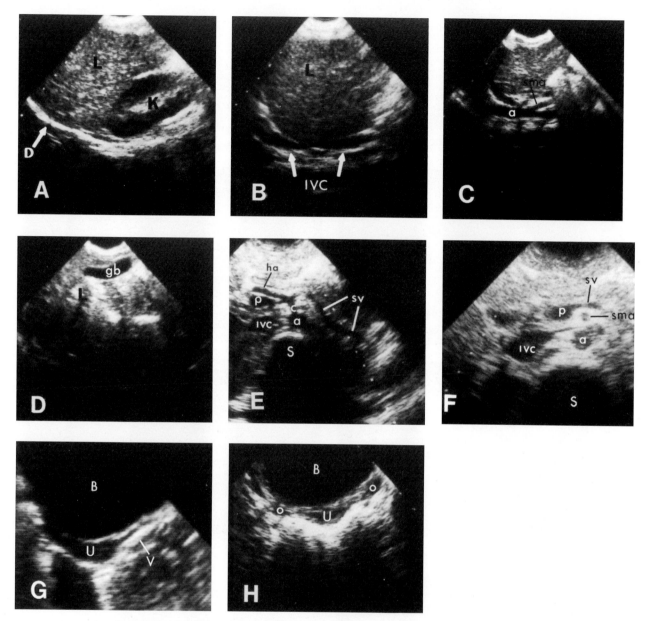

FIGURE 3.2. Normal abdomen: ultrasound. **(A)** Longitudinal scan on the right demonstrates the diaphragm (*D*), right kidney (*K*), and liver (*L*). **(B)** Longitudinal scan somewhat more medial demonstrates the inferior vena cava (*IVC*) and liver (*L*). **(C)** Longitudinal scan over the aorta demonstrates the aorta (*A*) and the superior mesenteric artery (*sma*) branching from it. **(D)** Another longitudinal scan demonstrates the liver (*L*) and gallbladder (*gb*). **(E)** Transverse scan demonstrates the spine (*S*), the aorta (*A*), the celiac artery (*C*), and the hepatic artery (*ha*). In addition, note the inferior vena cava (*ivc*), portal vein confluence (*p*), and the splenic vein (*sv*). **(F)** Another transverse cut demonstrating the spine (*S*), the aorta (*A*), and the superior mesenteric artery (*sma*). Characteristically, the superior mesenteric artery is surrounded by a collar of echogenicity. Also note the portal-vein confluence (*p*), the inferior vena cava (*ivc*), and the splenic vein (*sv*). **(F)** Another transverse cut demonstrating the spine (*S*), the aorta (*A*), and the superior mesenteric artery (*sma*). Characteristically, the superior mesenteric artery is surrounded by a collar of echogenicity. Also note the portal-vein confluence (*p*), the inferior vena cava (*ivc*), and the splenic vein (*sv*). The thin sonolucent steak heading medially from the inferior vena cava is the left renal vein. The pancreas lies above the splenic vein but is not clearly delineated here. **(G)** Longitudinal scan in the pelvis demonstrates the bladder (*B*), the uterus (*U*), and the vagina (*V*). The thin, sonolucent channel in the vagina is the vaginal lumen. **(H)** Transverse scan in the pelvis demonstrates the urinary bladder (*B*), the uterus (*U*), and both ovaries (*o*).

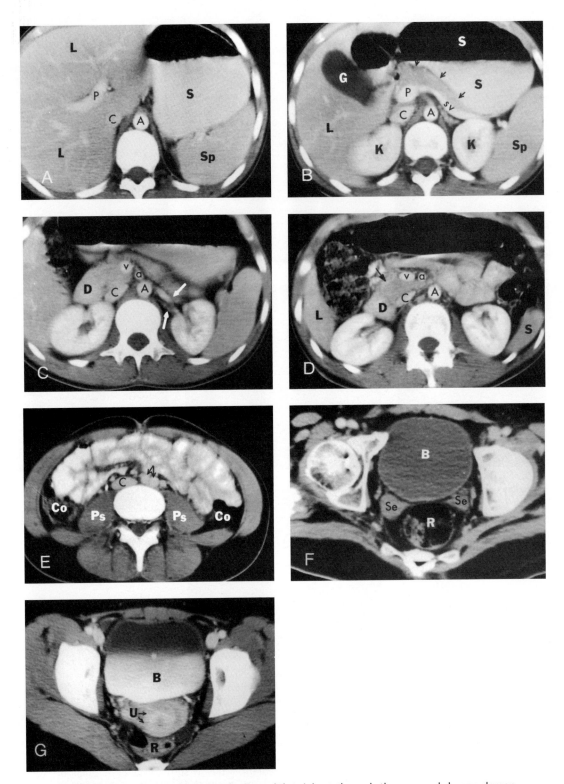

FIGURE 3.3. Normal abdomen: CT findings. **(A)** Axial cut through the upper abdomen demonstrates the liver (*L*), the spleen (*Sp*), the stomach (*S*), the aorta (*A*), the inferior vena cava (*C*) and the intrahepatic portal vein (*P*). **(B)** Slightly lower cut demonstrates many of the same structures, but, in addition, note the gallbladder (*G*), kidneys (*K*), the portal vein (*p*), and the body and tail of the pancreas (*arrows*) lying just anterior to the splenic vein (*sv*). **(C)** Lower cut demonstrates the duodenum (*D*), the aorta (*a*), the inferior vena cava (*C*), the left renal artery and vein (*arrows*), the superior mesenteric artery (*a*), and the superior mesenteric vein (*v*). **(D)** Many of the previously noted structures are again demonstrated, but specifically note the relationship of the superior mesenteric artery (*a*) and the superior mesenteric vein (*v*). Duodenum, *D*; head of the pancreas (*arrow*). **(E)** Axial cut just above the iliac wings demonstrates the inferior vena cava (*C*), the iliac arteries (*arrows*), the ascending and descending colon (*Co*), and the psoas muscles (*Ps*). **(F)** Pelvis in male. Note the bladder (*B*), rectum (*R*), and the prominent seminal vesicles (*Se*). **(G)** Axial pelvic cut in female demonstrates the bladder (*B*), rectum (*R*), and uterus (*U*).

REFERENCES

1. Carrico CW, Fenton LZ, Taylor GA, DiFore JW, Soprano JV. Impact of sonography on the diagnosis and treatment of acute lower abdominal pain in children and young adults. *AJR* 1999; 172:513–516.
2. Duran JD, Beidle TR, Perret R, Higgins J, Pfister R, Letourneau JG. Pictorial essay: CT imaging of acute right lower quadrant disease. *AJR* 1997;168:411–416.
3. Hendrick EP, Chong-Han C, Swischuk LE, John SD. Accuracy of ultrasound in acute right lower quadrant problems in children. *Emerg Radiol* 1999;6:350–354.
4. Mendelson RM, Lindsell DRM. Ultrasound examination of the paediatric "acute abdomen:" Preliminary findings. *Br J Radiol* 1987;60:414–416.
5. Nosaka S, Miyasaka M, Miyazaki O, Hayakawa M, Nakada K, Nakajima Y, Ishikawa T. Ultrasound in pediatric patients with suspected acute appendicitis: Value in establishing alternative diagnoses. *Emerg Radiol* 1999;4:207–211.
6. Rao PM, Turner MA. Right lower quadrant pain: Imaging with computed tomography. *Emerg Radiol* 1995;2:345–366.
7. See CC, Glassman M, Berezin S, Inamdar S, Newman LJ. Emergency ultrasound in the evaluation of acute-onset abdominal pain in children. *Pediatr Emerg Care* 1988;4:169–171.
8. Seibert JJ, Williamson SL, Golladay ES, Mollitt DL, Seibert RW, Sutterfield SL. The distended gasless abdomen: A fertile field for ultrasound. *J Ultrasound Med* 1986;5:301–308.

ACUTE ABDOMINAL PROBLEMS

Examination of the acute abdomen, regardless of cause, requires supine and upright views of the abdomen, and a posteroanterior view of the chest. This combined examination should never be cut short, and if the patient's condition is such that upright films cannot be obtained, cross-table lateral or decubitus views should be substituted. There is no room for a compromise, and the physician who cuts the examination short will regret it sooner or later. A lesser examination (1) has no place in the evaluation of the acute abdomen in infants and children.

After evaluation of these plain films, *one's best imaging tool is ultrasound, in which a negative study is as important as a positive study. Negative studies are helpful if clinical findings are equivocal, for they add support to the final impression that not much of significance is going on.*

REFERENCE

1. Mirvis SE, Young JWR, Keramati B, McCrea ES, Tarr R. Plain film evaluation of patients with abdominal pain: Are three radiographs necessary? *AJR* 1986;147:501–503.

ABNORMAL INTRALUMINAL GAS PATTERNS

Airless Abdomen

An airless abdomen usually is abnormal and most often results from excessive vomiting or diarrhea (Fig. 3.4). Many times this occurs with gastroenteritis, but an airless abdomen also can be seen in the early stages of acute appendicitis.

Paralytic Ileus

Generalized paralytic ileus can be seen with gastroenteritis, intestinal ischemia, neurogenic spinal shock, and conditions such as sepsis and hypokalemia (2). Paralytic ileus differs from mechanical ileus (mechanical obstruction) in that there is no differential distension of the gastrointestinal tract. *In other words, all portions of the gastrointestinal tract dilate in proportion to each other, and in the classic case the colon remains larger than the small bowel* (Fig. 3.5). Furthermore, the picture of dilated intestinal loops is much less orderly than in mechanical obstruction. In many cases, dilated, disorganized, sluggish intestinal loops seem to be present from top to bottom and side to side. On upright view, numerous air–fluid levels are seen, but the majority appear rather "inactive" and tend to extend over long lengths of bowel. In this regard, they are quite different from the short fluid levels seen in the acute, inverted, hairpin loops of the distended bowel seen with classic mechanical obstruction (Fig. 3.6).

Mechanical Ileus

Compared with paralytic ileus, the pattern of distended intestinal loops in mechanical obstruction is much more orderly, especially if one is dealing with small bowel obstruction. With low colonic obstruction, if ileocecal valve incompetence is present, there may be less orderliness and more difficulty in differentiating the findings from those of paralytic ileus, but in the classic case of small-bowel obstruction, the findings are rather typical (Fig. 3.6). The number of dilated loops visualized depends on the level of obstruction, but, in any case, the loops are visualized discretely and are rather orderly in appearance. If, as often occurs on the supine view, the loops are stacked one over the other, the term "stepladder" is applied to the configuration. In those cases in which obstruction has existed for a long period of time, no gas is seen distal to the obstruction, but if the duration of obstruction is short, or if the obstruction is incomplete, some gas may be seen in loops of intestine distal to the site

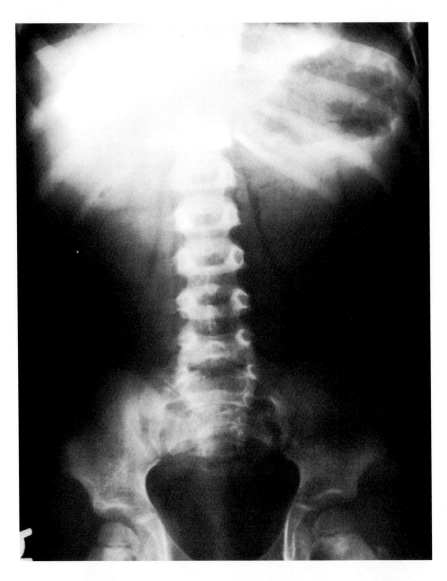

FIGURE 3.4. Airless abdomen. Gas is present in the stomach only (left upper quadrant). Most often, an airless abdomen is seen with gastroenteritis or acute appendicitis; this patient had gastroenteritis.

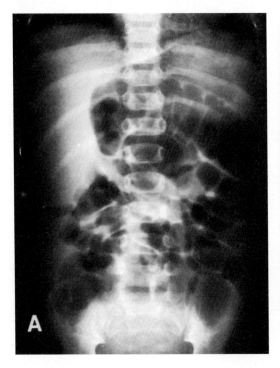

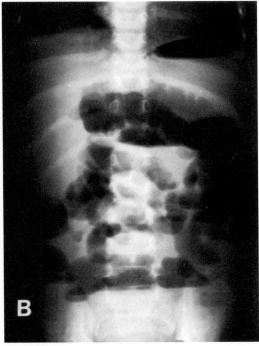

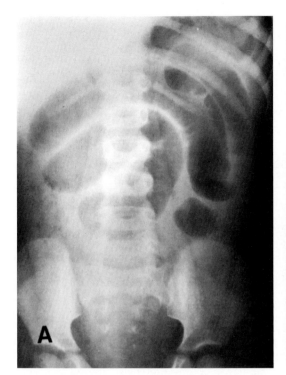
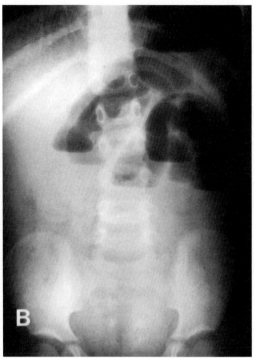

FIGURE 3.6. Mechanical ileus. **(A)** Note the well-organized loops of distended small bowel in the upper abdomen. No gas is seen distal to these loops, which are arranged in the so-called stepladder configuration. **(B)** Upright view showing persistence of the orderly pattern with acute inverted U- or hairpin-shaped loops characteristic of mechanically obstructed intestine. Also note that the air–fluid levels within any given loop are short and at different heights.

of obstruction. Of course, these intestinal loops are not distended.

On upright view, the loops of intestine form acute, hairpin loops with short air–fluid levels visible in both limbs of any given loop (Fig. 3.6). In addition, these fluid levels usually are at different heights in the two limbs of any given loop of intestine. This clearly demonstrates that mechanical obstruction is an active or dynamic process. In other words, in their effort to overcome the obstruction, the loops show hyperperistalsis, and as the intestinal contents churn back and forth, the air–fluid levels are captured at different heights in each limb of a loop.

One other point regarding obstructed loops of intestine is in order: In some cases, very little air is present in the distended intestinal loops, for they are filled with fluid. The loops of intestine may be seen as vague, opaque, sausagelike structures in the abdomen. On upright views, as the small amount of gas becomes trapped between the valvulae con-

niventes, a "string-of-beads" sign results (Fig. 3.7). On ultrasonography, such fluid-filled loops may be seen as markedly dilated, anechoic circular or sausagelike hyperperistaltic structures (Fig. 3.8A). With paralytic ileus, more uniform, circular, and less-dilated loops are seen, and peristalsis is diminished (Fig. 3.8B).

After determining that an intestinal obstruction is present, the second job for the radiologist is to determine its level. This is relatively easily accomplished with gastric and duodenal obstructions, but with small bowel and colonic obstructions it may be more difficult. Generally speaking, however, the number of loops visualized in these cases is the best clue to the level of obstruction: the lower the obstruction, the more loops one sees. In those cases of low small-bowel obstruction in which differentiation from colonic obstruction is difficult, one should not waste time trying to make the decision from plain films alone. A contrast study of the colon is most helpful in these cases and can identify problems such

FIGURE 3.5. *Paralytic ileus.* **(A)** Distended loops of intestine are present everywhere, but proportional distension persists, and the transverse colon (uppermost loop of distended intestine) remains larger than the numerous loops of distended small bowel. **(B)** Upright view showing numerous sluggish, long air–fluid levels scattered throughout the abdomen. Compare this adynamic appearance with the dynamic appearance of mechanical obstruction seen in Figure 3.6.

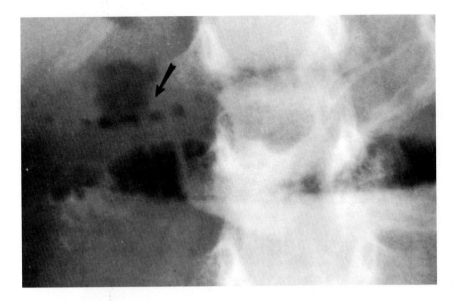

FIGURE 3.7. "String-of-beads" sign. On this upright view, note the string-of-beads effect of air trapped in between the valvulae conniventes (*arrow*).

as sigmoid volvulus, intussusception, Hirschsprung's disease, and so forth. Intussusception, however, in more and more cases now can be identified with confidence with ultrasound before contrast enema reduction is attempted. One of the reasons for performing an ultrasound study is that it can exclude the presence of intussusception and thus avoid any further investigation including a contrast enema (3).

Closed Loop Obstruction

If a loop of intestine is obstructed at both ends, it is termed a *closed loop* or *strangulated obstruction.* In many of these cases, the intestinal loop becomes gangrenous before the obstruction is diagnosed. Consequently, a closed loop obstruction is one of the most serious forms of mechanical obstruction of the intestinal tract, and the condition must

be recognized early. Closed loop obstructions can occur with colonic or small bowel volvulus or internal hernias, or if loops of intestine twist around congenital peritoneal bands or postoperative adhesions.

Roentgenographically, the hallmark of closed loop obstruction is the presence of a fixed, dilated loop of bowel, frequently assuming the shape of the letter U or a coffee bean. If such a loop is all that is visualized, the diagnosis is relatively easy (Fig. 3.9), but if a more classic small bowel obstruction begins to develop behind the strangulated loop, the loop itself may be difficult to isolate. In other cases, the loop is full of fluid, and although it still may retain its coffee-bean shape, more often it produces a less-specific mass on the abdominal roentgenogram. The closed loop, as a fixed loop with edematous walls, also is clearly visible on a CT scan (1).

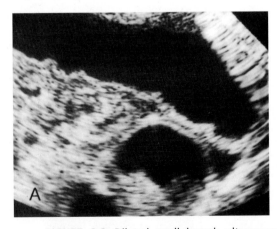 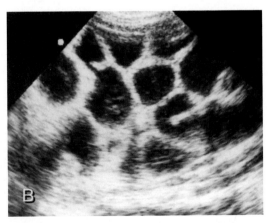

FIGURE 3.8. Dilated small bowel: ultrasonographic demonstration. **(A)** With small bowel obstruction, the fluid-filled loops are large and show considerable peristalsis. **(B)** With paralytic ileus, the fluid-filled loops are more numerous and of more uniform size and show far less in the way of peristalsis.

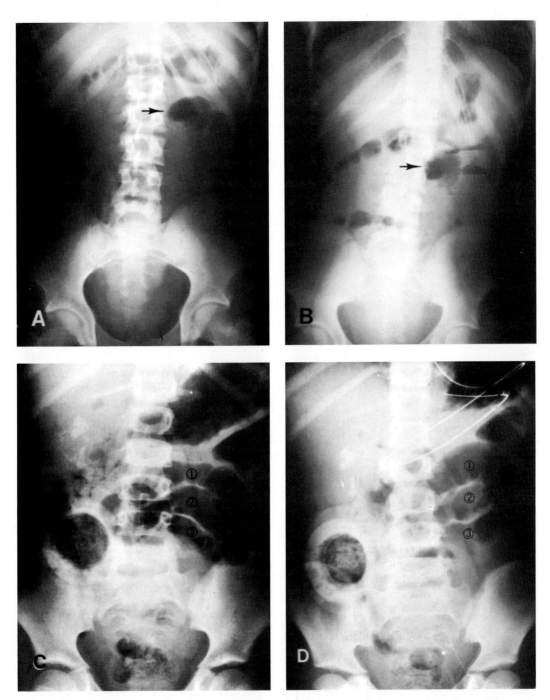

FIGURE 3.9. *Closed-loop obstruction: single and multiple loops.* (**A**) Note a single loop of distended jejunum (*arrow*) in this child with a closed-loop obstruction. A nasogastric tube is present in the stomach. (**B**) On upright view, note that the loop does not change position or configuration (*arrow*), and that its tapered end suggests a twisted or volved loop. One or two other loops of distended intestine with air–fluid levels are visualized, but it is the unchanging loop identified by the *arrow* that is most significant in indicating the presence of a closed-loop obstruction. (**C**) Another patient with postoperative adhesions leading to a closed-loop obstruction. Note the 1-2-3 arrangement of the distended loops of small bowel. (**D**) On upright view, the arrangement is essentially the same (i.e., fixed loops). Also note the colostomy bag and calculi in the right kidney.

Sentinel Loop

The term *sentinel loop* usually refers to a segment of intestine that becomes paralyzed and dilated as it lies next to an inflamed intraabdominal organ (3). It represents short segment paralytic ileus, and because it alerts one to the presence of an adjacent inflammatory process, it has been termed the sentinel loop. In the *right upper quadrant*, the sentinel loop can be seen with cholecystitis, pyelonephritis, and hepatic inflammatory or traumatic disease; in the *left upper quadrant*, it usually is seen with pancreatitis, pyelonephritis, or splenic injury. In the *right lower quadrant*, the sentinel loop classically occurs with appendicitis and mesenteric adenitis. Less often it is seen with regional enteritis and Meckel's diverticulitis. Sentinel loops in the left lower quadrant are much less common, but in the lower abdomen in female patients, genital problems such as salpingitis and hemorrhagic or torsed ovarian cysts or tumors also can produce a sentinel loop. In the upper midabdomen, most sentinel loops are seen with pancreatitis or trauma to the duodenum.

Roentgenographically, sentinel loops are visualized as isolated loops of distended intestine (Fig. 3.10A). It is most important, however, that if a sentinel loop is suspected it be demonstrated to remain in one position from film to film. This is most important, for it is not usual to see isolated loops of dilated intestine transiently and fortuitously on a single film of a patient (Fig. 3.10B). Such loops can appear in perfectly normal individuals or in patients with problems such as gastroenteritis, and thus *it is only if a sentinel loop persists that it is significant.*

A special form of the sentinel loop occurs as the so-called colon cutoff sign. Most often this sign has been believed to occur in the left transverse colon with pancreatitis, but it probably is more commonly seen on the right side with perforated appendicitis (see Fig. 3.50). A sentinel loop also can be seen in early intestinal obstruction (Fig. 3.9). In such cases, the visualized loop is the leading (sentinel) loop of an early intestinal obstruction and as such is quite valuable. Often it is overlooked, however, for it can be difficult to detect.

Acute Gastric Dilatation

Acute gastric dilatation can be seen in extremely sick individuals and reflects a profound degree of localized paralytic ileus. It can be a lethal condition, for it induces a vagal response that may result in cardiorespiratory arrest. Consequently, prompt treatment with nasogastric tube decompression is in order. Not all cases of a grossly dilated stomach, however, represent acute gastric dilatation. Indeed, dilatation of the stomach commonly is seen in gastroenteritis, some normal infants, and in infants and children with respiratory distress. In these latter cases, the finding results from excessive air swallowing. In addition, it has been noted that acute gastric dilatation can occur in emotionally neglected children (2). In these cases, gastric dilatation usually occurs after the first full meal. Evidently the stomach is not able to handle this unusually large food load, perhaps because there is some atrophy of the gastric muscle in these children (2). Once they get over the acute episode, they usually do not have further problems.

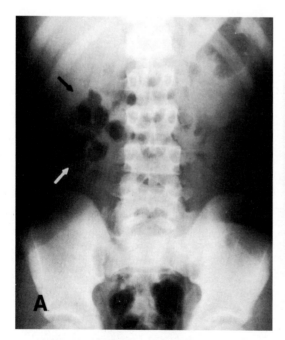
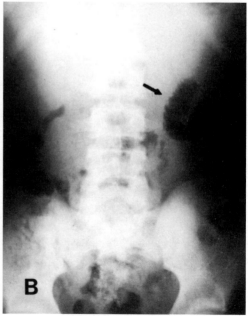

FIGURE 3.10. *Sentinel loops.* **(A)** Sentinel loops adjacent to intraabdominal inflammation. In this patient with suspected appendicitis, note the presence of a number of dilated loops of intestine in the right flank (*arrows*). These are sentinel loops lying adjacent to an inflamed appendix. **(B)** Pseudosentinel loop: fortuitous demonstration of an isolated loop of distended intestine. Note the single loop of distended jejunum on the left side of the abdomen (*arrow*) of this patient with gastroenteritis. Such fortuitous demonstration of a transiently dilated loop (or loops) of small bowel is not uncommon in gastroenteritis.

REFERENCES

1. Balthazare EK, Birnbaum BA, Megibow AJ, Gordon RB, Whelan CA, Hlnick DH. Closed-loop and strangulating intestinal obstruction: CT signs. *Radiology* 1992;185:769–775.
2. Franken EA Jr., Fox M, Smith JA, Smith WL. Acute gastric dilatation in neglected children. *AJR* 1978;130:297–299.
3. Young BR. Significance of regional or reflex ileus in roentgen diagnosis of cholecystitis, perforated ulcer, pancreatitis and appendiceal abscess, as determined by survey examination of acute abdomen. *AJR* 1957;78:581–586.

ABNORMAL EXTRALUMINAL GAS PATTERNS

Extraluminal air may lie in the intestinal wall itself (intramural) or, more often, completely outside the intestine. In the latter case, such air may be seen in the peritoneal cavity or retroperitoneal space and signifies the presence of a gastrointestinal perforation. Extraluminal, intramural air (pneumatosis cystoides intestinalis) usually is associated with a loss of intestinal mucosal integrity secondary to intestinal ischemia or severe inflammation with resulting necrotizing enterocolitis. Pneumatosis cystoides intestinalis also is seen in the absence of these problems, however, and in that case is termed "benign pneumatosis."

Portal vein gas most often occurs in association with intestinal infarction or necrotizing enterocolitis. Biliary-tree air usually is seen with intestinal obstructions of the duodenum distal to the ampulla of Vater.

Pneumoperitoneum (Free Peritoneal Air)

Pneumoperitoneum usually signifies the presence of gastrointestinal tract perforation but also occasionally can be seen secondary to pneumomediastinum. Gastrointestinal perforations usually occur with peptic ulcer disease, and occasionally with inflammatory disease such as Meckel's diverticulitis and appendicitis. They also can be seen with foreign body ingestion but most often are seen with abdominal trauma. Roentgenographically, the findings are virtually the same as in adults, but, in general, perforations resulting from nontraumatic causes are not nearly as common in children as in adults.

In the supine position, it is surprising to see how large a collection of free air may remain undetected. Such collections are most likely to occur in neonates and very young infants with gastric or colonic perforation, but the problem also can occur with small intestinal perforation associated with obstruction. In any of these cases, one may note an extremely sharp, almost diagrammatic appearance to a generally hyperlucent abdomen (Fig. 3.11). In addition, the fal-

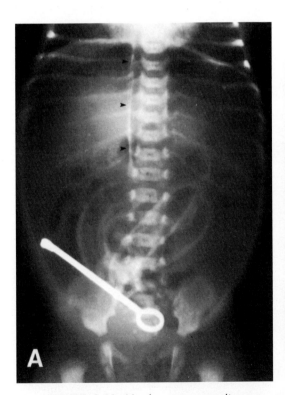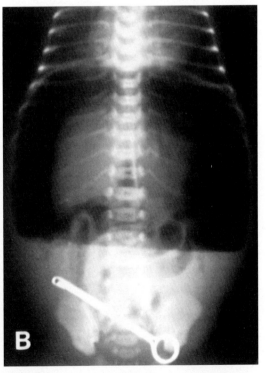

FIGURE 3.11. *Massive pneumoperitoneum: supine film findings.* **(A)** Note the hyperlucent appearance of the entire abdomen. Both aspects of the walls of the loops of intestine clustered in the center of the abdomen are well visualized. Because of this they appear as discrete linear and curvilinear white stripes. A similar phenomenon is seen along the falciform ligament (*arrows*). This aesthetically pleasing, almost diagrammatic appearance of the roentgenogram is characteristic of massive pneumoperitoneum but is overlooked with surprising regularity. **(B)** Upright view confirms the presence of a massive volume of free air in the peritoneal cavity. Note how the liver, spleen, and stomach have been compressed centrally.

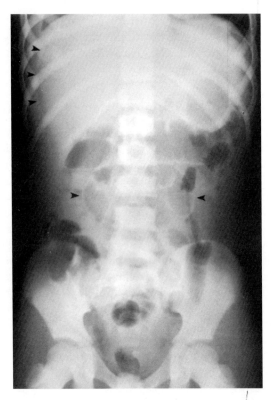

FIGURE 3.12. *Small-volume pneumoperitoneum: supine film findings.* Note the fine white line representing intestinal wall (*lower arrows*), visualized in this manner because air is present both inside the lumen of the intestine and along its outer surface in the peritoneal cavity. Also note the presence of free air overlying the liver anteriorly (*upper arrows*).

ciform ligament, urachus (6), or as an inverted V, the inferior epigastric arteries and lateral umbilical ligaments (1,14) can be outlined by air. Air also can collect in the fossa for the ligamentum teres as a vertical stripe of air over the liver (3). The overall configuration of massive pneumoperitoneum, as it appears on the supine roentgenogram of these infants, often is called the "saddlebag" or "football" sign (10).

In addition to the findings just noted, one usually sees loops of intestine with their walls outlined by air on both their serosal and mucosal surfaces (Fig. 3.11A). It is this finding that becomes most useful in the older child with lesser volumes of free air who is examined in the supine position. Before proceeding to this problem, one or two more points regarding massive pneumoperitoneum in the young infant might be considered: In some of these infants, air may extend into the scrotum or groin, for the processus vaginalis is patent in male infants of this age. In other infants, the abdominal viscera, especially the liver and spleen, become compressed toward the center of the abdomen. This finding often is more readily appreciated on upright or cross-table lateral views (Fig. 3.11B).

In the older child with lesser volumes of free air in the peritoneal cavity, the most useful finding on the supine film is visualization of both the outer and inner surfaces of a dilated loop of intestine (Fig. 3.12). A word of caution is in order regarding this sign, however, for it also can be present in the absence of pneumoperitoneum in children with grossly distended intestines. In such cases, one loop is visualized through another (4), and because these loops contain so much air, segments of the bowel wall appear to be outlined by air on both sides (Fig. 3.13). In other cases of

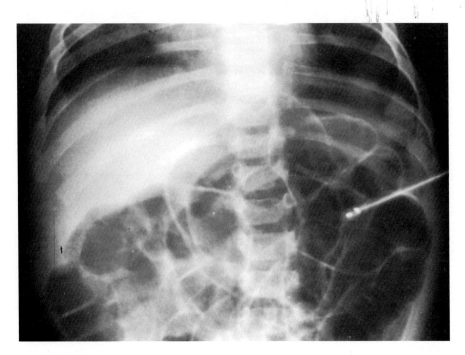

FIGURE 3.13. *Pseudofree air on supine film.* The grossly distended intestines in this patient cause the walls of each loop to be projected through other loops. This being the case, the walls appear to be outlined by air on both sides. No free air is present, but the finding is misleading and often misinterpreted as free air.

pneumoperitoneum, air is seen to collect over the anterior surface, or along the inferior aspect, of the liver (9), and as such appears as a variety of formless or linear parahepatic collections of air (Fig. 3.14A).

On *upright view,* of course, free intraperitoneal air characteristically collects beneath the diaphragmatic leaflets (Fig. 3.14B), but if upright positioning is impossible to accomplish because of the patient's condition, crosstable lateral or decubitus views demonstrate the same findings (Fig. 3.15). Indeed, with proper upright or decubitus positioning, it is said that as little as 1 mL of free air can be detected. Of course, the patient must remain in one of these positions for more than just a few seconds, for otherwise the air does not trickle up to the uppermost portion of the abdomen. In addition to these considerations, in adults it recently has been demonstrated that the upright lateral is more sensitive than the upright posteroanterior film for the detection of free intraperitoneal air (17).

Small collections of air beneath the diaphragmatic leaflet (Fig. 3.16A) must be differentiated from certain normal, almost artifactual findings. One of these occurs if a diaphragmatic leaflet is visualized just over the lower edge of a rib (Fig. 3.16B); another occurs if the gastric bubble is visualized under the left diaphragmatic leaflet (Fig. 3.16C). In differentiating the stomach bubble from pneumoperitoneum, it should be noted that the combined thickness of the distended stomach and diaphragm usually is thicker than that of the diaphragm alone (Fig. 3.16C).

Most cases of pneumoperitoneum eventually are associated with peritonitis, for they result from perforation of the gastrointestinal tract, but occasionally one can encounter pneumoperitoneum without peritonitis. This can occur with pneumatosis cystoides intestinalis, with pneumomediastinum, and after laparotomy. With regard to pneumatosis cystoides intestinalis, it is not the intestine that perforates but merely the outer serosal surface, and thus free air may escape into the peritoneal cavity but no intestinal content escapes.

The mechanism of pneumoperitoneum in cases of pneumomediastinum is poorly understood, but it has been suggested that air may track into the abdomen along the aorta and abdominal vessels, or that there actually may be a congenital pleural–peritoneal communication present. At any rate, whatever the precise cause, massive amounts of peri-

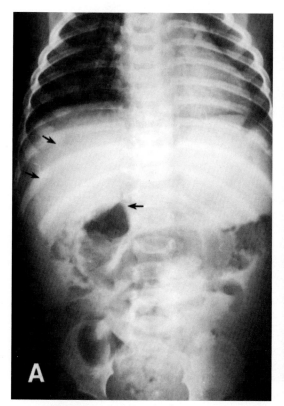 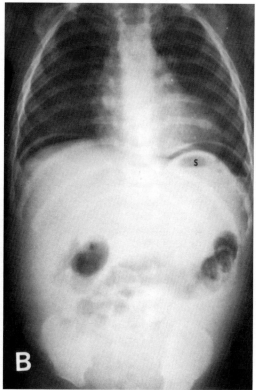

FIGURE 3.14. *Free peritoneal air: utilizing the upright view.* **(A)** On this supine view, it may be difficult to detect that free air is present. Some is present, however, over the anterior aspect of the liver (*upper arrows*), and some can be seen under the liver along its inferior medial aspect (*lower arrow*). This air probably outlines the gallbladder. **(B)** Upright positioning clearly identifies the presence of free air as it accumulates in characteristic fashion under both diaphragmatic leaflets. Stomach air bubble (*S*).

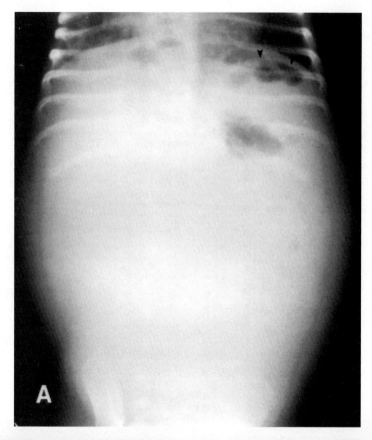

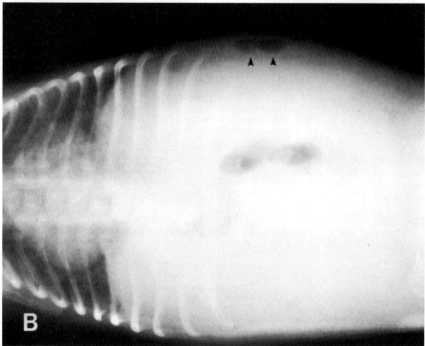

FIGURE 3.15. *Free peritoneal air: value of decubitus views.* **(A)** In this patient with intestinal perforation and peritonitis, the presence of free air in the abdominal cavity may be difficult to detect. The air demarcated by the arrows, however, turns out to be free air on the decubitus view. **(B)** Decubitus view demonstrating how the collection of free air has shifted in position and come to lie just below the abdominal wall (*arrows*).

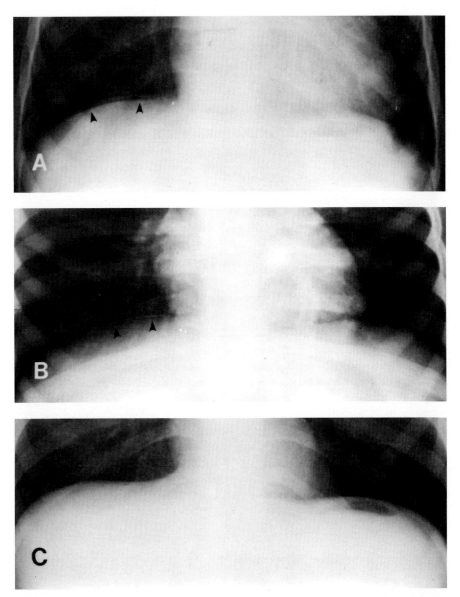

FIGURE 3.16. Small-volume pneumoperitoneum versus artifact. (**A**) Note the thin sliver of free air under the right diaphragmatic leaflet (*arrows*). Note how thin the diaphragmatic leaflet appears. (**B**) Pseudo–free air resulting from superimposition of the top of the right diaphragmatic leaflet over the lower aspect of the underlying rib (*arrows*). (**C**) Pseudopneumoperitoneum produced by gas in the stomach. Note that the white line (*arrows*) above the collection of gas in the stomach is thicker than that seen in **A**. It is thicker because it represents both the gastric wall and the diaphragmatic leaflet. The bolus of food present in the stomach further adds to the illusion that free air is present under the diaphragmatic leaflet.

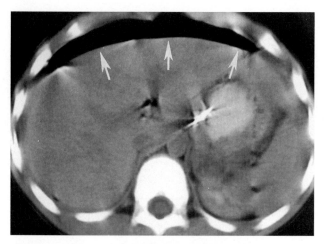

FIGURE 3.17. *Free air: CT demonstration.* Note the large collection of free air anteriorly (*arrows*).

toneal air can accumulate this way, and it is remarkable that both the pneumomediastinum and the pneumoperitoneum so incurred can remain rather silent. In addition, in some of these cases the presence of the initial lesion, that is, pneumomediastinum, may be difficult to detect, and only the pneumoperitoneum is seen. Free air also is clearly demonstrable with CT scanning but must be differentiated from normal fat (Fig. 3.17).

Retroperitoneal Free Air

Free air in the retroperitoneal space is much less commonly encountered than is free intraperitoneal air. Often such air layers itself against the psoas muscles or kidneys (Fig. 3.18), and in the more subtle cases it can be missed even by the experienced observer. Retroperitoneal free air can be seen with perforation of the duodenum, retrocecal appendicitis, or perforation of the rectum (Fig. 3.18B). It also can be seen with pneumomediastinum (Fig. 3.18A).

On supine view, if retroperitoneal air collects beneath the diaphragmatic leaflet, the leaflet itself is outlined (Fig. 3.18A). In addition, one also may visualize the inferior aspect of the heart border as a clear, distinct line (7). Retroperitoneal air also is vividly demonstrable on CT studies (Fig. 3.19).

Intramural Air (Pneumatosis Cystoides Intestinalis)

"Pneumatosis cystoides intestinalis" is a term utilized to designate the presence of intramural intestinal gas. Most frequently such gas is seen with loss of mucosal integrity as incurred by extensive inflammatory or ischemic disease of the intestine (13), and classically it is a feature of necrotizing enterocolitis of the premature or newborn infant. Pneumatosis cystoides intestinalis secondary to enterocolitis also is seen in some infants with Hirschsprung's disease, and is a feature of ischemia induced by mechanical catastrophes such as closed-loop strangulation or intestinal volvulus. Pneumatosis cystoides intestinalis also can be seen in older infants and children (15) in association with intestinal obstruction, collagen vascular diseases (5,11), cystic fibrosis (5,16), leukemia, or steroid or other immunosuppressive therapy (5,8) and occasionally with gastroenteritis (2).

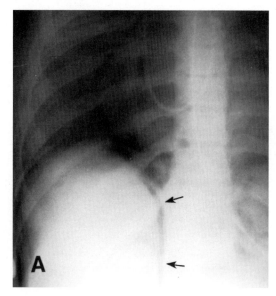
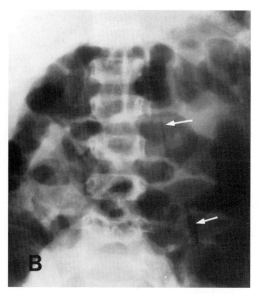

FIGURE 3.18. *Retroperitoneal air.* **(A)** Note air outlining the liver, right diaphragmatic leaflet, and right kidney (*arrows*). This air tracked from a pneumomediastinum resulting from ventilator therapy in a patient with a closed head injury. **(B)** Another patient with retroperitoneal air along the left psoas muscle (*arrows*). This resulted from a rectal perforation in a battered child.

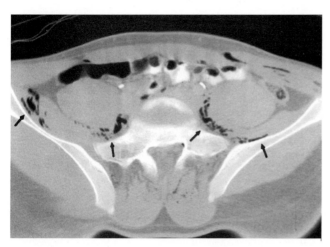

FIGURE 3.19. *Retroperitoneal free air: CT demonstration.* Note extensive retroperitoneal free air (*arrows*) surrounding the kidneys and in between the iliac bones and muscles.

With obstruction, simple intestinal overdistension is believed to lead to mucosal tears and leakage of intraluminal gas into the bowel wall (12). Most often, this is seen with chronic small bowel obstructions. Dilatation with loss of integrity of the mucosa also is believed to lead to pneumatosis cystoides intestinalis in children with collagen vascular diseases, but it should be noted that some of these patients also develop pneumatosis cystoides intestinalis secondary to intestinal ischemia and necrotizing enterocolitis.

Pneumatosis cystoides intestinalis in cystic fibrosis and in children on steroids or other immunosuppressive therapy is of unknown cause. With immunosuppressive therapy, it has been suggested that atrophy of submucosal lymphoid tissue may render the mucosa prone to tear more easily with overdistension. Pneumatosis cystoides intestinalis secondary to pneumomediastinum, with or without obstructive emphysema, is uncommonly seen in children. Because pneumatosis in many of these children is not related to intestinal ischemia, it is a relatively benign finding.

The classic roentgenographic appearance of pneumatosis cystoides intestinalis consists of linear or curvilinear collections of gas within the bowel wall (Fig. 3.20).

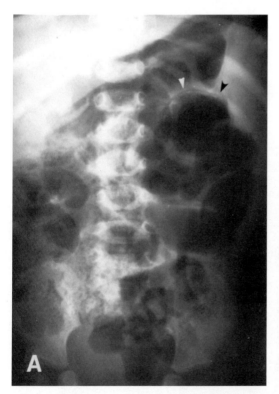
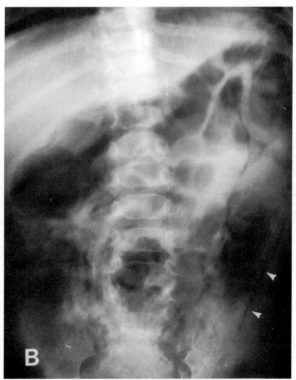

FIGURE 3.20. *Pneumatosis cystoides intestinalis (intramural air).* **(A)** Note classic curvilinear collections of air within distended loops of intestine (*arrows*). The bubbly pattern over the remainder of the abdomen often is misinterpreted as feces mixed with air but actually represents another configuration of pneumatosis cystoides intestinalis. **(B)** Typical curvilinear collections of free air are seen in the ascending colon, and linear collections of air are noted in the descending colon (*arrows*). *(continued on next page)*

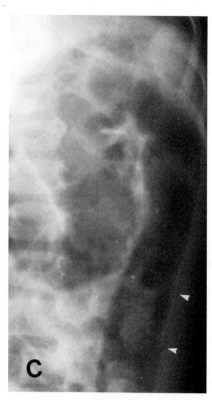

FIGURE 3.20. (continued) (C) Normal properitoneal fat line mimicking pneumatosis cystoides intestinalis. In this normal infant, the properitoneal fat line (*arrows*) might be misinterpreted as pneumatosis cystoides intestinalis.

Unfortunately, not all patients present with this configuration, and in others the collection of gas appears so bubbly that it is difficult to differentiate it from food in the stomach, fecal material in the colon, or an intraabdominal abscess (Fig. 3.20). Linear air collections must be differentiated from the normal properitoneal fat stripe (Fig. 3.20C).

Pneumatosis cystoides intestinalis occasionally can be limited to the stomach, and although in most such cases it merely is a part of more generalized, widespread enterocolitis, in others it truly is an isolated phenomenon. In these latter cases, it is believed to result from chronic overdistension of the stomach, such as is seen with infantile pyloric stenosis.

Portal Vein and Biliary Tract Gas

Portal vein gas is a common finding in necrotizing enterocolitis of infancy but can be seen with small bowel necrosis resulting from any number of causes. For this reason, it usually is seen hand-in-hand with pneumatosis cystoides intestinalis. Presumably, in these cases, gas enters the portal circulation from the intestinal wall, either through the veins or lymphatics, and then passes into the liver (Fig. 3.21). Biliary tract gas is quite uncommon and usually is seen with duodenal obstructions distal to the entrance of the common bile duct.

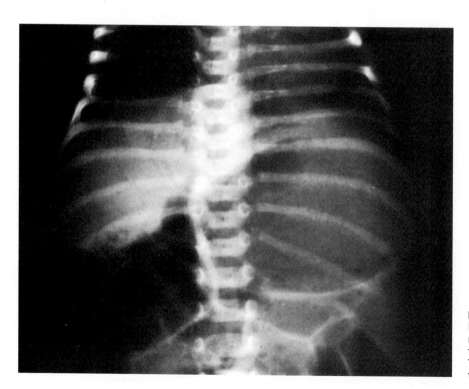

FIGURE 3.21. *Portal vein gas.* Note the linear collections of gas in the portal vein radicles of the liver. Characteristically, they radiate toward the porta hepatis. This patient had necrotizing enterocolitis.

REFERENCES

1. Bray JF. The "inverted V" sign of pneumoperitoneum. *Radiology* 1984;151: 45–46.
2. Capitanio MA, Greenberg SB. Pneumatosis intestinalis in two infants with rotovirus gastroenteritis. *Pediatr Radiol* 1991;21: 361–362.
3. Cho KC, Baker SR. Air in the fissure for the ligamentum teres: New sign of intraperitoneal air on plain radiographs. *Radiology* 1991;178:489–492.
4. De Lacey G, Bloomberg T, Wignall BK. Pneumoperitoneum: The misleading double wall sign. *Clin Radiol* 1977;28:445–448.
5. Gupta A. Pneumatosis intestinalis in children. *Br J Radiol* 1978; 51:589–595.
6. Jelasco DV, Schultz EH Jr. The urachus: An aid to the diagnosis of pneumoperitoneum. *Radiology* 1969;92: 295–296.
7. Klein DL. Visibility of the inferior heart border in pneumoperitoneum. *AJR* 1981;137:622–623.
8. Kleinman PK, Brill PW, Winchester P. Pneumatosis intestinalis: Its occurrence in the immunologically compromised child. *Am J Dis* Child 1980;134:1149–1151.
9. Menuck L, Siemers PT. Pneumoperitoneum: Importance of right upper quadrant features. *AJR* 1976;127:753–756.
10. Miller RE. Perforated viscus in infants: A new roentgen sign. *Radiology* 1960;74:65–67.
11. Mueller CF, Morehead R, Alter AJ, Michener W. Pneumatosis intestinalis in collagen disorders. *AJR* 1972;115:300–305.
12. Richmond JA, Mikity V. Benign form of necrotizing enterocolitis. *AJR* 1975;123:301–306.
13. Touloukian RJ, Posch JN, Spencer R. The pathogenesis of ischemic gastroenterocolitis of the neonate: Selective gut mucosal ischemia in asphyxiated neonatal piglets. *J Pediatr Surg* 1972;7: 194–205.
14. Weiner CI, Diaconis JN, Dennis JM. The "inverted V:" A new sign of pneumoperitoneum. *Radiology* 1973;197:47–48.
15. West KW, Rescorla FJ, Grosfeld JL, Vane DW. Pneumatosis intestinalis in children beyond the neonatal period. *J Pediatr Surg* 1989;24:818–822.
16. Wood RE, Herman CJ, Johnson KW, di Sant Agnese PA. Pneumatosis coli in cystic fibrosis. *Am J Dis Child* 1975;129: 246–248.
17. Woodring JH, Heiser MJ. Detection of pneumoperitoneum on chest radiographs: comparison of upright, lateral and posteroanterior projections. *AJR* 1995;165:45–47.

THICKENED AND PSEUDOTHICKENED BOWEL WALLS

True thickening of the intestinal wall can be seen with any type of inflammatory disease of the intestine, chronic intestinal obstruction, and intestinal ischemia or infarction (Fig. 3.22A). Bowel wall thickening now usually is more clearly visible with ultrasound (Fig. 3.22B).

Pseudothickening of the bowel wall is seen with ascites or peritonitis, or if loops of distended intestine contain

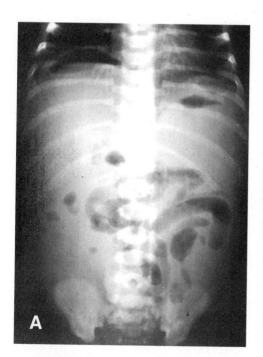
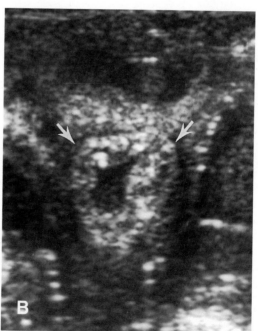

FIGURE 3.22. *True thickening of intestinal wall.* **(A)** Note that on this upright view the space between the air-filled loops of intestine is increased. False intestinal thickening would not persist on the upright view. This infant had necrotizing enterocolitis, and the intestine was thickened. **(B)** Ultrasound demonstration of circumferential mucosal thickening (*arrows*) in a segment of small bowel in a patient with gastroenteritis.

more fluid than air (1). In the first instance, as the loops of air-filled bowel float in the peritoneal fluid, they become separated to such a degree that bowel wall thickening is suggested (Fig. 3.23A). In the second case, bowel wall thickening is suggested if small amounts of gas collect at the top of a primarily fluid-filled loop of intestine. The cap of free air in each such loop is so small that an optical illusion suggesting thickened bowel wall occurs (Fig. 3.23B and C). All of these findings are summarized in Fig. 3.24, but it should be noted that if true bowel wall thickening is present, it tends to persist on the upright or other gravity-dependent view (Fig. 3.22A).

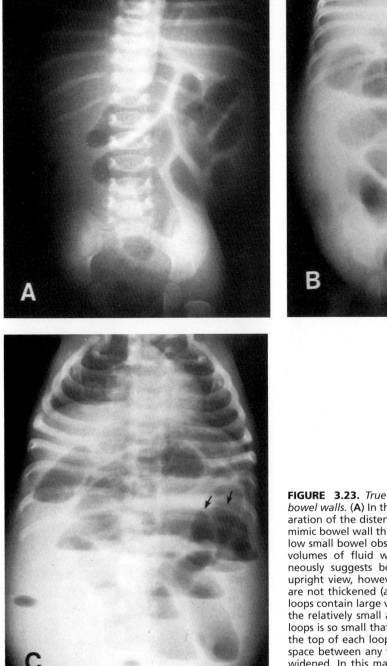

FIGURE 3.23. *True versus pseudothickening of bowel walls.* **(A)** In this infant, ascites is causing separation of the distended loops of intestine so as to mimic bowel wall thickening. **(B)** In this infant with low small bowel obstruction, the presence of large volumes of fluid within the dilated loops erroneously suggests bowel wall thickening. **(C)** On upright view, however, note that the bowel walls are not thickened (*arrows*), but that the intestinal loops contain large volumes of fluid. In these cases, the relatively small amount of air in the intestinal loops is so small that on supine view, as it floats to the top of each loop, the fluid under it causes the space between any two given air collections to be widened. In this manner, bowel-wall thickening is suggested but actually is not present (see Fig. 3.24A for diagrammatic depiction of this phenomenon).

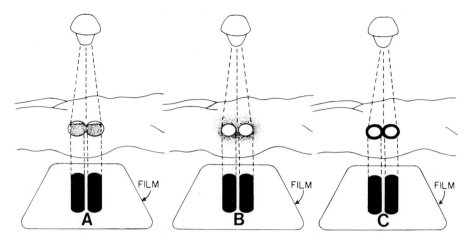

FIGURE 3.24. *True versus pseudothickening of bowel walls: diagrammatic representation.* **(A)** If large volumes of fluid are present in intestinal loops and only small amounts of gas float on top of this fluid, the resultant roentgenographic image is such that the space between the loops of intestine appears widened, and bowel wall thickening is suggested. The bowel wall, however, is not thickened. **(B)** With ascitic fluid between the bowel loops, the loops themselves are separated, and because the space between them is widened, bowel wall thickening once again is suggested erroneously. **(C)** True thickening of the bowel wall. The widened space between the loops of air-filled intestine truly represents thick intestinal walls. (From Hoffman RB, Wankmuller R, Rigler LG. Pseudoseparation of bowel loops: A fallacious sign of intraperitoneal fluid. *Radiology* 1966;87:845–847, with permission.)

REFERENCE

1. Hoffman RB, Wankmuller R, Rigler LG. Pseudoseparation of bowel loops: A fallacious sign of intraperitoneal fluid. *Radiology* 1966;87:845–847.

ABDOMINAL FLUID COLLECTIONS (ASCITES, PERITONITIS, HEMOPERITONEUM)

The roentgenographic findings of fluid in the abdomen are much the same from case to case and depend primarily on the volume, not the type, of fluid present (2). Types of fluid that might be encountered include serous effusions, chyle, urine, bile, blood, and pus. With massive fluid collections the diagnosis is relatively easy, for the abdomen becomes distended and opaque, and the normally visible liver edge and retroperitoneal structures become obscured (Fig. 3.25A). If distended loops of intestine also are present, they tend to float toward the center of the abdomen (Fig. 3.25B) and in so doing result in the clinically percussible "tympanic cap." In addition to these findings, in many cases one is able to delineate the edge of the medially displaced liver (Fig. 3.25B). This subtle finding is present more often than is generally appreciated and results from the fact that the densities of the liver and adjacent fluid are just different enough that a roentgenographically perceptible interface between them develops (4,7).

With lesser volumes of fluid, the findings on supine views of the abdomen often are subtle, and in this regard it should be noted that fluid first accumulates in the pelvis in the peritoneal cul-de-sac (Fig. 3.26A). If enough fluid accumulates here the cul-de-sac bulges laterally; the term "dog ears" has been used for this finding (Fig. 3.27A). It is not an easy finding to note, however, and in young infants it is almost impossible to detect. This is no longer a problem, however, because ultrasonography and CT scanning are far superior for the detection of peritoneal fluid in its various nooks and crannies of the abdomen.

With larger fluid collections, fluid accumulations tend to pass upward between the abdominal wall and both the ascending and descending portions of the colon (Figs. 3.26B and 3.27B). Eventually fluid reaches the liver, and as it collects along the inferior aspect of this organ its entire inferior edge become invisible (Figs. 3.25 and 3.26C). At the same time, fluid accumulates between the abdominal wall and liver and causes medial displacement of the liver (Figs. 3.25 and 3.26). Meanwhile, the accumulating fluid also tends to gather in between and cause separation of the centrally floating loops of intestine (Fig. 3.25). Currently, ultrasonography is the best tool for detecting the presence of peritoneal fluid of any volume. It is especially useful in detecting small fluid collections in and around the liver, in the lesser sac, and in the peritoneal cul-de-sac. Various configurations of such free abdominal fluid are presented in Figs. 3.28 through 3.30. If the fluid is dirty (echogenic),

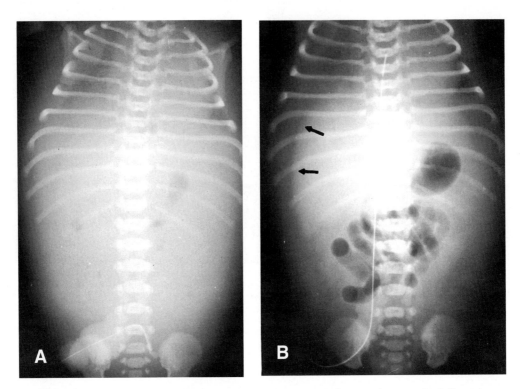

FIGURE 3.25. *Massive ascites.* **(A)** Massive ascites in a young infant produces marked distension and opacity of the abdomen, obliteration of the inferior liver edge, and obliteration of all the retroperitoneal structures. In the right upper quadrant, one can see a slight difference in density between the medially displaced liver and the adjacent ascitic fluid. **(B)** With more penetration of the abdomen, the interface between the liver and ascitic fluid is visualized more clearly (*arrows*). In addition, note that some air is now present in the intestines and that the air-filled loops of intestine cluster and float in the center of the abdomen.

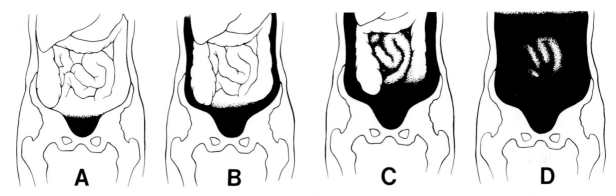

FIGURE 3.26. *Peritoneal fluid accumulation: sequence of findings.* **(A)** In early cases, in the supine position, fluid accumulates in the cul-de-sac. **(B)** With larger volumes, fluid begins to track upward and accumulates primarily between the abdominal wall and the ascending colon on the right, and the abdominal wall and descending colon on the left. **(C)** With even greater volumes of fluid, displacement of the ascending and descending colon medially becomes more pronounced, and fluid begins to accumulate beneath and around the liver. **(D)** With massive peritoneal fluid accumulations, the entire abdomen becomes filled with fluid, gas is forced out of the ascending and descending colon, and the few remaining air-filled loops of small bowel cluster and float in the center of the abdomen.

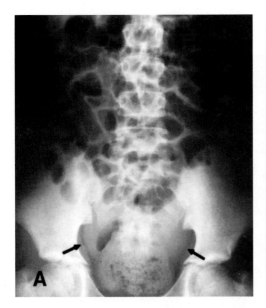
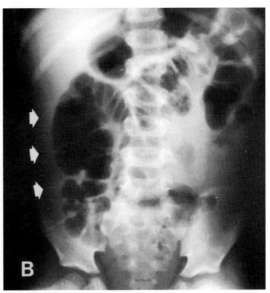

FIGURE 3.27. (A) Fluid in peritoneal cul-de-sac: the so-called dog-ears sign. Fluid first accumulates in the peritoneal cul-de-sac, and if the cul-de-sac bulges laterally, a dog ear-like configuration is suggested (*arrows*). **(B)** Fluid collecting between ascending colon and abdominal wall. This patient was in an automobile accident and had hemoperitoneum. The best evidence for the presence of peritoneal blood (fluid) lies in the increased distance between the right abdominal wall and the ascending colon (*arrows*).

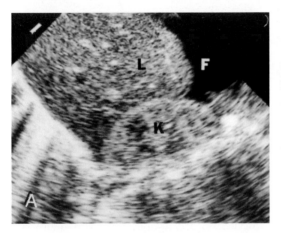
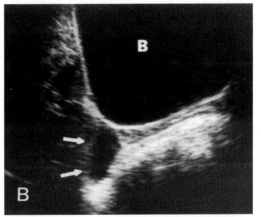

FIGURE 3.28. *Abdominal fluid: ultrasonographic findings.* **(A)** Note fluid (*arrows*) anterior to the liver (*L*) and kidney (*K*) in this young infant. **(B)** Adolescent girl with ruptured ovarian cyst, demonstrating fluid in the cul-de-sac (*arrows*). *B*, bladder.

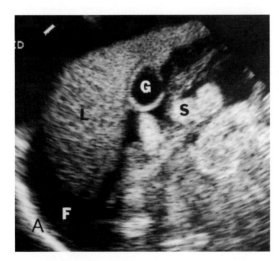
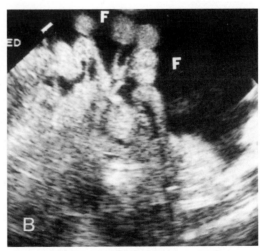

FIGURE 3.29. *Ascites: ultrasonographic findings.* **(A)** Free fluid (*F*) virtually surrounds the liver (*L*). There also is fluid between the gallbladder (*G*) and the echogenic small intestine (*S*). **(B)** Another view through the midabdomen demonstrates massive ascitic fluid (*F*), with the mesentery and loops of bowel floating in the fluid.

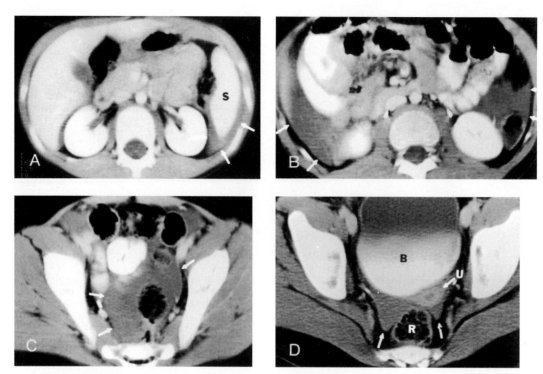

FIGURE 3.30. *Abdominal fluid: CT demonstration.* **(A)** Note hypodense fluid (*arrows*) around the spleen (*S*). There also is a little fluid between the liver and the kidney on the other side. **(B)** Large volume of paracolic fluid on both sides. **(C)** Same patient demonstrating a large collection of fluid (*arrows*) in the pelvis separating the various contrast and air-filled loops of intestine. **(D)** Classic fluid in the cul-de-sac (*arrows*) between the bladder (*B*) and rectum (*R*). The uterus (*U*) lies just off midline.

one should consider perforation or purulent exudate. CT study also vividly displays these fluid collections, but a problem can be encountered with fluid over the liver and its differentiation from pleural fluid (Fig. 3.31). This does not occur with ultrasound, for in the sagittal plane fluid is clearly defined to be either above or below the diaphragm.

Serous ascitic effusions in children can be seen with many conditions including (a) renal disease, (b) liver disease with portal hypertension, (c) portal vein obstruction, (d) hypoproteinemia, (e) protein-losing enteropathy, (f) congestive heart failure, and (g) pancreatitis (2,9). Chylous ascites usually occurs on a congenital basis and results from congenital

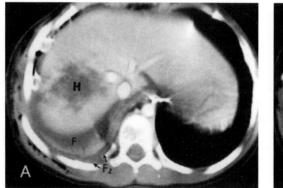
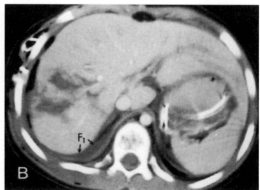

FIGURE 3.31. *Pleural versus peritoneal fluid: CT findings.* **(A)** Note the liver contusion–hematoma (*H*) and free abdominal fluid (*F*) between the liver and diaphragm. Also note pleural fluid (*F2*) above the diaphragm and some periportal tracking of blood along the portal vein branches. **(B)** Lower cut again demonstrates the liver contusion. In addition, note fluid (*F1*) between the diaphragmatic leaflet and liver.

defects or obstructions of the thoracic duct (2), but it also can occur secondary to abdominal trauma, and with intestinal lymphangiectasia. In any of these cases, if fat content is high enough, the chylous fluid may appear more radiolucent than the adjacent liver, both on plain films and CT scans.

Urine ascites is another cause of peritoneal fluid accumulation and most commonly occurs with urinary tract obstruction (2,3), but of course it also can be seen with renal or urinary bladder injuries secondary to abdominal trauma. If peritoneal fluid accumulation results from rupture of the urinary tract with urinary tract obstruction, it is believed that there is extravasation of urine into the perirenal space and then, through normal congenital defects, into the peritoneal cavity. Bile ascites can occur on a congenital basis from obstruction, tears, or defects of the bile ducts (1,5,9), but it also can result from bile duct injuries secondary to abdominal trauma.

Peritonitis in childhood may occur secondary to gastrointestinal perforations or as a primary infection. In the latter cases, the causative organism often, but not always, is *Streptococcus pneumoniae,* and these primary infections are especially likely to develop in children with the nephrotic syndrome (9). Tuberculous peritonitis uncommonly is seen in childhood in the United States, but if it occurs it tends to produce a more adhesive peritoneal reaction; consequently, the loops of bowel, instead of floating freely in the fluid, tend to remain more fixed from view to view. Peritonitis secondary to ascaris infection (6,8) also is uncommon in the United States, and meconium peritonitis, of course, is a problem of neonates.

Hemoperitoneum is seen most often secondary to abdominal trauma with splenic or liver injury. It also can be seen, however, with injuries to the mesenteric vessels and aorta. The clinical setting, of course, is what alerts one to the diagnosis, for the roentgenographic findings are similar to those of any other abdominal fluid collection.

Very few conditions can mimic the presence of free peritoneal fluid, but in some patients with voluminous collections of fluid in the bowel the findings at first might suggest free peritoneal fluid. This can occur with severe viral gastroenteritis, infection with *Shigella* sp, or small-bowel obstruction, and ultrasonography is excellent in demonstrating the fluid-filled intestinal loops (Fig. 3.8).

In addition to these situations, it should be mentioned that in some patients with large, extremely thin-walled mesenteric or lymphangiectatic cysts, the cysts may be so fluctuant that peritoneal fluid is mimicked both clinically and roentgenographically (2). Even paracentesis, the final tool in the investigation of any abdominal fluid collection, may not solve the problem. This occurs because as the cyst is drained it becomes so flaccid that no residual "mass" remains, and it appears that ascites was the problem. Unfortunately, such fluid almost always recurs, and it may require numerous paracenteses before one realizes that the real problem is a thin-walled lymphangiectatic mesenteric cyst.

REFERENCES

1. Esposito G. Biliary peritonitis in a child due to spontaneous perforation of the bile duct. *Ann Chir Inf* 1972;13:339–346.
2. Franken EA. Ascites in infants and children: Roentgen diagnosis. *Radiology* 1972;102:393–398.
3. Friedland GW, Tune B, Mears EM. Ascites due to spontaneous rupture of the renal pelvis in an 11-month-old infant with uretero-pelvic junctional obstruction. *Pediatr Radiol* 1974;2: 263–264.
4. Love L, Demos TC, Reynes CJ, Williams V, Shkoinik A, Gandhi V, Zerofos N. Visualization of the lateral edge of the liver in ascites. *Radiology* 1977;122:619–622.
5. Moore TC. Massive bile peritonitis in infancy due to spontaneous bile duct perforation with portal vein occlusion. *J Pediatr Surg* 1975;10:537–538.
6. Parashar SK, Nadkarni SV, Varma RA. Primary roundworm peritonitis. *Indian J Surg* 1974;36:200–201.
7. Porto AV, Lane EJ. Visualization of differences in soft-tissue densities: The liver in ascites. *Radiology* 1976;121:19–23.
8. Rao PLNG, Satyanarayana G, Venkatesh A. Intraperitoneal ascariasis. *J Pediatr Surg* 1988;23:936–938.
9. Rubin M, Blau EB, Michaels RH. Hemophilus and pneumococcal peritonitis in children with the nephrotic syndrome. *Pediatrics* 1975;56:598–601.

ABDOMINAL ABSCESS

Most abdominal abscesses are not visible on plain films. In the classic case an abdominal abscess has a bubbly, amorphous pattern, but in other instances only a mass displacing adjacent intestines is seen (Fig. 3.32). The granular appearance must be differentiated from a somewhat similar appearance seen in normal patients if gas is mixed with (a) fecal material in the colon, (b) food in the stomach, or (c) a bezoar in the gastrointestinal tract. Abscesses in the right lower quadrant usually result from perforation of the appendix or a Meckel's diverticulum and are dealt with in the section of this chapter on appendicitis. In the right upper quadrant, an abscess may be subhepatic or intrahepatic. Intrahepatic abscesses may be bacterial or amebic in origin and currently are best imaged with ultrasound or CT scanning. On plain films, one may be presented with a large liver, elevated right diaphragmatic leaflet, and associated changes in the right lung base (Fig. 3.33). Pyogenic abscesses may be encountered in totally normal children, but it also should be noted that one of the classic presentations of children with chronic granulomatous disease of childhood (neutrophil dysfunction) is liver abscess. Amebic liver abscess also can be seen in children, but liver abscess secondary to ascaris infection is uncommon. Subhepatic abscesses can develop after perforation of a retrocecal appendix, a duodenal ulcer, or the gallbladder.

Abscesses in the upper midabdomen usually are located in the lesser sac or in, and around, the pancreas. Lesser sac abscesses may result from perforation of duodenal ulcers; pancreatic abscesses result from more fulminant forms of

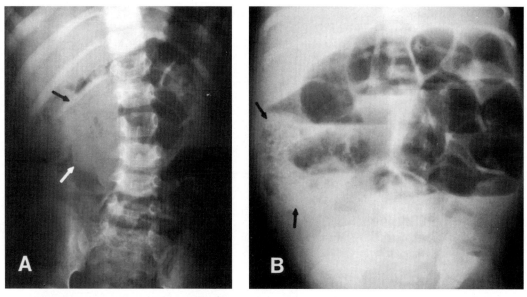

FIGURE 3.32. *Abdominal abscess: varying plain film configurations.* **(A)** Masslike effect of "walled-off" abdominal abscess (*arrows*) secondary to perforated appendicitis. Note pronounced ipsilateral scoliosis secondary to spasm of the psoas muscle. **(B)** Typical granular appearance of an abscess (*arrows*) in the right lower quadrant secondary to intestinal perforation in a young infant.

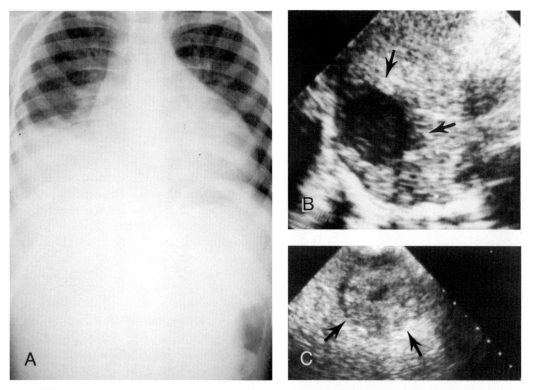

FIGURE 3.33. *Hepatic abscess.* **(A)** Plain film findings. Note the elevated right diaphragmatic leaflet and enlargement of the liver. Also note secondary changes in the right lung base. **(B)** Ultrasonogram in a patient with a liver abscess demonstrating a relatively hypoechoic amebic abscess (*arrows*). **(C)** Another patient with an almost solid, highly echogenic staphylococcal abscess (*arrows*).

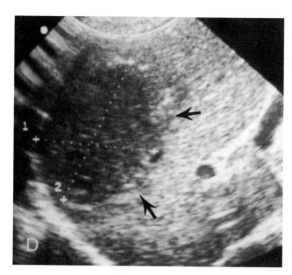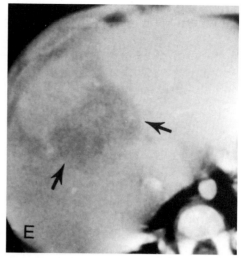

FIGURE 3.33. *(continued)* **(D)** Still another patient with a large liver abscess (*arrows*) of mixed echoes. **(E)** CT study in this patient demonstrates the hypodense abscess (*arrows*).

pancreatitis. Abscesses in the pelvis usually result from appendiceal perforation but also can be seen with salpingitis or bladder perforations.

A subphrenic abscess often elevates the diaphragmatic leaflet and is associated with pulmonary changes such as atelectasis and pleural effusion (Fig. 3.34). On the right, such an abscess often displaces the liver downward; on the left it displaces the stomach and splenic flexure medially or downwardly (7). Perinephric abscesses produce masslike configurations in the retroperitoneal area (1), obliteration of the retroperitoneal soft tissues, and, on intravenous pyelography, decreased function or displacement of the kidney. They are, however, relatively uncommon in children, as are intrarenal abscesses. Perinephric abscesses and renal infections, in general, are dealt with in a later section. Abscesses along, or in the psoas muscle may be tuberculous or nontuberculous in origin (3,4,7) and are best demonstrated with CT scanning (Fig. 3.35).

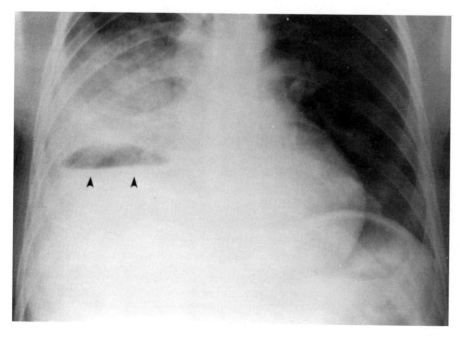

FIGURE 3.34. *Subphrenic abscess.* Note the elevated right diaphragmatic leaflet, gas accumulation beneath it (*arrows*), and associated changes in the right lung base. This patient had a right subphrenic abscess secondary to a perforated retrocecal appendix.

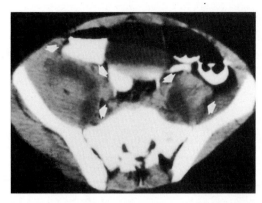

FIGURE 3.35. *Psoas abscess.* Bilateral psoas abscesses (*arrows*). The right is much larger than the left. Loculated fluid is seen within the abscesses.

Ultrasonography, as the screening imaging modality in the investigation of abdominal abscess, is virtually indispensable. Characteristically, with ultrasound, abscesses present with a sonolucent center and an irregular or well-defined wall, but more solid figurations also occur (Fig. 3.36). CT scanning also is excellent in delineating abscesses and usually is more informative than ultrasound as far as precise abscess localization is concerned (Fig. 3.36).

Liver abscesses may be pyogenic or amebic in origin (2,5,6,8), and amebic abscesses, more than pyogenic liver abscesses, tend to be strikingly anechoic (5). Amebic abscesses also may erode the diaphragm and extend into the chest or even the pericardial cavity (Fig. 3.37). Demonstration of these complications is extremely important, and if such an abscess is demonstrated to be near the diaphragmatic leaflet or the pericardium, penetration should be considered a real possibility. For this reason, the abscess should be drained immediately.

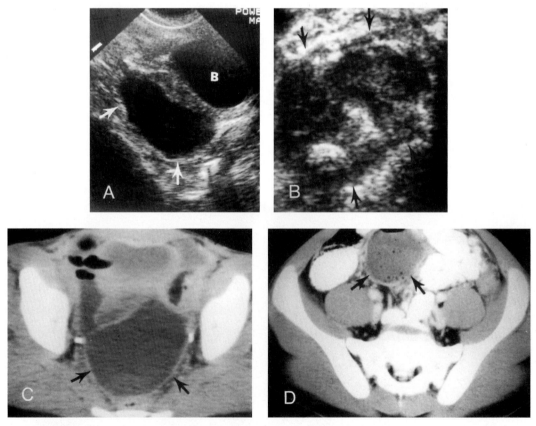

FIGURE 3.36. *Abdominal abscess: ultrasonographic and CT configurations.* **(A)** Patient with basically sonolucent pelvic abscess (*arrows*). *B,* Urinary bladder. **(B)** Another patient with an abscess (*arrows*) demonstrating heterogeneous echogenicity. **(C)** CT demonstration of another pelvic abscess (*arrows*) posterior to the bladder. **(D)** Another patient with an abscess demonstrating gas bubbles scattered throughout its substance and a bubble of air at the top of the abscess (*arrows*).

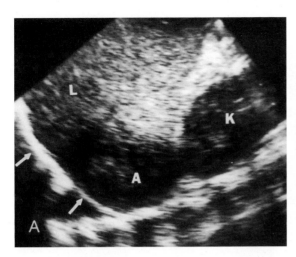

FIGURE 3.37. *Amebic abscess penetrating into the pleural space.* **(A)** Note the sonolucent liver abscess (*A*). *L,* liver; *K,* kidney; *arrows,* diaphragmatic leaflet. **(B)** Later, with penetration through the diaphragm, note accumulation of fluid (*F*) in the pleural space and a defect in the diaphragmatic leaflet (*arrows*). The abscess (*A*) now is much smaller.

REFERENCES

1. Bliznak J, Ramsey J. Emphysematous pyelonephritis. *Clin Radiol* 1972;23:61–64.
2. Foster SC, Schneider B, Seaman WB. Gas-containing pyogenic intrahepatic abscesses. *Radiology* 1970;94:613–618.
3. Graves VB, Schreiber MH. Tuberculous psoas muscle abscess. *Can J Assoc Radiol* 1973;24:268–271.
4. Hardcastle JD. Acute non-tuberculous psoas abscess. *Br J Surg* 1970;57:10.
5. Hayden CK Jr., Toups M, Swischuk LE, Amparo EG. Sonographic features of hepatic amebiasis in childhood. *Can J Assoc Radiol* 1984;35:279–282.
6. Newlin N, Silder TM, Stuck KJ, Sandler MA. Ultrasonic features of pyogenic liver abscess. *Radiology* 1981;139:155–159.
7. Parbhoo A, Govendel S. Acute pyogenic psoas abscess in children. *J Pediatr Orthop* 1992;12:663–666.
8. Ralls PW, Colletti PM, Quinn MF, Halls J. Sonographic findings in a hepatic amebic abscess. *Radiology* 1982;145:123–126.

ACUTE INFLAMMATORY PROBLEMS

Pneumonia Causing Acute Abdomen

Pneumonia, usually pneumococcal in origin, is notorious for producing symptoms suggesting an acute abdominal problem (1–3). Very often (3), but not always, the pneumonia is in the base of one of the lungs, and interestingly enough these pneumonias often are best seen on abdominal films (Fig. 3.38). The reason for this is that the higher-voltage technique utilized for abdominal roentgenography tends to accentuate the density of the pneumonia, and, in addition, because many of these pneumonias are hidden

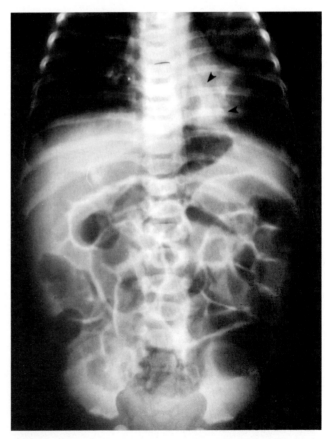

FIGURE 3.38. *Acute abdomen: pneumonia in the left base.* Note the extensive paralytic ileus in this patient with an acute abdomen. Also note, however, the area of increased density behind the left side of the heart (*arrows*), representing a pneumonia in the left lower lobe.

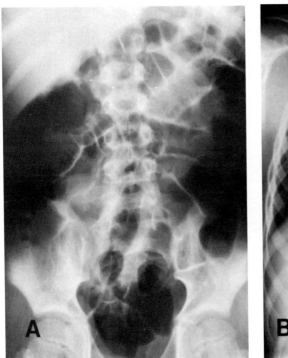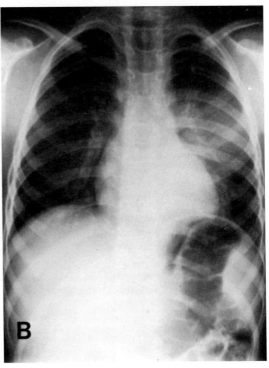

FIGURE 3.39. *Acute abdomen: value of chest film.* **(A)** Note extensive paralytic ileus in this patient presenting with an acute abdomen and suspected appendicitis. **(B)** Chest film demonstrates a large consolidating pneumonia in the left midlung.

behind the left or right side of the heart, a relatively over-penetrated roentgenographic technique actually is desirable. On the other hand, it should be remembered that not all such pneumonias are located in this area; indeed, many are located higher in the lungs and are missed if a chest roentgenogram is not obtained (Fig. 3.39).

Most often if a pneumonia produces symptoms referable to the abdomen, a condition such as appendicitis is at first suspected, but unlike appendicitis, roentgenographic examination of the abdomen usually is normal. On occasion, however, one can encounter both appendicitis and pneumonia in the same patient (1,2).

REFERENCES

1. Baechli D, Braun P. Concomitant pneumonia and acute appendicitis in a child. *Z Kinderchir* 1978;23:409–411.
2. Gongaware RD, Weil R III, Santulli TV. Right lower lobe pneumonia and acute appendicitis in childhood: A therapeutic disorder. *J Pediatr Surg* 1973;8:33–35.
3. Jona JZ, Belin RP. Basilar pneumonia simulating acute appendicitis in children. *Arch Surg* 1976;111:552–553.

Acute Gastroenteritis

Gastroenteritis is the most common childhood abdominal inflammatory problem, and most often one is dealing with a viral infection. The clinical symptoms of vomiting and diarrhea are well known, and dehydration, especially in young infants, is a common and potentially serious complication. Roentgenographically, dehydration commonly is reflected on the chest films by the presence of markedly overaerated lungs, decreased pulmonary vascularity, and a small cardiac silhouette.

In the abdomen, abnormal roentgenographic patterns are extremely variable and, to say the least, frequently very puzzling. The most common pattern, however, is that of many loops of air-filled, distended intestine. Both large and small bowel are involved, but so gross are the findings that frequently it is difficult to differentiate one from the other. Indeed, one frequently first believes that mechanical obstruction is present (Fig. 3.40). In other cases of gastroenteritis, only a portion of the gastrointestinal tract may be dilated. In such cases, if the stomach shows predominant dilatation, a gastric outlet obstruction may be suggested (Fig. 3.41); if one or two loops of small bowel predominate,

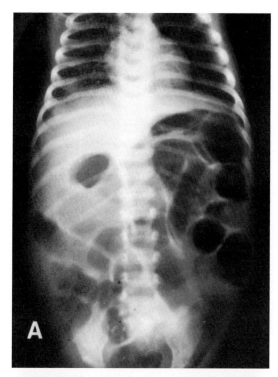

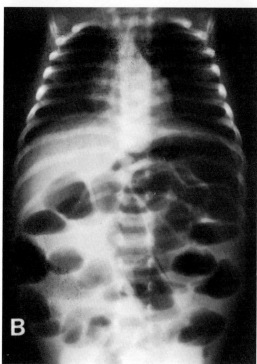

FIGURE 3.40. *Gastroenteritis.* **(A)** Note extensive dilatation of the intestines in this infant presenting with signs and symptoms of gastroenteritis. **(B)** Upright film demonstrates numerous air–fluid levels in the intestines. Although the characteristic dynamic, inverted U- or hairpin-shaped configuration of obstructed intestinal loops is absent, these findings still often are mistaken for intestinal obstruction.

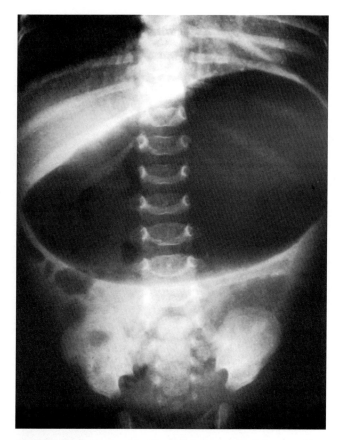

FIGURE 3.41. *Gastroenteritis: isolated gastric distension.* The isolated gastric distension in this infant with gastroenteritis could be misinterpreted as a gastric outlet obstruction.

a small bowel obstruction may be diagnosed erroneously (Fig. 3.42A); and if the findings are confined to the colon, colon obstruction is suggested (Fig. 3.42B). Finally, it should be noted that early in the course of gastroenteritis, when vomiting is the basic problem, one also may see a totally airless abdomen (Fig. 3.4). In still other instances, a locally dilated loop of small intestine (pseudosentinel loop) may be encountered (Fig. 3.10B). With ultrasound, gastroenteritis presents with dilated loops of intestine, hyperperistalsis, and, in many cases, muscosal thickening (Fig. 3.43). The findings are nonspecific for mucosal thickening; they also can be seen with Henoch–Schönlein purpura and other mucosal problems. In addition, gastroenteritis often is part and parcel of mesenteric adenitis, and in many cases it is difficult to separate the two. The findings in mesenteric adenitis are discussed subsequently in this chapter, but it should be noted that many cases of gastroenteritis also demonstrate mesenteric lymph-node enlargement in the right lower quadrant and in the mesentery around the aorta.

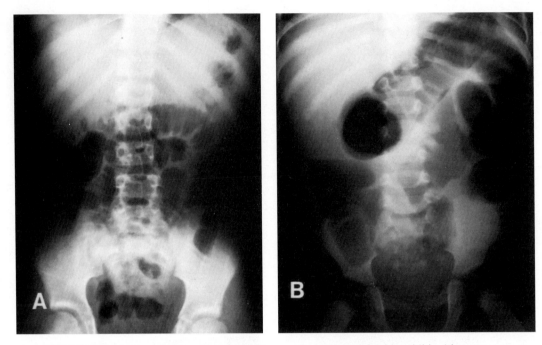

FIGURE 3.42. *Gastroenteritis: other misleading configurations.* **(A)** Older child with gastroenteritis demonstrating a picture suggesting jejunal obstruction. **(B)** Infant with gastroenteritis showing distension of the colon only.

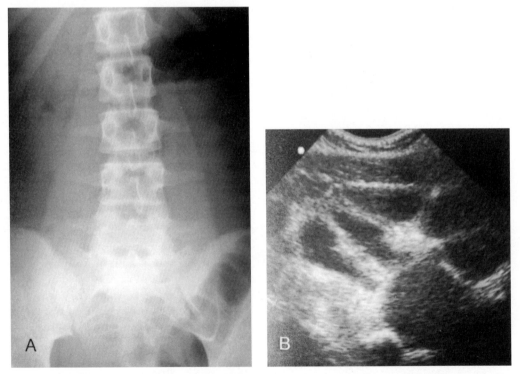

FIGURE 3.43. *Gastroenteritis: value of ultrasound.* **(A)** Note the virtually airless abdomen. **(B)** Ultrasonogram, however, demonstrates numerous loops of hyperperistaltic fluid-filled intestine.

Appendicitis

After gastroenteritis, *appendicitis is the most common acute abdominal inflammatory problem in childhood, and its accurate diagnosis remains as challenging as ever.* Many times the diagnosis is not secured until 24 to 48 hr have passed, and by that time perforation often occurs. It was demonstrated that observation in a hospital environment can significantly remedy this problem and result in a greater yield of positive laparotomies (44). The authors who did so, however, underscore the fact that such patients must be observed in the hospital and not on an outpatient basis. This is still true today, because, as is discussed here subsequently, even though ultrasound reduces the incidence of negative laparotomies, some patients still need observation in the hospital setting. In this regard we recommend, and practice, a 23 hr observation period in patients with difficult problems. These patients can be watched and not explored immediately. By the same token, it has been suggested that these patients may not need to be operated in the middle of the night (41). This notwithstanding, however, *the problem still is acute, and most often diagnosis and treatment will occur when the patient presents to the physician.*

The classic clinical findings of appendicitis are well known but, of course, are not always present in any one patient. In addition, there is the controversial problem of recurrent appendicitis and spontaneously resolving appendicitis (20). Because of this, the clinician often looks for help, and in this regard the additional studies and tests most often obtained in the past were the white blood cell count and the abdominal radiograph. Currently, however, a very valuable additional imaging study is ultrasonography. Indeed, it has become the most sensitive imaging indicator of appendicitis in infants and children. It is, however, quite operator-dependent, and it does take some time for one to become adept at performing and interpreting the study. Nonetheless, once this is accomplished, the vast majority of cases of appendicitis in children can be diagnosed accurately with ultrasound. In our institution the accuracy rate for all problems presenting with acute lower abdominal, and specifically right lower quadrant, pain is 98% (11). *Although there are those who still claim that the diagnosis of appendicitis is clinical (9), with experience one comes to the conclusion that ultrasound is much more sensitive.* To be sure, we have experienced many cases in which the diagnosis was seriously in doubt clinically and yet clearly evident ultrasonographically.

It has been suggested that a white blood cell count less than 10,000 per milliliter of blood is virtually incompatible with the diagnosis of acute appendicitis (15). By the same token, it can be stated that a count of greater than 20,000 per milliliter of blood also is unlikely to result from appendicitis, but of course neither limit completely excludes the diagnosis (15). The latter is true, but the former, now that ultrasound is playing a key role in the evaluation of appendicitis, is not true. The reason for this is that early in the disease process the white blood cell count is not elevated, because it does take some time for this response to occur. In addition, from the clinical standpoint it has been suggested that if two of four of the following findings are present appendicitis can be highly suspected (32,33): vomiting, guarding, right lower quadrant tenderness, and right lower quadrant pain. This is not to say that the presence of two or four of these findings is always diagnostic, but certainly it is highly suspicious.

Many still consider the abdominal roentgenogram valid only for the demonstration of a fecalith, free air, or some other complication of acute appendicitis. There is no question, however, that the study is of far more value than this, but the relationship of the pathology of perforated and nonperforated appendicitis to the roentgenographic findings must be understood. In this regard, it should first be noted that most children with acute nonperforated appendicitis show diminished air in the gastrointestinal tract. Indeed, in some cases the abdomen is airless (Fig. 3.44), but in others sentinel loops are seen on the right in the right lower quadrant or in the pelvis (22) (Fig. 3.45). In explaining the paucity of intestinal gas in these children, one merely must recall that acute nonperforated appendicitis usually is associated with one or all of the following: anorexia, nausea, vomiting, and diarrhea. In any combination, these findings readily lead to a paucity of air in the gastrointestinal tract. Of course, in those cases in which symptoms have not been present for a long enough period of time, usually less than 12 to 18 hours, the airless gas pattern may not have had enough time to develop and the roentgenograms are normal, except perhaps for the presence of scoliosis. On the other hand, seldom if ever is the gas pattern increased, and if in a patient with suspected appendicitis intestinal gas is abundant and the bowel dilated, perforation should be suspected. The reasons for this change in the intestinal gas pattern with appendiceal perforation are multiple. First of all, *just after perforation there is a relatively quiet clinical period,* and as the acute anorexia and nausea settle down, more air is swallowed and retained in the gastrointestinal tract. At the same time the inflammatory process in the right lower quadrant causes a partial, functional obstruction (16,30). In many cases the degree of resulting intestinal dilatation and gas accumulation is startling (Fig. 3.46), and if the findings are considered in the absence of clinical correlation, confusion with gastroenteritis can occur (i.e., compare Fig. 3.46 with Fig. 3.40).

It should be realized that perforation of the appendix may result in a variety of clinical and roentgenographic pictures. First, as already alluded to, very often there is a quiet clinical period in which the patient in fact seems to feel better. In these patients, if findings remain focal, slowly but surely right lower quadrant inflammation pro-

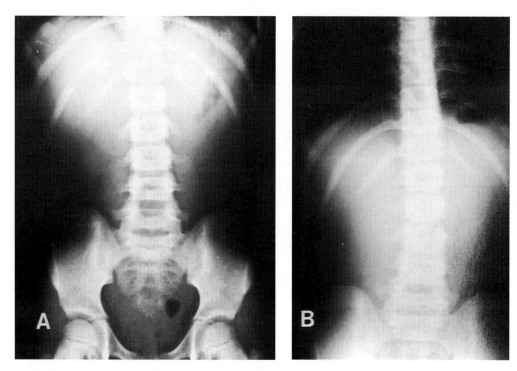

FIGURE 3.44. *Acute appendicitis: airless abdomen and scoliosis.* **(A)** Supine film showing abdomen in which gas is virtually absent. There is a minimal degree of scoliosis present. **(B)** On the upright film, however, note how much more pronounced the degree of scoliosis has become. Only a little gas is seen in the stomach.

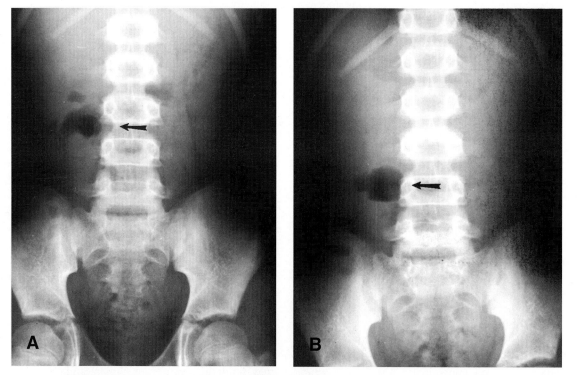

FIGURE 3.45. *Acute appendicitis: localized right-sided gas collections, indistinct right psoas shadow, and pelvic bowel loops.* **(A)** Supine film showing a few isolated loops of distended intestine in the right flank (*arrow*). The right psoas shadow is less distinct than the left. **(B)** On upright view, air–fluid levels are seen in the isolated loops of distended intestine (*arrow*). Indistinctness of the right psoas muscle is more apparent. No real scoliosis is present.

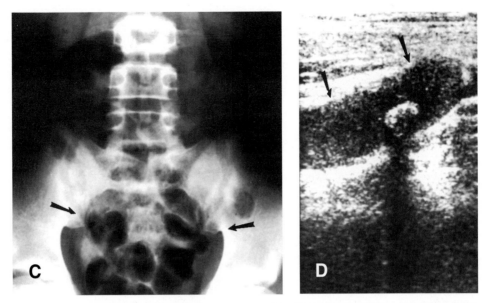

FIGURE 3.45. *(continued)* **(C)** Note the dilated loops of air-filled intestine in the pelvis *(arrows)*. **(D)** Ultrasound demonstrates the fluid-filled appendix *(arrows)* with an echogenic, shadowing fecalith.

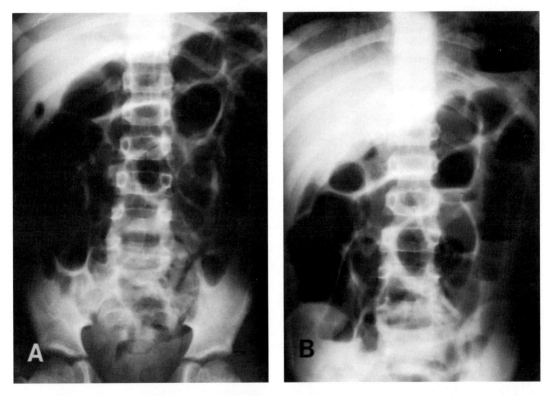

FIGURE 3.46. *Perforated appendicitis: large volumes of gas in the intestine.* **(A)** Note large volumes of gas present in both the large and small bowel in this patient with perforated appendicitis. The findings are distinctly different from those seen with nonperforated acute appendicitis as demonstrated in Figures 3.44 and 3.45. **(B)** Upright view showing numerous air–fluid levels scattered throughout both the large and small intestine. On the supine view, there is a small fecalith visualized just to the right of the midsacral spine, and there may be some suggestion of fluid displacing the cecum medially from the right abdominal wall, but otherwise the findings easily could be misinterpreted as gastroenteritis.

gresses and results in functional intestinal obstruction as seen in Fig. 3.46. On the other hand, if the problem results in diffuse peritonitis, there is extreme rigidity of the abdomen, and the patient is taken to surgery immediately. No further imaging studies are necessary. In the other patients, however, because the clinical picture may be quite confusing, it is not uncommon for one to utilize ultrasound and CT studies for final diagnosis. In infants and children, however, ultrasound usually suffices and is easier to obtain.

Other roentgenographic signs of acute appendicitis consist of the following: (a) lumbosacral scoliosis with concavity to the right; (b) absence or indistinctness of the right psoas muscle margin; (c) localized loops of dilated intestine in the right lower quadrant, flank, or pelvis (22); (d) air in the appendix; and (e) the presence of a calcified fecalith in the appendix.

Scoliosis with concavity to the right results from splinting of the paraspinal and psoas muscles, and the curve produced usually involves the lumbar spine or the lumbosacral junction. Scoliosis should be assessed on both the supine and upright views, for minimal degrees of scoliosis often become more apparent on upright views (Fig. 3.44). ***Scoliosis, albeit a very nonspecific finding, still is the most common finding seen on plain films (22).***

Absence or indistinctness of the right psoas muscle margin also is a common finding in acute appendicitis and in the past has been attributed to adjacent edema. Another more likely explanation, however, is distortion of the muscle edge resulting from spasm of the muscle (45). With spasm, the psoas muscle changes its cross-sectional shape, and the normal sharp outer edge is lost (Fig. 3.47). Localized right lower quadrant loops of distended intestine are sentinel loops and result from paralytic ileus of the terminal ileum and cecum secondary to the adjacent inflammatory process in the appendix.

Air in the appendix is a relatively rare finding in acute appendicitis (Fig. 3.48) but generally is suggestive of the condition. On the other hand, it has been pointed out that air may be present in the appendix of patients with profound paralytic ileus (16). Nevertheless, in a case of suspected acute appendicitis, the persistent presence of air in the appendix should be taken as a positive finding. This is especially true if the abdomen is airless and the appendix overdistended or its lumen increased in diameter (Fig. 3.48A and B). If these additional criteria are absent, however, one should be cautious about one's interpretation of air in the appendix.

In acute appendicitis, gas accumulates in the appendix because it is occluded and because gas-producing organisms grow within it. Occlusion can be secondary to a fecalith (calcified or uncalcified), inspissated feces, or inflammatory lymphadenopathy. ***Inflammatory lymphadenopathy may be more common than generally***

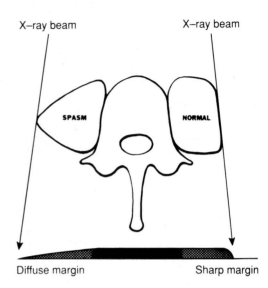

Effect of Psoas Angle on Radiographic Visualization

FIGURE 3.47. *Explanation of lack of psoas margin visualization.* Spasm of the psoas muscle distorts its contour and makes its outer edge appear more angled. As a result, the flat outer surface of the muscle is lost and the incidental beam (*arrows*), as it passes through the muscle and along the angled edge, does not produce a sharp margin. (From Williams SM, Harned RK, Hultman SA, Qualfe MA. The psoas sign: A reevaluation. *Radio-Graphics* 1985;5:525–536, with permission.)

appreciated and probably is the most common cause of obstruction. Such adenopathy probably occurs within the wall of the appendix and not around the appendix. Support for this concept lies in the fact that now that ultrasound is used so frequently in the diagnosis of appendicitis, many fecaliths seen in a distended, fluid-filled, inflamed appendix are not present in the neck of the appendix but rather in the body or even at the tip. Therefore, it seems that although the fecalith may predispose to the development of appendicitis (i.e., foreign body), it may not be the actual cause of obstruction in most cases.

A calcified fecalith in the right lower quadrant, pelvis, or right side of the abdomen (Fig. 3.49) in a patient with acute right lower quadrant pain virtually assures the diagnosis of acute appendicitis. This is not to say, however, that calcified fecaliths are seen only in patients with acute appendicitis; occasionally one encounters a calcified fecalith in a totally asymptomatic child. However, because it is generally held that over 50% of cases of perforated appendicitis are accompanied by fecaliths, the presence of this finding certainly does place even the asymptomatic patient in a higher-risk category. To be sure, there is continued debate as to whether prophylactic appendectomy is warranted in such cases, because there is the strong likeli-

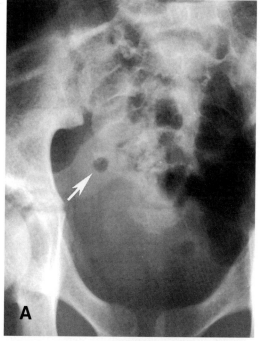

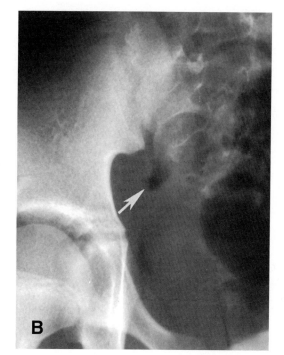

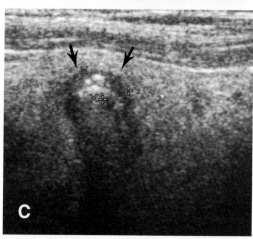

FIGURE 3.48. *Air in the appendix: acute appendicitis.* **(A)** Note air in the appendix (*arrow*). In addition, note absence of intestine in the right lower quadrant. **(B)** Another view showing the air-filled appendix (*arrow*). **(C)** Ultrasound shows the echogenic arc of air (*arrows*) obscuring the appendix.

hood that acute appendicitis will develop in these individuals sooner or later.

Roentgenographic signs of perforated appendicitis may consist of any of the following: (a) right-side colon cutoff sign (42), (b) functional small bowel obstruction with or without a paucity of gas in the right lower quadrant, (c) inflammatory mass or abscess in the right lower quadrant or pelvis, (d) positive flank stripe sign, (e) obliteration of the properitoneal fat line on the right, and (f) free intraperitoneal air. Many times, more than one of the findings are present in any one patient, but free air is relatively rare.

The right side colon cutoff sign (42) often is the first roentgenographic sign of perforation. It results from a combination of spasm of the cecum and ascending colon, induced by the adjacent inflammatory process, and reflex paralytic ileus of the transverse, and in some cases the ascending, colon. As a result, the two areas of the colon are demarcated by a sharp cutoff of gas in the right upper quadrant. This finding is best assessed on the supine view, for on upright view shifting gas and fecal material in the colon can totally obscure its presence (Fig. 3.50). It is most important that if the colon cutoff sign is present on supine films it be determined that right-side ascending colon gas is diminished because of spasm and not because the cecum and ascending colon are full of feces. If gas is present in the transverse colon and absent in the ascending colon because it is full of fecal material, the colon cut-

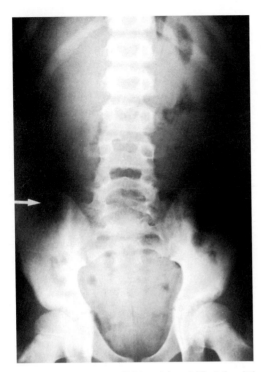

FIGURE 3.49. *Acute appendicitis with calcified fecalith.* Note that the abdomen shows virtual absence of intestinal gas. In addition, however, note the presence of a calcified fecalith in the right lower quadrant (*arrow*).

off sign is invalid (Fig. 3.51). Therefore, in any such case, if there is doubt about the validity of the sign, a decubitus film, with right side up, can be employed. If one is dealing with a false cutoff sign, the ascending colon should fill on the decubitus view (Fig. 3.52).

The right sided colon cutoff sign, of course, is not seen in all cases of perforated appendicitis, and actually one more commonly encounters a picture suggestive of low small bowel obstruction (Figs. 3.53 and 3.54). This type of obstruction has been termed "functional obstruction," for it probably represents a combination of mechanical and paralytic ileus (18,35). The mechanical component results from the obstructive effects of the progressive inflammatory process developing in the right lower quadrant; the paralytic aspect represents reflex paralysis of the small bowel (35). Together these factors lead to varying degrees of obstruction, and in some cases the picture of obstruction is so distracting that, unless one were cognizant of the phenomenon, one would not consider perforated appendicitis as the primary diagnosis. Other radiographic findings associated with perforated appendicitis include signs of peritonitis, a positive flank-stripe sign, and obliteration of the properitoneal fat line.

Signs of peritonitis include fluid in the abdomen (Fig. 3.55); a positive flank-stripe sign consists of an increase in

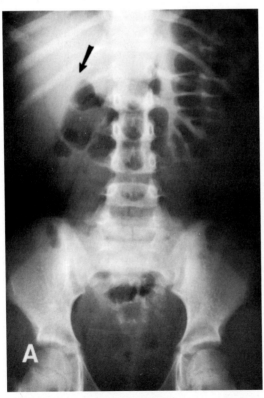
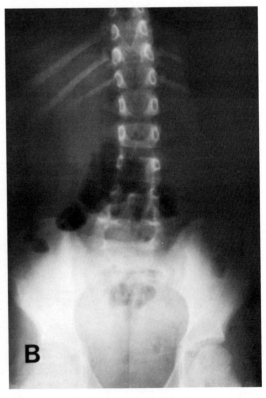

FIGURE 3.50. *Acute appendicitis: colon cutoff sign.* **(A)** Note gas in the transverse colon. The transverse colon is not unduly dilated, but gas terminates abruptly in the region of the hepatic flexure (*arrow*). This is the colon cutoff sign. The ascending colon and cecum are virtually empty, but there are one or two locally distended sentinel loops of intestine in the right lower quadrant. **(B)** Upright view demonstrating the development of significant scoliosis, loss of the colon cutoff sign, and confirmation of the presence of locally distended loops of dilated intestine in the right lower quadrant.

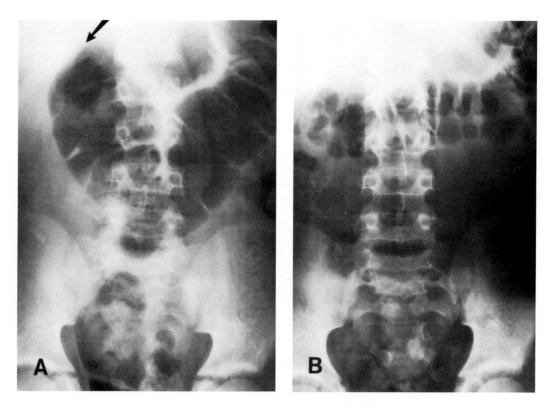

FIGURE 3.51. *Acute appendicitis: colon cutoff sign.* **(A)** Note the colon cutoff sign (*arrow*) and the presence of a fecalith. **(B)** Two years earlier the patient had symptoms suggestive of appendicitis; The fecalith was present and a colon cutoff sign was suggested. However, note feces in the ascending colon and lack of dilatation of the transverse colon. This negates the colon cutoff sign, but a decubitus film was not obtained. The patient was not operated upon at this time but returned 2 years later with perforated appendicitis as demonstrated in **A**.

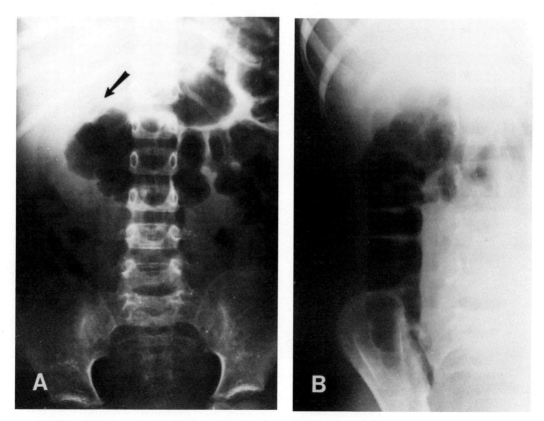

FIGURE 3.52. *Acute abdomen: pseudocolon cutoff sign.* **(A)** On this supine view, note that a colon cutoff sign is suggested (*arrow*). **(B)** Decubitus film shows the ascending colon to readily fill with air. This negates the original suggestion of a colon cutoff sign.

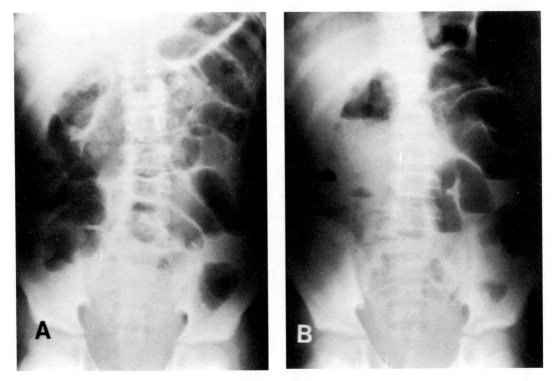

FIGURE 3.53. *Perforated appendicitis with early functional obstruction.* **(A)** Note moderate scoliosis and three of four loops of distended small bowel just to the left of the spine. **(B)** Upright view showing the same loops, but this time with air–fluid levels. These findings represent early functional obstruction secondary to perforated appendicitis.

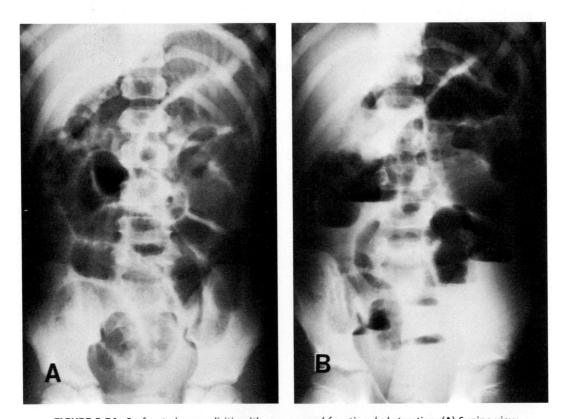

FIGURE 3.54. *Perforated appendicitis with pronounced functional obstruction.* **(A)** Supine view demonstrating numerous loops of distended intestine. However, note that the loops of jejunum are disproportionately distended, compared with gas in the colon. **(B)** The findings are visualized with greater clarity on the upright view, in which numerous acute-appearing air–fluid levels are noted within the distended loops of jejunum. These findings represent pronounced functional obstruction secondary to perforation of the appendix.

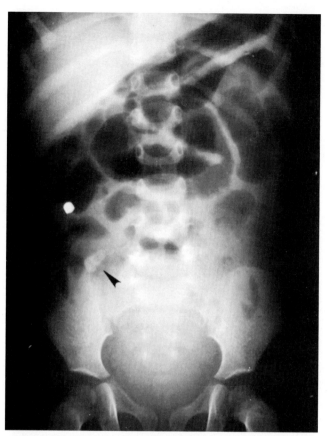

FIGURE 3.55. *Perforated appendicitis with abscess, fecalith, and peritonitis.* First note that there are numerous loops of distended intestine in the abdomen (i.e., functional obstruction). Note, however, that the space between the individual loops is thickened. This indicates the presence of intraperitoneal fluid (pus) and, hence, the presence of peritonitis. Also note the calcified fecalith (*arrow*) and surrounding inflammatory mass (abscess). Increased density and whiteness of the lower abdomen and pelvic regions are caused by the presence of intraperitoneal pus. An incidental colonic foreign body is seen above the calcified fecalith.

the soft tissue distance between the abdominal wall and air-filled descending colon or cecum. The soft tissue space is widened by inflammatory edema or frank abscess formation. If the finding is present it is very useful, but it is rare, and often so many other findings of perforated appendicitis also are present that its practical value is diminished (Fig. 3.56). Absence of the right properitoneal fat line also is seen in advanced cases of appendiceal perforation, but as with the positive flank-stripe sign, absence of the properitoneal fat line often is a superfluous finding, for other findings of perforation usually are present (Fig. 3.56). The presence of free air is the least common finding in perforated appendicitis, and if present the air usually is of small volume and more difficult to detect.

An abscess clearly reflects an underlying perforation, and although in some cases the abscess may appear classi-

cally granular or dense and well defined, more often it is less well organized (Figs. 3.55 and 3.56). In still other instances, fixed, formless air bubbles are present within the generalized opacity of the abscess (Fig. 3.57), and finally, in some cases massive accumulations of air are seen in abscess cavity (Fig. 3.58).

Ultrasonography is now commonly used for the evaluation of acute appendicitis (1,4,5,12,19,24–26,36–38, 43,46), especially in the pediatric population. Generally, the criteria utilized for the ultrasonic diagnosis of acute appendicitis include focal tenderness over the inflamed appendix, lack of compressibility of the appendix, fluid in the appendiceal lumen, and a transverse diameter of 6 mm or more (25). This diameter is quite reliable, but one occasionally encounters appendices that are up to 6 mm or slightly greater in diameter whose enlargement is not caused by acute purulent appendicitis. In such cases the appendix is inflamed secondary to some other problem, and the increase in diameter results from appendiceal wall thickening rather than a distended, fluid-filled appendix (Fig. 3.59). These appendices also are compressible and tend to be seen in association with adjacent inflammation, such as mesenteric adenitis or intestinal ischemia in patients with sickle cell disease. It should be remembered, however, that in cases of acute appendicitis, in the early stages the appendix can be slightly compressible but does not compress completely. Graded compression is important in equivocal cases of appendicitis (24,47), but in most cases the findings are initially so classic that graded compression is not needed. *This, of course, is important, because with compression pain can be a problem, and if compression can be avoided it is more comfortable for the patient.*

The normal appendix usually measures no more than 4 mm in diameter and is not distended with fluid (Fig. 3.60). Some normal appendices may contain fluid, but these do not measure more than 6 mm in diameter (Fig. 3.59). This is important, because some of these appendices are tender and are seen in association with mesenteric adenitis, pelvic inflammatory disease, and sickle cell abdominal crisis. All of this can lead to some subjectivity in the evaluation of the appendix with ultrasound, but this occurs only in a minority of cases. *In most cases the diagnosis is relatively straightforward once one becomes proficient with ultrasound. However, it does take some time to become proficient, and it has been documented that unless such proficiency is achieved the study is quite unreliable (23).*

Very often the patient can point exactly to the location of the inflamed appendix; this self-localization is quite helpful (6). In most cases the appendix lies just under the abdominal wall and is easy to find. If it is retrocecal, however, it is much more difficult to identify, and in such cases graded compression becomes more useful, for it may take

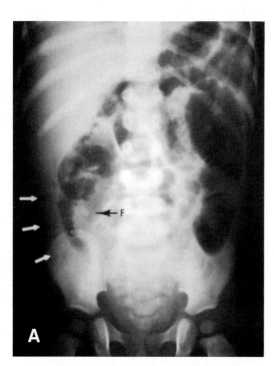
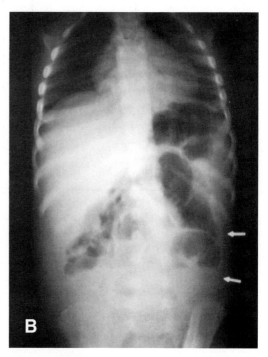

FIGURE 3.56. *Perforated appendicitis–calcified fecalith, abscess, positive flank-stripe sign, and absent properitoneal fat stripe.* (**A**) Supine view demonstrating abundant gas within dilated intestines, a calcified fecalith (*F*), and medial displacement of the contracted cecum (*C*). The cecum is displaced medially because of the presence of fluid and edema between it and the abdominal wall. This constitutes a positive flank-stripe sign (*arrows*). (**B**) Upright view showing the presence of a few distended loops of jejunum with air–fluid levels, but in addition clear-cut evidence that the properitoneal fat stripe on the right is absent. The properitoneal fat stripe on the left (*arrows*) is present. In addition, note that the gas-filled intestine on the right continues to be displaced medially from the abdominal wall (i.e., positive flank-stripe sign).

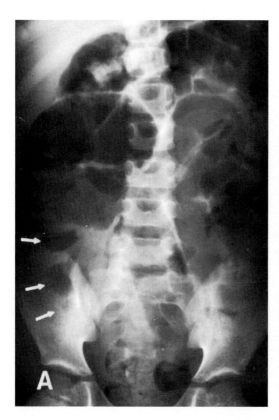
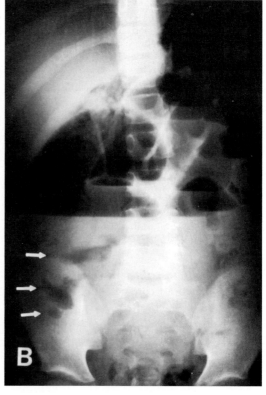

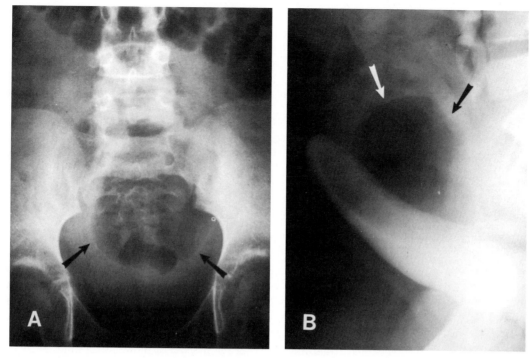

FIGURE 3.58. *Appendiceal abscess.* (**A**) Note the large gas-filled abscess (*arrows*). (**B**) Lateral view showing the same abscess (*arrows*) behind the contrast-filled bladder.

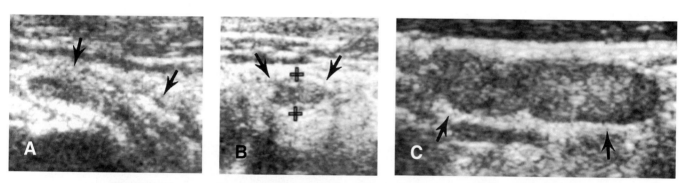

FIGURE 3.59. *Appendiceal enlargement not caused by acute appendicitis.* (**A**) Note the enlarged appendix (*arrows*). The mucosa shows some thickening, but there is a little fluid in the lumen. This patient did not have acute appendicitis but had gastroenteritis with mesenteric adenitis. (**B**) Cross-sectional view demonstrates the compressed, oval-shaped appendix (*arrows*). (**C**) Adjacent enlarged lymph nodes (*arrows*).

FIGURE 3.57. *Perforated appendicitis with abscess: fixed bubbles.* (**A**) Supine view demonstrating numerous loops of distended small bowel in the abdomen and two or three formless loops of gas in the right lower quadrant. In addition, a soft tissue inflammatory mass around these latter air collections is suggested (*arrows*). (**B**) Upright view shows the development of numerous air–fluid levels in the distended loops of small bowel. A functional obstruction is present. Note, however, that the formless collections of gas in the right lower quadrant (*arrows*) have not changed significantly in configuration or position. This lack of change in the appearance of the bubbles from supine to upright view can be taken as presumptive evidence for the presence of an abscess (which was surgically confirmed).

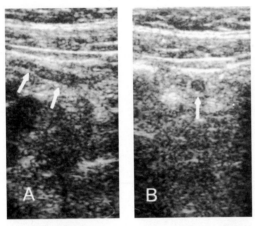

FIGURE 3.60. *Normal appendix.* **(A)** Longitudinal view demonstrating the normal appendix (*arrows*). **(B)** Cross-sectional view showing the appendix (*arrow*).

identified, and such fecaliths may not be calcified. For this reason more fecaliths are identified with ultrasound than on plain films. Fluid may be seen around the appendix but does not necessarily indicate frank perforation (10). Localized adenopathy also occasionally can be seen but is not nearly as common or profound as with mesenteric adenitis.

Color flow Doppler has been shown to demonstrate increased flow to the wall of the inflamed appendix (17,21,25) (Fig. 3.62). This finding can be useful in some cases, but it should be appreciated that if the appendix is very edematous or gangrenous, while periappendicular blood flow is increased, none is seen in the appendiceal wall itself.

As mentioned previously, most cases of acute appendicitis present with rather typical findings, but still there is considerable variability from patient to patient (Fig. 3.63). Appendicitis may involve only the tip of the appendix, and the remainder of the appendix may appear relatively normal (28). With gangrenous appendicitis, the entire appendiceal wall can appear thick and hypoechoic, with no delineation of the mucosa or intraluminal fluid. Such appendices may be associated with small fluid collections around them. All of these variations are demonstrated in Figs. 3.63 and 3.64.

With perforated appendicitis, ultrasound may demonstrate the presence of free peritoneal fluid, which is frequently echogenic and dirty (Fig. 3.65), a fluid collection in juxtaposition to the appendix, periappendiceal fat echogenicity, or actual abscess formation. One of the most important and problematic features of perforated appendicitis in our experience, however, is that the appendix itself collapses (10) and becomes more difficult to identify

more time to find the more deeply located appendix (5). In the usual case, however, the classic appearance of an inflamed appendix is that of a relatively small, fluid-filled, noncompressible or barely compressible tubular structure resembling a small sausage (Fig. 3.61). In some cases the intraluminal fluid is relatively sonolucent, but in other cases it contains debris and is more echogenic (Fig. 3.61). Adjacent mesenteric fat is echogenic, but this finding is more evident and extensive once the appendix has become gangrenous or undergoes frank perforation. The appendiceal mucosa is variably intact and in some cases is virtually destroyed. In these cases gangrenous appendicitis should be considered. Of course, a fecalith frequently is

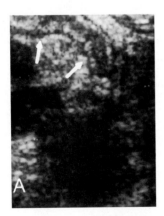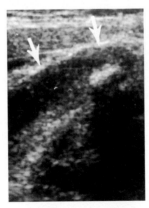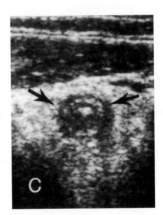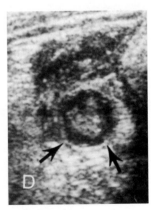

FIGURE 3.61. *Acute appendicitis: ultrasonographic features.* **(A)** Note the distended, fluid-filled appendix (*arrows*). The echogenic mucosa is still intact. **(B)** Another patient with a distended appendix (*arrows*), but with the mucosa less intact. There is an echogenic fecalith in the tip of the appendix. **(C)** Cross-sectional view in another patient of a swollen, distended appendix (*arrows*). Note the concentric ring configuration. An echogenic but nonshadowing fecalith is present in the center. **(D)** Another patient with a markedly distended appendix (*arrows*) with a sonolucent rim and a great deal of echogenic debris within its lumen.

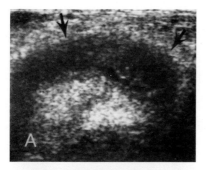
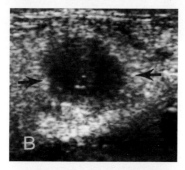
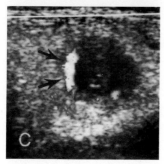

(Fig. 3.65). This also has been noted by others (13). Color flow Doppler, with its ability to show increased blood flow to the inflamed appendiceal wall and periappendiceal tissues, is useful in these cases. Overall, however, imaging the perforated appendix is more difficult than imaging the nonperforated appendix.

The appendix also can be located almost anywhere in the right side of the abdomen and pelvis. Although most reside in the general vicinity of the right lower quadrant, an inflamed appendix can be encountered as high as the liver. In other cases, the appendix is retrocecal and, as mentioned previously, is more difficult to identify. Consequently, perforation and delay in diagnosis are common. In addition, because the disease process is more longstanding, more inflammation is seen in the structures around the appendix such as the terminal ileum and cecum (Fig. 3.66). In addition, adenopathy may be more pronounced than in the usual case of appendicitis. This is important, because in such cases one may come to the erroneous conclusion that mesenteric adenitis is the problem.

Abscesses after perforation can be located in a variety of places and have a number of configurations ranging from oval to round to lobulated. They may have a sonolucent center, contain debris, be virtually solid, or show a hyperechoic rim (Fig. 3.67). CT scanning, of course, is also very useful in the detection of postperforation abscesses (Fig. 3.68) and in addition can clearly identify the presence of free fluid in the abdomen, especially in the cul-de-sac. An important clinical feature of completely walled-off abscesses is that they do not present with acute findings. The patient usually is obviously not completely healthy but yet not seriously ill. In addition, in many cases, perforation results in an inflammatory mass called a ***phlegmon*** rather than a frank abscess (Fig. 3.69). The point is moot, however, because both findings are completely abnormal, and

FIGURE 3.62. *Acute appendicitis: color flow Doppler ultrasonographic findings.* **(A)** Note the swollen appendix *(arrows)* on longitudinal view. There is very little residual echogenic mucosa. **(B)** Cross-sectional view shows the distended appendix *(arrows)*. **(C)** Color flow Doppler ultrasonography demonstrates excessive flow to the appendiceal wall *(arrows)*.

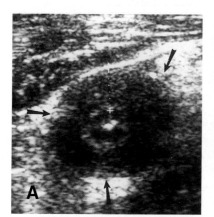
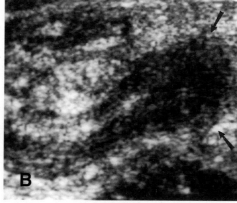
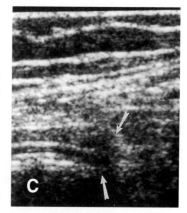

FIGURE 3.63. *Acute appendicitis: variations.* **(A)** Note the large edematous appendix *(arrows)* measuring nearly 2 cm in diameter. **(B)** Fluid-filled long appendix with a gangrenous tip *(arrows)*. **(C)** In this patient the appendix is normal and collapsed, except for the tip which is edematous *(arrows)*.

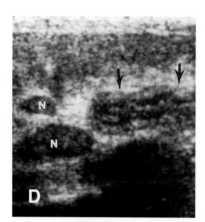
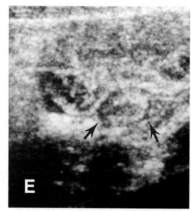
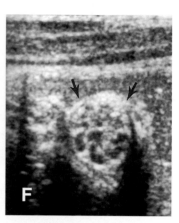

FIGURE 3.63. *(continued)* (D) Inflamed appendix (*arrows*), surrounded by echogenic mesanteric fat. Note two small lymph nodes (*n*). Adenopathy is not a prominent feature of acute non-perforated appendicitis. (E) Same patient demonstrating the appendix in cross-section (*arrows*). Above it lies the terminal ileum demonstrating tortuous thickening of the mucosal folds. (F) Cross-section of the terminal ileum (arrows) demonstrates the edematous mucosal fluids (secondary inflammation).

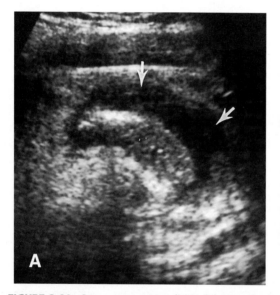
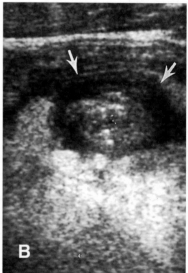

FIGURE 3.64. *Gangrenous appendicitis.* (A) Note the large inflamed appendix (*arrows*). At first hypoechoic fluid is suggested. (B) On cross-sectional view, the central echogenic debris is noted, and the markedly edematous appendiceal wall produces a circumferential halo of hypogenicity (*arrows*). In other cases, actual adjacent fluid is seen (see Fig. 3.66).

although it might be difficult to differentiate one from the other, there is no question that the patient should be subject to surgical intervention.

The use of CT, especially helical CT scanning with or without contrast material introduced into the colon, is becoming popular in the evaluation of acute appendicitis in adults, and to some degree in children (2,7,14,27–31,34). The inflamed appendix is easy to identify in adults, because

they usually have more surrounding fat (Fig. 3.70). ***However, all of the findings present in cases of mesenteric adenitis are not as easy to demonstrate with CT study as they are with ultrasound. This is important, because mesenteric adenitis is a common affliction of children and because mesenteric adenitis is easier to identify with ultrasound, it probably will remain the dominant imaging modality in children.*** This is especially true if all of this is coupled with

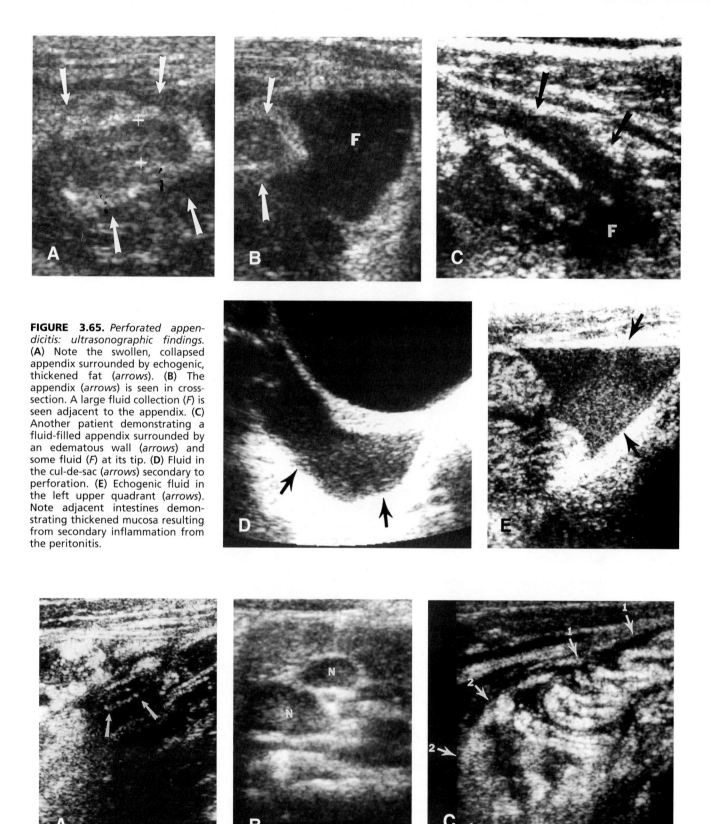

FIGURE 3.65. *Perforated appendicitis: ultrasonographic findings.* (**A**) Note the swollen, collapsed appendix surrounded by echogenic, thickened fat (*arrows*). (**B**) The appendix (*arrows*) is seen in cross-section. A large fluid collection (*F*) is seen adjacent to the appendix. (**C**) Another patient demonstrating a fluid-filled appendix surrounded by an edematous wall (*arrows*) and some fluid (*F*) at its tip. (**D**) Fluid in the cul-de-sac (*arrows*) secondary to perforation. (**E**) Echogenic fluid in the left upper quadrant (*arrows*). Note adjacent intestines demonstrating thickened mucosa resulting from secondary inflammation from the peritonitis.

FIGURE 3.66. *Retrocecal appendicitis with perforation.* (**A**) Note the small appendix (*arrows*) with surrounding fluid. It lies deep to the abdominal wall and just over the psoas muscle. (**B**) Lymph node enlargement (*n*) with surrounding echogenic mesantry in the general area. (**C**) Adjacent thickening of the mucosa of the terminal ileum (1) and cecum (2). Such widespread inflammatory change is common with perforated retrocecal appendicitis.

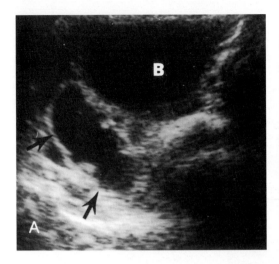

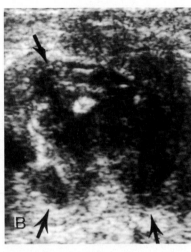

FIGURE 3.67. *Perforated appendicitis with abscess: ultrasound findings.* **(A)** Note the sonolucent irregular abscess (*arrows*) behind the urinary bladder (*B*). **(B)** Another abscess (*arrows*) basically sonolucent but with echogenic debris and a central fecalith.

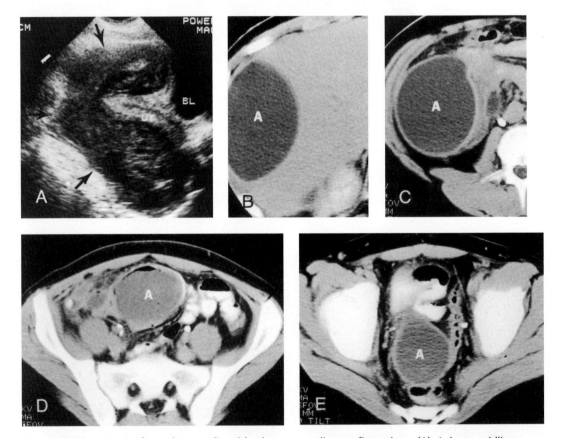

FIGURE 3.68. *Perforated appendix with abscess: peculiar configurations.* **(A)** A large midline abscess (*arrows*) surrounding the uterus. *bl*, bladder. **(B)** Another patient 3 weeks after perforation demonstrates a well-circumscribed abscess (*A*) adjacent to the liver. The abscess appears intrahepatic but was extrahepatic. **(C)** A little lower in the abdomen one can see the well-defined abscess (*A*) with a slightly hyperintense rim. **(D)** Low in the pelvis another abscess (*A*) is demonstrated. Some air is present in this abscess. There is also adjacent soft-tissue edema on the right. **(E)** Lower, this same abscess (*A*) extends in front of the rectum. These abscesses were drained percutaneously.

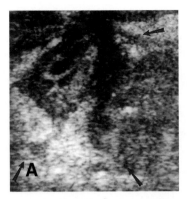
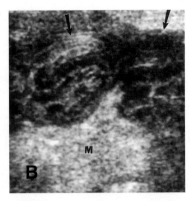
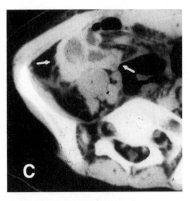

FIGURE 3.69. *Phlegmon.* **(A)** Note the featureless inflammatory mass (*arrows*) consisting of echogenic mesenteric fat, a central nonspecific area of mixed heterogenicity. Some fluid is present and a fluid-filled appendix is suggested in the center. **(B)** Just adjacent to the area one sees more echogenic mesenteric fat (**M**) and in addition, two loops of small bowel (*arrows*) which are becoming engulfed by the inflammatory mass. The mucosa of these loops is thickened. **(C)** CT study in another patient demonstrates a phelgmon (*arrows*). Note surrounding stranding into the mesenteric fat. Three fluid-filled loops of intestine are becoming engulfed in the phlegmon.

the fact that children tend to have less fat and then, the appendix is more difficult to identify on CT scans. Nonetheless, both studies have merit, and in certain cases CT scanning may be preferred. Magnetic resonance imaging also has been shown to be valuable in the identification of acute appendicitis (12), but its expense makes it rather prohibitive.

Other interesting features of acute appendicitis include the following: (a) Appendiceal foreign bodies can lead to appendiceal inflammation (39); (b) urinary tract disease can present as appendicitis or vice versa (3); and (c) an inflamed or perforated appendix can lie in an inguinal or femoral hernia, or in the scrotum of a young male infant (8,18). In the latter cases, the infant may present with an acute abdomen, intestinal obstruction, or a mass in the inguinal region or scrotum. With urinary tract involvement, symptoms such as pyuria, hematuria, and right-flank pain may render the problem virtually indistinguishable from that of true urinary tract infection. Liver abscess also can be seen as a complication of perforated appendicitis (39).

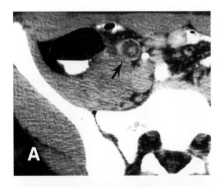
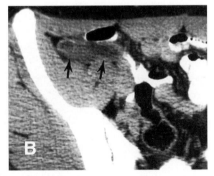
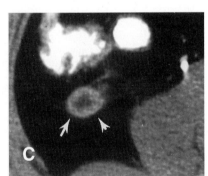
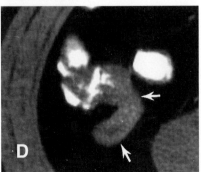

FIGURE 3.70. *Appendicitis: CT findings.* **(A)** Note the inflamed appendix (*arrow*). There is some associated periappendiceal stranding of fat. **(B)** Another view demonstrating the inflamed appendix (*arrows*). **(C and D)** In this adult the inflamed appendix (*arrows*) is clearly visible because there is so much surrounding fat. Note that in the child illustrated in **A** and **B**, intraabdominal fat is much less abundant.

REFERENCES

1. Allbery SM, McNees SW, Swischuk LE, John SD. Ultrasound in the acute pediatric abdomen: How accurate is it for surgical conditions? *Emerg Radiol* 1996;3:102–104.

2. Balthazar EJ, Birnbaum BA, Yee J, Megibow AJ, Roshkow J, Gray C. Acute appendicitis: CT and US correlation in 100 patients. *Radiology* 1994;190:31–35.

3. Buckley K, Buonoma C. Bilateral ureteral obstruction and renal failure due to a perforated appendix. *Pediatr Radiol* 1994;24: 308–309.

4. Carrico CW, Fenton LZ, Taylor GA, DiFore JW, Soprano JV. Impact of sonography on the diagnosis and treatment of acute lower abdominal pain in children and young adults. *AJR* 1999; 172:513–516.

5. Ceres L, Alonso I, Lopez P, Parra G, Echeverry J. Ultrasound study of acute appendicitis in children with emphasis for the diagnosis of retrocecal appendicitis. *Pediatr Radiol* 1990;20:258–261.

6. Chesbrough RM, Burkhard TK, Balsara ZN, Goff WB II, Davis DJ. Self-localization in US of appendicitis: An addition to graded compression. *Radiology* 1993;187:349–351.

7. Friedland JA, Siegel MJ. CT appearance of acute appendicitis in childhood. *AJR* 1997;168:439–442.

8. Friedman SC, Sheynkin YR. Acute scrotal symptoms due to perforated appendix in children: case report and review of the literature. *Pediatr Emerg Care* 1995;11:181–182.

9. Haln HB, Hoepner FU, Kalle TV, et al. Sonography of acute appendicitis in children: 7 years' experience. *Pediatr Radiol* 1998; 28:147–151.

10. Hayden CK Jr., Kuchelmeister J, Lipscomb TS. Sonography of acute appendicitis in childhood: Perforation vs. nonperforation. *J Ultrasound Med* 1992;11:209–216.

11. Hendrick EP, Chung-Han C, Swischuk LE, Juhr SD. Accuracy of ultrasound in acute right lower quadrant problems in children. *Pediatr Radiol* 2000;6:350–354.

12. Hormann M, Paya K, Eibenberger K, Dorffner R, Lang S, Kreeuzer S, Metz VM. MR imaging in children with non-perforated acute appendicitis: Value of unenhanced MR imaging in sonographically selected cases. *AJR* 1998;171:467–470.

13. Jeffrey RB, Jain KA, Nghiem HV. Pictorial essay: Sonographic diagnosis of acute appendicitis. Interpretive pitfalls. *AJR* 1994; 162:55–59.

14. Lane MJ, Katz DS, Ross BA, Clautice-Engle TL, Mindelzun RE, Jeffrey RB Jr. Unenhanced helical CT for suspected acute appendicitis. *AJR* 1997;168:405–409.

15. Lee PWR. The leukocyte count in acute appendicitis. *Br J Surg* 1973;60:618.

16. Lim MS. Gas-filled appendix: Lack of diagnostic specificity. *AJR* 1977;128:209–210.

17. Lim HK, Lee WJ, Kim TH, Namgung S, Lee SJ, Lim JH. Appendicitis: Usefulness of color Doppler US. *Radiology* 1996; 201:221–225.

18. Melamed M, Melamed JL, Rabushka SE. Appendicitis: "Functional" bowel obstruction associated with perforation of the appendix. *AJR* 1967;99:112–117.

19. Nosaka S, Miyasaka M, Miyazaki O, Hayakawa M, Nakada K, Nakajima Y, Ishikawa T. Ultrasound in pediatric patients with suspected acute appendicitis: Value in establishing alternative diagnoses. *Emerg Radiol* 1997;4:207–211.

20. Migraine S, Atri M, Bret PM, Lough JO, Hinchey JE. Spontaneously resolving acute appendicitis: clinical and sonographic documentation. *Radiology* 1997;205: 55–58.

21. Patriquin HB, Garcier JM, Lafortune M, Yazbeck S, Russo P, Jequier S, Ouimet A, Filiatrault D. Appendicitis in children and young adults: Doppler sonographic-pathologic correlation. *AJR* 1996;166: 629–633.

22. Phillpott JW, Swischuk LE, John SD. Appendicitis in the era of ultrasound: Are plain radiographs still useful? *Emerg Radiol* 1997; 4:68–71.

23. Pohl D, Golub R, Schwartz GE, Stein HD. Appendiceal ultrasonography performed by nonradiologists: Does it help in the diagnostic process? *J Ultrasound Med* 1998;17:217–221.

24. Puylaert JBCM, Rutgers PH, Lalisang RI, deVries BC, van der Werf SDJ, Dorr JPJ, Blok RAPR. A prospective study of ultrasonography in the diagnosis of appendicitis. *N Engl J Med* 1987; 317:666–669.

25. Quillin SP, Siegel MJ. Appendicitis: Efficacy of color Doppler sonography. *Radiology* 1994;191:557–560.

26. Ramachandran P, Sivit CJ, Newman KD, Schwartz MZ. Ultrasonography as an adjunct in the diagnosis of acute appendicitis: A 4-year experience. *J Pediatr Surg* 1996;31:164–169.

27. Rao PM. Technical and interpretative pitfalls of appendical CT imaging. *AJR* 1998;171:413–425.

28. Rao PM, Rhea JT, Novelline RA. Distal appendicitis: CT appearance and diagnosis. *Radiology* 1997;204:709–712.

29. Rao PM, Rhea JT, Novelline RA. Focused helical appendiceal computed tomography: Technique and interpretation. *Emerg Radiol* 1997;4:268–275.

30. Rao PM, Rhea JT, Novelline RA, McCabe CJ, Lawrason JN, Berger DL, Sacknof R. Helical CT technique for the diagnosis of appendicitis: Prospective evaluation of a focused appendix CT examination. *Radiology* 1997;202:139–144.

31. Rao PM, Rhea JT, Novelline PA, Mostafavi AA, Lawrason JN, McCabe CJ. Helical CT combined with contrast material administered only through the colon for imaging of suspected appendicitis. *AJR* 1997;169:1275–1280.

32. Reynolds SL. Missed appendicitis in a pediatric emergency department. *Pediatr Emerg Care* 1993;9:1–3.

33. Reynolds SL, Jaffe DM. Diagnosing abdominal pain in a pediatric emergency department. *Pediatr Emerg Care* 1992;8: 126–128.

34. Rhea JT, Rao PM, Novelline PA, McCabe CJ. A focused appendiceal CT technique to reduce the cost of caring for patients with clinically suspected appendicitis. *AJR* 1997;169:113–118.

35. Riggs W, Parvey LS. Perforated appendix presenting with disproportionate jejunal distention. *Pediatr Radiol* 1976;5:47–49.

36. Sivit CJ. Pictorial essay: Diagnosis of acute appendicitis in children. Spectrum of sonographic findings. *AJR* 1993;161: 147–152.

37. Sivit CJ, Newman KD, Boenning DA, et al. Appendicitis: Usefulness of US in diagnosis in a pediatric population. *Radiology* 1992;185:549–552.

38. Skaane P, Amland PR, Nordshus T, Solheim K. Ultrasonography in patients with suspected acute appendicitis: A prospective study. *Br J Radiol* 1990;63:787–793.

39. Slovis TL, Haller JO, Cohen HL, Berdon WE, Watts FB Jr. Complicated appendiceal inflammatory disease in children: Pylephlebitis and liver abscess. *Radiology* 1989;171:823–825.

40. Sukhotnik I, Klin B, Siplovich L. Foreign-body appendicitis. *J Pediatr Surg* 1995;30:1515–1516.

41. Surana R, Quinn G, Puri P. Is it necessary to perform appendicectomy in the middle of the night in children? *Br Med J* 1993;306:1168.

42. Swischuk LE, Hayden CK Jr. Appendicitis with perforation: The dilated transverse colon sign. *AJR* 1980;135: 687–689.

43. Vignault F, Filiatrault D, Brandt ML, Garel L, Grignon A, Ouimet A. Acute appendicitis in children: Evaluation with US. *Radiology* 1990;176: 501–504.

44. White JJ, Santillana M, Haller JA Jr. Intensive in-hospital obser-

vation: A safe way to decrease unnecessary appendectomy. *Ann Surg* 1975;41:793–798.

45. Williams SM, Harned RK, Hultman SA, Qualfe MA. The psoas sign: A reevaluation. *RadioGraphics* 1985;5:525–536.

46. Worrell JA, Drolshagen LF, Kelly TC, Hunton DW, Durmon GR, Fleischer AC. Graded compression ultrasound in the diagnosis of appendicitis: A comparison of diagnostic criteria. *J Ultrasound Med* 1990;9:145–150.

47. Wong ML, Casey SO, Leonidas JC, Elkowitz SS, Becker J. Sonographic diagnosis of acute appendicitis in children. *J Pediatr Surg* 1994;29:1356–1360.

Conditions Mimicking Acute Appendicitis

The most common right lower quadrant conditions mimicking the clinical and roentgenographic findings of acute appendicitis are (a) mesenteric adenitis, (b) ileocolitis caused by infection with *Yersinia* sp (c) Crohn's disease or regional enteritis, and (d) the so-called ileocecal syndrome or typhlitis in children with leukemia. In addition, occasionally one encounters a case of Meckel's diverticulitis or infarction of the appendices epiploicae. It also should be remembered that some cases of urinary tract disease, pelvic inflammatory disease, and noninflammatory adnexal disease also mimic appendicitis.

Mesenteric Adenitis

The cause of mesenteric adenitis usually is a virus (e.g., rotovirus), but the condition also can be seen with infection with *Yersinia enterocolitis, Helicobactor jejuni, Shigella* sp, and *Salmonella* sp (7,9,10,15,16). In the past this condition usually was diagnosed by exclusion. It commonly mimics, both clinically and on plain films, the findings of appendicitis, but

more recently ultrasonographically documented adenopathy, along with other findings present in these patients, has made the diagnosis of this condition more definitive (10,16). Initially, the findings in mesenteric adenitis were believed to be restricted to right lower quadrant adenopapthy and inflammation of the terminal ileum (8), but we have determined that many, if not most, of these cases have findings that go far beyond this presentation (16).

The ultrasonographic constellation of findings seen in patients with mesenteric adenitis may vary from case to case, but adenopathy is the mainstay of the diagnosis. Such adenopathy occurs in both the right lower quadrant and the upper mesenteric (paraaortic) region (16). Indeed, lymphadenopathy is the hallmark of mesenteric adenitis, but such adenopathy should be associated with tenderness of the lymph nodes, because nontender lymph nodes are commonly seen in apparently normal children (11,13). The scenario in these cases probably is much the same as it is in cases of cervical adenopathy in children. Many children have cervical adenopathy that is nontender and is the aftermath of some previous infection. It never seems to disappear, yet if another infection occurs the lymph nodes enlarge and become tender. Such residual adenopathy is also seen in the groin, and therefore, ***this phenomenon should be expected to occur in the abdomen.***

Adenopathy in the right lower quadrant or along the superior mesenteric artery in the paraaortic region appears the same, but the latter often is best visualized from the left upper quadrant. Regardless, however, the lymph nodes may be less than 1 cm or as large as 2 cm in diameter (16). Size notwithstanding, such nodes are tender and usually surrounded by echogenic, inflamed mesentery (Fig. 3.71). In addition to being tender, the inflamed lymph nodes often can be demonstrated to show increased blood flow with

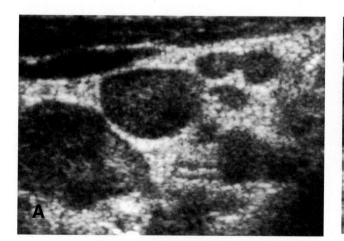
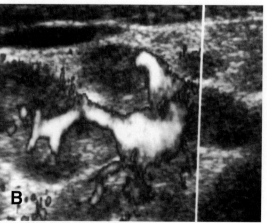

FIGURE 3.71. *Mesenteric adenitis: adenopathy.* **(A)** Note numerous enlarged, tender nodes in the right lower quadrant. **(B)** Color flow Doppler ultrasonography demonstrates increased flow to the nodes.

(continued on next page)

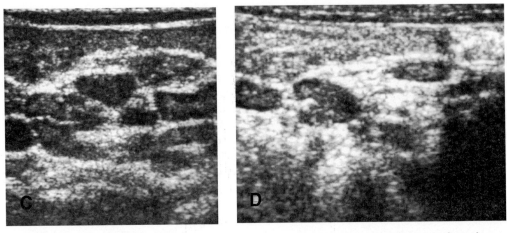

FIGURE 3.71. *(continued)* **(C)** These enlarged nodes are located in the upper abdomen along the mesentery. **(D)** Another patient with fewer nodes but more echogenic inflamed mesentery.

color flow Doppler imaging (Fig. 3.71B). In terms of differentiating the adenopathy from that seen with acute appendicitis, it has been our experience that with acute appendicitis, adenopathy is not as profound and usually amounts to nothing more than one, two, or three small lymph nodes in and around the appendix. On the other hand, with retrocecal appendicitis, because inflammation of the appendix may be more longstanding before diagnosed, adenopathy resembling that seen with mesenteric adenitis is more common. Otherwise, *in the usual case of appendicitis, adenopathy, in our experience, is not a predominant imaging feature of the condition.*

Because mesenteric adenitis often is associated with enteritis, hyperperistaltic fluid-filled loops of intestine commonly are present (Fig. 3.72). In addition, segmental thick-

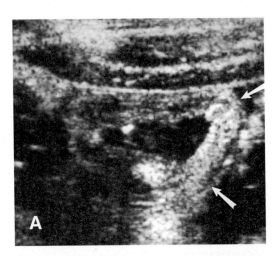

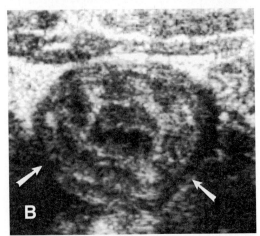

FIGURE 3.73. *Mesenteric adenitis–enteritis: circumferential mucosal thickening.* **(A)** Note circumferential thickening of the mucosa in a loop of intestine (*arrows*). Some fluid is present in the center. **(B)** In this loop, more collapsed, thickened mucosa virtually fills the lumen (*arrows*). (From Swischuk LE, and John SD. Mesenteric adenitis-acute ileitis: A constellation of findings definable with ultrasound. *Emerg Radiol* 1998;5:210–218, with permission.)

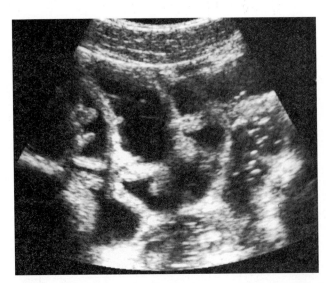

FIGURE 3.72. *Mesenteric adenitis: hyperperistaltic fluid-filled loops.* Note numerous fluid-filled loops, all demonstrating peristalsis.

ening of the mucosa throughout the course of the small bowel (best seen in the left upper quadrant in the jejunum) occurs. Mucosal thickening can take one of two forms: circumferential thickening (Fig. 3.73) or tortuous, nodular thickening of the mucosal folds (Fig. 3.74). *If combined with hyperperistalsis, the tortuously thickened mucosal folds have the appearance of a churning "bag of worms" (16).* With color flow Doppler ultrasound, increased blood flow to the inflamed, thickened intestinal wall can be demonstrated.

Circumferential or nodular thickening of the mucosal folds also can be seen in the terminal ileum, but the nodular pattern is more common (Fig. 3.75).

Another interesting feature of mesenteric adenitis is that in some cases it is associated with an inflammatory mass (3) consisting of enlarged tender lymph nodes, thickened echogenic mesentery, and a thickened terminal ileum or fluid-filled appendix (Fig. 3.76). In some cases actual suppuration of the lymph nodes occurs (3), and in other cases the resultant mass may be suggestive of the phlegmon or abscess of perforated appendicitis (Fig. 3.76). This finding was present in 11% of our cases (16).

Free fluid also can be a feature of mesenteric adenitis (Fig. 3.77A) but was not nearly as commonly seen in a study done at our institution (13) as has been reported by others (12). In a few cases, edematous thickening of the cecum also can

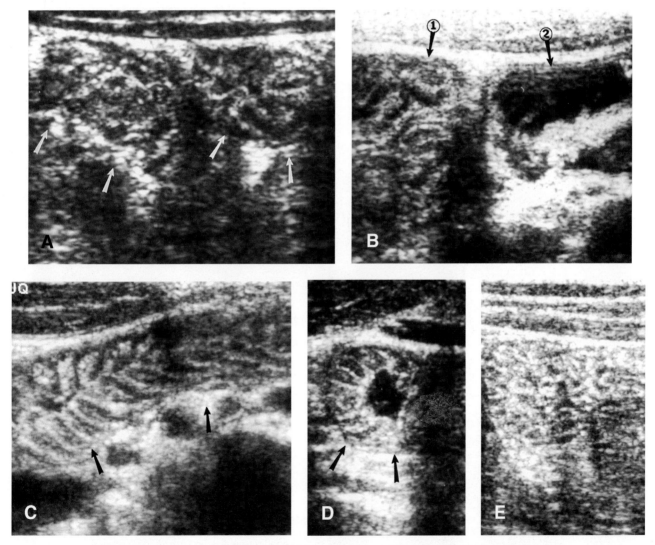

FIGURE 3.74. *Mesenteric adenitis–enteritis: tortuous mucosal thickening.* **(A)** Note marked nodular thickening of the mucosa (*arrows*) in two loops of intestine in the left upper quadrant. **(B)** In this patient one loop of intestine (*1*) demonstrates thickened nodular folds; the other is fluid-filled and the mucosa is less thickened. **(C)** Longitudinal view of a loop of intestine with thickened mucosal folds (*arrows*). **(A–C** are from Swischuk LE, John SD. Mesenteric adenitis-acute ileitis: A constellation of findings definable with ultrasound. *Emerg Radiol* 1998;5:210–218, with permission.) **(D)** Cross-sectional view of the same loop (*arrows*). **(E)** Normal mucosal folds for comparison.

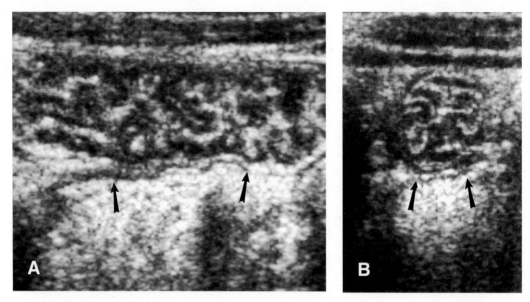

FIGURE 3.75. *Mesenteric adenitis–enteritis: terminal ileal thickening.* (**A**) Note nodular thickening of the mucosa of the terminal ileum (*arrows*). (**B**) Cross-section demonstrates the same finding (*arrows*). (From Swischuk LE, John SD. Mesenteric adenitis-acute ileitis: A constellation of findings definable with ultrasound. *Emerg Radiol* 1998;5:210–218, with permission.)

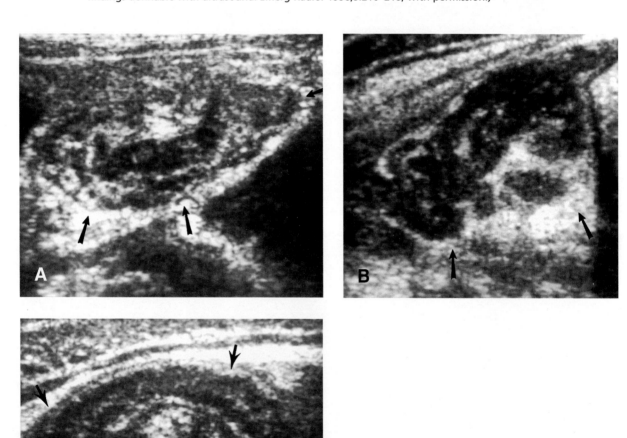

FIGURE 3.76. *Mesenteric adenitis–enteritis: masslike configuration.* (**A**) Note the masslike configuration of the thickened terminal ileum, surrounding echogenic inflamed mesentery and some adenopathy. (**B**) In this patient adenopathy is more profound, but the same pseudomass configuration is present (*arrows*). (**C**) In this patient the appendix (*upper arrows*) is draped over a pseudomass configuration (*lower arrow*). (From Swischuk LE, John SD. Mesenteric adenitis-acute ileitis: A constellation of findings definable with ultrasound. *Emerg Radiol* 1998;5:210–218, with permission.)

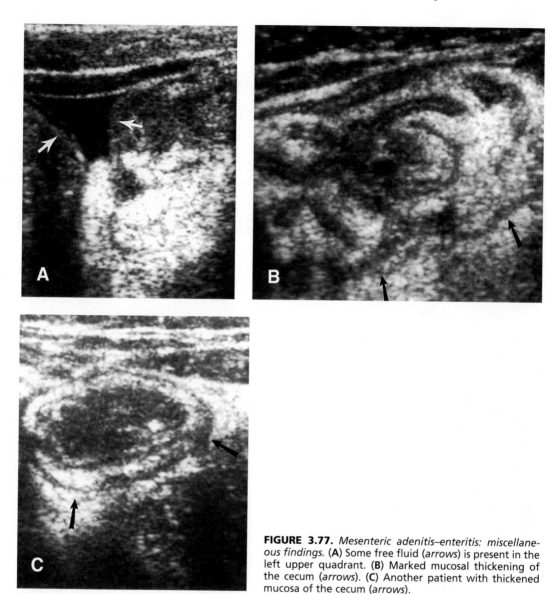

FIGURE 3.77. *Mesenteric adenitis–enteritis: miscellaneous findings.* **(A)** Some free fluid (*arrows*) is present in the left upper quadrant. **(B)** Marked mucosal thickening of the cecum (*arrows*). **(C)** Another patient with thickened mucosa of the cecum (*arrows*).

be seen (Fig. 3.77B and C), but more commonly (27% of our cases) a fluid-filled appendix can be visualized (16). This finding must be treated with caution, so as not to misinterpret it as being representative of acute appendicitis. In this regard, only 1 of 16 patients in our study demonstrated an appendix with a diameter greater than 6 mm. Another problematic finding is that the appendix may be tender in these patients, but it also usually is compressible (Fig. 3.78). It is tender because of surrounding inflammation, and it is compressibility that differentiates it from the appendix that is distended secondary to purulent appendicitis.

Finally it should be noted that mesenteric adenitis also can be demonstrated with CT imaging (11). Although not commonly utilized in children because ultrasound is so successful, CT scans can demonstrate enlarged lymph nodes,

and associated inflammation can be seen (Fig. 3.79). The other intestinal findings demonstrable with ultrasound, however, are not as clearly delineated with CT studies, ***and thus in children ultrasound is preferred.***

Crohn's Disease or Regional Enteritis

This condition is notorious for first presenting with findings suggestive of acute appendicitis (5,6). There is no real way to get around this dilemma, except to remember that such patients are going to be seen in the emergency room from time to time. Even so, they might be operated upon for acute appendicitis. Ultrasonographically, regional enteritis presents with edematous thick bowel, which then is confirmed with barium studies (Fig. 3.80).

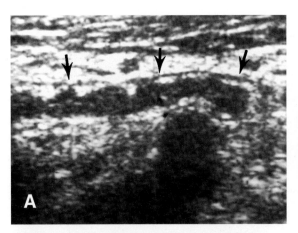
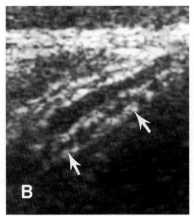
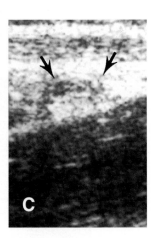

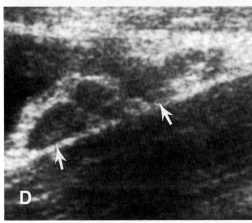

FIGURE 3.78. *Mesenteric adenitis–enteritis: fluid-filled appendix.* **(A)** Note the fluid-filled appendix (*arrows*) in this patient with mesenteric adenitis. The appendix was slightly tender but compressible. (From Swischuk LE, John SD. Mesenteric adenitis-acute ileitis: A constellation of findings definable with ultrasound. *Emerg Radiol* 1998;5:210–218, with permission.) **(B)** Another patient with a fluid-filled appendix and extensive mucosal wall thickening (*arrows*). **(C)** On cross-sectional view the appendix is completely compressible (*arrows*). **(D)** Adjacent adenopathy (*arrows*) is present.

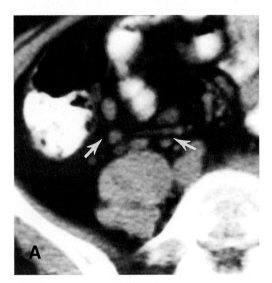
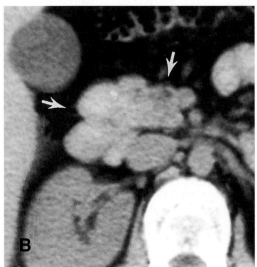

FIGURE 3.79. *Mesenteric adenitis–enteritis: CT findings.* **(A)** Note numerous small lymph nodes in the right lower quadrant (*arrows*). **(B)** Somewhat higher a large group of lymph nodes is seen in the mesentery (*arrows*).

Meckel's Diverticulitis

Meckel's diverticulitis also can mimic acute appendicitis, and findings on right lower quadrant imaging are similar to those seen in acute appendicitis. Other manifestations of Meckel's diverticulitis include right lower quadrant or lower abdominal air- or fluid-filled mass (with larger diverticula) and stone formation (4). Torsion of a Meckel's diverticulum also can occur (7), and then the findings mimic those of appendicitis.

Typhlitis

This condition, also referred to as the ***ileocecal syndrome,*** is an affliction of patients with leukemia (1,2,8,14). It is char-

acterized by a profound necrotizing inflammation of the terminal ileum, appendix, and cecum and often is a fatal event. Just why it occurs, however, is not known. The clinical findings mimic those of acute appendicitis, and the key to proper diagnosis is knowledge that the patient is suffering from leukemia. Ultrasonographically, the large, swollen cecum can be seen as an echogenic but disorganized segment of thickened bowel (Fig. 3.81). Intramural air (i.e., pneumotosis cystoides intestinalis) also has been documented with typhlitis (8).

Idiopathic infarction or torsion of the appendices epiploicae is not particularly common in childhood but in some cases can mimic the findings of acute appendicitis.

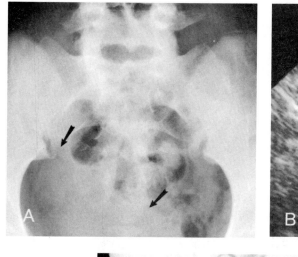
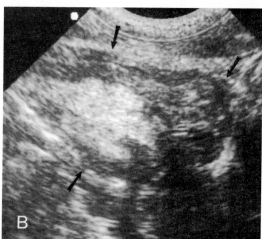
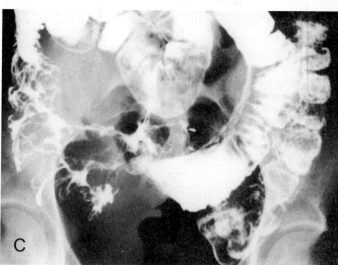

FIGURE 3.80. *Regional enteritis.* **(A)** Note the soft-tissue mass in the right pelvis (*arrows*). **(B)** Longitudinal ultrasonographic scan through the mass demonstrates a large, oval-shaped heterogeneous soft tissue mass (*arrows*). **(C)** Upper gastrointestinal series with follow-through demonstrates an extensive inflammatory mass resulting from regional enteritis. There are extensive mural thickening and sinus formation.

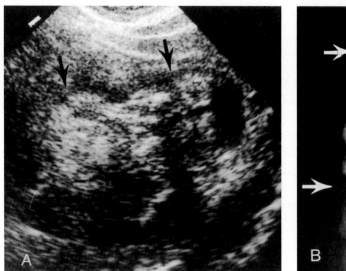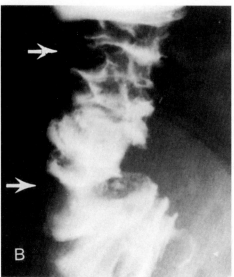

FIGURE 3.81. *Typhlitis.* **(A)** Sonogram demonstrates an oval, heterogeneous mass (*arrows*). **(B)** Barium enema demonstrating the cecal involvement consisting of spasm and intramural thickening with considerable thumbprinting (*arrows*).

REFERENCES

1. Alexander JE, Williamson SL, Seibert JJ, Golladay ES, Jimenez JF. The ultrasonographic diagnosis of typhlitis (neutropenic colitis). *Pediatr Radiol* 1988;18:200–204.
2. Abramson SJ, Berdon WE, Baker DH. Childhood typhlitis: Its increasing association with myelogenous leukemia. Report of five cases. *Radiology* 1983;146:61–64.
3. Alvear DT, Kain TM. Suppurative mesenteric lymphadenitis, a forgotten clinical entity. *J Pediatr Surg* 1975;10:969–970.
4. Baldero J. Calculi in a Meckel's diverticulum. *J Fac Radiol* 1958;9:157–160.
5. Cohen WN, Denbesten L. Crohn's disease with predominant involvement of the appendix. *AJR* 1970;113: 361–363.
6. Ewen SWB, Anderson J, Galloway JMD, et al. Crohn's disease initially confined to the appendix. *Gastroenterology* 1971;60: 853–857.
7. Gallego-Herrero C, del Pozo-Garcia G, Marin-Rodriguez C, Ibarrola de Andres C. Torsion of a Meckel's diverticulum: Sonographic findings. *Pediatr Radiol* 1998;28:599–601.
8. Kamsal M, Wilkinson AG, Gibson B. Radiological features of fungal typhlitis complicating acute lymphoblastic leukaemia. *Pediatr Radiol* 1997;27:18-19.
9. Martin HCO, Goon HK. Salmonella ileocecal lymphadenitis masquerading as appendicitis. *J Pediatr Surg* 1986;21:377–378.
10. Puylaert JB. Mesenteric adenitis and acute terminal ileitis: ultrasound evaluation using graded compression. *Radiology* 1986;161: 691–695.
11. Rao PM, Rhea JT, Novelline RA. CT diagnosis of mesenteric adenitis. *Radiology* 1997;202:145–149.
12. Sivit CJ. Significance of peritoneal fluid identified by ultrasonographic examination in children with acute abdominal pain. *J Ultrasound Med* 1993;12:743–746.
13. Sivit CJ, Newman KD, Chandra RS. Visualization of enlarged mesenteric lymph nodes at Us examination: Clinical significance. *Pediatr Radiol* 1993;23:471–475.
14. Sherman NJ, Woolley MW. Ileocecal syndrome in acute childhood leukemia. *Arch Surg* 1973;107:39–42.
15. Sue K, Nishimi T, Yamada T, Matsuo Y, Tanaka N. A right lower abdominal mass due to Yersinia mesenteric lymphadenitis. *Pediatr Radiol* 1994;24:70–71.
16. Swischuk LE, John SD. Mesenteric adenitis-acute ileitis: A constellation of findings definable with ultrasound. *Emerg Radiol* 1998;5:210–218.

OTHER INTRAABDOMINAL INFLAMMATIONS OR INFECTIONS

These include pancreatitis, hepatitis, cholecystitis, cholelithiasis, renal infections, salpingitis, and a variety of colon inflammations.

Pancreatitis

Pancreatitis is not as common in childhood as in adults but is seen with cholecystitis and viral infections such as mumps and infectious mononucleosis, and after blunt abdominal trauma (4,9). The latter is especially common in the battered child syndrome (14). In addition, pancreatitis can occur with cystic fibrosis, juvenile diabetes mellitus, hyperparathyroidism, refeeding in malnourished children (3), drug and toxic substance (especially steroid) ingestion (16), organic acidemias (5), and on a hereditary basis in certain families (1).

Abdominal roentgenograms in acute pancreatitis most often are entirely normal, but in a few instances one sees so-called sentinel loops of distended intestine overlying the inflamed pancreas. These loops may take the form of (a) a dilated portion of the transverse colon (colon cutoff sign), (b) a dilated duodenum, or (c) dilated loops of small bowel in the upper midabdomen or left upper quadrant (12). In

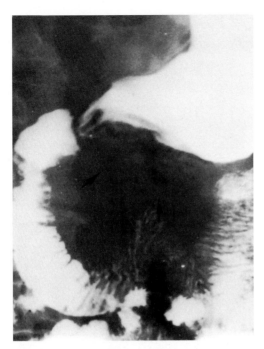

FIGURE 3.82. *Emphysematous pancreatitis.* Note the widened duodenal loop, elevated antrum of the stomach, and collection of bubbles in the region of the pancreas (*arrows*). These bubbles are gas collections in the pancreas.

all of these cases, the findings represent paralytic ileus of the loop of intestine lying next to the inflamed pancreas. *In most cases, however, the plain films are normal.* If pancreatic inflammation is so severe that pancreatic necrosis occurs, a gas abscess of the pancreas can develop (Fig. 3.82).

In most cases, pancreatitis is suspected and diagnosed clinically. Confirmation frequently is sought with ultra-

sonography or CT scanning, and although these studies often are normal, if enlargement of the pancreas is seen the diagnosis should be suspected (Fig. 3.83). On ultrasound images, increased lucency of the pancreas (Fig. 3.83A) may be seen (2), and in addition to this finding, one may see fluid in or around the pancreas (7) and increased echogenicity in and around the right kidney and liver caused by lipolysis of fat (15) (Fig. 3.83B). On CT scans, enlargement of the pancreas and peripancreatic fluid collections can be seen (Fig. 3.84). If a pseudocyst is present, a large cystic cavity with or without debris is seen (Fig. 3.84). Traumatic pancreatitis in childhood can be seen with any type of blunt abdominal trauma but is most common in the battered child syndrome. In these cases, the pancreas simply may be enlarged and edematous, but in other cases an actual fracture or laceration of the pancreas can be seen. These fractures can be identified with ultrasonography or CT (see Fig. 3.140). Initially the lesion may appear rather innocuous, but pseudocyst formation is a very likely possibility. It is interesting, however, that more recently conservative therapy of this lesion in cases of trauma has proved to be satisfactory (8).

It is important to realize that although pancreatitis is an abdominal problem, many extraabdominal clinical and roentgenographic manifestations also can be seen. These findings can distract one's attention from the main problem, and thus one must be aware of all of these findings. First, it should be noted that associated pleural effusions (Fig. 3.85) are very common (10,13), and that occasionally even pericardial effusions can be seen. In addition, if pancreatic enzymes are liberated into the bloodstream, pulmonary edema and profound respiratory insufficiency can result (10). In other instances, hypocalcemia resulting from the binding of calcium to these same pancreatic enzymes

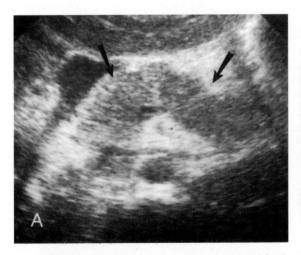
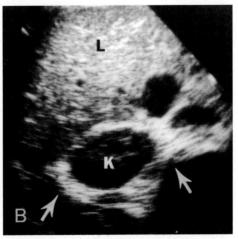

FIGURE 3.83. *Acute pancreatitis: ultrasound findings.* **(A)** Note the enlarged and slightly hypoechoic pancreas (*arrows*). **(B)** Another patient with an echogenic expanded fat compartment (*arrows*) around the kidney (*K*). This finding is due to lipolysis. Most often, however, the pancreas looks normal. *L*, liver.

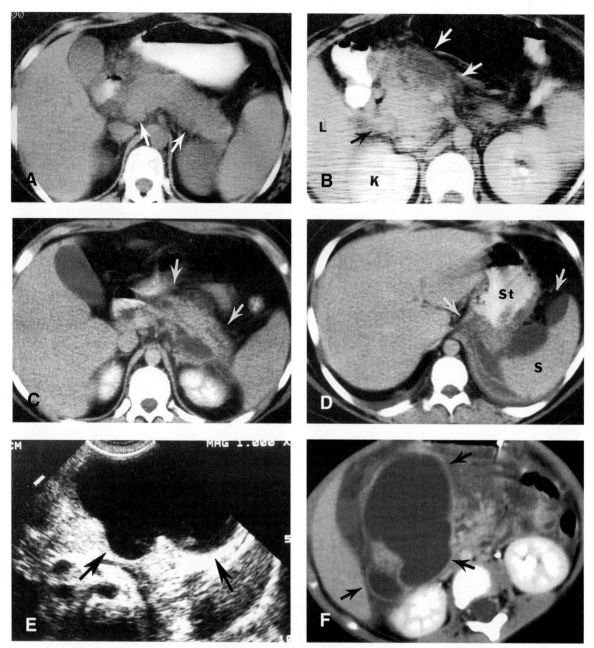

FIGURE 3.84. *Pancreatitis and complications: CT findings.* **(A)** Note the enlarged, swollen pancreas (*arrows*) with ragged edges. There appears to be some fluid accumulating around the pancreatic head. **(B)** Slightly lower slice demonstrates the large, inflammatory fluid collection (*white arrows*). Some of the fluid has extended into the space (*black arrow*) between the liver (*L*) and kidney (*K*). Such an inflammatory reaction causes lipolysis of the fatty tissue, as seen in Figure 3.83**B**. **(C)** In this patient the pancreas is indistinct, and there is suggestion of visualization of the pancreatic duct. Surrounding edema and fluid also are present. A discrete fluid collection is present between the tail of the pancreas and the left kidney. **(D)** Peripancreatic fluid has extended between the stomach (*ST*) and spleen (*S*). Both indistinct and discrete fluid collections are present (*arrow*). **(E)** Pseudocyst: Ultrasonographic findings. Note the basically anechoic, lobulated pancreatic pseudocyst (*arrows*). **(F)** CT findings. Note the multilobulated pancreatic pseudocyst (*arrows*). On both ultrasound and CT imaging, some cysts may contain more debris.

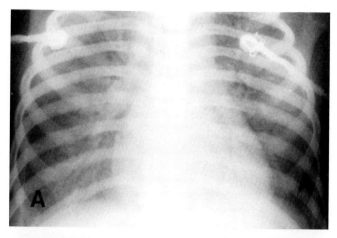

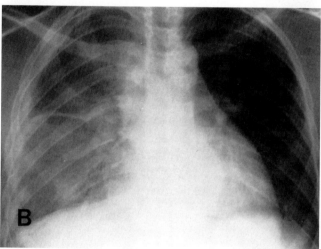

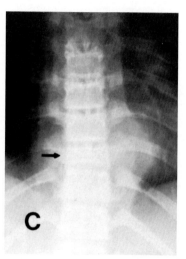

FIGURE 3.85. *Pancreatitis with chest findings.* **(A)** Note bilateral interstitial pulmonary edema causing haziness of the lungs in this patient with acute pancreatitis. **(B)** Another patient with a semi-opacified right hemithorax caused by a pleural effusion secondary to pancreatitis. Pulmonary edema of the right lung also probably is present, and a paraspinal mass is present on the left. **(C)** A week or two later this paraspinal mass was determined to result from a compression fracture of a thoracic vertebra (*arrow*). The findings were believed to represent vertebral collapse secondary to osteolysis resulting from fat necrosis.

can lead to electrocardiographic changes suggesting myocardial ischemia (6). Hypocalcemia also can lead to neurologic manifestations, and fat necrosis from the liberation of lipase into the bloodstream can produce subcutaneous nodules (11), widespread necrosis of the fat of the mesentery, and in some cases fat necrosis; induced lytic lesions in the bones (3,6,14). These latter lesions can mimic osteomyelitis and usually are seen 2 or 3 weeks after the acute episode of pancreatitis.

REFERENCES

1. Crane JM, Amoury RA, Hellerstein S. Hereditary pancreatitis: Report of a kindred. *J Pediatr Surg* 1973;8: 893–900.
2. Fleischer AC, Parker P, Kirchner SG, James AE Jr. Sonographic findings of pancreatitis in children. *Radiology* 1983;146:151–155.
3. Gryboski J, Hillemeier C, Kocoshis S, Anyan W, Seashore JS. Refeeding pancreatitis in malnourished children. *J Pediatr* 1980; 97:441–443.
4. Haddock G, Coupar G, Youngson GG, MacKinlay GA, Raine PAM. Acute pancreatitis in children: A 15-year review. *J Pediatr Surg* 1994;29:719–722.
5. Kahler SG, Sherwood WG, Woolf D. Pancreatitis in patients with organic acidemias. *J Pediatr* 1994;124:239–243.
6. Keating JP, Shackelford GD, Shackelford PG, Ternberg JL. Pancreatitis and osteolytic lesions. *J Pediatr* 1972;81:350–353.
7. King LR, Siegel MJ, Balie DM. Acute pancreatitis in children: CT findings of intra and extrapancreatic fluid collections. *Radiol* 1995;195:196–200.
8. Lucaya J, Vazquez E, Caballero F, Chair PG, Daneman A, Wesson D. Non-operative management of traumatic pancreatic pseudocysts associated with pancreatic duct laceration in children. *Pediatr Radiol* 1998;28:5–8.
9. Mader TJ, McHugh TP. Acute pancreatitis in children. *Pediatr Emerg Care* 1992;8:157–161.
10. Rovner AJ, Westcott JL. Pulmonary edema and respiratory insufficiency in acute pancreatitis. *Radiology* 1976;118:513–520.
11. Schrier RW, Melmon KL, Fenster LF. Subcutaneous nodular fat necrosis in pancreatitis. *Arch Intern Med* 1965;116:832–836.
12. Schwartz S, Nadelhaft J. Simulation of colonic obstruction at the splenic flexure by pancreatitis: Roentgen features. *AJR* 1957; 78:607–616.
13. Simmons MZ, Miller JA, Zurlo JV, Levine CD. Pleural effusions associated with acute pancreatitis: Incidence and appearance based on computed tomography. *Emerg Radiol* 1997;4:287–289.
14. Slovis TL, Berdon WE, Haller JO, Baker DH, Rosen L. Pancreatitis and the battered child syndrome: Report of two cases with skeletal involvement. *AJR* 1975;125:456–461.
15. Swischuk LE, Hayden CK. Pararenal space hyperechogenicity in childhood pancreatitis. *AJR* 1985;145:1085–1086.
16. Weizman Z, Sofer S. Acute pancreatitis in children with anticholinesterase insecticide intoxication. *Pediatrics* 1992;90:204–206.

Cholecystitis and Cholelithiasis

Cholecystitis and cholelithiasis are more common in childhood than is generally appreciated (1,2,4), and although it once was generally believed that cholelithiasis most often was secondary to hemolytic blood disorders, it has become increasingly apparent that most cases, perhaps two thirds or more, have other causes (2,4). Indeed, many are idiopathic, and, just as in the adult, more cases occur in females than in males.

Clinical features are much the same as in adults, but in infancy the diagnosis may be difficult. Jaundice may be present, and in those cases of empyema or hydrops of the gallbladder (1,3), a mass may be palpable. Indeed, an enlarged gallbladder may be visible roentgenographically (Fig. 3.86). If calcified gallstones are present, they may be seen on plain films (Fig. 3.87A), and if gangrene or abscess formation

develops in the gallbladder, one may see air in the gallbladder or within its wall (i.e., emphysematous cholecystitis). Otherwise, the diagnosis of most cases of cholecystitis and cholelithiasis is relegated to ultrasonography and, to some extent, nuclear scintigraphy. Ultrasound can identify acute cholecystitis, the presence of gallstones, a hydropic gallbladder, and dilated intrahepatic ducts. Nuclear scintigraphy, utilizing one or the other of the IDA isotopes, also can be utilized to identify acute cholecystitis, a hydropic gallbladder, or an obstructed biliary tract.

Gallstones, on ultrasound images, are strongly echogenic with pronounced, distal acoustic shadowing (Fig. 3.87B). Shadowing, however, is not always present (Fig. 3.87C) and probably depends on the amount of calcium in the stone. Acute cholecystitis may show nothing more than a distended gallbladder, but edema of the wall also can be seen (Fig. 3.88A). Such edema is not present in every case and

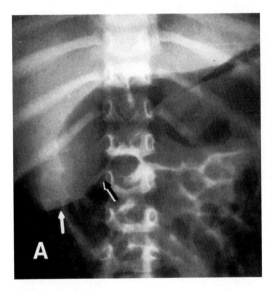

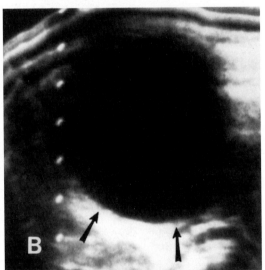

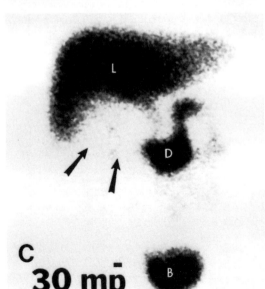

FIGURE 3.86. *Acute hydrops of the gallbladder.* **(A)** Note the large, distended gallbladder (*arrows*). **(B)** Ultrasound study demonstrating a hydropic gallbladder in another patient (*arrows*). **(C)** Isotope technetium–HIDA study demonstrates no isotope activity in the gallbladder (*arrows*). Isotope, however, has passed into the duodenum (*D*) and is being excreted into the urinary bladder (*B*).

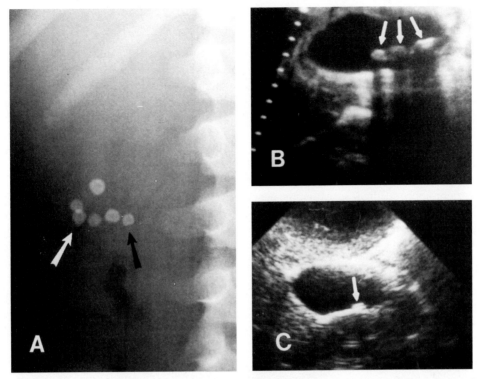

FIGURE 3.87. *Cholelithiasis.* **(A)** Note calcified gallstones (*arrows*) in this patient with sickle cell disease. **(B)** Ultrasonography demonstrates the gallbladder and numerous hyperechoic gallstones (*arrows*), with distal acoustical shadowing. **(C)** Another patient with a single gallstone (*arrow*).

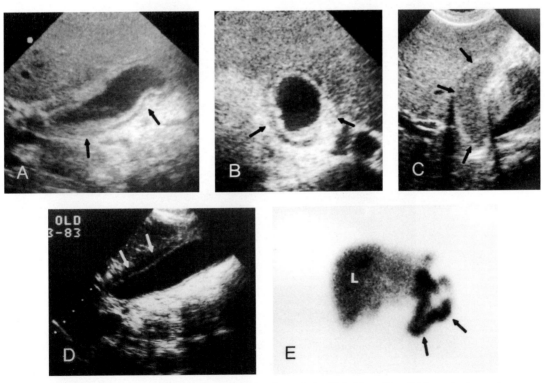

FIGURE 3.88. *Acute cholecystitis.* **(A)** Note the distended gallbladder with a thickened echogenic mucosa and a thickened hypoechoic muscular wall (*arrows*). **(B)** View in cross-section demonstrates the same findings (*arrows*). **(C)** Another patient with acalculus cholecystitis demonstrating a distended gallbladder full of sludge (*arrows*). **(D)** Another patient with a distended gallbladder and some fluid (*arrows*) around its wall. **(E)** Scintigram in the same patient demonstrates no accumulation of isotope material in the gallbladder. Isotope, however, is seen in the small bowel (*arrows*). *L*, liver.

also is nonspecific (5,6). In this regard, it can be seen with generalized anasarca and ascites. In most cases, however, it is seen with inflammatory disease of the gallbladder, and although it is nonspecific it is a valuable positive finding. Currently it is a common finding in patients with AIDS.

If a hydropic gallbladder is present, it is easily identified as a large, cystic, anechoic structure (Fig. 3.86B). A normal, nondistended gallbladder is not identified. This is important, for with choledochal cysts, another condition presenting as a large cystic right upper quadrant structure, the normal gallbladder usually is identified. Dilated intra- and extrahepatic bile ducts also can be identified with ultrasound (Fig. 3.89), as well as obstructing stones in the common bile duct (Fig. 3.89C).

Gallbladder sludge, ever since ultrasonography has come to be commonplace, has been identified frequently in a variety of patients. For the most part, gallbladder sludge is secondary to stasis, and such sludge can be a precursor of gallstone formation. Gallbladder sludge is a common finding in fasting patients and patients on hyperalimentation, but it also is seen in patients with acute cholecystitis and obstructive pathology of the biliary tract (Figs. 3.88 and 3.89). It also is commonly seen in patients with sickle cell disease. Indeed, it recently has been demonstrated that such sludge in these patients frequently goes on to frank gallstone formation (1).

In terms of nuclear scintigraphy, a technetium–IDA study often is very useful. Normally there is progression of the isotope from the liver into the bile ducts, the gallbladder, and then the intestines. If obstruction is present, this sequence of events is interrupted. For example, with acute cholecystitis, because the cystic duct is obstructed, the gallbladder usually is not visualized (Fig. 3.88). Similarly, if hydrops of the gallbladder is present, the gallbladder does

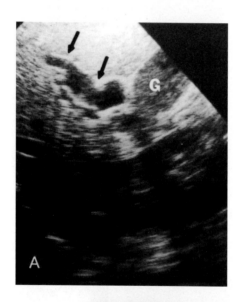
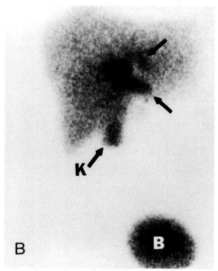
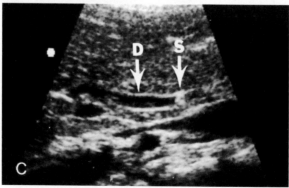

FIGURE 3.89. *Acute cholecystitis with obstruction.* **(A)** Note the distended gallbladder (*G*) containing some echogenic sludge. Also note the dilated hepatic duct (*arrows*). **(B)** Technetium–IDA study demonstrates isotope in the dilated, obstructed bile ducts (*arrows*), but none in the gallbladder. In addition, none has passed into the gastrointestinal tract. Some is being excreted, as would be expected, into the kidney (*K*) and the bladder (*B*).**(C)** Another patient with an obstructing stone (*S*) in a dilated common bile duct (*D*).

not accept any of the isotope. If the biliary tract is obstructed, accumulation of the isotope can be seen in the dilated biliary ducts (Fig. 3.89).

REFERENCES

1. Al-Salem AH, Quaisruddin S. The significance of biliary sludge in children with sickle cell disease. *Pediatr Surg Int* 1998;13:14–16.
2. Harned RK, Babbitt DP. Cholelithiasis in children. *Radiology* 1975;117:391–393.
3. Kumari S, Lee WJ, Baron MG. Hydrops of the gallbladder in a child: Diagnosis by ultrasonography. *Pediatrics* 1979;63:295–297.
4. Newman DE. Gallstones in children. *Pediatr Radiol* 1973;1: 100–104.
5. Patriquin HB, DePietro M, Barber FE. Sonography of thickened gallbladder wall: Causes in children. *AJR* 1983;141:57–60.
6. Teefey SA, Baron RL, Bigler SA. Sonography of the gallbladder: Significance of striated (layered) thickening of the gallbladder wall. *AJR* 1991;156:945–947.

Urinary Tract Infection

Acute pyelonephritis and cystitis are common in childhood, especially in girls. With ultrasound, however, cystitis now is seen commonly in males, and in many cases it is secondary to viral infection. Clinical findings in these patients consist of lower abdominal pain and hematuria, and on ultrasound images thickening of the bladder mucosa is seen (see Fig. 3.96). For the most part, however, plain film findings in patients with acute urinary tract infection usually are normal. On the other hand, in a few cases, sentinel loops may be seen over the infected kidney or bladder, and if a unilateral problem such as a renal carbuncle or perinephric abscess exists, evidence of perirenal inflammation or an actual mass with scoliosis to the ipsilateral side may be noted (Fig. 3.90). In these cases, pyelographic findings may demonstrate a displaced kidney with variably decreased renal function (Fig. 3.90B), but in acute pyelonephritis without these complications, except for mild to moderate

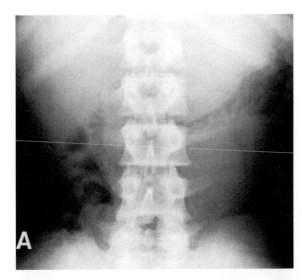

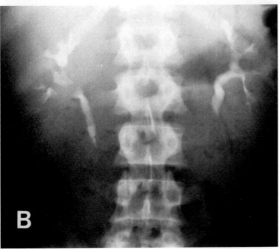

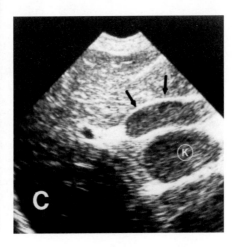

FIGURE 3.90. *Perinephric abscess.* **(A)** Note sentinel loops and absence of the psoas shadow on the right. The normal psoas shadow is visible on the left. Also note that the inferior edge of the liver is obliterated. **(B)** Intravenous pyelogram demonstrating poorly defined right renal margins and a right kidney that appears a little larger than the left. **(C)** Ultrasonographic findings in another patient demonstrate an echogenic abscess (*arrows*) just above the kidney (*K*).

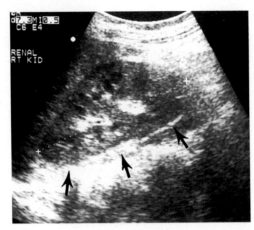

FIGURE 3.91. *Pyelonephritis: ultrasonographic findings.* Note the enlarged kidney demonstrating increased echogenicity.

calyceal dilatation and blunting in some cases, the pyelographic findings are normal. Similarly, ultrasound studies usually are normal. Occasionally, generalized renal enlargement with increased echogenicity (Fig. 3.91) and mild caliectasis can be seen (3), but unless a complication such as an abscess occurs, the findings usually are normal.

Renal or perirenal abscesses, in general, can be liquid or solid on ultrasonographic examination and are readily demonstrable with CT imaging (Fig. 3.92). Many of these abscesses now are drained percutaneously. Lobar nephronia or focal nephritis also can be detected with ultrasound (5). Generally, these inflamed areas present as round or oval areas in the kidney that are echogenic (Fig. 3.93). It has been suggested that echogenicity is a result of focal hemorrhage secondary to the vasculitis induced by the infection (4). These lesions also are readily demonstrable with cortical imaging agents such as technetium-99–DMSA or glucoheptonate (1).

Color flow Doppler also can be utilized in the evaluation of renal infections (2,5). Generally, blood flow is increased with diffuse parenchymal infection, but this finding is seen only in advanced cases. Lobar nephronia, because the inflammatory process is so intense that there is compression of the blood vessels in the involved area shows absence of blood flow to the area of lobar nephronia.

Finally, a note regarding infection associated with hydronephrosis is in order. It is well known that obstructive uropathy predisposes one to urinary tract infection. In most such cases only the obstructed urinary tract is detected, but in some cases the entire tract may become filled with purulent material. This can occur both with bacterial and fungal infections and can lead to anuria. In these profound cases, ultrasonography readily demonstrates the purulent material in the dilating collecting system (Fig. 3.94).

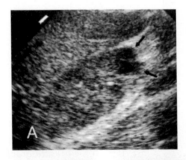
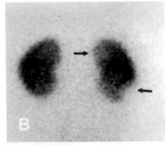
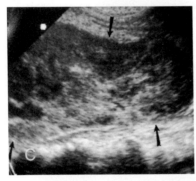
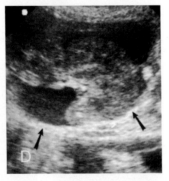
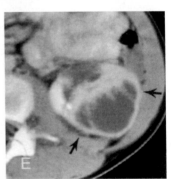

FIGURE 3.92. *Renal abscess.* **(A)** Note the small sonolucent abscess (*arrows*) in the inferior pole of the right kidney. **(B)** Technetium-99m glucoheptenate study demonstrates the focal defect in the lower pole of the right kidney (*lower arrow*) but also demonstrates another suspicious defect in the upper pole (*upper arrow*). This second defect was not visible ultrasonographically. **(C)** Another patient with a markedly enlarged and completely distorted kidney (*arrows*) resulting from pyonephrosis. **(D)** Cross-sectional view demonstrates the distorted kidney and a sonolucent subcapsular fluid (pus) collections (*arrows*). **(E)** CT study shows the enlarged left kidney (*arrows*) demonstrating a complete loss of normal architecture and the subcapsular fluid collections noted in **(D)**.

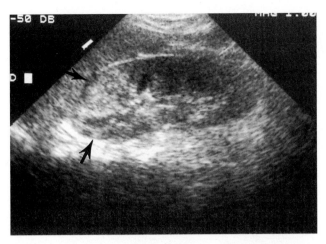

FIGURE 3.93. *Lobar nephronia.* Note the echogenic area in the upper pole of the right kidney (*arrows*).

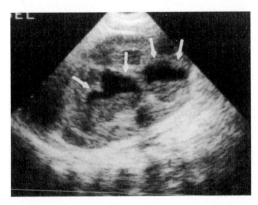

FIGURE 3.94. *Hydropyonephrosis.* Note the dilated calyces with numerous fluid debris levels (*arrows*).

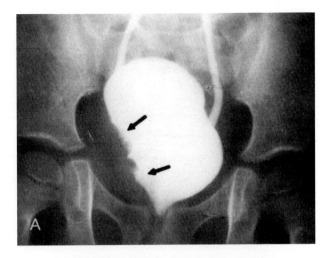

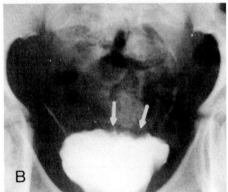

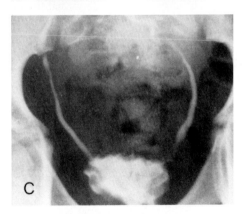

FIGURE 3.95. *Cystitis: various configurations.* **(A)** Note irregularity and masslike indentation of the right side of the bladder (*arrows*) in this patient presenting with bleeding from the urinary tract. This patient had cytoxan cystitis. **(B)** Note irregularity over the top of the bladder (*arrows*) in this patient with symptoms of cystitis. **(C)** Postvoid film demonstrates marked mucosal irregularity and thickening of the bladder.

REFERENCES

1. Bjorgvinsson E, Majd M, Eggli KD. Diagnosis of acute pyelonephritis in children: Comparison of sonography and 99mTc-DMSA scintigraphy. *AJR* 1991;157:539–543.
2. Eggli KD, Eggli D. Color Doppler sonography in pyelonephritis. *Pediatr Radiol* 1992;22:422–425.
3. Pickworth FE, Carlin JB, Ditchfield MR. Sonographic mneasurement of renal enlargement in children with acute pyelonephritis and time needed for resolution: Implications for renal growth assessment. *AJR* 1995;165:405–408.
4. Rigsby CM, Rosenfield AT, Glickman MG, Hodson J. Hemorrhagic focal bacterial nephritis: Findings on gray-scale sonography and CT. *AJR* 1986;146:1173–1177.
5. Winters WD. Power Doppler sonographic evaluation of acute pyelonephritis in children. *J Ultrasound Med* 1996;15:91–96.

Cystitis

Cystitis usually is seen in combination with pyelonephritis, although it can occur as an isolated infection. Most often, it is of bacterial origin, but viral infections can occur (2,3). In most cases of cystitis, one notes a spastic, irregular bladder, secondary to spasm and mucosal edema (Fig. 3.95). If

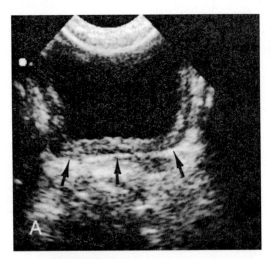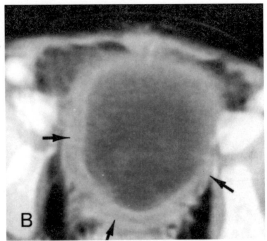

FIGURE 3.96. *Cystitis: various ultrasonographic and CT findings.* **(A)** Note the markedly thickened echogenic mucosa (*arrows*). **(B)** CT study in another patient again demonstrates markedly thickened mucosa (*arrows*).

blood clots are present, they may be seen as radiolucent filling defects in the bladder. Another form of cystitis in children is cyclophosphamide (Cytoxan) cystitis, but this problem is seen exclusively in patients with blood dyscrasias or other tumors requiring therapy with that agent (Fig. 3.95C).

Generally, urinary bladder abnormalities are best demonstrated with the bladder fully distended, but often edema and irregularity of the mucosa are demonstrated more clearly on the postvoiding or partially filled study (Fig. 3.95C). In addition, now that ultrasonography is available, thickening of the bladder mucosa in cases of cystitis is readily detected (Fig. 3.96A). In some of these cases mucosal thickening can be profound and mimic the findings of a bladder tumor (1,4). Cystitis cystica is one such condition. Thickening of the bladder mucosa also is demonstrable on CT studies (Fig. 3.96B).

REFERENCES

1. Harris VJ, Javapour N, Fizzotti G. Cystitis cystica masquerading as a bladder tumor. *AJR* 1974;120:410–412.
2. Mufson MA, Zallar LM, Mankad VN, Manalo D. Adenovirus infection in acute hemorrhagic cystitis. *Am J Dis Child* 1971;121: 281–285.
3. Numazaki Y, Shigeta A, Kumasaka K, Miyazawa T, Yamanaka M, Yano N, Takai S, Ishida N. Acute hemorrhagic cystitis in children: Isolation of adenovirus II. *N Engl J Med* 1968;278:700–704.
4. Rosenberg HK, Eggli KD, Zerin M, Ortega W, Wallach M, Kolberg H., Lebowitz RL, Snyder HM. Benign cystitis in children mimicking rhabdomyosarcoma. *J Ultrasound Med* 1994;13:921–932.

Salpingitis

Salpingitis occurs in adolescent girls (2,4) and has a real propensity to produce localizing, sentinel loops over the lower abdomen or profound paralytic ileus mimicking mechanical obstruction (Fig. 3.97). These findings result from the diffuse peritonitis induced by pus extruding into the peritoneal cavity from the fallopian tubes. In other cases, masslike configurations representing pus collections in the lower abdomen and pelvis can be seen. These pus collections can represent true pelvic abscesses, pyosalpinx, or tuboovarian abscesses. In any of these cases, the clinical findings may mimic acute appendicitis, and, to be sure, this also can be a problem with ultrasonography (3). Ultrasound, however, probably still is the best imaging modality for detecting all of these findings. Currently, transvaginal ultrasound tends to produce clearer and more definitive studies (1), but transabdominal ultrasound still is useful as the first study. Ultrasonographically, one may see a variety of findings including dilated, pus-filled fallopian tubes, a tuboovarian abscess, fluid in the cul-de-sac, and fluid in the peritoneal cavity. Although all of these findings generally are nonspecific, in the proper clinical setting they are highly suggestive (Fig. 3.97 and 3.98).

In other cases one may encounter focally inflamed segments of small bowel, and then differentiation from acute appendicitis may be difficult. The reason this occurs is that

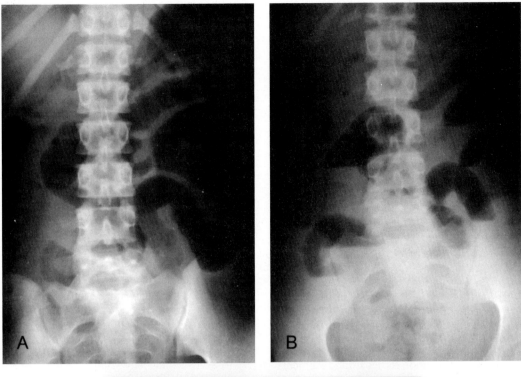

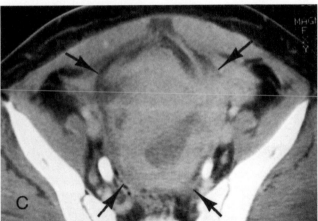

FIGURE 3.97. *Salpingitis and pelvic inflammatory disease.* **(A)** Young adolescent with acute abdomen. Findings suggest peritonitis or obstruction. **(B)** Upright film suggests intestinal obstruction. After antibiotic treatment, these findings disappeared in 24 hours. **(C)** Another patient whose CT study shows a large pelvic mass with mixed densities (*arrows*). The findings are nonspecific.

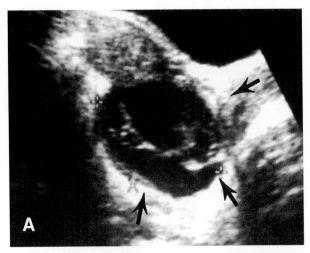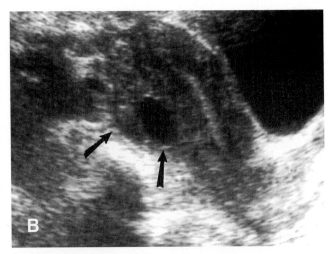

FIGURE 3.98. *Tuboovarian abscess.* **(A)** Note the basically hypoechoic mass (*arrows*) with some internal echogenic debris. **(B)** In this case an oval-shaped mass (*arrows*) is seen. It has a thick wall and a central collection of fluid. It most likely represents an inflamed fallopian tube constituting pyosalpinx.

with pelvic inflammatory disease diffuse peritonitis occurs, and if the subsequent inflammation settles around segments of the intestine, persistent pain and positive physical findings persist. Ultrasonographically it can be determined that all of this results from segmentally inflamed intestine.

REFERENCES

1. Bulas DI, Ahlstrom PA, Sivit CJ, Nussbaum AR, O'Donnell RM. Pelvic inflammatory disease in the adolescent: Comparison of transabdominal and transvaginal sonographic evaluation. *Radiology* 1992;183:435–439.
2. Golden N, Cohen H, Gennari Q, Neuhobb S. The use of ultrasonography in the evaluation of adolescents with pelvic inflammatory disease. *Am J Dis Child* 1987;141:1235–1238.
3. Terry J, Forrest T. Sonographic demonstration of salpingitis: Potential confusion with appendicitis. *J Ultrasound Med* 1989;8:39–41.
4. Shafer MAB, Irwin CE, Sweet RL: Acute salpingitis in the adolescent female. *J Pediatr* 1982;100:339-350.

Inflammatory Bowel Disease and Colitis

More and more conditions considered to represent inflammatory bowel disease are being identified with ultrasound (6). The most common, of course, is simple viral gastroenteritis, but any number of inflammatory diseases can be encountered. For the most part, two patterns exist: diffuse or segmental mucosal thickening resulting from mucosal disease and transmural intestinal thickening caused by diseases such as regional enteritis (Fig. 3.99). Overall, however, except for viral gastroenteritis, inflammatory problems of the gas-

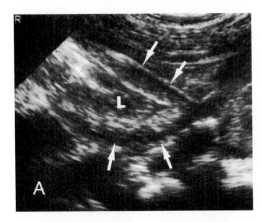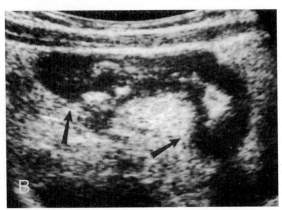

FIGURE 3.99. *Inflammatory bowel disease.* **(A)** Characteristic mucosal thickening (*arrows*) producing echogenic thickening of the mucosa. *L*, intestinal lumen. **(B)** Transmural thickening resulting from late-stage regional enteritis produces more uniform hypoechoic thickening of the intestinal wall (*arrows*).

trointestinal tract usually involve the colon or teminal ileum. Focal mucosal thickening in the stomach also can be seen with acute gastritis and gastric ulcer disease (5). Color flow Doppler demonstrates increased blood flow in these inflammatory conditions and can differentiate inflammatory from ischemic bowel disease (8).

Colitis, on an acute basis, can be seen with shigellosis, ulcerative colitis (Fig. 3.100B and C), pseudomembranous colitis (4) (Fig. 3.100A), typhlitis, granulomatous colitis (Crohn's disease), amebiasis, and food (milk) allergy in infants (2,6,10). Colitis also can be seen with the hemolytic–uremic syndrome (1,7).

For the most part, plain-film findings in colitis are lacking, except in those patients with toxic megacolon. Most often, this complication is seen with ulcerative colitis, and in such cases the colon (usually the transverse colon) is distended and paralyzed. It is void of haustral markings and its wall may be smooth, coarsely serrated, or thumbprinted (Fig. 3.101). The latter configurations result from extensive

mucosal inflammation and edema. Toxic megacolon also can be seen with granulomatous colitis and amebic colitis (11).

In some cases of gastroenteritis, massive volumes of fluid in the small intestine or colon can lead to plain film findings that might at first suggest more serious problems such as ascites, peritonitis, or bowel obstruction (Fig. 3.102A). Every so often one ends up performing a barium enema in such a patient, and the intense colonic spasm demonstrated can be striking (Fig. 3.102B). Organisms likely to produce these findings include shigella and rotovirus.

Necrotizing enterocolitis is primarily an affliction of premature infants but also can be seen in older infants with any type of ischemic insult of the intestine (9). Intestinal ischemia also can occur after cocaine ingestion (3). In any case, the findings consist of (a) pronounced abdominal distension secondary to paralytic ileus of the intestine, (b) pneumatosis cystoides intestinalis, (c) portal vein gas, (d) free air in the peritoneal cavity when perforation occurs, and (e) peritonitis.

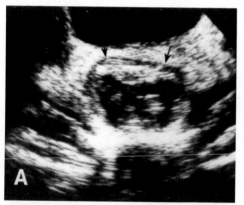
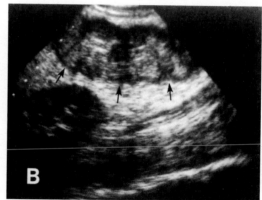
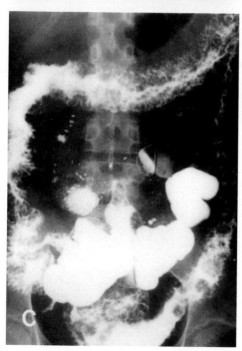

FIGURE 3.100. *Colitis: ultrasonographic findings.* **(A)** Note the sonolucent rim of thickened rectal wall (*arrows*) in this patient with pseudomembranous colitis. Sonolucent fluid is present in the lumen and there are areas of echogenicity caused by debris and thickened mucosa. **(B)** Another patient with ulcerative colitis. Note the sonolucent rim of thickened colon wall (*arrows*) and numerous echoes from the thickened mucosa within. **(C)** Barium enema in the same patient.

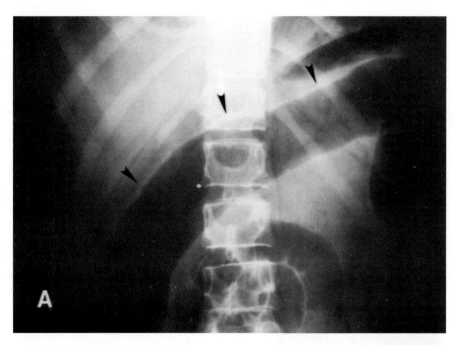

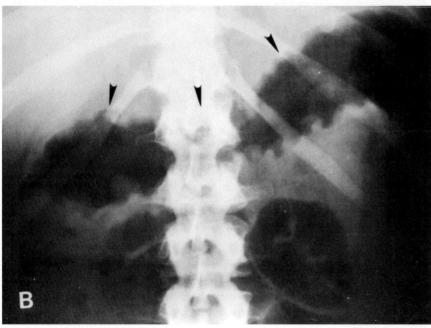

FIGURE 3.101. *Toxic megacolon.* **(A)** Note the dilated but smooth transverse colon with no haustral markings (*arrows*). **(B)** Another patient with a dilated colon, but in this case note the nodular projections into the lumen of the dilated colon (*arrows*). The findings represent thickening, edema, and pseudopolyp formation of the colon. (Courtesy of Virgil B. Graves, M.D.)

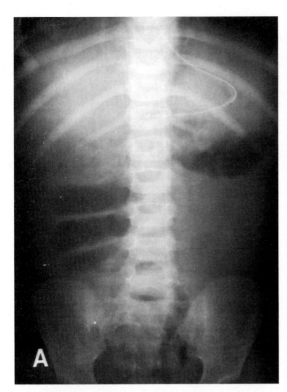 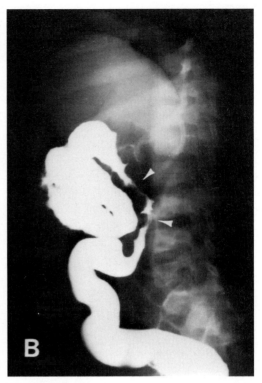

FIGURE 3.102. *Shigellosis.* **(A)** Supine film demonstrating diffuse opacity throughout the abdomen and three sentinel loops on the right. The findings could be misinterpreted as peritonitis, small bowel obstruction, or some other intraabdominal problem. The patient had a shigella infection of the gastrointestinal tract. **(B)** Barium enema in another patient demonstrating extreme spasm with thumbprinting of the descending colon (*arrows*).

REFERENCES

1. Bar-Ziv J, Ayoub J, Fletcher B. Hemolytic uremic syndrome: Case presenting with acute colitis. *Pediatr Radiol* 1974;2: 203–205.
2. Bloom DA, Buonomo C, Fishman SJ, Furuta G, Nurko S. Allergic colitis: A mimic of Hirschsprung disease. *Pediatr Radiol* 1999; 29:37–41.
3. Endress C, Gray DGK, Wollschlaeger G. Case report: Bowel ischemia and perforation after cocaine use. *AJR* 1992;159:73–75.
4. Han SJ, Jung PM, Kim H, Kim JE, Hong J, Hwang EH, Seong I. Multiple intestinal ulcerations and perforation secondary to Methicillin-resistant staphylococcus aureus enteritis in infants. *J Pediatr Surg* 1999;34:381–386.
5. Hayden CK Jr., Swischuk LE, Rytting JE. Gastric ulcer disease in infants: US findings. *Radiology* 1987;164:131–134.
6. Hill SM, Milla PJ. Colitis caused by food allergy in infants. *Arch Dis Child* 1990;65:132–133.
7. Peterson RB, Meseroll WP, Shrago GG, et al. Radiographic features of colitis associated with the hemolyticuremic syndrome. *Radiology* 1976;118:667–671.
8. Siegel MJ, Friedland JA, Hildebolt CF. Bowel wall thickening in children: Differentiation with US. *Radiology* 1997;203:631–635.
9. Takayanagi K, Kapila L. Necrotizing enterocolitis in older infants. *Arch Dis Child* 1981;56:468–471.
10. Swischuk LE, Hayden CK. Barium enema findings (segmental colitis) in four neonates with bloody diarrhea: Possible cow's milk allergy. *Pediatr Radiol* 1985;15:34–37.
11. Vargas M, Pena A. Toxic amoebic colitis and amoebic colon perforation in children: An improved prognosis. *J Pediatr Surg* 1976; 11:223–225.

MISCELLANEOUS ACUTE ABDOMINAL PROBLEMS

Systemic Conditions Presenting with an Acute Abdomen

An acutely painful abdomen can be seen in patients with diabetes mellitus (1), sickle cell anemia, abdominal migraine, and pneumonia. For the most part, the abdominal roentgenograms in these patients are normal or merely show paralytic ileus. In diabetes mellitus the problem usually is ketoacidosis or electrolyte imbalance; in sickle cell disease the problem is sludging of the blood and ischemia of the intestine. Abdominal migraine is a matter of vasospasm; with pneumonia the problem is referred pain.

REFERENCE

1. Valerio D. Acute diabetic abdomen in childhood. *Lancet* 1977;1: 66–67.

Peptic Ulcer Disease and Gastritis

A thorough, complete discussion of these entities is beyond the scope of this book, but it is worth noting that both conditions are more common in childhood than is generally appreciated. In some children, acute abdominal pain clearly suggestive of duodenal ulcer disease can be seen, but many children present with little in the way of abdominal pain, and vomiting is the predominant feature. In still other cases, bleeding may be the problem.

Roentgenographically, the actual ulcer may be seen (Fig. 3.103A), but most cases of peptic ulcer disease do not demonstrate an actual ulcer. More often, spasm of the antrum and duodenal bulb along with edema of the mucosa

of these structures is seen. In addition, in some cases of gastritis, one may see a diffuse cobblestone appearance to the edematous mucosa (Fig. 3.103B). Ultrasound also can demonstrate the presence of gastritis (2). In these cases, the gastric wall is thickened and there is disruption of the normal layers of the wall (Fig. 3.103C). It is difficult to visualize an actual ulcer with ultrasound, but if the ulcer is large it may be seen.

Gastritis and peptic ulcer disease also can be seen secondary to steroid therapy (1), and more recently *Helicobacter pylori* infections have been invoked as a causal organism. Although originally this organism was believed to be the cause of both antral gastritis and duodenal ulcer disease (4), there is growing opinion that the problem most often is gastritis (3,5).

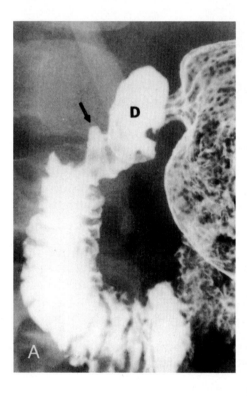

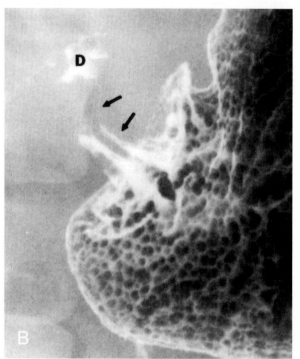

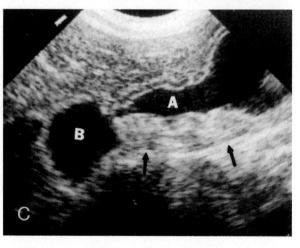

FIGURE 3.103. *Peptic ulcer disease and gastritis.* **(A)** Note the postapical ulcer crater (*arrow*). There are edematous folds radiating from its base and marked spasm of the postapical portion of the duodenum. *D*, duodenal bulb. **(B)** Gastritis. Note the diffuse mucosal nodularity throughout the stomach. In addition, note spasm of the antrum (*arrows*) and duodenal bulb (*D*). **(C)** Ultrasonogram demonstrating gastritis with marked thickening of the gastric wall (mucosa and submucosa) along the inferior curvature of the antrum (*arrows*). Note the normal layers on the opposite side. *B*, duodenal bulb; *A*, antrum.

REFERENCES

1. Bickler SW, Harrison MW, Campbell JR. Perforated peptic ulcer disease in children: Association of corticosteroid therapy. *J Pediatr Surg* 1993;28:785–787.
2. Deckelbaum RL, Roy CC, Lussier-Lazaroff J, Morin CL. Peptic ulcer disease: A clinical study in 73 children. *Can Med Assoc J* 1974;111:225–228.
3. Gormally SM, Prakash N, Durnin MT, et al. Association of symptoms with Helicobacter pyulori infection in children. *J Pediatr* 1995;126:753–756.
4. Hayden CK Jr., Swischuk LE, Rytting JE. Gastric ulcer disease in infants: US findings. *Radiology* 1987;164:131–134.
5. Israel DM, Hassall E. Treatment and long-term follow-up of Helicobacter pylori–associated duodenal ulcer disease in children. *J Pediatr* 1993;123:53–58.
6. Marks MP, Lanza MV, Kahlstrom EJ, et al. Pediatric hypertrophic gastropathy. *AJR* 1986;147:1031–1034.

Hiatus Hernia and Esophagitis

The symptoms of a hiatus hernia and gastroesophageal reflux are well known to all, and if one takes the time, a strongly suggestive history can be extracted from an older child if the problem is present. In younger infants the problem is more difficult, and vomiting may be the only symptom. Associated problems such as resistant asthma (2), sudden infant death syndrome (3,4), and apnea (6) have been attributed to gastroesophageal reflux. Although all of these problems do occur, they are not nearly as common as generally believed. Certainly our experience suggests that gastroesophageal reflux is not a very common cause of refractory asthma or the sudden infant death syndrome.

Esophagitis secondary to the ingestion of corrosive materials is dealt with subsequently in this chapter. Rarely, esophagitis caused by a virus (herpes [1,5]) or infection with *Candida* sp is encountered in childhood. These infec-

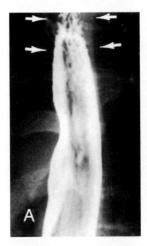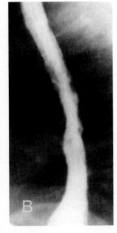

FIGURE 3.104. *Esophagitis.* **(A)** Herpes. Note the fine nodularity and mucosal fold thickening (*arrows*) in the upper esophagus. **(B)** Monilia. Note extensive spasm of the esophagus and irregularity of the mucosa of the esophagus.

tions are seen more often now that HIV-infected patients have become commonplace. The findings usually involve the mucosa with diffuse edema, often manifesting in cobblestoning or edematous striation of the esophagus (Fig. 3.104). Of course, pronounced spasm is present, and with esophagitis caused by *Candida* sp, such spasm can be profound. Solitary ulcers are less common, for the problem usually is one of diffuse, superficial ulceration.

REFERENCES

1. Bastian JF, Kaufman IA. Herpes simplex esophagitis in a healthy 10-year-old boy. *J Pediatr* 1962;100:426–427.
2. Danus O, Casar C, Larrain A, Pope CE II. Esophageal reflux: An unrecognized cause of recurrent obstructive bronchitis in children. *J Pediatr* 1976;89:220–224.
3. Herbst JJ, Book LS, Bray PF. Gastroesophageal reflux in the "near miss" sudden infant death syndrome. *J Pediatr* 1978;92:73–75.
4. Leape LL, Holder TM, Franklin JD, Amoury RA, Ashcraft KW. Respiratory arrest in infants secondary to gastroesophageal reflux. *Pediatrics* 1977;60:924–928.
5. Meyers C, Durkin MG, Love L. Radiographic findings in herpetic esophagitis. *Radiology* 1976;119:21–22.
6. Walsh JK, Farrell MK, Kennan WJ, Lucas M, Kramer M. Gastroesophageal reflux in infants: Relation to apnea. *J Pediatr* 1981; 99:197–201.

Intestinal Infarction and Intramural Bleeding or Edema

Intestinal infarction in children is uncommon, except with mechanical problems such as volvulus or intussusception, or after blunt abdominal trauma causing injury to the blood vessels of the gut. Plain films may show sentinel loops, generalized paralytic ileus, or edematous loops of infarcted intestine. Extremely edematous loops of the intestine may show so-called thumbprinting of the bowel wall, and on ultrasound, thickening of the intestinal wall is seen.

Bleeding into the intestinal wall can occur in hemophilia or Henoch–Schönlein purpura or after trauma. Edema can occur with hypoproteinemia, portal hypertension, and angioneurotic edema. Usually there is little to see on the plain films of these patients, but if the bleeding or edema is extensive, thumbprinting or a masslike configuration of the intestine can be noted. Most often, these changes are demonstrated more clearly with barium studies of the upper gastrointestinal tract, but bowel thickening now is initially readily demonstrable with ultrasound.

Henoch–Schönlein purpura is not an uncommon cause of intestinal bleeding, and the findings of bleeding in an acute abdomen may precede the classic purpuric skin rash (6). The condition is believed to be a virus-induced hypersensitivity problem leading to small vessel thrombosis and subsequent bleeding. If the gastrointestinal tract is involved, the main clinical manifestation is abdominal pain (5,9). The thickened hemorrhagic mucosa can be identified readily with ultrasound (1–4) (Fig. 3.105) and usually man-

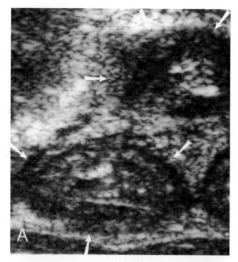

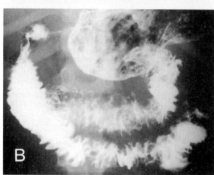

FIGURE 3.105. *Henoch–Schönlein purpura.* **(A)** Note concentric thickening of the intestinal wall primarily caused by echogenic mucosa (*arrows*). A number of loops of intestine are involved. **(B)** Another patient whose upper gastrointestinal series demonstrates extensive edema and thickening of the intestinal wall, producing marked spiculation and thumbprinting of the involved segments of the intestine.

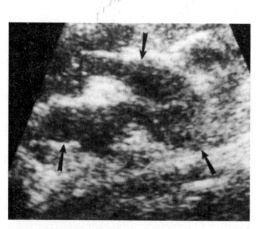

FIGURE 3.106. *Henoch–Schönlein purpura: pseudointussusception.* Note the pseudokidney appearance of this liquified hematoma (*arrows*). The findings resemble those of intussusception. This patient was not obstructed and had a normal barium enema.

ifests as concentric thickening of the intestinal wall (6). In other cases, it may be more eccentric (3). Free peritoneal fluid also can be seen in small amounts, and intussusception is a known complication of the condition (8,9). The ultrasonographic appearance of the intussusception is no different than with other causes of intussusception, but we have noted that a liquified hematoma can produce ultrasonographic findings similar to those seen with intussusception (Fig. 3.106). If a gastrointestinal barium study is performed (7, 10), the appearance of the thickened intestinal loops can be quite striking (Fig. 3.105B). Urinary tract involvement also can be seen. In many cases this consists of a hemorrhagic nephritis (6), but hemorrhagic stenotic ureteritis also has been described (10).

REFERENCES

1. Agha FP, Nostrat TT, Keren DF. Leucocytoplastic vasculitis (hypersensitivity angiitis) of the small bowel presenting with severe gastrointestinal hemorrhage. *Am J Gastroenterol* 1986;81: 195–198.
2. Bomelburg T, Claasen U, von Lengerke HJ. Intestinal ultrasonographic findings in Schonlein syndrome by high frequency ultrasound. *Eur J Pediatr* 1991;150:158–160.
3. Couture A, Veyrac C, Baud C, Galifer RB, Armelin I. Evaluation of abdominal pain in Henoch-Schonlein syndrome by high frequency ultrasound. *Pediatr Radiol* 1992;22:12–17.
4. Demirci A, Cengiz K, Baris S, Karagoz F. CT and ultrasound of abdominal hemorrhage in Henoch-Schonlein purpura. *J Comput Assist Tomogr* 1991;15:143–145.
5. Glasier CM, Siegel MJ, MacAlister WH, Schakelford GD. Henoch-Schonlein syndrome in children: Gastrointestinal manifestations. *AJR* 1981;136:1081–1085.
6. John SD, Swischuk LE, Hayden CK Jr. Gastrointestinal sonographic findings in Henoch-Schonlein purpura. *Emerg Radiol* 1996;3:4–8.
7. Martinez-Frontanilla LA, Haase GM, Ernster JA, Bailey CW. Surgical complications in Henoch-Schonlein purpura. *J Pediatr Surg* 1984;19:434–436.
8. Martinez-Frontanilla LA, Silverman L, Meagher DP Jr. Intussusception in Henoch-Schonlein purpura: Diagnosis with ultrasound. *J Pediatr Surg* 1988;23:375–376.
9. Rodriquez-Erdman F, Levitan R. Gastrointestinal and roentgenological manifestations of Henoch-Schonlein purpura. *Gastroenterol* 1968;54:260–264.
10. Smet MH, Marchal G, Oyen R, Breysem L. Stenosing hemorrhagic ureteritis in a child with Henoch-Schonlein purpura: CT appearance. *J Comput Assist Tomogr* 1991;15:326–328.

Hepatitis

With hepatitis, as the liver enlarges it stretches its capsule, and abdominal pain can be the presenting problem. Hepatitis usually is viral in origin but also can be toxic in origin. There are few imaging findings with hepatitis. In most cases, ultrasonographically the liver merely is enlarged. In some cases of acute liver necrosis, however, edema of the liver can produce a sonolucent-appearing liver, with marked periportal echogenicity (1,2) (Fig. 3.107A and B).

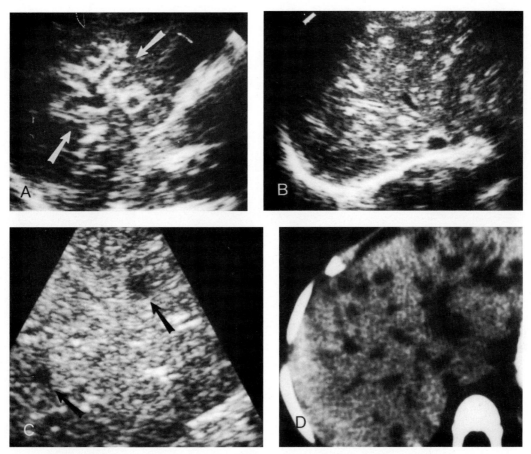

FIGURE 3.107. *Acute hepatic necrosis.* **(A)** Note the relatively hypoechoic liver parenchyma and marked periportal echogenicity (*arrows*). **(B)** Another view demonstrating similar findings. **(C)** Cat-scratch disease granulomas. Note the two hypoechoic areas in the liver (*arrows*). **(D)** CT scan demonstrates numerous low-density lesions scattered throughout the liver. (From Port J, Leonidas JC. Granulomatous hepatitis in cat-scratch disease. *Pediatr Radiol* 1991;21:598–599, with permission.)

In addition, it has been noted that in cat-scratch disease, multiple sonolucent granulomas may be seen in the liver and spleen (3–5). These also are demonstrable with CT imaging (Fig. 3.107C and D).

REFERENCES

1. Blane CE, Jongeward RH, Silver TM. Sonographic features of hepatocellular disease in neonates and infants. *AJR* 1983;141: 1313–1316.
2. Kurtz AB, Rubin CS, Cooper HS, Nisenbaum HL, Cole-Beuglet C, Medoff J, Goldberg BB. Ultrasound findings in hepatitis. *Radiology* 1980;136:717–723.
3. Larsen CE, Patrick LE. Abdominal (liver, spleen) and bone manifestations of cat-scratch disease. *Pediatr Radiol* 1992;22:353–355.
4. Port J, Leonidas JC. Granulomatous hepatitis in cat-scratch disease. *Pediatr Radiol* 1991;21:598–599.
5. Rappaport DC, Cumming WA, Ros PR. Case report: Dissemi-
nated hepatic and splenic lesions in cat-scratch disease. Imaging features. *AJR* 1991;156:1227–1228.

Renal Colic

Renal colic is not as great a problem in children as it is in adults, but it does occur. The clinical symptoms are exactly the same as in adults, and imaging of these patients centers around plain films, ultrasonography, and intravenous pyelography. More recently, however, spiral CT imaging has proven to be quite accurate in the detection of renal calculi (1,4,5). For the most part, this has occurred in the adult population, but it also should be applicable to older children (Fig. 3.108).

Plain films may reveal an enlarged renal silhouette and a calcified stone (Fig. 3.108). Ultrasound can demonstrate hydronephrosis, hydroureter, intrarenal stones, or an echogenic calculus in the ureter (Fig. 3.108). Intravenous

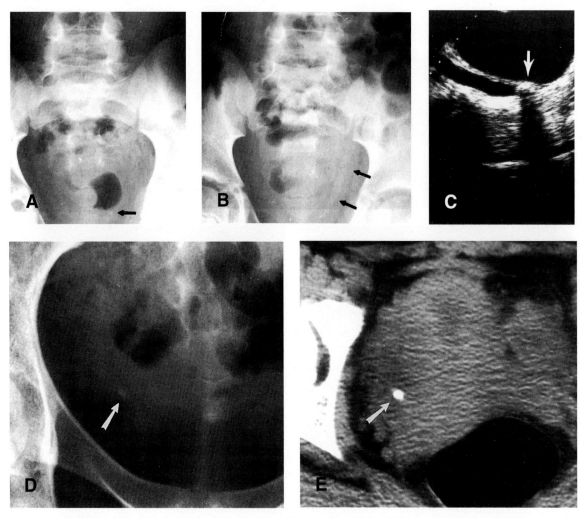

FIGURE 3.108. *Renal colic, imaging findings.* **(A)** Note the small calcified renal calculus (*arrow*) in the pelvis of this patient who presented with renal colic. **(B)** Subsequent intravenous pyelogram demonstrates moderate dilatation of the distal ureter on the left (*arrows*). The small calcified calculus is visualized again. **(C)** Ultrasound demonstrates a renal stone (*arrow*) producing distal shadowing, embedded in the distal ureter. **(D)** Another patient. Note the calcified renal calculus in the right pelvis (*arrow*). **(E)** Helical CT scanning clearly demonstrates the calculus (*arrow*).

pyelography often still is used to diagnose renal colic, because it more clearly demonstrates the level and the degree of obstruction. With acute obstruction, one sees a delayed nephrogram and diminished renal function of the involved kidney. Urethral stones also can be a problem and cause obstruction of the urinary tract. Ultrasonography can identify such stones, and clinically the findings are hematuria and dysuria (2,3).

REFERENCES

1. Dobbins JM, Novelline RA, Rhea JT, Rao PM, Prien EL Jr., Dretler SP. Helical computed tomography of urinary tract stones: Accuracy and diagnostic value of stone size and density measurements. *Emerg Radiol* 1997;4:303–308.
2. Kessler A, Rosenberg HK, Smoyer WE, Blyth B. Urethral stones: US for identification in boys with hematuria and dysuria. *Radiology* 1992;185:767–768.
3. Seltzer LG, Fischer WW, Miller SZ. Pediatric bladder outlet obstruction due to urethral calculus: Case report and review of the literature. *Pediatr Radiol* 1993;23:549–550.
4. Smith RC, Rosenfield AT, Choe KA, Essenmacher KR, Verga M, Glickman MG, Lange RC. Acute flank pain: Comparison of noncontrast-enhanced CT and intravenous urography. *Radiology* 1995;194:789–794.
5. Sommer FG, Jeffrey RB Jr., Rubin GD. Detection of ureteral calculi in ptients with suspected renal colic: Value of reformatted noncontrast helical CT. *AJR* 1995;165:509–513.

Adnexal Problems in Girls

The most common problem in this group of abnormalities is a simple ovarian cyst. Small follicular cysts 1 cm or smaller in diameter commonly are found in adolescent girls (Fig. 3.109A). If any of these cysts enlarge (Fig. 3.109B), they can cause lower abdominal and pelvic pain. Furthermore, bleeding into these cysts or into a corpus lutean cyst (Fig. 3.101) can produce considerable pain. Roentgenographically, simple cysts are anechoic, for they are fluid-filled (Fig. 3.109C), but once hemorrhage occurs, the pattern becomes mixed (Fig. 3.109D). It is often difficult to differentiate a hemorrhagic cyst from an ovarian tumor such as a teratoma or dermoid (Fig. 3.110). Normal ovaries and ovaries with cysts also can undergo torsion and hemorrhage (1,3,4), and if a cyst undergoes hemorrhage, the deposition of fibrin along the cyst wall may mimic the rim sign of a duplication cyst (1). Torsion of a fallopian tube also can occur (2).

With any of these pelvic problems, fluid often is present in the cul-de-sac. This fluid can be blood or simply reactive fluid. Normal fluid in the cul-de-sac is not as common in girls as it is in women, and thus in children it should be treated with more suspicion. Consequently, if a patient is encountered with pelvic pain, a few small cysts in an ovary, and fluid in the cul-de-sac, the clinician should become suspicious that one of these cysts may have hemorrhaged. ***Cysts do not have to be large to produce local hemorrhage.*** This is especially important to note if no other cause for the abdominal pain is detected. This is not to say that the findings are pathognomonic, but only that they are highly suggestive in the proper clinical setting.

Ultrasound is best for detecting all of these problems but, as mentioned previously, differentiating one from another is difficult. For the most part, most of these lesions present as a round or oval mass with a mixed pattern of echogenicity, and frequently associated fluid in the cul-de-sac. Calcification, of course, is the hallmark of a dermoid or teratoma. In addition, spontaneous detorsion of an ovary can be observed ultrasonographically (5), much like spontaneous detorsion of a torsed testicle.

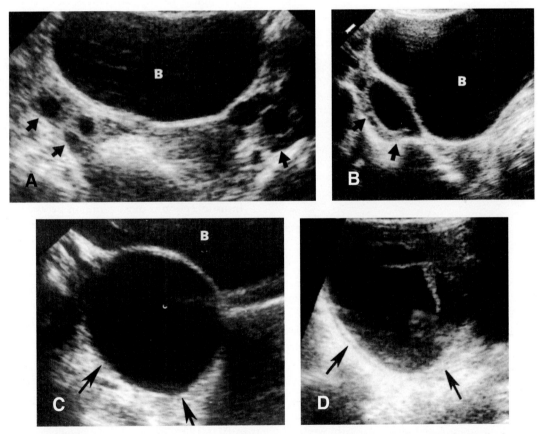

FIGURE 3.109. *Ovarian cysts.* **(A)** Note bilateral numerous small cysts in both ovaries (*arrows*) of this adolescent girl. *B,* bladder. **(B)** Another patient whose sagittal view of one of the adnexal regions demonstrates one large cyst and numerous smaller cysts (*arrows*). *B,* bladder. **(C)** Another patient with a large sonolucent cyst (*arrows*). *B,* bladder. **(D)** Hemorrhage in this cyst produces echogenic debris and fibrin strands. Fibrin also layers the wall of the cyst, producing an echogenic inner layer.

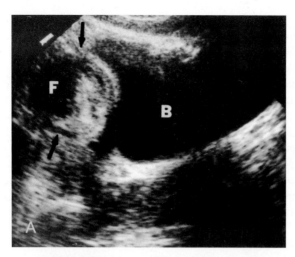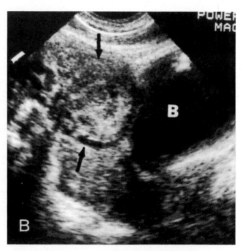

FIGURE 3.110. *Hemorrhagic corpus lutean cyst.* **(A)** Sagittal view demonstrates the large cyst (*arrows*) with a heterogeneous center. Fluid (*F*) in the cyst is suggestive but not totally diagnostic of a hemorrhagic corpus lutean cyst. *B*, bladder. **(B)** Cross-section through the hemorrhagic cyst (*arrows*) reveals the heterogeneous but virtually solid appearance of the cyst. These findings are difficult to differentiate from torsion of normal ovaries or tumors of ovaries. B, bladder.

REFERENCES

1. Godfrey H, Abernethy L, Boothroyd A. Torsion of an ovarian cyst mimicking enteric duplication cyst on transabdominal ultrasound: Two cases. *Pediatr Radiol* 1998;28:171–173.
2. Kurzbart E, Mares AJ, Cohen Z, Mordehai J, Finaly R. Isolated torsion of the fallopian tube in premenarcheal girls. *J Pediatr Surg* 1994;29:1384–1385.
3. Meyer JS, Harmon CM, Harty MP, Markowitz RI, Hubbard AM, Bellah RD. Ovarian torsion: Clinical and imaging presentation in children. *J Pediatr Surg* 1995;30:1433–1436.
4. Stark JE, Siegel MJ. Ovarian torsion in prepubertal and pubertal girls: sonographic findings. *AJR* 1995;163:1479–1482.
5. Warnock NG, Brown BP, Barloon TJ, Hermann LS. Spontaneous detorsion of the ovary demonstrated by ultrasonography. *J Ultrasound Med* 1994;12:57–59.

ACUTE MECHANICAL PROBLEMS

Entities discussed in this section include intussusception, volvulus, hernia, and visceral torsion. Any of these conditions can present with acute, even catastrophic, clinical pictures, and the radiologist should be aware of them all and the pertinent plain film findings with which they might present.

Intussusception

The clinical findings of classic intussusception are well known and include (a) crampy abdominal pain, (b) vomiting, (c) bloody (currant-jelly) stools, and (d) either a palpable mass or palpable emptiness in the right flank or lower quadrant. Not all of these findings need be present at the same time, and furthermore, in many patients they are intermittent. Indeed, it is becoming more and more apparent that many cases of intussusception are atypical in their presentations. To be sure, the classic triad of crampy abdominal pain, a palpable abdominal mass, and rectal bleeding, in our experience, occurs in less than one half of cases. This also has been the experience of others.

Altered consciousness and apathy (6,38) also have been documented as manifestations of intussusception, but it is not precisely known why these phenomena occur. It is postulated, however, that intestinal ischemia may lead to release of endotoxins, which then could alter the blood–brain barrier and lead to central nervous system depression (6). ***Overall, then, one should realize that a good many cases of intussusception present with less than classic findings.***

Intussusception is most common between the ages of 6 months and 2 years but, of course, can be seen in the older child or even the neonate. In most cases, intussusception is idiopathic, although mesenteric lymph node enlargement or redundant, edematous, intestinal mucosa (i.e., as part of a viral infection) probably accounts for the lead point in most cases. Indeed, now that ultrasound is available, adenopathy, in our experience, is encountered rather routinely. A more discrete leading lesion such as polyp, Meckel's diverticulum, duplication cyst, appendix, or hemangioma is found in less than 10% of cases, usually in older children or neonates (11,16,20,32).

Most cases of intussusception are ileocolic, with ileo–ileo and ileo–ileocolic intussusceptions accounting for no more than 10 to 12% of cases (30). Generally speaking, these latter intussusceptions are more difficult to diagnose and tend to be present for longer periods of time before definitive treatment is accomplished. Consequently, complications such as bowel necrosis and perforation are more common and, because of this, these intussusceptions generally are considered more serious. When all of the foregoing is considered, it can readily be seen why intussusception can be so problematic, both clinically and on imaging.

Plain-film roentgenographic findings of intussusception are variable (46) and in one series (42) were useful in only 50% of cases. In early cases, a normal gas pattern is usual, but the longer the intussusception is present, the more likely one is to see a pattern of small-bowel obstruction (Fig. 3.111A). In other cases, one can see the actual head of the intussusception on plain films (Fig. 3.111B and D), but this generally occurs in less than 50% of cases. Visualization

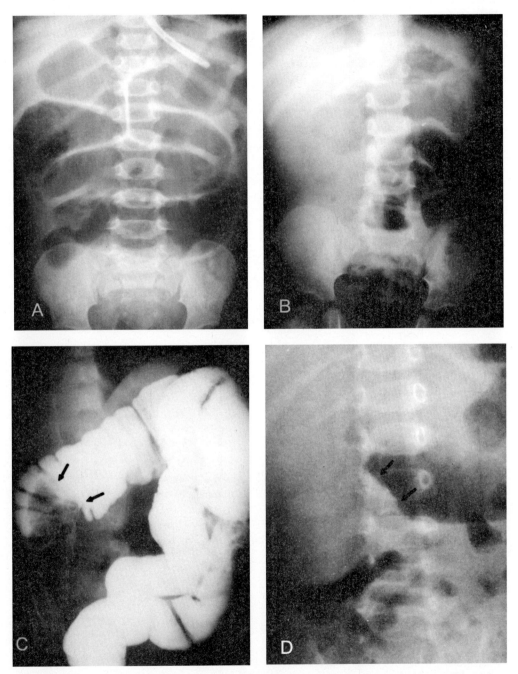

FIGURE 3.111. *Intussusception: plain film findings.* **(A)** In this patient, classic low small bowel obstruction is present. **(B)** Classic configuration of intussusception consisting of paucity of gas in the right flank and two or three loops of distended (obstructed) small bowel just to the left of the lower lumbar spine. In addition, a soft-tissue defect is vaguely apparent in the transverse colon just to the left of the hepatic flexure. Could this be the head of the intussusception? **(C)** Subsequent barium enema demonstrates that the head of the intussusception (*arrows*) corresponds to its suspected location on the plain abdominal film seen in **B**. **(D)** Note, in another patient, a clear-cut mass (*arrows*) in the transverse colon. Otherwise the abdominal gas pattern is completely normal.

of the head of the intussusception is said to be enhanced and increased in likelihood to 60% by the use of decubitus views (57), but such views generally are not obtained. Perhaps more commonly than the head of the intussusception, one sees interruption of the air column in the transverse colon (24). Another useful but relatively rare finding is the visualization of ringlike fat densities on the plain film (25,39) (Fig. 3.112). Pneumatosis cystoides intestinalis also has been described with intussusception (31) but is rare.

Absence of gas in the right lower quadrant or flank (Fig. 3.111B) also is a useful finding. Absence of gas in the right lower quadrant or flank results from the fact that as an intussusception develops the air is squeezed out of the intestine. Failure of visualization of the liver edge (18) occurs because if right upper quadrant bowel gas is absent, the natural contrasting effect of liver against adjacent air-filled bowel is lost. Of course, if bowel necrosis and perforation ensue, the findings of peritonitis and free peritoneal air supervene. All of these points notwithstanding, however, it should be noted that many cases still demonstrate normal or near normal abdominal films. However, this should not dissuade one from pursuing the diagnosis of intussusception if it is suspected at all clinically. ***It is here that ultrasound becomes very useful (17).*** We now perform ultrasound in all cases of suspected intussusception, and especially those in which clinical findings are equivocable.

Ultrasound is very effective in detecting intussusception and increasingly has become the next imaging modality after plain films (9,37,43,51,54,55). False negative studies are few, and although some suggest that ultrasound should be used for clinically atypical cases only, its usefulness goes far beyond this. Color flow Doppler also is of some use, because if blood flow is not seen to the head of an intussusception, (see Fig. 3.116) nonsurgical reduction is more difficult to accomplish (21,23,26). Color flow Doppler, however, is not foolproof, and one can be surprised in any given case. Nonetheless, it generally is utilized if intussusception is investigated with ultrasound.

In the earlier years of ultrasonography, resolution of the various intestinal layers was not possible, and thus the overall findings led to the terms "sonolucent donut" and "pseudokidney" signs (51). With high-resolution linear transducers, however, visualization of the individual layers of the intussusception has become possible and commonplace. As a result, the findings now are a layered oval mass on longitudinal view, and a round mass with concentric rings on cross-sectional view (Fig. 3.113). Lymph nodes, as noted previously, always have been considered a lead point for intussusception, and most likely they represent the most common lead point. This is especially true if they are associated with mucosal edema and thickening. In our experience, lymph nodes now commonly are seen in intussuceptions (Fig. 3.114A and B) and clearly can be seen to be part

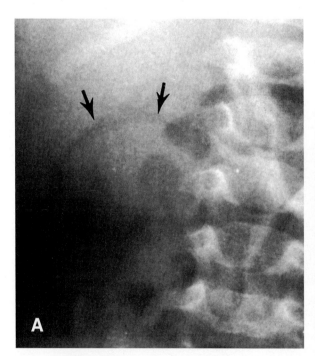
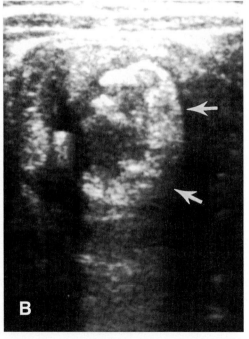

FIGURE 3.112. *Intussusception: ring-of-fat sign.* **(A)** Note the ring of radiolucent fat (*arrows*) in the right upper quadrant. **(B)** Ultrasound study demonstrates the echogenic fat in a crescent shape (*arrows*).

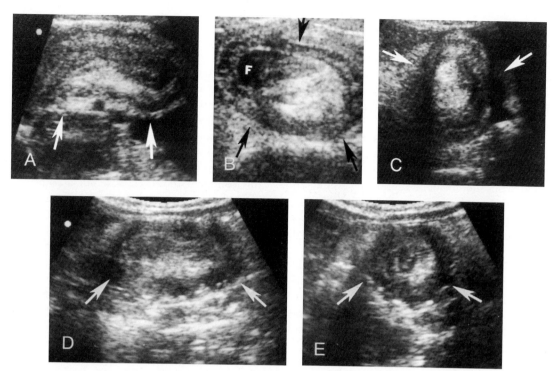

FIGURE 3.113. *Intussusception: ultrasonographic findings.* **(A)** Longitudinal section through the intussusception demonstrates an oval, somewhat layered mass (*arrows*) with an echogenic center. **(B)** Slightly oblique view through the intussusception (*arrows*) demonstrates the various layers more clearly and also shows some fluid (*F*) in the lumen. **(C)** Cross-sectional view of the intussusception shows the echogenic center and the relatively hypoechoic rim (*arrows*). **(D)** Another patient with a more uniform sonolucent rim to the generally oval-shaped intussusception (*arrows*). **(E)** Cross-sectional view in the same patient demonstrates a sonolucent donut configuration (*arrows*).

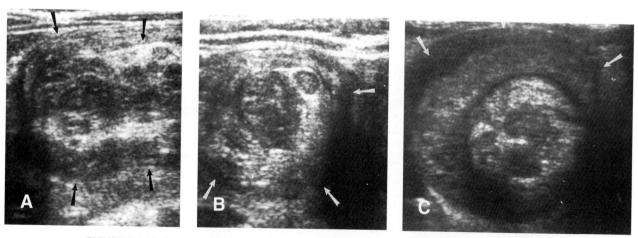

FIGURE 3.114. *Intussusception with lymph nodes and echogenic mesentery.* **(A)** Note the head of the intussusception (*arrows*). In the center, echogenic fat with sonolucent lymph nodes is seen. **(B)** Cross-sectional view demonstrates similar findings (*arrows*). One large node is seen in the right upper quadrant. **(C)** Somewhat more proximally the central echogenic intussusception with hypoechoic lymph nodes is seen within a loop of bowel showing marked mucosal thickening (*arrows*).

of the head of the intussusception. Trapped fluid within an intussusception also can be seen and has been demonstrated to be peritoneal fluid (10). This finding is considered a sign indicative of difficulty with nonsurgical, hydrostatic reduction.

In addition to the foregoing findings, a small amount of free peritoneal fluid (53) can be seen in some cases of intussusception (Fig. 3.115). This is important to note, so as not to interpret this finding as resulting from intestinal perforation or bowel necrosis. Indeed, free fluid in small amounts is seen not uncommonly at surgical exploration of these patients, and thus this should not be a surprising finding on ultrasound. If fluid is more voluminous, however, and especially if it is echogenic and associated with fibrinous bands, perforation or impending perforation should be considered (Fig. 3.116C).

Almost all patients with intussusceptions should undergo contrast enema reduction. Those patients to be excluded, for the most part, are those demonstrating signs of peritonitis or perforation (2). The fact that the intussusception may have been present for 24 hr or more is no longer generally considered a contraindication to nonsurgical reduction (2,49). In addition, the presence of the so-called crescent sign (contrast coating the head of the intussusception) is not considered a contraindication (2,49).

In the more remote past, barium was used almost exclusively for the nonsurgical hydrostatic reduction of intussusception, but currently the preferred contrast agents are air

(9,13,14,19,48) and positive contrast aqueous solutions (2). Air is favored, and the end result is that barium eventually will cease to be used. Barium still tends to be used by radiologists not trained recently (27,29,50), but eventually it should pass from the scene. It is questionable whether it should be used at all, because the complications associated with perforation if barium is used are well known.

Carbon dioxide as a substitute for air also has been used (33), and hydrostatic ultrasound-guided reduction of intussusceptions also has been advocated (5,34,41,47,56). On this continent, however, it is not a common method of reduction of intussusception. Furthermore, it does not appear to be as effective as air reduction; it is about as effective as barium reduction (14). CT scanning also can demonstrate intussusception (7), but often the finding is incidental when the abdomen is being investigated for abdominal pain. This is especially true of postoperative intussusceptions (1). In these cases the possibility of intussusception usually is initially not considered, but still it is a relatively common problem (Fig. 3.117).

Proponents of gas reduction list the following as the major advantages of utilizing either air, carbon dioxide, or oxygen: higher reduction rates, no ionizing radiation (35), and shorter studies. All of this is true, and the aftermath of this is that science entered into the how and why of reduction of intussusception. It was demonstrated by Kuta and Benator (22) that to generate the pressures of 120 mm Hg obtained with air systems, one had to raise a barium column to 3.5 ft, and a column of aqueous material to 5 ft. We have used the aqueous method for more than a decade and have had a success rate of around 80%. We have used gastrografin diluted 5:1 with normal saline to render it isotonic and have had no difficulty with visualization. We have not used other aqueous contrast agents but do not see why they would not be as effective.

Success rates are variable, and in the past, when barium was the sole agent used for hydrostatic reduction, many times they were quite low. However, now that air, or aqueous contrast agents are utilized, however, success rates generally hover around 70 to 85%, with most studies reporting a rate close to 80% (27,28,30). In terms of air reduction, it has been demonstrated that pressures of 60 mm Hg are required to move an intussusception and 100 mm Hg to reduce it (41). Intramural pressures should not exceed 120 mm Hg for prolonged periods of time, for perforation becomes more likely, and in piglets normal colons have been demonstrated to perforate at 200 mm Hg (44).

If air is being used, the study must be monitored very closely, and actually some form of safety valve to avoid going over the prescribed limits of pressure should be included in the system. All of this notwithstanding, however, what the use of air has done is to encourage a generally more aggressive approach to the reduction of intussusception. Once barium is removed from the picture, perforation is not such a devastating problem, whether one

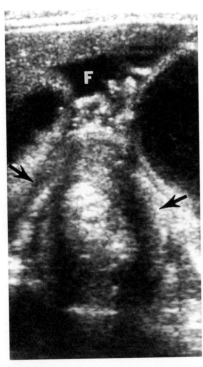

FIGURE 3.115. *Intussusception with free fluid.* Note the classic intussusception (*arrows*). Some clean, free fluid (*F*) is seen above it.

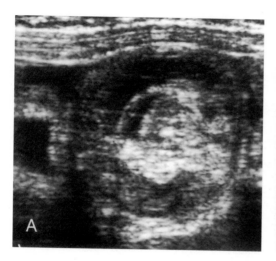

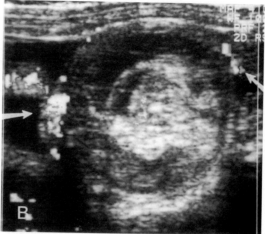

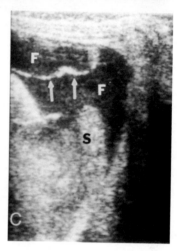

FIGURE 3.116. *Intussusception with color flow Doppler ultrasonography.* **(A)** Note the characteristic cross-sectional appearance of the intussusception. **(B)** On color flow Doppler ultrasonography, flow is seen around the periphery (*arrows*), but none is seen within the center. This was not reducible. **(C)** Same patient. Considerable fluid (*F*) is seen just around the tip of the spleen (*S*). Note the fibrinous strand within the fluid (*arrows*). At surgery, this patient showed areas of necrosis with impending perforation.

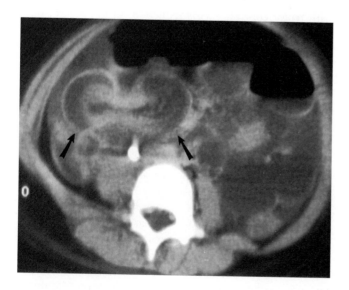

FIGURE 3.117. *Intussusception: CT findings.* Note the typical concentric ring configuration of an intussusception (*arrows*).

uses air or aqueous contrast agents. Furthermore, all who work with intussusception know that if the colon becomes distended, no matter what the contrast agent, the infant becomes irritable and more awake. In keeping with this, it has been demonstrated that Valsalva maneuvers so induced in the infant during this excitable state can transiently raise the intracolonic pressure from 120 to 140 mm Hg above prescribed limits (3). In the end, this has been determined to be a positive factor that enhances reduction (3,45,58).

It has been demonstrated that colonic perforation most likely is secondary to bowel necrosis and not simply to excessive pressures (4). Perforation rates with nonsurgical reduction generally run around 1 to 3% (2,48). If perforation occurs one should cease the study. Perforations with air are cleaner than those with aqueous contrast agents or barium, but barium is the only real problem. Fortunately in any case, the colon in these patients is not full of fecal material, because diarrhea commonly is present. The problem with barium is that it induces so-called barium peritonitis, but if one does not use barium, perforation is not a major complication. In addition to these considerations, although in the past manual compression and massaging of the intussusception were considered inappropriate, recently it has been demonstrated that manual compression can be helpful (12). We have attempted this on a few occasions, but *we believe that it is important that manual massage be used only if the pressures used for reducing intussusception have been decompressed.*

The consequences of perforation still are incompletely answered with air reduction, but massive pneumoperitoneum can be a serious problem necessitating immediate needle decompression. The reason for this is that massive pneumoperitoneum can lead to a vasovagal response culminating in cardiac arrest. This is important, for it is not as easy to visualize air leaking into the peritoneal cavity as it is to detect positive contrast material leaking into the peritoneal cavity. On the other hand, if air or some comparable agent is being used, if perforation occurs there is an abrupt loss of pressure in the system being used. Once this occurs, the system should be shut down and decompressed immediately.

In the past, glucagon was advocated in stubborn cases, but it never really proved effective and now generally is not used. Sedation also once was popular and seemed to help. Recently, however, as mentioned previously, proponents of air reduction, now able to monitor pressures more closely, suggest that without sedation the infant is able to generate, through straining (Valsalva's maneuver), greater transient, but beneficial, pressures in the colon. All of this is interesting, but over the years *I have come to the conclusion that in the end, most depends on just how well one seals off the anus. It must be totally occluded.*

Total occlusion of the anus usually is best accomplished by tight taping of the buttocks with abundant quantities of cloth adhesive tape of good quality. Transparent adhesive tape is not good for this job; this is important because inadequate taping leads to repeat studies and lower reduction rates. In addition, we utilize a Foley bulb in the rectum, and although not all agree with this maneuver, we have found it indispensable in obtaining total occlusion. We inflate the bulb under fluoroscopic control after the colon is filled and the intussusception identified. The balloon is inflated to near the diameter of the contrast-filled rectum, and then it is pulled down as a plunger against the sealed anus. We have found this to be the most important part of reduction, for *if the anus is not totally occluded, reduction is impaired.*

The configuration of intussusceptions, on any contrast study, generally are similar and typical (Fig. 3.117). The retrograde progress of the head of the intussusception as it is pushed around the colon is easy to detect and document fluoroscopically. Often it tends to "hang up" at the splenic and hepatic flexures and also at the ileocecal valve. At any of these sites, if maximal pressures are reached and no progress is made, no matter which method one uses, it is best to decompress the system and try again. With aqueous contrast agents one simply lowers the bag to the floor and drains the contents back into the bag. Thereafter, one raises the bag to the appropriate level (5 ft) and tries again. With air reduction, simple decompression by "leaking off" the system can be accomplished. With aqueous contrast material, we have repeated this decompressive maneuver five to seven times, although in most cases three attempts suffice (2). At any site, if no progress is made after 5 min with any contrast agent, it probably is wise to stop.

With final reduction through the ileocecal valve, the filling defect of the intussusception disappears, and contrast material rushes into the dilated, obstructed small bowel (Fig. 3.118). This is a most important observation, for otherwise one cannot say that reduction is complete. In addition, although contrast may enter the terminal ileum with ileo–ileocolic intussusceptions, it is only if the contrast material reaches the dilated small bowel proximal to the obstruction that one can say reduction is complete. It is easier to see this with aqueous contrast agents than with air. In addition, it has been noted that air can rapidly gush into, and fill, the dilated small bowel before reduction actually occurs (15). This is not a problem with positive contrast agents, but these agents can unveil a variety of potentially confusing postreduction pseudotumoral, cecal, and distal small bowel configurations (36). These changes probably are multifactorial in origin but most likely are caused by inflammation and edema of the intestine. They are not a cause for concern and also may be seen, although perhaps not as clearly, with air reduction enemas. A postevacuation film should be obtained after reduction is complete, and a follow-up film can be made after 24 hr in problem cases to determine whether the intussusception has remained reduced or has recurred. If the intussusception is not fully reduced, small bowel obstruction does not disappear, and the colon distal to the intussusception will remain spastic.

Recurrence rates after nonsurgical reduction range from 4 to 10% (2,40), and the first recurrence should be treated with repeat contrast enema reduction. In this regard, now that nonsurgical reduction of intussusception is so easily accomplished, it has been suggested that recurrent intussusception should be treated nonsurgically, even if it recurs more than once (8).

Recurrent intussusceptions occur more commonly in those cases in which a definite leading point is seen and, by the same token, are more difficult to reduce in the first place. In addition, the longer the intussusception remains untreated or the lower it is in the colon, the more difficult is the reduction. Perforation rates, as mentioned previously, hover at around 1 to 3% but may become a little higher with the general trend toward more aggressive approaches to reduction. However, now that barium is being used less and less, perforation is a more acceptable complication, and if it is detected the case immediately becomes surgical.

Spontaneous reduction of intussusception (52) is encountered more commonly now and the reason for this is that the phenomenon can be documented with ultrasound studies. It is not unusual to have a patient present with find-

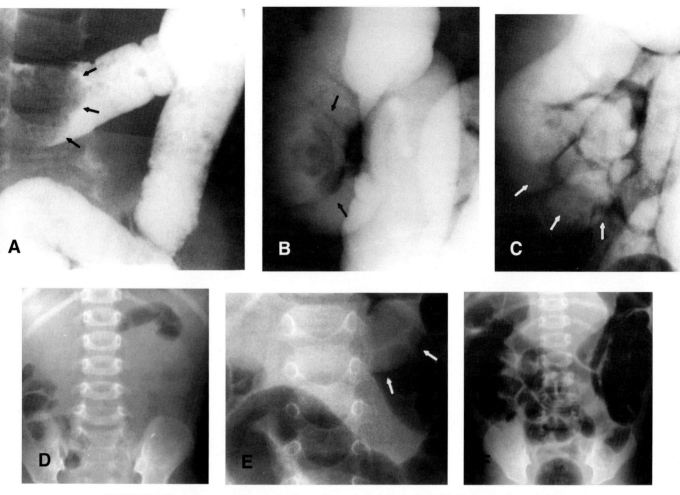

FIGURE 3.118. *Intussusception: reduction with gastrografin and air.* **(A)** *Gastrografin reduction.* Note the typical appearance of the head of the intussusception (*arrows*). **(B)** Later the intussusception is at the ileocecal valve (*arrows*). **(C)** With full reduction, contrast material (gastrografin) floods the small bowel (*arrows*). **(D)** *Reduction with air.* Note the preliminary abdominal film demonstrating scattered loops of slightly dilated intestine. **(E)** The head of the intussusception is outlined clearly (*arrows*). **(F)** With reduction, air fills the small bowel.

ings very suggestive of intussusception, to demonstrate its presence with ultrasound, and yet to not be able to find the intussusception with subsequent contrast enemas. In such cases, one should be cognizant of the fact that the intussusception has reduced spontaneously (52). One may even see this in real time when one is performing the ultrasound study (i.e., the intussusception is seen to induce and then reduce).

In conclusion, it should be mentioned that intussusception can be a presenting feature of cystic fibrosis in older children (meconium ileus equivalent). In these patients, fecal impactions and redundancy and thickening of the intestinal mucosa predispose to intussusception. In addition, it should be noted that although the appendix can act as a lead point for intussusception, isolated intussusception of the appendix also can occur and may be seen in totally asymptomatic individuals.

REFERENCES

1. Albery SM, Swischuk LE, John SD, Angel C. Post-operative intussusception: Often an elusive diagnosis. Case Report. *Pediatr Radiol* 1998;28:271.
2. Barr LL, Stansberry SD, Swischuk LE. Significance of age, duration, obstruction and the dissection sign in intussusception. *Pediatr Radiol* 1990;20:454–456.
3. Bramson RT, Shiels WE II, Eskey CJ, Hu SY. Intraluminal colon pressure dynamics with valsalva maneuver during air enema study. *Radiology* 1997;202:825–828.
4. Bramson RT, Blickman JG. Perforation during hydrostatic reduction of intussusception: Proposed mechanism and review of the literature. *J Pediatr Surg* 1992;27:589–591.
5. Chan KL, Saing H, Peh WCG, Mya GH, Cheng W, Khong PL, Lam C, Lam WWM, Leong LLY, Low LCK. Childhood intussusception: Ultrasound-guided Hartmann's solution hydrostatic reduction or barium reduction? *J Pediatr Surg* 1997;32:3–6.
6. Conway EE Jr. Central nervous system findings and intussusception: How are they related? *Pediatr Emerg Care* 1993;9:15–18.

7. Cox TD, Winters WD, Weinberger E. CT of intussusception in the pediatric patient: Diagnosis and pitfalls. *Pediatr Radiol* 1996;26:26–32.

8. Daneman A, Alton DJ, Lobo E, Gravett J, Kim P, Ein SH. Patterns of recurrence of intussusception in children: A 17 year review. *Pediatr Radiol* 1998;28:913–919.

9. del-Pozo G, Albillos JC, Tejedor D, Calero R, Rasero M, de-la-Calle U, Lopez-Pacheco U. Intussusception in children: current concepts in diagnosis and enema reduction. *RadioGraphics* 1999; 19:299–319.

10. del-Pozo G, Gonzalez-Spinola J, Gomez-Anson B, Serrano C, Miralles M, Gonzalez-deOrbe G, Cano I, Martinez A. Intussusception: Trapped peritoneal fluid detected with US. Relationship to reducibility and ischemia. *Radiology* 1996;201:379–383.

11. Eklof OA, Johanson L, Lohr G. Childhood intussusception: Hydrostatic reducibility and incidence of leading points in different age groups. *Pediatr Radiol* 1980;10:83–86.

12. Grasso SN, Katz ME, Presberg HJ, Croitoru DP. Transabdominal manually assisted reduction of pediatric intussusception: Reappraisal of this historical technique. *Radiology* 1994;191:777–779.

13. Gu L, Alton DJ, Daneman A, Stringer DA, Liu P, Wilmot DM, Reilly BJ. Intussusception reduction in children by rectal insufflation of air. *AJR* 1988;150:1345–1348.

14. Hadidi AT, El Shal N. Childhood intussusception: A comparative study of nonsurgical management. *J Pediatr Surg* 1999;34: 304–307.

15. Hedlund GL, Johnson JF, Strife JL. Ileocolic intussusception: Extensive reflux of air preceding pneumatic reduction. *Radiology* 1990;174:187–189.

16. Hutchinson IF, Olayiwola B, Young DG. Intussusception in infancy and childhood. *Br J Surg* 1980;67:209–212.

17. John SD. The value of ultrasound in children with suspected intussusception. *Emerg Radiol* 1998;5:297–305.

18. Jorulf H. Tip of the liver in intussusception of the bowel in infancy and childhood. *Acta Radiol* 1974;14:26–32.

19. Katz H, Phelan E, Carlin JB, Beasley SW. Gas enema for the reduction of intussusception: Relationship between clinical signs and symptoms and outcome. *AJR* 1993;160:363–366.

20. Kim G, Daneman A, Alton DJ, Myers M, Sandler A, Superina R. The appearance of inverted Meckel diverticulum with intussusception on air enema. *Pediatr Radiol* 1997;27:647–650.

21. Kong MS, Wong HG, Lin SL, Chung JL, Lin JN. Factors related to detection of blood flow by color Doppler ultrasonography in intussusception. *J Ultrasound Med* 1997;16:141–144.

22. Kuta AJ, Benator RM. Intussusception: Hydrostatic pressure equivalents for barium and meglumine sodium diatrizoate. *Radiology* 1990;175:125–126.

23. Legalla R, Caruso G, Novara V, Derchi LE, Cardinale AE. Color Doppler ultrasonography in pediatric intussusception. *J Ultrasound Med* 1994;13:171–174.

24. Lazar L, Rathaus V, Erez I, Katz S. Interrupted air column in the large bowel on plain abdominal film: A new radiological sign of intussusception. *J Pediatr Surg* 1995;30:1551–1553.

25. Lee JM, Kim H, Byun JY, Lee H, Kim CY, Shinn KS, Bahk YW. Intussusception: Characteristic radiolucencies on the abdominal radiograph. *Pediatr Radiol* 1994;24:293–295.

26. Lim HK, Bae SH, Lee KH, Seo GS, Yoon GS. Assessment of reducibility of ileocolic intussusception in children: Usefulness of color Doppler sonography. *Radiology* 1994;191:781–785.

27. McAlister WH. Intussusception: Even Hippocrates did not standardize his technique of enema reduction. *Radiology* 1998;206: 595–598.

28. Meyer JS, Dangman BC, Buonomo C, Berlin JA. Air and liquid contrast agents in the management of intussusception: A controlled, randomized trial. *Radiology* 1993;188:507–511.

29. Meyer JS. The current radiologic management of intussusception: A survey and review. *Pediatr Radiol* 1992;22:323–325.

30. Mok PM, Humphry A. Ileo-ileocolic intussusception: Radiological features and reducibility. *Pediatr Radiol* 1982;12:127–131.

31. Navarro O, Daneman A, Alton DJ, Thorner P. Colo-colic intussusception associated with pneumatosis cystoides intestinalis. *Pediatr Radiol* 1998;28:515–517.

32. Ong NT, Beasley DW. The leadpoint in intussusception. *J Pediatr Surg* 1990;25:640–643.

33. Paterson CA, Langer JC, Somers S, Stevenson G, McGrath FP, Malone D, Winthrop AL. Pneumatic reduction of intussusception, using carbon dioxide. *Pediatr Radiol* 1994;24:296–297.

34. Peh WCG, Khong PL, Chan KL, Lam C, Cheng W, Lam WWM, Mya GH, Saing H, Leong LLY, Low LCK. Sonographically guided hydrostatic reduction of childhood intussusception using Hartmann's solution. *AJR* 1996;167:1236–1241.

35. Persliden J, Schuwert P, Mortensson W. Comparison of absorbed radiation doses in barium and air enema reduction of intussusception: A phantom study. *Pediatr Radiol* 1996;26:329–332.

36. Pokorny WJ, Wagner ML, Harberg FJ. Lateral wall cecal filling defects following successful hydrostatic reduction of cecalcolic intussusceptions. *J Pediatr Surg* 1980;15:156–159.

37. Pracros JP, Tran-Minh VA, Morin DeFinfe CH, Desfrenne-Pracros P, Louis D, Basset T. Acute intestinal intussusception in children: Contribution of ultrasonography (145 cases). *Ann Radiol* 1987;30:525–530.

38. Rachmel A, Rosenbach Y, Amir J, Dinari G, Shoenfeld T, Nitzan M. Apathy as an early manifestation of intussusception. *Am J Dis Child* 1983;137:701–702.

39. Ratcliffe JF, Fong S, Cheong L, O'Connell P. Plain film diagnosis of intussusception: Incidence of the target sign. *AJR* 1991; 158:619–621.

40. Renwick AA, Beasleuy SW, Phelan E. Intussusception: Recurrence following gas (oxygen) enema reduction. *Pediatr Surg Int* 1993;7:361–363.

41. Riebel TW, Nasir R, Weber K. US-guided hydrostatic reduction of intussusception in children. *Radiology* 1993;188:513–516.

42. Sargent MA, Babyn P, Alton DJ. Plain abdominal radiography in suspected intussusception: A reassessment. *Pediatr Radiol* 1994; 24:17–20.

43. Shanbhouge RLK, Hussain SM, Meradji M, Robben SGF, Vernooij JEM, Molenaar JC. Ultrasonography is accurate enough for the diagnosis of intussusception. *J Pediatr Surg* 1994;29: 324–328.

44. Shiels WE II, Kirks DR, Keller GL, Ryckman FR, Daugherty CC, Specker BL, Summa DW. John Caffey Award: Colonic perforation by air and liquid enemas. Comparison study in young pigs. *AJR* 1993;160:931–935.

45. Shiels WE II, Maves CK, Hedlund GL, Kirks DR. Air enema for diagnosis and reduction of intussusception: Clinical experience and pressure correlates. *Radiology* 1991;181:169–172.

46. Smith DS, Bonadio WA, Losek JD, Walsh-Kelly CM, Hennes HM, Glaeser PW, Melzer-Lange M, Rimm AA. The role of abdominal x-rays in the diagnosis and management of intussusception. *Pediatr Emerg Care* 1992;8:325–327.

47. Soon OC, Park WH, Wo SK. Ultrasound-guided water enema: An alternative method of non-operative treatment for childhood intussusception. *J Pediatr Surg* 1994;29:498–500.

48. Stein M, Alton DJ, Daneman A. Pneumatic reduction of intussusception: 5-year experience. *Radiology* 1992;183:681–684.

49. Stephenson CA, Seibert JJ, Strain JD. Intussusception: Clinical and radiographic factors influencing reducibility. *Pediatr Radiol* 1989;20:57–60.

50. Swischuk L.E. The current radiology management of intussusception: A survey and review. *Pediatr Radiol* 1992;22:317.

51. Swischuk LE, Hayden CK, Boulden T. Intussusception: Indications for ultrasonography and an explanation of the donut and pseudokidney signs. *Pediatr Radiol* 1985;15:388–391.

52. Swischuk LE, John SD, Swischuk PN. Spontaneous reduction of

intussusception: Verification with ultrasound. *Radiology* 1994; 192:269-271.

53. Swischuk LE, Stansberry SD. Ultrasonographic detection of free peritoneal fluid in uncomplicated intussusception. *Pediatr Radiol* 1991;21:350–351.

54. Tran-Minh VA, Pracros JP, Massard PE, Louis D, Pracros-Deffrenne P. Diagnosis of acute intestinal intussusception (AII) by real-time ultrasonography: Evaluation of 176 children with suspicion of AII. *Pediatr Radiol* 1985;15:267–268.

55. Verschelden P, Filiatrault D, Garel L, Grignon A, Perreault G, Boisvert J, Dubois J. Intussusception in children: Reliability of US in diagnosis. A prospective study. *Radiology* 1992;184:741–744.

56. Wang G, Liu S. Enema reduction of intussusception by hydrostatic pressure under ultrasound guidance: A report of 377 cases. *J Pediatr Surg* 1988;23:814–818.

57. White SJ, Blane CE. Intussusception: Additional observations on the plain radiograph. *AJR* 1982;139:511–513.

58. Zambuto D, Bramson RT, Blickman JG. Intracolonic pressure measurements during hydrostatic and air contrast barium enema studies in children. *Radiology* 1995;196:55–58.

Volvulus

Conditions considered under the broad topic of volvulus include midgut volvulus, segmental small bowel volvulus, volvulus of the colon, and gastric volvulus.

Midgut Volvulus

Midgut volvulus is associated with obstructing duodenal bands and intestinal malrotation. Usually it is a problem of the neonate, but it also can present in older infants and children. In such cases, the presentation often is atypical, both clinically and roentgenographically (5,8,10,11).

In the classic case of midgut volvulus in the neonate, there is acute onset of bilious vomiting, crampy abdominal pain, and varying degrees of abdominal distension. If vascular compromise is severe, signs of shock also are evident and, as the bowel undergoes necrosis, perforation with peritonitis may supervene. Most such cases declare themselves in the first month of life, but in the older child symptoms usually are atypical and confusing. These children frequently first are considered to have chronic abdominal problems such as malabsorption ulcer disease or protein-losing enteropathy or simply continue to be treated for undiagnosed recurrent abdominal pain. It requires an astute physician to reach the diagnosis under these conditions. In this regard, Bonadio et al. (2) have shown that although bilious vomiting was seen in 97% of their patients with midgut volvulus, blood in the stool was present in only 16%. On physical examination, no abnormal abdominal findings were seen in 76% of their cases.

Roentgenographically, a wide spectrum of abnormality is seen in midgut volvulus, and unfortunately, in some cases the abdominal roentgenograms can appear near normal. In those cases demonstrating abnormality, however, one of the most helpful findings is that of obstruction of the duodenum in its third and fourth portions (Fig. 3.119). In these

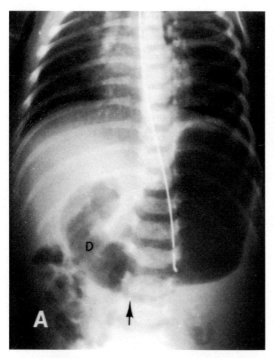
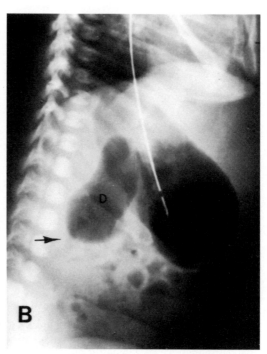

FIGURE 3.119. *Duodenal obstruction with malrotation.* **(A)** Supine film demonstrating distended stomach and descending duodenum **(D)**. The site of obstruction in the third and fourth portions of the duodenum is demarcated by the *arrow*. **(B)** Lateral view demonstrating site of obstruction (*arrow*) in the dilated descending duodenum **(D)** to better advantage. This level of obstruction is typical for the complex of malrotation, duodenal band, and midgut volvulus. (From Swischuk LE. *Radiology of the newborn infant and young child,* ed. 4. Baltimore: Williams and Wilkins, 1997, with permission.)

cases, obstruction may result from the associated duodenal bands only or from complicating midgut volvulus. With midgut volvulus, however, obstruction often is more pronounced. In those infants in whom the obstructed duodenum is full of fluid and a supine film only is obtained, air in the distended stomach erroneously suggests a gastric-outlet obstruction (Fig. 3.120).

Other patients with midgut volvulus may show evidence of a classic small bowel obstruction (Fig. 3.121) or a small bowel obstruction in association with a soft tissue mass (Fig. 3.122). In these latter cases, the mass represents fluid-filled, volved bowel, or, in other words, a form of closed loop obstruction. The volved mass of intestine frequently is located in the right lower quadrant (9) but can be seen anywhere in the abdomen.

Because of the high obstruction present in these patients, one would think that all of them would show deficient abdominal gas patterns. This is not so, however; some infants show considerable volumes of gas in distended loops of intestine. The reason for this seeming paradox is that once venous compromise occurs, intestinal gas absorption is severely compromised (6). Consequently, the presence of numerous loops of distended intestine in patients with sus-

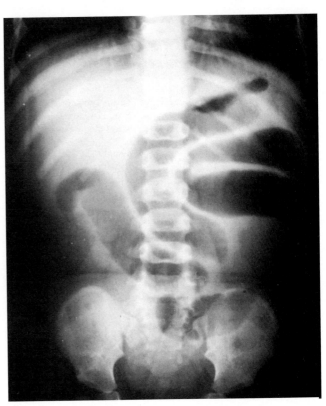

FIGURE 3.121. *Midgut volvulus: small bowel obstruction pattern.* Note the numerous loops of distended small intestine in this patient with midgut volvulus and obstruction.

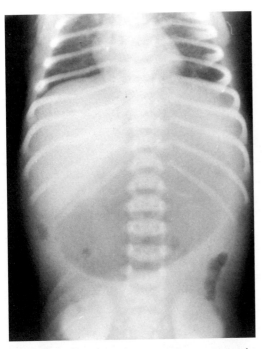

FIGURE 3.120. *Midgut volvulus appearing as a gastric outlet obstruction.* Note the distended stomach. There is no visible gas in the duodenum, and very little is scattered throughout the remainder of the gastrointestinal tract. A gastric-outlet obstruction might be suspected, but actually, this patient had midgut volvulus with descending duodenal obstruction. In the supine position, however, the duodenum is filled with fluid and thus is invisible roentgenographically. (From Swischuk LE. *Radiology of the newborn infant and young child*, ed. 4. Baltimore: Williams and Wilkins, 1997, with permission.)

pected midgut volvulus should be considered an ominous sign. Of course, if bowel necrosis occurs, pneumatosis cystoides intestinalis may be seen, and if perforation occurs, signs of peritonitis and free air develop.

Either the upper gastrointestinal series or barium enema can be used to confirm the presence of midgut volvulus and should be performed immediately (11). In our institution we prefer the upper gastrointestinal series. With barium enema examinations, one can be totally certain that midgut volvulus is present only if the cecum is misplaced high into the midabdomen, behind the transverse colon (Fig. 3.123). In such cases, as the intestine volves, the cecum is drawn tightly behind the transverse colon and the findings are pathognomonic. If the cecum simply is out of place, however, that is, if it is medial in position and not in its normal right lower quadrant location (14), one cannot assume that midgut volvulus is present. Furthermore, a normally placed cecum does not exclude underlying malrotation, and hence the possibility that midgut volvulus could develop. Because of these points, the upper gastrointestinal series basically has replaced the barium enema as the initial investigative procedure in patients with suspected midgut volvulus.

In midgut volvulus, the upper gastrointestinal series shows either obstruction of the third portion of the duodenum or obstruction of the duodenum and associated,

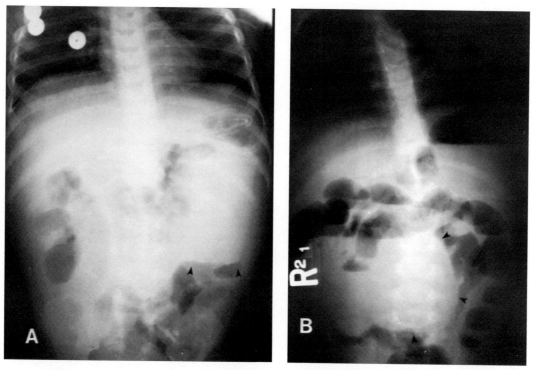

FIGURE 3.122. *Midgut volvulus with abdominal mass.* **(A)** Note soft tissue mass on the left side of the abdomen (*arrows*). **(B)** Upright view demonstrates that the mass has shifted to a new position (*arrows*). Note also that a small bowel obstruction is suggested. This patient was being investigated for malabsorption and one night developed severe crampy abdominal pain. At laparotomy, he had midgut volvulus. The soft tissue mass on the abdominal films represented fluid trapped in some of the volved loops.

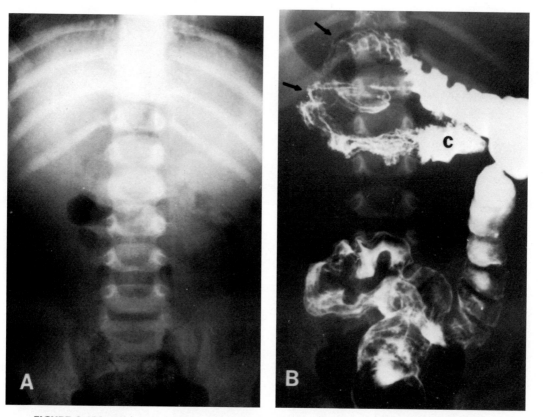

FIGURE 3.123. *Midgut volvulus, barium enema findings.* **(A)** Abdominal film revealing a misleadingly near normal appearance. Note, however, that although some gas is present in the stomach, the remainder of the abdomen shows a paucity of gas. If these findings are considered with the fact that this patient had acute onset of bilious vomiting and crampy abdominal pain, one should think of some underlying acute mechanical problem. In this case, both midgut volvulus and intussusception were considered, and because of this a barium enema was obtained. **(B)** Barium enema demonstrating the typical, totally abnormal position of the volved cecum (*C*) and the twisted colon (*arrows*).

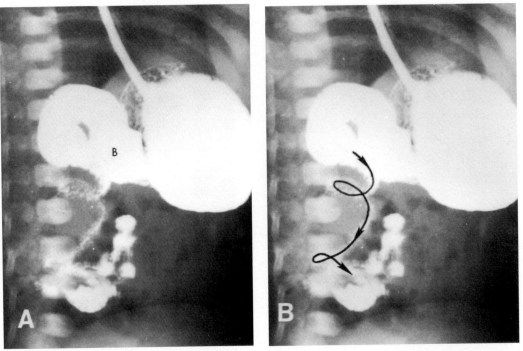

FIGURE 3.124. *Midgut volvulus: duodenal obstruction and spiraling of small bowel.* **(A)** Note the distended duodenal bulb (*B*) and descending duodenum. Also note spiraling of the small bowel distal to the site of obstruction of the duodenum. **(B)** Diagrammatic representation of spiraling of the small bowel.

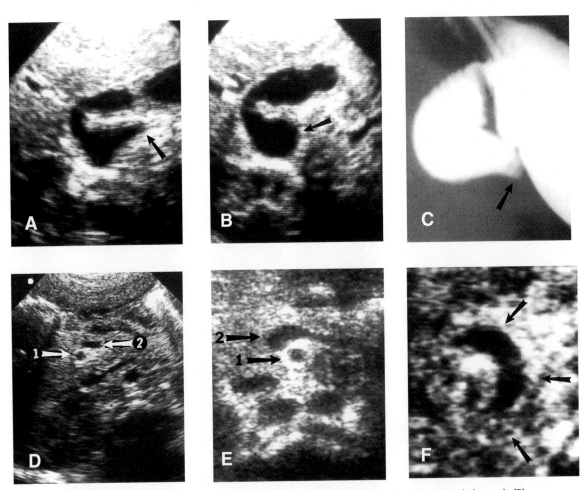

FIGURE 3.125. *Midgut volvulus: ultrasonographic findings.* **(A)** Note the typical beak (*arrow*). **(B)** Later, note a bulbous configuration (*arrow*) of the obstructed duodenum. **(C)** Upper gastrointestinal series demonstrates the typical beak (*arrow*). **(D)** Reversal of the SMA (*1*) and SMV (*2*) signifies the presence of volvulus. **(E)** Normal SMA (*1*) and SMV (*2*). **(F)** Twisted mesentery demonstrates curvilinear blood vessels (*arrows*), constituting the whirlpool sign. (Courtesy of Kenneth Martin, M.D.).

pathognomonic spiraling of the small intestine around the superior mesenteric artery (Fig. 3.124). In addition, the point of duodenal obstruction lies over the right pedicles of the spine. The small bowel after this point passes on to an abnormal midabdominal or right side position. All of this reflects the presence of malrotation and poor intestinal fixation, including absence of the ligament of Treitz, which normally fixes the bowel to the left of the spine. If edema of the loops of intestine distal to the area of spiraling also is noted, vascular compromise can be assumed with certainty.

Ultrasonography also can demonstrate findings of midgut volvulus (Fig. 3.125A and B), similar to those seen on an upper gastrointestinal series (3,4). In addition, the twisted pedicle of the mesentery and reversal of the normal relationship of the superior mesenteric artery and vein (15) can be seen (Fig. 3.125C). It has been noted that this reversal can be mimicked by distal ileocolic intussusception (7).

On the other hand, it is a reasonably reliable sign of malrotation. The twisted pedicle, on ultrasound, leads to the so-called whirlpool sign (9), and color flow Doppler can significantly enhance the findings of this sign (Fig. 3.125D).

In older children, however, as mentioned previously, clinical and roentgenographic findings usually are atypical. Considering that one may have apparently normal intestinal position with poor development of the mesentery (6) and incomplete rotation of the intestine with normal cecal position (12), one can understand why such atypia arises. Nonetheless, it is just this type of case that passes into older childhood, and then one must look for every possible clue (13) on the upper gastrointestinal series, barium enema, or ultrasound study for proper diagnosis. In this regard, any bizarre configuration of the duodenum, small bowel, or cecum should be treated with suspicion (1) (Fig. 3.126).

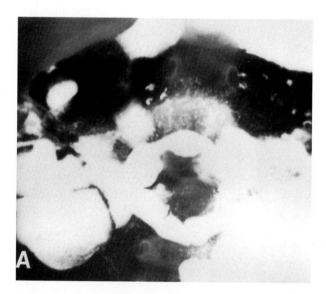

FIGURE 3.126. *Abnormal fixation of intestine.* **(A)** In this patient with chronic intermittent abdominal pain, note the peculiarly spiraled and generally abnormal configuration of the upper small bowel. **(B)** Same patient shows unusual position of terminal ileum (*arrows*). **(C)** Another patient with abnormal positioning of the cecum and compression by a band (*arrow*). All of these configurations should make one suspect abnormal intestinal fixation. (Courtesy of the late Sue Jacobi, M.D.)

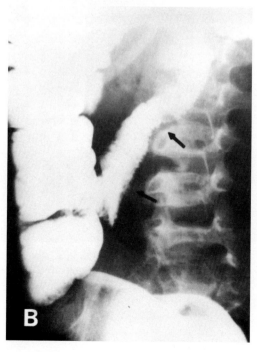

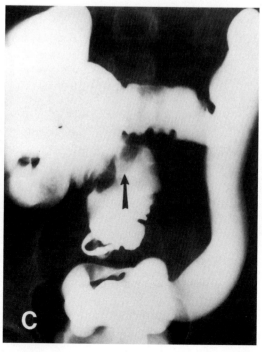

REFERENCES

1. Ablow RC, Hoffer FA, Seashore JH, Touloukian RJ. Z-shaped duodenojejunal loop: Sign of mesenteric fixation anomaly and congenital bands. *AJR* 1983;141:461–464.
2. Bonadio WA, Clarkson T, Naus J. The clinical features of children with malrotation of the intestine. *Pediatr Emerg Care* 1991;7:348–349.
3. Dufour D, Delaet MH, Dassonville M, Cadranel S, Perlmutter N. Midgut malrotation, the reliability of sonographic diagnosis. *Pediatr Radiol* 1992;22:21–23.
4. Hayden CK Jr, Boulden TF, Swischuk LE, Lobe TE. Sonographic demonstration of duodenal obstruction with midgut volvulus. *AJR* 1984;143:9–10.
5. Janik JS, Ein SH. Normal intestinal rotation with non-fixation: A cause of chronic abdominal pain. *J Pediatr Surg* 1979;14:670–674.
6. Kassner EG, Kottmeier PK. Absence and retention of small bowel gas in infants with midgut volvulus: Mechanisms and significance. *Pediatr Radiol* 1975;4:28–30.
7. Papadopoulou F, Effremidis SC, Raptopoulou A, Tryfonas GI, Tsikopoulos G. Distal ileocolic intussusception: another cause of inversion of superior mesenteric vessels in infants. *AJR* 1996;167:1243-1246.
8. Pochaczevski R, Ratner H, Leonidas JC, Naysan P, Feraru F. Unusual forms of volvulus after the neonatal period. *AJR* 1972;114:390–393.
9. Pracros JP, Sann L, Genin G, Tran-Minh VA, Morin XX, de Finfe CH, Foray P, Louis D. Ultrasound diagnosis of midgut volvulus: The "whirlpool" sign. *Pediatr Radiol* 1992;22:18–20.
10. Long FR, Kramer SS, Markowitz RI, Taylor GI, Liacouras CA. Intestinal malrotation in children: Tutorial on radiographic diagnosis in difficult cases. *Radiology* 1996;198:775-780.
11. Simpson AJ, Leonidis JC, Krasna IH, Becker JM, Schneider KM. Roentgen diagnosis of midgut malrotation: Value of upper gastrointestinal radiographic study. *J Pediatr Surg* 1972;7:243–252.
12. Slovis TL, Klein MD, Watts FB Jr. Incomplete rotation of the intestine with a normal cecal position. *Surgery* 1980;87:325–330.
13. Spigland N, Brandt ML, Yazbeck S. Malrotation presenting beyond the neonatal period. *J Pediatr Surg* 1990;25:1139–1142.
14. Steiner GM. The misplaced caecum and the root of the mesentery. *Br J Radiol* 1978;51:406–413.
15. Zerin JM, DiPietro MA. Superior mesenteric vascular anatomy at US in patients with surgically proved malrotation of the midgut. *Radiology* 1992;183:693–694.

Segmental Volvulus

Segmental volvulus of the small bowel represents a classic cause of closed loop obstruction and often is associated with anomalous peritoneal bands, congenital mesenteric defects, internal hernias, incomplete malrotation problems, or postoperative adhesions. As with all closed-loop obstructions, diagnosis may be late in coming.

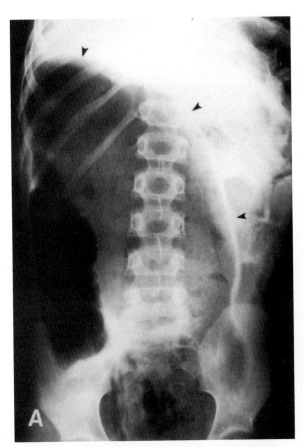 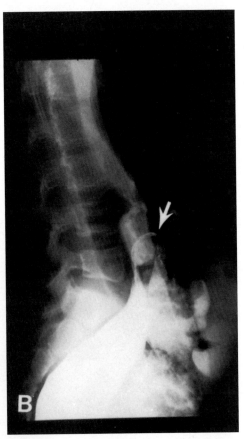

FIGURE 3.127. *Sigmoid volvulus.* **(A)** Note the large dilated loop of sigmoid colon, in its typical right-sided position (*arrows*). **(B)** Barium enema showing narrowing at site of volvulus (*arrow*). (From Campbell JR, Blank E. Sigmoid volvulus in children. *Pediatrics* 1974;53:702–705, with permission.)

Volvulus of the Colon

Volvulus of the colon is not a common problem in childhood, but it does occur, most often in the sigmoid colon (2,4). In some of these cases, the U-shaped loop of the volved sigmoid colon appears typical, lying far to the right of the spine and having its apex pointing toward the liver (Fig. 3.127). This does not always occur, however, and overall the findings of sigmoid volvulus in children are less specific than in adults. In addition, it should be noted that the normally redundant but nonvolved sigmoid colon can present with findings mimicking sigmoid volvulus (Fig. 3.128A). If, in such cases, the child is asymptomatic and volvulus is not suspected, the finding can be treated as being strictly fortuitous. In other cases, however, it may be difficult to discard the finding without barium enema verification (Fig. 3.128B). Cecal volvulus is less common than sigmoid volvulus (5), and the roentgenographic findings are different. With cecal volvulus, the dilated, volved cecum is located in the upper midabdomen or left upper quadrant (Fig. 3.129). Volvulus of the transverse colon is very rare (1,3,8) but, if present, demonstrates the volved

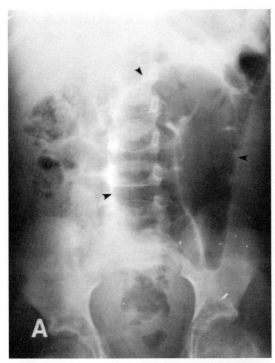

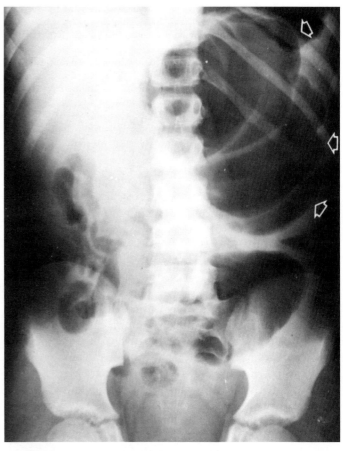

FIGURE 3.128. *Pseudovolvulus of sigmoid colon.* **(A)** Note the inverted U-shaped appearance of the sigmoid colon (*arrows*), which in this patient spuriously suggests sigmoid volvulus. This patient had no symptoms of obstruction, however, and was being investigated for painless rectal bleeding. **(B)** Subsequent barium enema demonstrates normal, but very redundant, sigmoid colon. This, of course, is not to say that such a loop will not volve, for indeed it could.

FIGURE 3.129. *Volvulus of the cecum.* Note the dilated cecum in its typical left upper quadrant position (*arrows*).

loop to be more central and in the upper abdomen. Volvulus of any type is more likely to occur in the bedridden child, and overall this and normal redundancy of the sigmoid colon in infants and children are the prime predisposing factors to the development of volvulus.

Once volvulus is suspected, a barium enema examination should be attempted (6), for not only does it demonstrate the typical beaking, narrowing, or twisting deformity of the volved segment of colon (Fig. 3.127B), it also often is therapeutic. If the barium enema does not relieve the obstruction, proctoscopy with insertion of a decompressing tube should be attempted. After reduction, the colon may show persistent narrowing or thumbprinting as a result of residual edema and spasm (7). The presence of such edema of the intestine also is demonstrable with ultrasound.

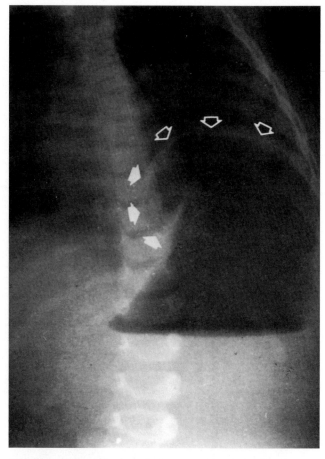

FIGURE 3.130. *Volvulus of the stomach.* Note the inverted stomach (*upper arrows*). The *solid arrows* demarcate the tapered tip of one end of the volved stomach. (From Campbell JB, Rappaport LN, Skerker LB. Acute mesentero-axial volvulus of the stomach. *Radiology* 1972;103:153–156, with permission.)

REFERENCES

1. Asano S, Konuma K, Rikimaru S, et al. Volvulus of the transverse colon in a four-year-old boy. *Z Kinderchir* 1982;35:21–23.
2. Campbell JR, Blank E. Sigmoid volvulus in children. *Pediatrics* 1974;53:702–705.
3. Houshian S, Sorensen JS, Jensen KEJ. Volvulus of the transverse colon in children. *J Pediatr Surg* 1998;33:1399–1401.
4. Hunter JG, Keats TE. Sigmoid volvulus in children. *AJR* 1970;108:621–623.
5. Kirks DR, Swischuk LE, Merten DF, Filston HC. Cecal volvulus. *AJR* 1981;136:419–422.
6. Mellor MFA, Drake DJ. Colonic volvulus in children: Value of barium enema for diagnosis and treatment in 14 children. *AJR* 1994;162:1157–1159.
7. Meyers MA, Ghahremani GG, Govoni AF. Ischemic colitis associated with sigmoid volvulus: New observations. *AJR* 1977;128:591–595.
8. Newton NA, Reines HD. Transverse colon volvulus: case reports and review. *AJR* 1977;128:69–72.

Gastric Volvulus

Gastric volvulus is a true surgical emergency (1–3), and symptoms of vomiting and severe abdominal pain often have sudden onset. Shock may supervene, and chest and abdominal films reveal a large, distended stomach causing the left diaphragmatic leaflet to be high in position (Fig. 3.130). In addition, one may note two air–fluid levels within the volved stomach (2). If barium is administered, it either stops at the gastroesophageal junction or passes into the inverted, rotated stomach. If the barium stops at the gastroesophageal junction, this infers that volvulus is so tight that complete obstruction has occurred at this level. Volvulus of the stomach also can be seen with congenital diaphragmatic hernias and in some cases may be a chronic, recurrent problem (1).

REFERENCES

1. Ash MJ, Sheiman NJ. Gastric volvulus in children: Report of two cases. *J Pediatr Surg* 1977;12:1059–1062.
2. Campbell JB, Rappaport LN, Skerker LB. Acute mesentero-axial volvulus of the stomach. *Radiology* 1972;103:153–156.
3. Honna T, Kamii Y, Tsuchida Y. Idiopathic gastric volvulus in infancy and childhood. *J Pediatr Surg* 1990;25:707–710.

Hernias

Internal hernias are difficult to diagnose. The clinical and roentgenographic findings usually are nonspecific and, at most, merely suggest an intestinal obstruction. These hernias often are paraduodenal in location but can be found anywhere along the mesentery or omentum. Hernias through the foramen of Winslow frequently involve the cecum, right colon, or terminal small bowel. In such cases, these structures herniate into the lesser sac behind the stomach (3,4), and at first the plain film findings might suggest cecal volvulus.

With lateral positioning, however, it is seen that the dilated loop or loops of intestine are located behind the stomach and not in front, as they would be with volvulus of the cecum.

Incarcerated inguinal hernias frequently are overlooked during physical examination of an infant with a distended abdomen secondary to the intestinal obstruction caused by the hernia. In such infants, in addition to the pattern of small bowel obstruction, one may see the incarcerated loops of air-filled intestine in the groin or scrotum (Fig. 3.131). If the loops of intestine do not contain air, one may see fullness of the cutaneous inguinal fold (2) on the involved side (Fig. 3.132A). In such cases, ultrasound (1) is of value in demon-

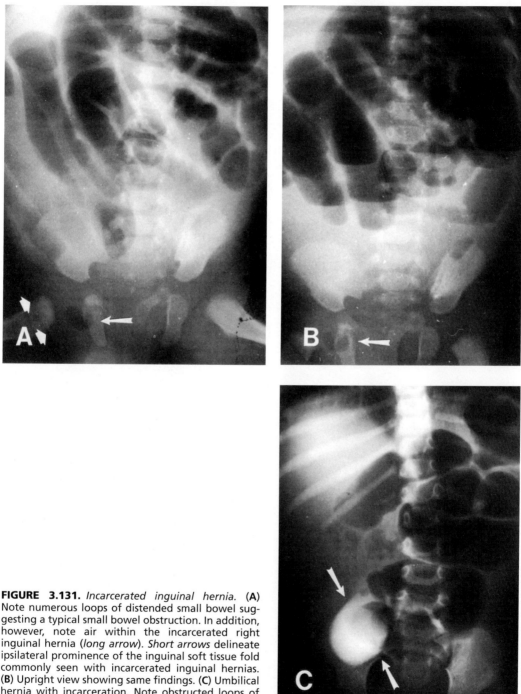

FIGURE 3.131. *Incarcerated inguinal hernia.* **(A)** Note numerous loops of distended small bowel suggesting a typical small bowel obstruction. In addition, however, note air within the incarcerated right inguinal hernia (*long arrow*). *Short arrows* delineate ipsilateral prominence of the inguinal soft tissue fold commonly seen with incarcerated inguinal hernias. **(B)** Upright view showing same findings. **(C)** Umbilical hernia with incarceration. Note obstructed loops of bowel and central umbilical hernia (*arrows*).

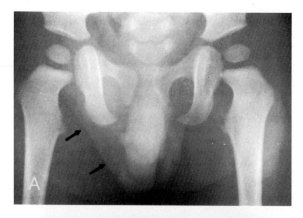

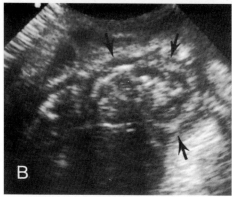

FIGURE 3.132. *Left incarcerated inguinal hernia; prominent inguinal soft tissue fold only.* **(A)** Note prominence of the right inguinal soft tissue fold (*arrows*). Compare with the normal appearance of the fold on the left. This patient had an incarcerated inguinal hernia on the right and presented with hip pain and restricted motion of the right leg. **(B)** Ultrasonographic findings in another patient. Note the layered appearance of incarcerated intestine (*arrows*).

strating that the mass in the inguinal canal or scrotum is a hernia (Fig. 3.132B). In addition, color flow Doppler can be used to demonstrate the presence or absence of blood flow to the hernia. Incarcerated umbilical hernias with obstruction also occur but are less common (Fig. 3.131C).

REFERENCES

1. Chen KC, Chu CC, Chow TY, Wu CJ. Ultrasonography for inguinal hernias in boys. *J Pediatr Surg* 1998;33:1784–1787.
2. Currarino G. Incarcerated inguinal hernia in infants: Plain films and barium enema. *Pediatr Radiol* 1974;2:247–250.
3. Henisz A, Matesanz J, Westcott J. Cecal herniation through the foramen of Winslow. *Radiology* 1974;112:575–578.
4. Zer M, Dintsman M. Incarcerated "foramen of Winslow" hernia in a newborn. *J Pediatr Surg* 1973;8:325.

Visceral Torsion

Visceral torsion usually involves the spleen or liver, but splenic torsion is more common (1–4,6–8). Torsion (volvu-

lus) of the stomach and colon have been discussed in previous sections. An unusual cause of visceral torsion is torsion of the gallbladder (5).

In splenic and liver torsion, the predisposing factor usually is a hypermobile, poorly fixed organ. Clinical findings, with torsion of either the spleen or liver, usually consist of acute, crampy abdominal pain which may or may not refer itself to the expected upper quadrant of the abdomen. Symptoms also may be chronic and intermittent.

Abdominal roentgenograms in torsion of the spleen usually show absence of the normal splenic or liver silhouette and replacement of the space by gas-filled colon or small bowel. The organ itself may be seen as a soft-tissue mass anywhere in the abdomen, but often the spleen lies on the left (Fig. 3.133). Small bowel obstruction also may occur. Ultrasonographically, clues to the diagnosis again consist of absence of the spleen in its normal location, but, in addition, color flow Doppler can show blood flow to the spleen and in the twisted pedicle to be diminished or absent. In more advanced cases, with splenic infarction, the spleen may show irregular sonolucent areas of hemorrhage. CT imaging also can identify the abnormal, torsed spleen and twisted pedicle (7) (Fig. 3.133). Of course, if blood flow is

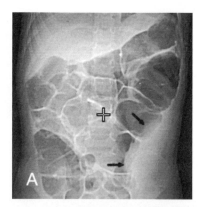

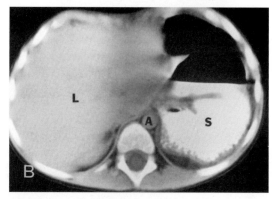

FIGURE 3.133. *Splenic torsion.* **(A)** CT topogram demonstrates diffuse paralytic ileus of the intestines and a mass (*arrows*) in the left lower quadrant. Note that the normal splenic silhouette is absent. **(B)** Scan through the upper abdomen demonstrates the liver (*L*), the aorta (*A*), and the stomach (*S*). There is no evidence of the spleen. The spleen should be visualized on this cut.

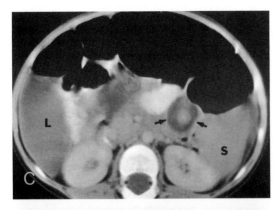

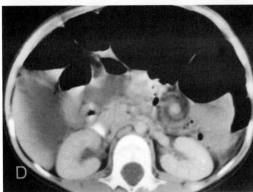

FIGURE 3.133. *(continued)* **(C)** Lower cut demonstrates the liver (*L*), both kidneys to either side of the spine, and the spleen (*S*). Also note a peculiar round structure with a dense center (*arrows*). This represents the twisted pedicle of the spleen, with some incorporated fat. **(D)** Slightly lower cut again demonstrates a whirl-like appearance of the twisted pedicle. (From Swischuk LE, Williams JB, John SD. Torsion of wandering spleen: New CT finding. *J Pediatr Radiol* 1993;23:pp #s, with permission.)

seriously compromised, the spleen does not enhance with contrast material.

Nuclear scintigraphic scans with chromium-51–labeled, heat-damaged, red blood cells show either totally absent uptake or partially absent uptake in the spleen. In splenic torsion, blood smear findings show Howell–Jolly bodies, burr cells, a leukocytosis with shift to the left, and thrombocytosis.

REFERENCES

1. Ali-Ali F, Macpherson RI, Ogthersen HB, Chavin K. A wandering liver in an infant. *Pediatr Radiol* 1997;27:287.
2. Broker FHL, Fellows K, Treves S. Wandering spleen in three children. *Pediatr Radiol* 1978;6:211–214.
3. Feins NR, Borger J. Torsion of the right lobe of the liver with partial obstruction of the colon. *J Pediatr Surg* 1972;7:724–725.
4. Herman TE, Siegel MJ. CT of acute splenic torsion in children with wandering spleen. Case report. *AJR* 1991;156:151–153.
5. Kitagawa H, Nakada K, Enami T, Yamaguchi T, Kawaguchi F, Nakada M, Yamate N. Cases of torsion of the gallbladder diagnosed preoperatively. *J Pediatr Surg* 1997;32:1567–1569.

6. Seo T, Ito T, Watanabe Y, Umeda T. Torsion of an accessory spleen presenting as an acute abdomen with an inflammatory mass. US, CT and MRI findings. *Pediatr Radiol* 1995;24:532–534.
7. Swischuk LE, Williams JB, John SD. Torsion of wandering spleen: New CT finding. *J Pediatr Radiol* 1993;23:
8. Thompson JS, Ross RJ, Pizzaro ST. The wandering spleen in infancy and childhood. *Clin Pediatr* 1980;19:221–224.

Omental Strangulation and Infarction

These problems are quite rare but do occur (1–4). They are very difficult to diagnose roentgenographically, but with the availability of ultrasound, one may be able to demonstrate an echogenic abdominal mass that would mitigate toward surgical exploration of the abdomen.

REFERENCES

1. Chew DKW, Holgersen LO, Friedman D. Primary omental torsion in children. *J Pediatr Surg* 1995;30:816–817.
2. Myers MT, Grisoni ER, Sivit CJ. Segmental omental infarction in a 9-year-old girl. *Emerg Radiol* 1997;4:112–114.
3. Puylaert JBCM. Right-sided segmental infarction of the omentum: Clinical, US and CT findings. *Radiology* 1992;185:169–172.
4. Rich RH, Filler RM. Segmental infarction of the greater omentum: A cause of acute abdomen in childhood. *Can J Surg* 1983;26:241–243.

ABDOMINAL TRAUMA

General Approach

In abdominal trauma, the abdominal roentgenogram now is used more as an initial screening examination than for specific diagnosis. Ultrasound and, even more so, CT scanning have supplanted this study. Spiral CT images are especially useful (2), and in the future portable CT scanning, as its technology evolves, also will come to play a significant part of the assessment of these patients (12). All of this notwithstanding, the plain film still has some use, and one should develop some type of general approach to its assessment.

In beginning assessment of the abdomen, one should note the lung bases, diaphragmatic leaflets, larger abdominal viscera, and overall gas pattern quickly. Then one should look at the pelvis, ribs, and vertebrae. One also should look at the spine for evidence of scoliosis, because scoliosis is very helpful in lateralizing abnormalities to one side or the other. Next, one should inspect the abdomen for evidence of free air, peritoneal fluid (blood, bile, and so forth), focally distended loops of intestine (i.e., sentinel loops), and, as mentioned, fractures of the ribs, bony pelvis, or spine.

Both ultrasound and CT imaging, as mentioned previously, now are utilized commonly in the investigation of abdominal trauma. Although some suggest that plain films and ultrasound should suffice in cases of minor trauma

(1,5,6,10,28), all agree that if intraabdominal injury is suggested seriously, CT scanning is much more informative and the preferred modality (2,3,7,14,22,24). The detection of large volumes of fluid (blood) with ultrasound has proven to be useful (8,9,13,15,17,23,29) but not foolproof, because it is operator-dependent and experience is necessary. If one is not experienced, errors are common (4,11,20,22,27).

In assessing the abdomen on a CT scan, if shock is present normal organs become hyperintense. Often this phenomenon is best seen in the kidneys, but it also frequently is visualized in the walls of shocked, fluid-filled, and paralyzed intestinal loops (Fig. 3.134). In addition, with hypovolemic shock the aorta is small (Fig. 3.134B). Also, if the hematocrit level is low secondary to hemorrhage, the aorta

is small and the blood low in density (Fig. 3.134C). Another finding of shock consists of nonenhancement of the spleen (18).

Another phenomenon often seen with abdominal trauma, and in the past believed to be associated with hepatic trauma and bleeding, is so-called periportal tracking of fluid. Although originally it was believed to be caused by blood tracking along the periportal space, there is now considerable data to suggest that this finding results from transudation of fluid into the periportal space from associated portal lymphatic obstruction (i.e., hematoma) or fluid overload from iatrogenic bolus intravenous fluid therapy (16,19,21,25,26). Actually the latter is probably what occurs most often (Fig. 3.134D).

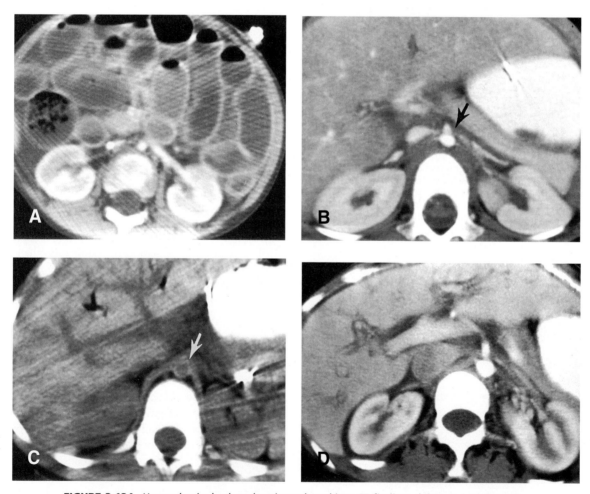

FIGURE 3.134. *Hypovolemic shock and periportal tracking: CT findings.* **(A)** Note how hyperintense the kidneys appear, and in addition note the hyperintense appearance of the intestinal walls. The intestines are dilated and filled with fluid and air. **(B)** The opacified aorta (*arrow*) is small in this patient with hypovolemic shock. Also note the hyperintense appearance of the kidneys. **(C)** In this patient, without contrast, the aorta also is small (*arrow*). It is hypointense because of a low hematocrit level. **(D)** Periportal tracking. Note the hypointense areas along the portal tracks. This is secondary to fluid extravasation after massive fluid resuscitation. Also note the hyperintense shocked kidneys

REFERENCES

1. Akgur FM, Tanyel FC, Akhan O, Buyukpamukdu N, Hicsonmez A. The place of ultrasonographic examination in the initial evaluation of children sustaining blunt abdominal trauma. *J Pediatr Surg* 1993;28:78–81.
2. Brody AS, Seidel FG, Kuhn JP. CT evaluation of blunt abdominal trauma in children: Comparison of ultrafast and conventional CT. *AJR* 1989;153:803–806.
3. Bulas DI, Taylor GA, Eichelberger MR. The value of CT in detecting bowel perforation in children after blunt abdominal trauma. *AJR* 1989;153:561–564.
4. Chiu WC, Cushing BM, Rodriguez A, Shiu M, Mirvis SE, Shanmuganathan K, Stein M. Abdominal injuries without hemoperitoneum: A potential limitation of focused abdominal sonograpny for trauma (FAST). *J Trauma* 1997;42:617–625.
5. Filiatrault D, Longpre D, Patriquin H, Perreault G, Grignon A, Pronovost J, Bosvert J. Investigation of childhood blunt abdominal trauma: A practical approach using ultrasound as the initial diagnostic modality. *Pediatr Radiol* 1987;17:373–379.
6. Katz S, Lazar L, Rathaus V, Erez I. Can ultrasonography replace computed tomography in the initial assessment of children with blunt abdominal trauma? *J Pediatr Surg* 1996;31:649–651.
7. Kretschjmer KH, Bohndorf K, Pohlenz OP. The role of sonography in abdominal trauma: The European experience. *Emerg Radiol* 1997;4:62–67.
8. Lentz KA, McKenney MG, Nunez DB Jr, Martin L. Evaluating blunt abdominal trauma: Role for ultrasonography. *J Ultrasound Med* 1996;15:447–451.
9. McGahan JP, Richards JR. Ultrasound, CT or DPL for evaluation of blunt abdominal trauma. *Appl Radiol* 1998;8:7–17.
10. McKenney KL, McKenney MG, Nunez DB, Martin L. Cost reduction using ultrasound in blunt abdominal trauma. *Emerg Radiol* 1997;4:3–6.
11. McKenney KL, Nunez DB, McKenney MG, Cohn S. Ultrasound for blunt abdominal trauma: Is it free fluid? *Emerg Radiol* 1998;5:203-209.
12. Mirvis SE, Shanmuganathan K, Donohue R, White WH, Fritz S, Hartsock R. Mobile computed tomography in the trauma/critical care environment: Preliminary clinical experience. *Emerg Radiol* 1997;4:212–217.
13. Mutabagani KH, Coley BD, Zumberge N, McCarthy DW, Besner GE, Caniano DA, Cooney DR. Preliminary experience with focused abdominal sonography for trauma (FAST) in children: Is it useful? *J Pediatr Surg* 1999;34:48–54.
14. Neish AS, Taylor GA, Lund DP, Atkinson CC. Effect of CT information on the diagnosis and management of acute abdominal injury in children. *Radiology* 1998;206:327–331.
15. Patel JC, Tepas JJ III. The efficacy of focused abdominal sonography for trauma (FAST) as a screening tool in the assessment of injured children. *J Pediatr Surg* 1999;34:44–47.
16. Patrick LE, Ball TI, Atkinson GO, Winn KJ. Pediatric blunt abdominal trauma: Periportal tracking at CT. *Radiology* 1992;183:689–691.
17. Patrick DA, Bensaard DD, Moore EE, et al. Ultrasound is an effective triage tool to evaluate blunt abdominal trauma in the pediatric population. *J Trauma* 1998;45:57–63.
18. Ramsdell MG, Rao PM. Splenic nonenhancement at computed tomography: A sign of the hypoperfusion complex. *Emerg Radiol* 1997;4:329–331.
19. Shanmuganathan K, Mirvis SE, Amoroso M. Periportal low density on CT in patients with blunt trauma: Association with elevated venous pressure. *AJR* 1993;160:279–283.
20. Sherbourne CD, Shanmuganathan K, Mirvis SE, Chiu WC, Rodriguez A. Visceral injury without hemoperitoneum: A limitation of screening abdominal sonography for trauma. *Emerg Radiol* 1997;4:349–354.
21. Siegel MJ, Herman TE. Periportal low attenuation at CT in childhood. *Radiology* 1992;183:685–688.
22. Sivit CJ, Frazier AA, Eichelberger MR. Computed tomography of pediatric blunt abdominal trauma. *Emerg Radiol* 1997;4:150–166.
23. Sivit CJ, Taylor GA, Bulas DI, Bowman LM, Eichelberger MR. Blunt trauma in children: Significance of peritoneal fluid. *Radiology* 1991;178:185–188.
24. Sivit CJ, Taylor GA, Bulas DI, Kushner DC, Potter BM, Eichelberger MR. Post-traumatic shock in children: CT findings associated with hemodynamic instability. *Radiology* 1992;182:723–726.
25. Sivit CJ, Taylor GA, Eichelberger MR, Bulas DI, Gotshall CS, Kushner DC. Significance of periportal low-attenuation zones following blunt trauma in children. *Pediatr Radiol* 1993;23:388–390.
26. Taylor GA, Fallat ME, Eichelberger MR. Hypovolemic shock in children: Abdominal CT manifestations. *Radiology* 1987;164:479–481.
27. Taylor GA, Sivit CJ. Posttraumatic peritoneal fluid: Is it a reliable indicator of intraabdominal injury in children? *J Pediatr Surg* 1995;30:1644–1648.
28. Thomas B, Falcone RE, Vasquez D, Santanello S, Townsend M, Hockenberry S, Innes J, Wanamaker S. Ultrasound evaluation of blunt abdominal trauma: Program implementation, initial experience, and learning curve. *J Trauma* 1997;42:384–390.
29. Thourani VH, Pettitt BJ, Schmidt JA, Cooper WA, Rozycki GS. Validation of surgeon-performed emergency abdominal ultrasonography in pediatric trauma patients. *J Pediatr Surg* 1998;33:322–328.

Specific Organ Injury

Spleen

One of the most commonly injured organs is the spleen. Clinically, upper abdominal, left upper quadrant, flank, or left-shoulder (referred from the diaphragm) pain provides a clue to the diagnosis. The roentgenographic findings associated with splenic injury often are difficult to evaluate, but one or more of the following findings should be sought: (a) medial displacement of the stomach, (b) downward or medial displacement of the splenic flexure, (c) elevation of the left diaphragmatic leaflet, (d) scoliosis of the spine with concavity to the left, (e) sentinel loops over the left upper quadrant, (f) pleural effusions or atelectasis in the left lung base (2), and in a few cases (g) associated rib fractures. Of course, not all these findings are present in any one patient, but being aware of all of them is most important (Fig. 3.135).

Splenic injuries are identified readily with CT scanning. Ultrasonography, initially employed in the investigation of splenic injury, is not as productive, and we have found that splenic hematomas can be missed with ultrasound. Consequently, we seldom perform ultrasonography for suspected splenic injury, for CT scanning usually clearly identifies all forms of splenic injury (Fig. 3.136). In terms of the CT

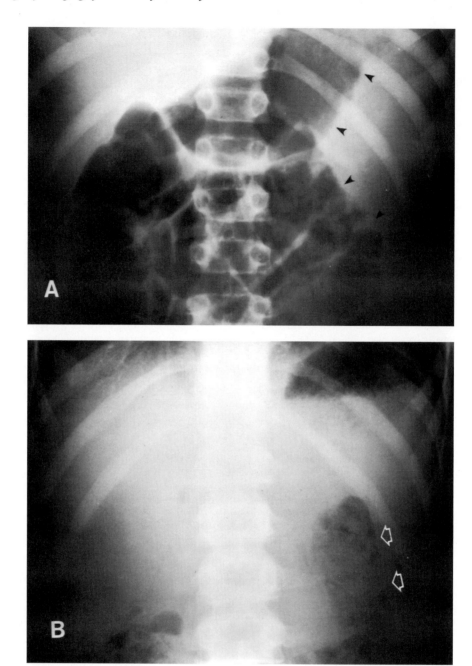

FIGURE 3.135. *Splenic trauma: plain film findings.* **(A)** Note the enlarged splenic silhouette displacing the stomach and intestines medially (*arrows*). **(B)** Another case showing a medially displaced splenic flexure (*arrows*). The spleen is difficult to identify as such, but the splenic space is increased in width.

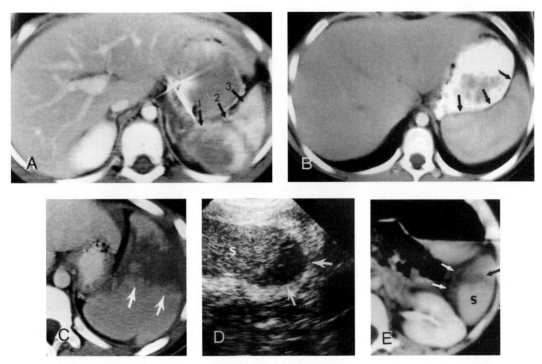

FIGURE 3.136. *Splenic trauma: CT findings.* **(A)** Note the completely abnormal spleen demonstrating a large hematoma *(1)*, a central laceration *(2)*, and residual, relatively normal splenic pulp *(3)*. There is a little free fluid (blood) between the splenic pulp and the abdominal wall. **(B)** Normal irregular opacification of the spleen *(arrows)* resulting from imaging early during a bolus injection. This is an important artifact, not to be misinterpreted as multiple splenic contusions. **(C)** Another patient with a splenic "fracture" *(arrows)*. **(D)** Subcapsular splenic hematoma *(arrows)* visualized with ultrasound. *S,* spleen. **(E)** CT findings in same patient demonstrate the spleen *(S)*, a central laceration *(black arrow)*, and the subcapsular collection of blood *(white arrows)*.

examination, one should be aware of the phenomenon of irregular contrast opacification of the spleen very early after the bolus contrast injection (1) (Fig. 3.136B).

REFERENCES

1. Donnelly LF, Foss JN, Frush DP, Bisset GS III. Heterogeneous splenic enhancement patterns on spiral CT images in children: Minimizing misinterpretation. *Radiology* 1999;210:493–497.
2. Kittredge RD, Finby N. Infrapulmonary effusion in traumatic rupture of the spleen. *AJR* 1964;91:891–895.

Liver, Gallbladder, and Bile Ducts

Liver injury with virtual exsanguinating hemorrhage is a true emergency, and often there is barely enough time to obtain abdominal roentgenograms. In such cases, emergency ligation or embolization of the hepatic artery frequently is performed. Intracapsular hematomas, a much more common problem, lead to enlargement of the liver, upward displacement of the right diaphragmatic leaflet, medial displacement of the duodenum and stomach, down-ward displacement of the hepatic flexure, and, in some cases, downward displacement and compression of the right kidney (Fig. 3.137). Of course, atelectasis and pleural effusions in the right lung base also may be noted, along with right-rib fractures. Intrahepatic air, probably forced into the liver from the intestinal tract, also has been described (1). If blood escapes into the peritoneal cavity, the finding is intraperitoneal fluid. Ultrasonography is more rewarding with liver injuries than with splenic injuries, but CT scanning is still the procedure of choice (7,8) (Fig. 3.138). Posttraumatic hepatic-artery aneurysms are uncommon (6).

Injury to the bile ducts or gallbladder often is difficult to diagnose and usually is accompanied by injury to other viscera in the area, mainly the liver. If the gallbladder or bile ducts are injured alone, however, bile peritonitis is the presenting feature (3,4). In such cases, the peritonitis produced often is of a smoldering nature, and it is not until paracentesis is performed that the diagnosis is substantiated. Prior to this one can utilize technetium–HIDA scans, which demonstrate isotope activity outside the hepatobiliary system and gastrointestinal tract. Posttraumatic gallbladder torsion (5) and gallbladder avulsion (2) are rare.

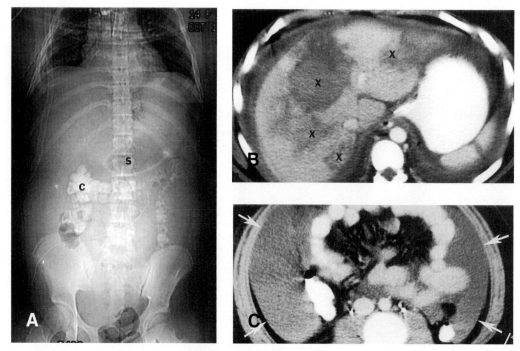

FIGURE 3.137. *Liver trauma.* **(A)** Note density in the right upper quadrant with downward displacement of the stomach (*s*) and colon (*c*). Fluid in the paracolic gutters is displacing the contrast-filled ascending and descending portions of the colon inward. **(B)** *CT.* Note extensive multiple contusions and hematomas of the liver (*x*). Fluid surrounds the liver and the spleen. **(C)** On a lower slice, fluid is seen in both paracolic gutters (*arrows*) displacing the colon inwards.

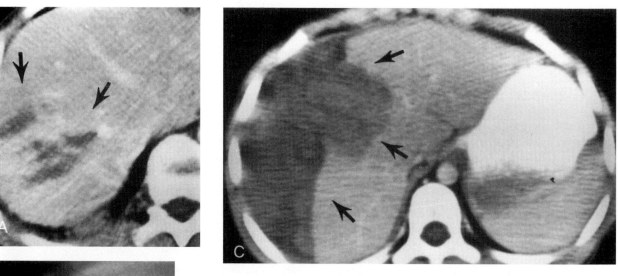

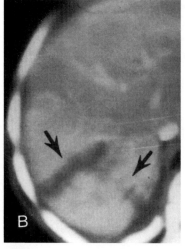

FIGURE 3.138. *Liver trauma: CT findings.* **(A)** Note numerous intrahepatic hypodense, irregular contusions (*arrows*). These areas represent small areas of hemorrhage. **(B)** Another patient with a laceration (fracture) through the right lobe of the liver (*arrows*). **(C)** Large subcapsular intrahepatic hematoma (*arrows*).

REFERENCES

1. Abramson SJ, Berdon WE, Kaufman RA, Ruzal-Shapiro C. Hepatic parenchymal and subcapsular gas after hepatic laceration caused by blunt abdominal trauma. *AJR* 1989;153:1031–1032.
2. Bindra PS, Dobbins JM, Novelline RA. Diagnosis of traumatic gallbladder avulsion: Role of sagittal and coronal computed tomographic reformations. *Emerg Radiol* 1998;5:256–258.
3. Evans JP. Traumatic rupture of the gallbladder in a three-year-old boy. *J Pediatr Surg* 1976;11:1033–1034.
4. Moulton SL, Downey EC, Anderson DS, Synch FP. Blunt bile duct injuries in children. *J Pediatr Surg* 1993;28:795–797.
5. Salman AB, Yildirgan MI, Gelebi F. Posttraumatic gallbladder torsion in a child. *J Pediatr Surg* 1996;31:1586.
6. Siduh MK, Shaw DWW, Daly CP, Waldhausen JH, Coldwell D. Post-traumatic hepatic pseudoaneurysms in children. *Pediatr Radiology* 1999;29:40–52.
7. Stalker HP, Kaufman RA, Towbin R. Patterns of liver injury in childhood: CT analysis. *AJR* 1986;147:1100–1205.
8. Vock P, Kehrer B, Tschaeppeler H. Blunt liver trauma in children: The role of computed tomography in diagnosis and treatment. *J Pediatr Surg* 1986;21:413–418.

Pancreatic Trauma

Pancreatic trauma in childhood is relatively common (2) and can occur with surprisingly mild injury. Most often it is seen with automobile accidents, bicycle-handlebar accidents, blows with the fist to the abdomen, falls on a blunt object, and seatbelt injuries in older children. It also commonly is seen in the battered child syndrome.

The roentgenographic findings are variable, and actually most often the abdominal roentgenograms are normal. In other cases, however, one may see telltale sentinel loops of dilated intestine over the area of the pancreas. In any given case, these loops may be of dilated small bowel, duodenum, or transverse colon (Fig. 3.139A). If the transverse colon is dilated (3), it results in the colon cutoff sign (Fig. 3.139B). In addition to these findings, one may see widening of the soft tissue space between the stomach and transverse colon as a result of bleeding or edema in this area. Each of these findings, however, is either rare or subtle, and thus suspected pancreatic injury is best assessed with CT scanning (2). Ultrasonography also can be useful but is not as rewarding as CT scanning.

In some cases the pancreas may be enlarged, and on ultrasound somewhat hypoechoic (edema). In other cases parapancreatic fluid collections are present, and occasionally an actual laceration or "fracture" of the pancreas is seen (Fig. 3.140A). These same findings are demonstrable with CT scanning (Fig. 3.140B), and both ultrasound and CT (1) can document clearly the presence of complicating post-traumatic pseudocysts.

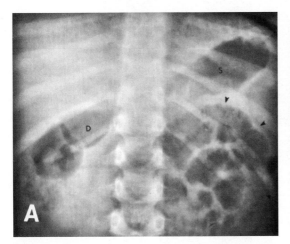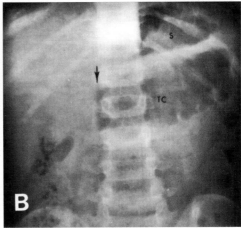

FIGURE 3.139. *Pancreatic trauma.* **(A)** Note the stomach (*S*), duodenum (*D*), and sentinel loops of dilated small bowel in the left abdomen (*arrows*). The stomach is displaced upward, and the soft-tissue space between the stomach and intestines is widened. The duodenal bulb is filled with air secondary to paralytic ileus. **(B)** Another case demonstrating the colon cutoff sign. Note the dilated transverse colon (*TC*), and the abrupt cutoff of gas just to the right of the spine (*arrow*). Also note that the soft-tissue space between the stomach (*S*) and the transverse colon is increased. (From Young LW, Adams JT. Roentgenographic findings in localized trauma to pancreas in children. *AJR* 1967;101:639–648, with permission.)

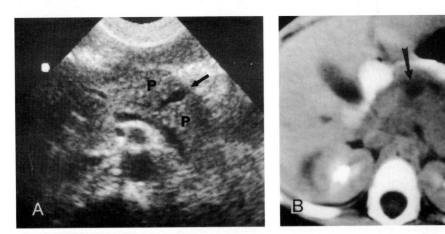

FIGURE 3.140. *Pancreatic fracture.* **(A)** Ultrasound study demonstrates a wedgelike fracture (*arrow*) through the pancreas (*P*). The pancreas is a little enlarged, and there is some peripancreatic fluid present. **(B)** CT study in another patient demonstrates a similar wedge-like fracture (*arrow*). A little peripancreatic fluid also is present. In other cases, the findings in pancreatic trauma are no different than in other cases of pancreatitis from other causes (Fig. 3.74).

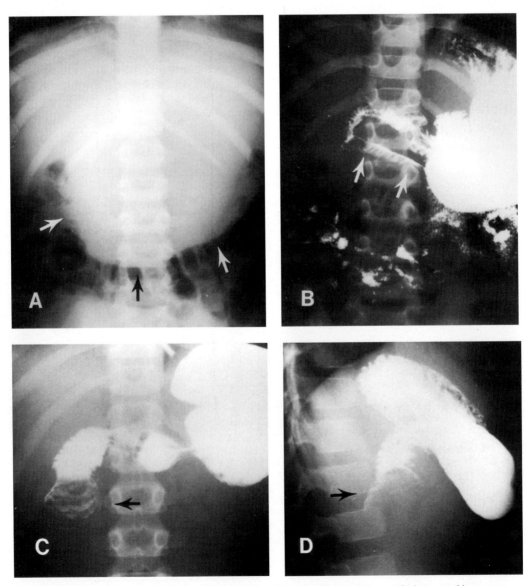

FIGURE 3.141. *Duodenal trauma.* **(A)** Note large distended stomach (*arrows*) obstructed because of a duodenal hematoma. **(B)** Typical appearance of the duodenal hematoma; an intramural lesion (*arrows*). **(C and D)** Another patient with classic findings of an intramural hematoma (*arrows*). (Courtesy of Virgil Graves, M.D.)

REFERENCES

1. Dahman B, Stephens CA. Pseudocysts of the pancreas after blunt abdominal trauma in children. *J Pediatr Surg* 1981;16:17–21.
2. Sivit CJ, Eichelberger MR, Taylor GA, Bulas DI, Gotschall CS, Kushner DC. Blunt pancreatic trauma in children: CT diagnosis. *AJR* 1992;158:1097–1100.
3. Young LW, Adams JT. Roentgenographic findings in localized trauma to pancreas in children. *AJR* 1967;101: 639–648.

Duodenum

Trauma to the duodenum often is seen in conjunction with pancreatic injury but, of course, can occur alone. It results from the same types of injuries responsible for pancreatic trauma, and also is seen in the battered child syndrome. Trauma to the duodenum may manifest in actual duodenal rupture, intramural duodenal tears, or intramural hematoma formation. The last injury, however, is most common. If duodenal rupture occurs, the usual site of perforation is along the posterior duodenal wall, and subsequently there is leakage of intestinal contents into the retroperitoneal space. Symptoms of such leakage may not become apparent immediately; they may take hours or days to develop. When they do develop, they include pain in the back or flank, and roentgenographically, if water-soluble contrast agents are administered to these patients, retroperitoneal extravasation can be demonstrated. On a CT scan, free air can be seen in the pararenal space (2). The duodenum, of course, also is deformed or even obstructed. Intraperitoneal rupture of the duodenum is rare.

With duodenal intramural hematoma formation, the plain films may show nothing abnormal, or they may show evidence of duodenal or gastric obstruction (Fig. 3.141A). Less commonly, the hematoma itself may be seen as an abdominal mass. If duodenal injury is suspected, however, ultrasound or an upper gastrointestinal series should be performed. The upper gastrointestinal series demonstrates the duodenal obstruction resulting from an intramural mass (Fig. 3.141B–D), and with intramural tears, barium is seen extravasating from the duodenum. Intramural hematomas eventually disappear, with the blood escaping into the bowel lumen and follow-up gastrointestinal studies usually showing a complete return to normal.

Duodenal hematomas are more likely to be first demonstrated with ultrasonography or CT scanning (1). CT findings are similar to those seen on upper gastrointestinal series, in that there is a mass present resulting from the hematoma and associated displacement or deformity of the duodenum. With ultrasonography, the early hematoma appears as an echogenic mass (Fig. 3.142), but with maturation the hematoma liquifies and becomes anechoic (see Fig. 3.143C).

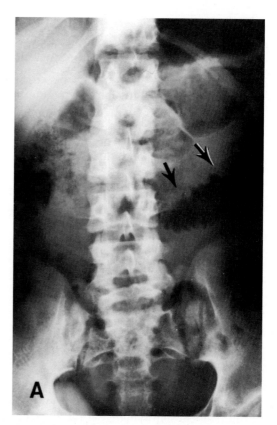

FIGURE 3.143. *Small bowel trauma.* **(A)** Note sentinel loop (*arrows*) secondary to jejunal injury. The next day the patient developed a classic small bowel obstruction.

(continued on next page)

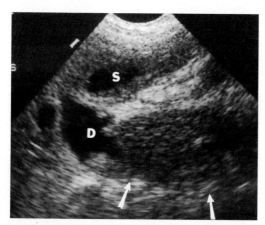

FIGURE 3.142. *Duodenal hematoma: ultrasonographic findings.* Note the echogenic, eccentric hematoma (*arrows*) located in the distal duodenum and producing some obstruction of the descending duodenum (*D*). *S*, stomach.

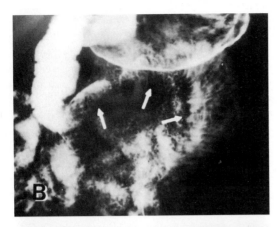

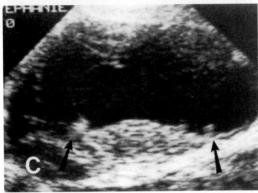

FIGURE 3.143. *(continued)* (B) Upper gastrointestinal series demonstrating a large intramural jejunal hematoma (*arrows*). **(C)** Ultrasonogram demonstrates a large, sonolucent hematoma (*arrows*). (B–C are from Kaufman RA, Babcock DS. An approach to imaging the upper abdomen in the injured child. *Semin Roentgenol* 1984;14:308–320, with permission.)

REFERENCES

1. Hayashi K, Futgagawa S, Kozaki S, Hirao K, Hombo Z. Ultrasound and CT diagnosis of intramural duodenal hematoma. *Pediatr Radiol* 1988;18:167–168.
2. Kunin JR, Korobkin M, Ellis JH, Francis IR, Kane NM, Siegel SE. Duodenal injuries caused by blunt abdominal trauma: Value of CT in differentiating perforation from hematoma. *AJR* 1993;160:1221–1223.

Stomach, Esophagus, Small Intestines, and Colon

Small intestinal injury has become more common as seatbelt injuries have increased in frequency (5,7,8,13), but, of course, any type of blunt trauma to the abdomen can cause small bowel injury. It is important to note that with seatbelt injuries concommittent spinal injury can coexist and may go undetected (5). Ecchymotic changes across the lower abdomen, however, should serve as a signal that internal or spinal injuries could be present in these patients (13). This is most important to appreciate, for in the rush of evaluat-

ing such patients these injuries may be overlooked. In terms of imaging, it is worthwhile to obtain a lateral view of the abdomen, which includes the spine, as part of the topogram for the inevitably performed CT study of the abdomen.

In terms of the specific type of injury incurred in the small bowel, perforation and hematoma formation probably are the most common. In either case, posttraumatic stenoses with obstruction of the intestines can result (4,8,10). In addition, protrusion of a loop of small bowel into an associated spinal fracture–dislocation can occur (11) , and internal or abdominal wall hernias also can be encountered (1,6,16).

With small bowel injuries the abdominal roentgenogram frequently is normal, but in some cases one or two sentinel loops of dilated, injured small bowel can be seen. If these loops appear thickened, intramural bleeding or edema should be suspected, but often this is a difficult finding to appreciate on plain films; it usually is best demonstrated with CT scanning. In some of these cases, the hematoma may extend into the mesentery or omentum (3), but in either case, if large enough, the hematoma may present as an abdominal mass on plain films. In most cases, however, ultrasonography or CT scanning is more productive in detecting these hematomas (Fig. 3.143).

As already noted, small bowel injury can be subtle. and it has been suggested that clinical evaluation of these patients is better than roentgenographic evaluation (2,9). The reason for this is that very little free air often is seen, even on CT scan

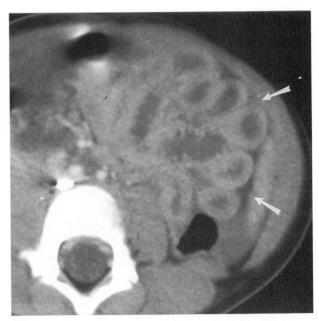

FIGURE 3.144. *Small bowel contusion.* There are numerous loops of small bowel on the left (*arrows*), with thickened walls. There is also some edema of the surrounding fat.

(3,12,15) and thus, following these patients clinically often is more rewarding than imaging them instantly. Small bowel injury can be suspected if thickened loops of small bowel are detected on the CT scan (Fig. 3.144).

Perforation of the stomach (7) or colon may lead to free air being visualized in the abdomen. With gastric or colonic perforations, such air usually is intraperitoneal and of such a volume that it is readily visualized. Rectal perforations may lead to air accumulations in the pelvic soft tissues, and both rectal and duodenal perforations can lead to retroperitoneal air collections.

Esophageal perforation (14) can present with widening of the mediastinum, air in the mediastinum, or hydropneumothorax. Esophageal perforations can be confirmed with the administration of contrast material; they usually result from acutely increased intraluminal pressures secondary to blunt trauma to the abdomen and lower chest. Perforation from foreign bodies is rare, as is perforation from vomiting.

REFERENCES

1. Ciftci AO, Salman B, Turken A, Senocak ME. Acute blunt traumatic abdominal hernia. *J Pediatr Surg* 1997;32: 1732–1734.
2. Ford EG, Senac MO Jr. Clinical presentation and radiographic identification of small bowel rupture following blunt trauma in children. *Pediatr Emerg Care* 1993;9:139–142.
3. Graham JS, Wong AL. A review of computed tomography in the diagnosis of intestinal and mesenteric injury in pediatric blunt abdominal trauma. *J Pediatr Surg* 1996;31:754–756.
4. Hardacre JM II, West KW, Rescorla FR, Vane DW, Grosfeld JL. Delayed onset of intestinal obstruction in children after unrecognized seat belt injury. *J Pediatr Surg* 1990;25:967–969.
5. Hoy GA, Cole WG. Concurrent paediatric seat belt injuries of the abdomen and spine. *Pediatr Surg Int* 1992;7:376–379.
6. Iuchtman M, Kessel B, Kirshon M. Trauma-related acute spigelian hernia in a child. *Pediatr Emerg Care* 1997;13:404–405.
7. Kimmins MH, Poenaru D, Kamal I. Traumatic gastric transection: A case report. *J Pediatr Surg* 1996;31:757–758.
8. Lynch JM, Albanese CT, Meza MP, Wiener ES. Intestinal stricture following seat belt injury in children. *J Pediatr Surg* 1996;31: 1354–1357.
9. Moss RL, Musemeche CA. Clinical judgment is superior to diagnostic tests in the management of pediatric small bowel injury. *J Pediatr Surg* 1996;31:1178–1182.
10. Shalaby-Rana E, Eichelberger MR, Kerzner B, Kapur S. Case report: Intestinal stricture due to lap-belt injury. *AJR* 1992;158: 63–64.
11. Silver SF, Nadel HR, Flodmark O. Case report: Pneumorrhachis after jejunal entrapment caused by a fracture dislocation of the lumbar spine. *AJR* 1988;150:1129–1130.
12. Sivit CJ, Eichelberger MR, Taylor GA. CT in children with rupture of the bowel caused by blunt trauma: Diagnostic efficacy and comparison with hypoperfusion complex. *AJR* 1994;163: 1195–1198.
13. Sivit CJ, Taylor GA, Newman KD, Bulas DI, Gotschall CS, Wright CJ, Eichelberger MR. Safety-belt injuries in children with lap-belt ecchymosis: CT findings in 61 patients. *AJR* 1991; 157:111–114.
14. Sartorelli KH, McBride WJ, Vane DW. Perforation of the intrathoracic esophagus from blunt tgrauma in a child: Case report and review of the literature. *J Pediatr Surg* 1998;34: 495–497.
15. Swischuk LE. Go-cart accident. *Pediatr Emerg Care* 1998;14: 441–443.
16. Wang SF, Tiu CM, Chou YH, Chang T. Obstructive intestinal herniation due to improper use of a seat belt: a case report. *Pediatr Radiol* 1993;23:200–201.

Urinary Tract

Injury to the *urinary tract* is one of the more common manifestations of abdominal trauma, and renal injury can range from simple renal parenchymal contusion to complete avulsion of the renal pedicle. A diagrammatic representation of these injuries is offered in Fig. 3.145. Interestingly, however, most of these lesions can be treated conservatively (1), and it is only the massive injury to the kidneys or their blood supply that requires immediate surgical intervention. In addition, initial studies, no matter what they consist of, usually are not useful in predicting future problems such as scarring (12) and systemic hypertension. Therefore, over the years, the approach to renal trauma generally has become quite conservative. In this regard, it has been shown that with renal trauma if the patient is normotensive and there are fewer than 50 urine red blood cells per high-power field, no investigation is necessary (11).

In the past, one relied almost solely on the intravenous pyelogram for the evaluation of renal trauma, but although the study is still occasionally utilized (8), CT scanning has provided a more definitive method with which to document and follow renal injury (9,14). Ultrasonography also can be utilized, but there is no comparison to the information yielded with contrast-enhanced CT scanning (Fig. 3.146). Indeed, small contusions and lacerations can be missed with ultrasound.

With simple *renal contusions, intrarenal hematomas, and renal infarctions* (7), the renal silhouette is intact, but the kidneys may be focally or generally enlarged. Intravenous pyelography usually demonstrates generalized or focal decreased renal function (Fig. 3.147A); ultrasound may show a focal echogenic lesion. CT scanning, however, most clearly identifies the noncontrast-enhancing contusion (Fig. 3.147B). Renal lacerations, transected kidneys, crushed kidneys, and perirenal fluid collections (blood, urine) also are best demonstrated with CT imaging (Fig. 3.148). If lacerations extend through the renal capsule, extravasation of contrast material and urine into the perinephric space may be seen (Fig. 3.148).

Injuries to the *renal pelvis* also lead to extravasation of urine and contrast material around the kidneys, and in some cases the urine collection leads to the development of

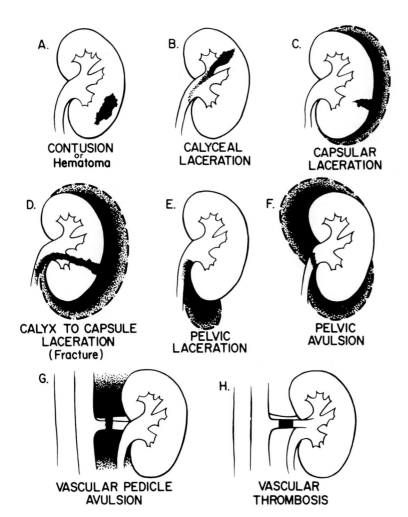

FIGURE 3.145. *Types of renal injury: diagrammatic representation.* Black areas represent areas of blood accumulation, except in **(H)**, in which the black area represents the area of thrombosis. (Modified from Macpherson RI, Decter A. Pediatric renal trauma. *Can J Assoc Radiol* 1971;22:10—21, with permission.)

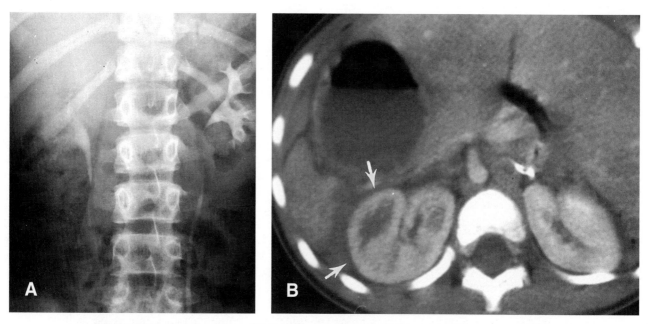

FIGURE 3.146. *Renal contusion.* **(A)** Note decreased function of the entire kidney in this patient with a right renal contusion. **(B)** CT study in another patient demonstrates an enlarged right kidney with slightly decreased function (*arrows*). There is some edema of the surrounding fat.

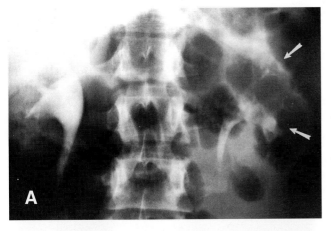

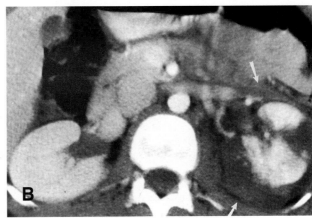

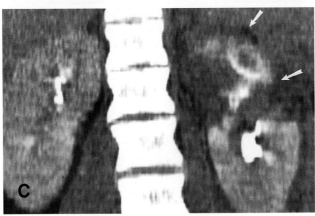

FIGURE 3.147. *Renal trauma: PF and CT findings.* **(A)** There is markedly decreased function of the left kidney (*arrows*). **(B)** CT study more clearly demonstrates the extent of the injury. The kidney is fractured and surrounded by fluid (blood; *arrows*). **(C)** Coronal reconstruction demonstrates the fractured upper pole (*arrows*) and the intact lower pole.

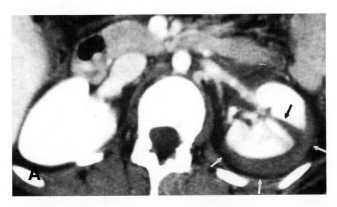

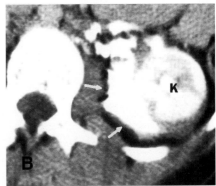

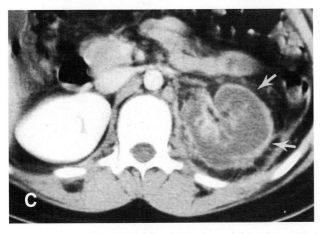

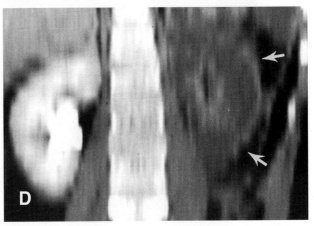

FIGURE 3.148. CT findings. **(A)** In this patient a complete fracture of the kidney has occurred (*black arrow*), and the kidney is surrounded by subcapsular blood (*arrows*). **(B)** Later, extravasation of contrast material (*arrows*) is seen. *K*, kidney. **(C)** This left kidney, in another patient, is totally underprofused (*arrows*). Only the capsule is visible. This represents a dead kidney secondary to vascular injury. **(D)** Coronal reconstruction showing similar findings (*arrows*).

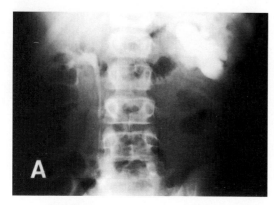
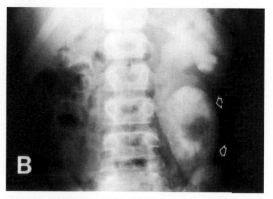

FIGURE 3.149. *Parapelvic urinoma.* **(A)** Early film demonstrating an elevated and obstructed left kidney. Note one or two curvilinear collections of contrast material below the left kidney. **(B)** Delayed films demonstrate filling of a large urinoma (*arrows*), which was obstructing the left kidney.

a so-called urinoma (4). This collection of urine may be visualized as a soft tissue mass on plain abdominal roentgenograms, and on intravenous pyelography it eventually fills with contrast material (Fig. 3.149). Associated obstruction of the upper urinary tract is common in these cases, and the urine collections may extend into the thorax (3). These urine collections usually are readily demonstrable with ultrasonography, for they are sonolucent. They are also readily visualized with CT scanning.

Vascular injury to the renal pedicle may range from traumatic avulsion of both the artery and vein to renal artery thrombosis (2). With total avulsion of the renal pedi-

cle, perinephric hematoma formation usually is profound, and nonfunction of the involved kidney is seen. With traumatic renal artery thrombosis, the kidney usually is not enlarged, and arteriography usually is required for demonstration of the obstructed artery (6).

Before leaving this discussion of renal trauma, a note regarding ***trauma to a previously unsuspected hydronephrotic kidney*** is in order. In some of these cases, trauma seems to be relatively mild, but pain and hematuria cause the child to seek medical attention. Indeed, one often is surprised at just how large these hydronephrotic kidneys are, and how they remain silent until the time of injury (Fig. 3.150). In

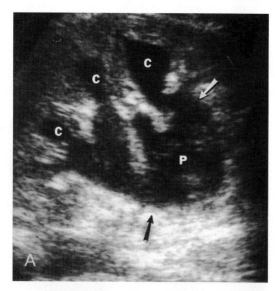
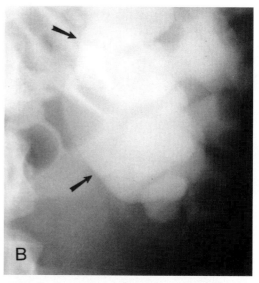

FIGURE 3.150. *Trauma to hydronephrotic kidney.* **(A)** This patient had abdominal trauma and subsequent hematuria. Abdominal ultrasound revealed a large hydronephrotic left kidney (*arrows*). Note the dilated renal pelvis (*P*) and calyces (*C*). **(B)** Subsequent intravenous pyelogram demonstrates the same findings, with a markedly hydronephrotic renal pelvis and calyces (*arrows*). The patient had a ureteropelvic-junction obstruction, which was unsuspected until the time of trauma.

these cases, one most often is dealing with an underlying ureteropelvic junction obstruction, but ureteral stenosis at a lower level also can be encountered. If such a kidney is injured, nothing more than hematuria may result, but in other instances, frank tears of the renal pelvis or calyces lead to extravasation of urine, blood, and contrast material.

Injuries to the ureter are rare, but ***bladder and urethral injury*** is rather common, especially in the presence of pelvic fractures. ***Urethral injury*** is most often seen in males, and as such usually involves the posterior urethra at its junction with the bladder neck. Tears of the nondistended bladder around the bladder neck and posterior ure-

thra lead to extravasation of urine into the extraperitoneal pelvic soft tissues. In such instances, plain films frequently demonstrate the presence of an accompanying pelvic fracture (Fig. 3.151) and obliteration of the soft tissue planes of the pelvis. Intravenous urography or retrograde cystography demonstrate extravasation of urine into the pelvic soft tissues. Ultrasonography and CT scanning, of course, also readily demonstrate these fluid collections.

In investigating a potential bladder or urethral injury, it is important to first perform a retrograde urethrogram. This yields information as to the condition of the urethra (Fig. 3.152); if the urethra and bladder neck are normal, a formal

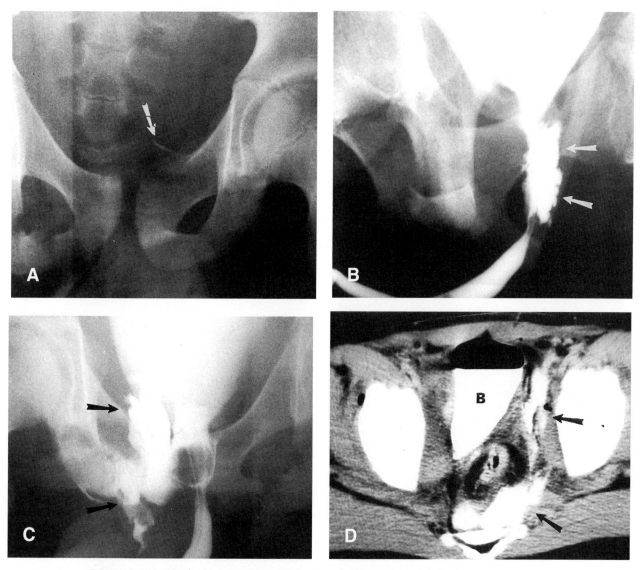

FIGURE 3.151. *Urethral injury with pelvic fracture.* **(A)** Numerous pelvic fractures are present on both sides. The most clearly visualized has occurred through the left superior pubic ramus (*arrow*). **(B)** After retrograde urethrography, extravasation of contrast material is seen from the posterior urethra (*arrows*). The Foley bulb is in the bladder. **(C)** Later, with retraction of the Foley bulb into the posterior urethra, extravasation of contrast material is seen into the adjacent soft tissues. **(D)** CT study demonstrates the displaced urinary bladder (*B*), extensive edema on the left and extravasation of contrast material into the soft tissues (*arrows*).

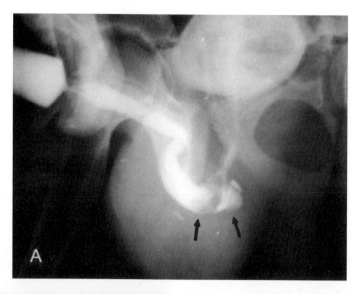

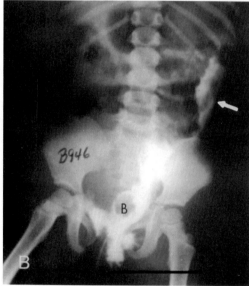

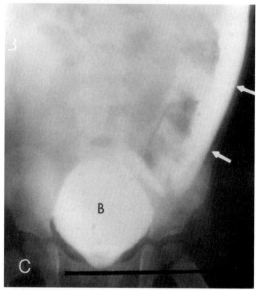

FIGURE 3.152. *Bladder and urethral trauma.* (**A**) Urethral tear resulting in extravasation of contrast material (*arrows*) on this retrograde urethrogram. (**B**) Patient with bladder trauma. Note the displaced urinary bladder (*B*). It is displaced to the left because of intrapelvic blood and urine accumulation. Below the bladder, note extravasation of contrast material into the pelvic soft tissues. Also note that there has been intraperitoneal leakage of contrast material (*arrow*). (Courtesy of Charles J. Fagan, M.D.) (**C**) Intraperitoneal rupture (*arrows*) of the bladder (*B*) in a battered child. (Courtesy of Theresa Stacy, M.D.)

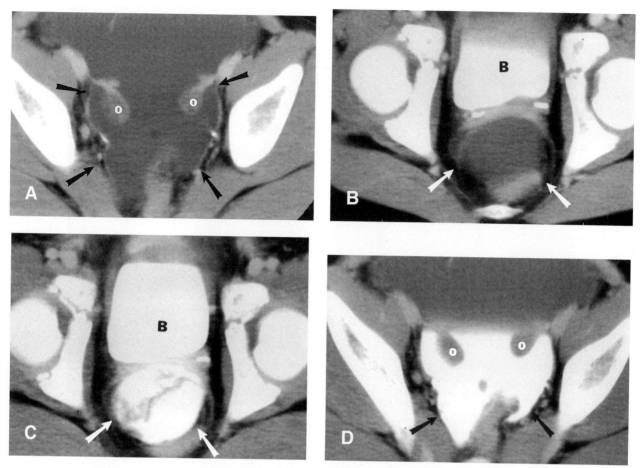

FIGURE 3.153. *Bladder perforation: delayed imaging findings.* **(A)** Note extensive pelvic fluid (*arrows*) The ovaries (*O*) are floating in the fluid. **(B)** Early-phase CT study demonstrates contrast material in the bladder (*B*) and a collection of fluid behind the bladder (*arrows*). **(C)** Later in the study, the fluid collection contains contrast material (*arrows*) indicating that a perforation has occurred. *B*, bladder. **(D)** Later study demonstrating the now opacified pelvic fluid (*arrows*). *O*, ovaries.

retrograde cystogram can be performed. If a Foley catheter is being utilized for this procedure, however, it should be placed in a position in which the inflated bulb does not occlude the bladder neck (Fig. 3.151). This is important, for if the bulb occludes the bladder neck, it also may occlude a nearby perforation. In cases in which a perforation is suspected but not demonstrated, oblique views of the bladder and bladder neck should be obtained, for these views often demonstrate smaller leaks. In addition, if CT studies are obtained, delayed images should be obtained if bladder perforation is suspected (10). Such delayed imaging can reveal a previously occult bladder perforation (Fig. 3.153).

Distended urinary bladders, if ruptured, often lead to urine extravasation into the peritoneal cavity. In such cases, plain films demonstrate the presence of abdominal fluid, and subsequent cystography demonstrates the site and extent of the leak (Fig. 3.152B and C). Ultrasonography (5) and CT scanning also can demonstrate these fluid collections around the bladder, but these studies have not replaced the cystogram (Fig. 3.154A and B). One reason is that the cystogram is performed under fluoroscopic control, and one can determine where the leak has occurred. With ultrasound, however, in some cases an actual defect in the bladder wall can be seen (13). Most often, however, this does not occur. Trauma to the bladder without perforation also can occur and is especially common with pelvic fractures. Such injury is difficult to document roentgenographically unless a pelvic hematoma surrounds the bladder. In these cases, the bladder may be minimally deformed or elevated, eccentrically deformed or elevated, or deformed in typical pear-shaped fashion (Fig. 3.154C and D).

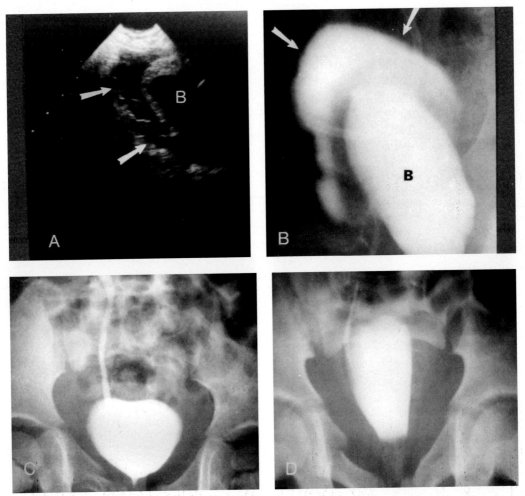

FIGURE 3.154. *Bladder trauma.* **(A)** Sagittal sonogram demonstrating the urinary bladder (*B*) and fluid with echogenic strands within it, surrounding the bladder (*arrows*). The bladder wall appears a little thickened. These findings constitute the so-called bladder within bladder sign (8). **(B)** Retrograde cystogram demonstrates the bladder (*B*) and extravasated contrast material (*arrows*). This patient had a perforation through the dome of the bladder. **(C)** Hematoma around bladder. Note the increased soft-tissue space between the contrast-filled bladder and surrounding bony pelvis. There is a fracture through the pubic bone on the right. **(D)** Typical elongated, almost pear-shaped bladder from extensive perivesical hematoma formation. Note multiple fractures of the pelvis.

REFERENCES

1. Abdalati H, Bula DI, Sivit CJ, Majd M, Rushton HG, Eichelberger MR. Blunt renal trauma in children: healing of renal injuries and recommendations for imaging follow-up. *Pediatr Radiol* 1994;24:573-576.

2. Barlow B, Gandhi R. Renal artery thrombosis following blunt trauma. *J Trauma* 1980;20:614–617.

3. Baron RL, Stark DD, McClennan BL, Shanes JG, Davis GL, Koch DD. Intrathoracic extension of retroperitoneal urine collections. *AJR* 1981;137:37–41.

4. Itoh S, Yoshioka H, Kaeriyama M, Taguchi T, Oka R, Oka T, Okamura Y. Ultrasonographic diagnosis of uriniferous perirenal pseudocyst. *Pediatr Radiol* 1982;12:156–158.

5. Kauzlaric D, Barmeir E. Sonography of traumatic rupture of the bladder: "Bladder within a bladder" appearance of extra-peritoneal extravasation. *J Ultrasound Med* 1986;5:97–98.

6. Kokihova E, Obenbergerova D, Apetaurova B. Total severance of renal pedicle caused by blunt trauma in children. *Pediatr Radiol* 1973;1:59–62.

7. Lewis DR Jr, Mirvis SE, Shanmuganathan K. Segmental renal infarction afrter blunt abdominal trauma: clinical significance and appropriate management. *Emerg Radiol* 1996;3:236-240.

8. Mayor B, Gudinchet F, Wicky S, Reinberg O, Schnyder P. Imaging evaluation of blunt renal trauma in children: diagnostic accuracy of intravenous pyelography and ultrasonography. *Pediatr Radiol* 1995;25:214-218.

9. Sandler CM, Toombs BD. Computed tomographic evaluation of blunt renal injuries. *Radiology* 1981;141:461–466.

10. Sivit CJ, Cutting JP, Eichelberger MR. CT diagnosis and localization of rupture of the bladder in children with blunt abdominal trauma significance of contrast material extravasation in the pelvis. *AJR* 1995;164:1243-1246.

11. Stalker HP, Kaufman RA, Stedje K. The significance of hematuria in children after blunt abdominal trauma. *AJR* 1990;154:569–571.

12. Surana R, Khan A, Fitzgerald RJ. Scarring following renal trauma in children. *Br J Urol* 1995;75:663-665.

13. Wan YL, Hsieh H, Lee TY, Tsai CC. Wall defect as a sign of urinary bladder rupture in sonography. *J Ultrasound Med* 1988;7:511–513.

14. Yale-Loehr AJ, Kramer SS, Quinlan DM, LaFrance ND, Mitchell SE, Gearfhart JP. CT of severe renal trauma in children: Evaluation and course of healing with conservative therapy. *AJR* 1989;152:109–113.

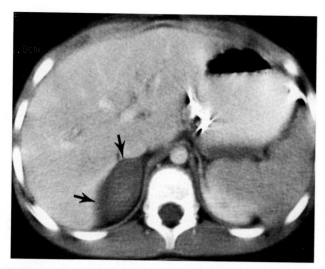

FIGURE 3.155. *Adrenal contusion–hematoma.* Note the hypodense hematoma—contusion of the right adrenal gland (*arrows*).

Adrenal Trauma

Adrenal trauma is not particularly common in childhood but can occur. In such cases the adrenal gland is seen to be enlarged no matter what the imaging study. This enlargement, however, is best demonstrated with CT scanning (Fig. 3.155).

Diaphragm

Rupture of a diaphragmatic leaflet secondary to blunt abdominal trauma is not exceptionally common in childhood, but by the same token it frequently is overlooked. Most often, such rupture occurs on the left, but because in many cases there is nothing more to see than a slightly elevated or obscured diaphragmatic leaflet, the findings are missed. Of course, if atelectasis or a pleural effusion exists on the ipsilateral side, more attention is focused on the diaphragmatic leaflet, and if loops of distended intestine or stomach are seen in the chest, the diagnosis is virtually assured (Fig. 3.156). In such cases, the findings are quite similar to those seen with delayed diaphragmatic hernia, and in either case, often a nasogastric tube can be seen to be heading into the chest rather than the abdomen (4).

On the right side, because the liver protects the right diaphragmatic leaflet, even with tears of the diaphragm one usually sees only elevation of the right diaphragmatic leaflet. Associated rib fractures can be seen on either side, and contrast studies may be necessary to determine that intestines or stomach are present in the chest. Currently, spiral CT with reconstruction is very effective at demonstrating this abnormality (2,3). Much more rarely, abdominal contents can herniate into the pericardial sac (1). Delayed herniation weeks or months after initial injury also can occur.

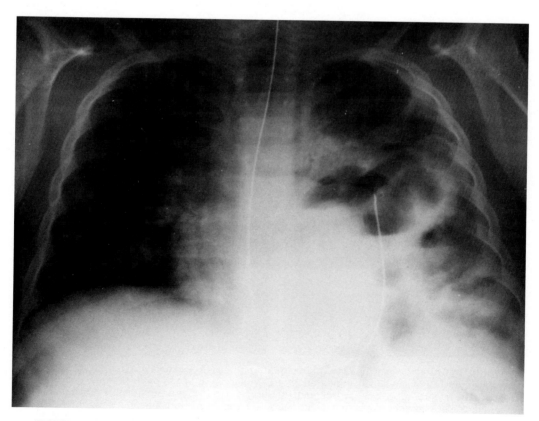

FIGURE 3.156. *Traumatic diaphragmatic hernia.* Note numerous collections of intestine in the left chest, and note the position of the nasogastric tube as it heads into the stomach, herniated into the chest.

REFERENCES

1. Gelman R, Mirvis SE, Gens D. Diaphragmatic rupture due to blunt trauma: Sensitivity of plain chest radiographs. *AJR* 1991; 156:51–57.
2. Hoy JF, Shortsleeve MJ. Diagnosis of diaphragmatic rupture utilizing spiral computed tomographic reconstruction. *Emerg Radiol* 1997;4:127–128.
3. Israel RS, Mayberry JC, Primack SL. Case report: Diaphragmatic rupture. Use of helical CT scanning with multiplanar reformations. *AJR* 1996;167:1201–1203.
4. Perlman SJ, Rogers LF, Mintzer RA, Mueller CF. Abnormal course of nasogastric tube in traumatic rupture of left hemidiaphragm. *AJR* 1984;142:85–87.

REFERENCE

1. Brown MA, Hauschildt JP, Casola G, Gosink BB, Hoyt DB. Intravascular gas as an incidental finding at US after blunt abdominal trauma. *Radiology* 1999;210:405–408.

Vascular Injury

Vascular injury often is catastrophic, and there is no time for roentgenograms to be obtained. In less severe cases in which such studies are obtained, the findings often are nonspecific and consist of nothing more than one or two loops of isolated, dilated intestine. Angiography, of course, is the procedure of choice in such cases. Intervascular air has been demonstrated with blunt abdominal trauma without vascular injury (1). In these cases it is believed that the high intraabdominal pressures frequently generated with blunt abdominal trauma lead to the phenomenon.

Battered Child Syndrome

Abdominal injury in the battered child syndrome usually is given less attention than it deserves. Very often, however, these children are dead on arrival to the emergency room and, interestingly, may show little in the way of skeletal injury (Fig. 3.157). One of the most commonly injured organs is the pancreas; acute pancreatitis and subsequent pseudocyst formation are very common in the battered child syndrome (1,6,7). Duodenal trauma, usually with duodenal hematoma formation (4,5), also is a common injury in the battered child syndrome and, interestingly, so is small intestinal trauma. In addition, colon injuries are probably more common than generally is appreciated. These can result from blunt trauma or insertion of various objects into the rectum with perforation (Fig. 3.158). Traumatic mesenteric avulsion also has been reported in a case of presumed battered child (1), and if one encounters a child with any abdominal injury that is explained inadequately, one should suspect that the child has been battered.

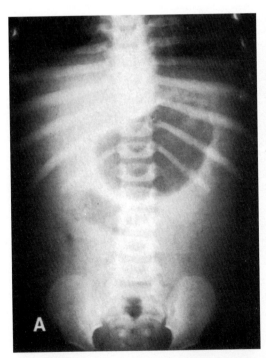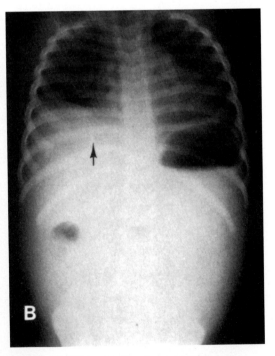

FIGURE 3.157. *Abdominal trauma: battered child syndrome.* **(A)** Supine film demonstrating generalized opacity of the abdomen and absence of visualization of the psoas shadows and liver edge. The findings suggest peritoneal fluid. **(B)** Upright view demonstrating similar findings and a slightly elevated right diaphragmatic leaflet. There was a small subpulmonic effusion on the right. Also note an almost invisible fresh rib fracture on the right (*arrow*). This was the only sign of skeletal injury in this battered child, who had peritonitis secondary to perforation of the colon.

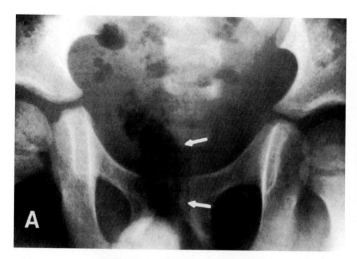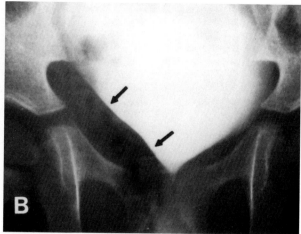

FIGURE 3.158. *Battered child syndrome: intestinal perforation.* **(A)** Note the bubbles of gas in the right groin area (*arrows*). This abscess resulted from a rectal perforation after insertion of an object into the rectum. **(B)** Cystogram demonstrates displacement of the bladder by the abscess (*arrows*).

Another interesting feature of the battered child syndrome, although it usually is not seen in the acute phase, is the post pancreatic trauma development of lytic lesions in the long bones secondary to fat necrosis. These lesions, although not particularly common, can be perplexing unless one is aware of the phenomenon (1,2–4,5,7).

REFERENCES

1. Fournemont E. Traumatic mesenteric avulsion: Case report of presumed battered child. *Ann Radiol* 1977;20:517–521.
2. Goluboff N, Cram R, Ramgotra B, Singh A, Wilkinson GW. Polyarthritis and bone lesions complicating traumatic pancreatitis in two children. *J Can Med Assoc* 1978;118:924–928.
3. Keating JP, Shackelford GD, Shackelford PG, Ternbert JL. Pancreatitis and osteolytic lesions. *J Pediatr* 1972;81:350–353.
4. Kleinman PK, Brill PW, Winchester P. Resolving duodenal–jejunal hematoma in abused children. *Radiology* 1986;160:747–750.
5. Kleinman PK, Raptopoulos VD, Brill PW. Occult nonskeletal trauma in the battered child syndrome. *Radiology* 1981;141:393–396.
6. Pena SDJ, Medovy H. Child abuse and traumatic pseudocyst of the pancreas. *J Pediatr* 1973;83:1026–1028.
7. Slovis TL, Berdon WE, Haller JO, Baker DH, Rosen L. Pancreatitis and the battered child syndrome: Report of 2 cases with skeletal involvement. *AJR* 1975;125:456–461.

INGESTED AND INSERTED FOREIGN BODIES AND MATERIALS

Corrosive Substance Ingestion

The most frequently ingested corrosive substance is lye (sodium hydroxide). Lye results in deep, full-thickness thermal burns, causing coagulation necrosis of the entire wall of the hypopharynx and/or esophagus (1). With such extensive tissue necrosis, perforation is not uncommon, and, in this regard, the most devastating corrosives are the highly concentrated liquid corrosives, some of which also contain potassium hydroxide. These substances produce the severest of burns (2,9,12), and because of their high specific gravity and slickness, can pass to the stomach with great rapidity. This being the case, it is not uncommon to have the entire esophagus involved and, in addition, to have associated gastric burns. In those cases where granular or pellet corrosives are ingested, focal, upper third, esophageal burns are more common.

Hypopharyngeal burns usually are detected clinically. In some cases, lye may spill over onto the vocal cords and produce edema of these structures. In some cases, on chest films, one may note a distended (paralyzed) air-filled esophagus or, if acute esophageal perforation occurs, mediastinal widening, with or without associated pneumomediastinum, pneumopericardium, or pneumatosis of the esophagus (Fig. 3.159). In other cases, tracheoesophageal fistulas (1) or communications to the pericardial sac can be seen (Fig. 3.159B).

Other corrosive fluids ingested include ammonium hydroxide and a variety of acids. These substances, however, unlike sodium and potassium hydroxide, usually do not produce a deep thermal burn to the esophagus; their damage is more superficial. In addition, because acids induce less esophageal and hypopharyngeal muscle spasm than does lye, the child is able to drink more, and because of this, gastric rather than esophageal burns are more common (4,7). This is especially true of substances such as sulfuric acid which possess a greater degree of slickness and a higher specific gravity. Often the end result is pyloric scarring and stenosis. Occasionally, with larger volumes of concentrated acids such

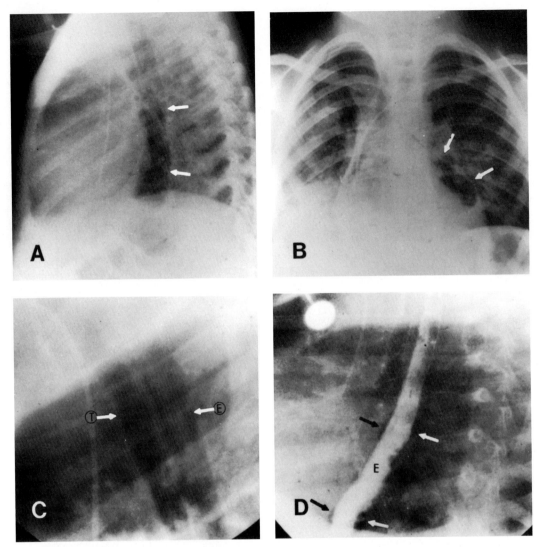

FIGURE 3.159. *Corrosive esophagitis.* **(A)** Note the paralyzed, distended, air-filled esophagus (*arrows*). **(B)** Same patient later with development of pneumopericardium (*arrows*). Also note that the mediastinum is widened, and that numerous infiltrates are present secondary to aspiration. **(C)** Preliminary barium-swallow film demonstrates the trachea (*T*) and dilated, air-filled esophagus (*E; arrows*). The central longitudinal density in the esophagus actually is the esophageal mucosa, and the air around results from pneumatosis of the esophagus. **(D)** Subsequent barium swallow demonstrates the esophageal lumen (*E*) and the presence of pneumatosis of the esophagus (*arrows*). Some contrast material is in the trachea secondary to aspiration.

as sulphuric acid, gastric wall damage can be more severe and the entire process can involve adjacent organs (3).

Other less common caustic agent burns to the esophagus are those sustained from the ingestion of Clinitest tablets (2) and, more recently, alkaline disk batteries (5,6). The latter, when impacted for prolonged periods of time, can lead to mucosal ulceration from sheer mechanical erosion, but it also has been determined that in some of these cases hydroxides within the battery are readily liberated into the esophagus and cause focal caustic burns. Interestingly enough, if these batteries pass into the stomach and distal gastrointestinal tract, little, if any, problem arises (6). How-

ever, with lodgement in the esophagus, acquired tracheoesophageal fistula can result (8,9).

The performance of a contrast study of the esophagus is of debatable value in the acute phase of a corrosive fluid ingestion problem. However, if perforation is suspected, a water-soluble contrast agent can be utilized to demonstrate the site of the leak. If no perforation is present, the contrast study of the esophagus shows little more than intense spasm and, in the more severe cases, evidence of mucosal ulceration. After a week or 10 days, a barium swallow can identify potential sites of stricture, for these sites will appear narrow, stiff, and aperistaltic.

REFERENCES

1. Amoury RA, Hrabovsky EE, Leonidas JC, Holder TM. Tracheoesophageal fistula after lye ingestion. *J Pediatr Surg* 1975;10: 273–276.

2. Burrington JD. Clinitest burns of the esophagus. *Ann Thorac Surg* 1975;20:400–404.

3. Canty TG Sr. Extensive multi-organ necrosis secondary to sulfuric acid ingestion. *J Pediatr Surg* 1988;23:848–849.

4. Gillis DA, Higgins G, Kennedy R. Gastric damage from ingested acid in children. *J Pediatr Surg* 1985;20:494–496.

5. Litovitz T, Schmitz BF. Ingestion of cylindrical and button batteries. *Pediatrics* 1992;89:747–757.

6. Maves MD, Lloyd TV, Carithers JS. Radiographic identification of ingested disc batteries. *Pediatr Radiol* 1986;16:154–156.

7. Muhletaler CA, Gerlock AJ Jr, deSoto L, Halter SA. Acid corrosive esophagitis: Radiographic findings. *AJR* 1980;134:1137–1140.

8. Pinna CD. Pyloric stenosis from acid burn in a six-year-old girl. *Riv Chir Pediatr* 1967;9:384–395.

9. Sigalet D, Lees G. Tracheoesophageal injury secondary to disc battery ingestion. *J Pediatr Surg* 1988;23:996–998.

10. Vaishnav A, Spitz L. Alkaline battery-induced tracheoesophageal fistula. *Br J Surg* 1989;76:1045.

Ingested Foreign Bodies

Hypopharyngeal foreign bodies have been discussed in Chapter 2, and the discussion of ingested foreign bodies in this section is confined to esophageal, gastric, and intestinal foreign bodies. If such a foreign body is radiolucent, it will not be detected roentgenographically unless secondary signs of inflammation or perforation are present. In this regard, this has become a problem with aluminum pop-top tabs from soft drink cans (3,8,12). However, it also is a problem with aluminum coins (10) and a wide variety of plastic objects (Fig. 3.160). Opaque foreign bodies, on the other hand, are readily detected roentgenographically (Fig. 3.161), and because of this a roentgenographic survey of the neck, chest, and abdomen is in order, indeed, mandatory (11). This is especially true of infants and young children, for unlike older children, they cannot tell the physician exactly where they think the foreign body has lodged.

Most round or oval foreign bodies pass down the esophagus into the stomach and through the intestine to cause little if any problem (7). On the other hand, larger or sharp foreign bodies and those of irregular shape may well become impacted somewhere along the course of the gastrointestinal tract. In the esophagus, foreign bodies commonly lodge at the level of the: (a) cricopharyngeal muscle, (b) aortic knob, or (c) gastroesophageal junction (Fig. 3.162). The least common site is at the gastroesophageal junction. If these foreign bodies are radiopaque they are not difficult to detect, but if they are radiolucent they will go undetected until a barium swallow is obtained. In this regard, some of these children have underlying esophageal strictures secondary to old tracheoesophageal fistula repairs, hiatus hernia problems, or lye burns (Fig. 3.163).

Animal bones impacted in the hypopharynx or esophagus are not as common in children as in adults. However, they still are encountered, and, in this regard, it should be noted that fishbones, although potentially visible (Table

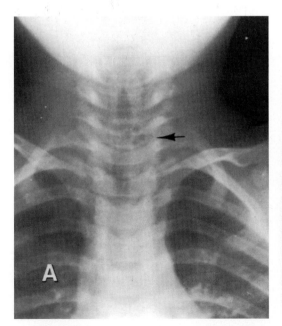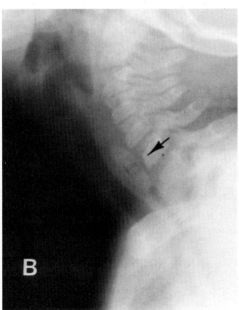

FIGURE 3.160. *Semiopaque button in upper esophagus.* **(A)** Note the four radiolucent holes in the button (*arrow*), lodged in the upper esophagus. **(B)** Lateral view demonstrates the button (*arrow*) and a mild degree of anterior displacement and compression of the trachea.

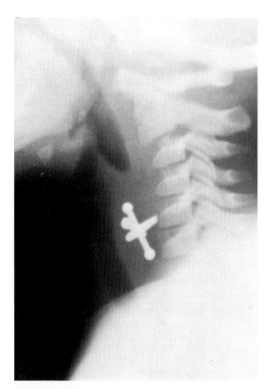

FIGURE 3.161. *Opaque foreign body (jack) in the upper esophagus.* Note the readily visible opaque jack in the upper esophagus of this infant.

3.1), usually are difficult to visualize with certainty (5). Chicken and turkey bones, on the other hand, often contain enough calcium to allow them to be visible roentgenographically (Fig. 3.164). In those cases where a foreign body such as a fishbone is suspected but not visible, one may administer a cotton ball pledget soaked with barium to the patient. In some of these cases, the pledget becomes impaled on the bone, and thus aids in its localization. However, this maneuver does not work nearly as often as one would first believe.

The misinterpretation of normally calcified laryngeal cartilages as a foreign body such as a chicken or fishbone is not a great problem in childhood. Apart from the hyoid bone, which ossifies early, about the only calcified cartilage presenting such a problem is the calcified cartilage triticei (Fig. 3.165). In teenagers and adults, of course, laryngeal calcifications are much more common and the problem of differentiating them from an opaque foreign body is much greater.

In the past, removal of coins and other foreign bodies from the esophagus generally had been accomplished endoscopically. More recently, however, Foley catheter removal has become popular (4,5,9,14,16,19). When the Foley catheter is utilized, the deflated bulb of the catheter is inflated under fluoroscopic control, and opaque aqueous contrast material is utilized to distend the bulb so that it is visible roentgenographically. After inflation of the bulb, the catheter is withdrawn and the foreign body is retrieved. One must be careful that the patient does not reswallow or inhale the foreign body, and, of course, this procedure should be restricted to foreign bodies of recent impaction and to those that are not pointed or impaled in the esophageal wall. In addition, periesophageal edema (see Fig. 3.170) is a contraindication to catheter removal (23), and of course the entire procedure is not without hazard (23). Esophageal perforation always is a potential problem. In this regard, an alternate approach has been suggested (1), consisting of pushing the foreign body down into the

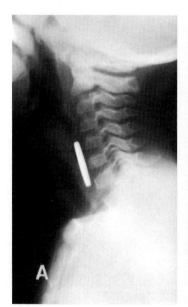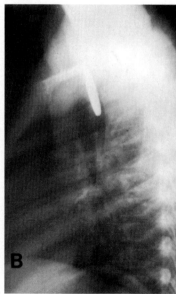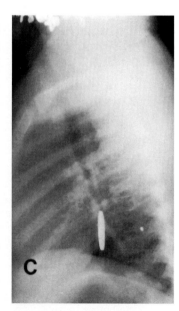

FIGURE 3.162. *Typical sites of foreign-body lodgement in the esophagus.* Foreign bodies in the esophagus usually lodge at one of the following sites: **(A)** just above the level of the cricopharyngeal muscle; **(B)** just above the level of the aortic knob; **(C)** just above the gastroesophageal junction.

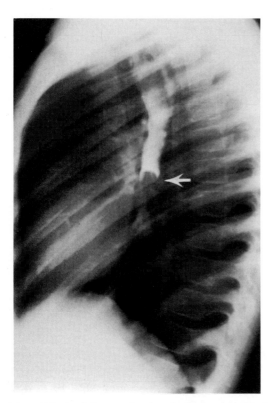

FIGURE 3.163. *Radiolucent foreign body in the esophagus.* Note the typical curvilinear filling defect (*arrow*) produced by a nonopaque foreign body in this barium-filled esophagus. This patient had underlying esophageal stenosis secondary to an old tracheoesophageal fistula repair. The obstructing foreign body was a kernel of corn.

TABLE 3.1. RADIOPACITY OF BONES OF VARIOUS FISH SPECIES[a]

Fish	No. Bones X-rayed	Definitely Diagnostic	Visible but Poorly Defined	Invisible
Bass	2	2		
Bluefish	4	3		1
Butterfish	3		3	
Codfish	5	5		
Flounder	3	3		
Fluke	2	2		
Fresh Salmon	4	4		
Gray sole	2	2		
Haddock	2	2		
Halibut	4	4		
Mackerel	4	1		3
Pompano	5		2	3
Porgie	3	3		
Red snapper	2	2		
Sea bass	2	2		
Smelt	1	1		
Smoked salmon	2	2		
Striped bass	2	2		
Trout	3		2	1
White Perch	2	2		
Yellow pike	3	3		

[a]Reproduced from Bachman, AL: Radiology of fish foreign bodies in the hypopharynx and cervical esophagus. *Mt Sinai J Med* 1981;48: 212–220.

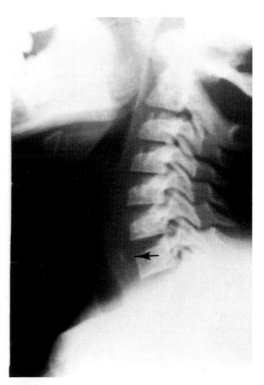

FIGURE 3.164. *Chicken bone in upper esophagus.* Note faint calcification in a chicken bone (*arrow*) lodged in the upper esophagus of this patient.

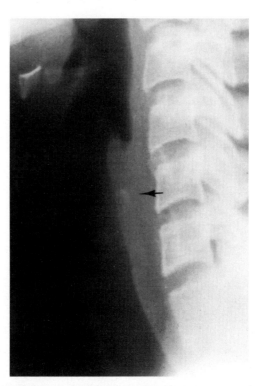

FIGURE 3.165. *Calcification in the cartilage triticei* (*arrow*) often is mistaken for an opaque foreign body.

esophagus rather than pulling it back (Fig. 3.166). Finally, it should be noted that metallic foreign bodies also can be retrieved with a magnet (24).

Those foreign bodies that pass into the stomach can pose a problem in terms of follow-up roentgenograms. However, if the foreign body is small or of such a shape that almost surely it should pass uneventfully, follow-up roentgenograms are not required. On the other hand, should such a foreign body not pass with normal stooling, one might obtain a follow-up roentgenogram on the slight possibility that one might be dealing with an underlying, previously unsuspected, obstructing lesion such as gastric or duodenal web or diverticulum (2,13,21) (Fig. 3.167). Obviously, this is a more remote consideration, but still one to be considered under the proper circumstances.

The problem is quite different with the pointed, jagged, or long foreign body, for impaction of this type of foreign body is more common. Follow-up roentgenograms are most important in these cases, and if the foreign body fails to make progress or, even more significantly, if it does not change its position at all, one should suspect impaction and consider surgical intervention (Fig. 3.168). Another time when a foreign body may cease to make progress is when it lodges in the appendix. In some of these cases, no symp-

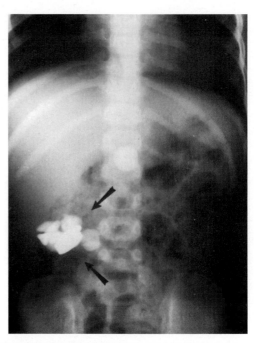

FIGURE 3.167. *Foreign bodies trapped in duodenal web.* Note numerous opaque foreign bodies on the right (*arrows*). These changed little in position from view to view and ultimately were demonstrated to be trapped behind a duodenal web. There also is a foreign body in the gastric antrum.

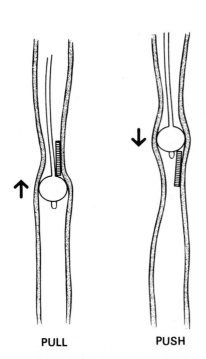

PULL   **PUSH**

FIGURE 3.166. *Foley-catheter foreign-body removal.* Two methods are available. Pulling the foreign body is more popular, but we have found that pushing the foreign body can be quite productive. (From Alexander AA, Hayden CE, Swischuk LE. Catheter removal of esophageal foreign bodies: Push or pull? *AJR* 1988;151:835, with permission.)

toms arise, but in others acute appendicitis eventually may develop.

Additionally, it should be noted that upper esophageal foreign bodies can present with stridor or pneumonia and little in the way of dysphagia (12,17,18,20,22). Many of these patients are young infants, and they seem to adapt to the esophageal obstruction with deceptive ease. They do this primarily by changing their diet to a more acceptable liquid one. Such a change often is so subtle that it eludes the parent and physician, and overall the presenting symptoms will cause one to focus on the respiratory tract (i.e., stridor, wheezing, cough, etc.). It is only with the knowledge that this can occur, and adequate examination of the lateral neck, chest, and esophagus that many of these foreign bodies are finally discovered (Fig. 3.169). In some cases ulceration or actual perforation of the esophagus eventually results (20). However, initially only periesophageal edema occurs, and it is interesting to see how quickly such edema can develop. It is this edema that produces compression of the adjacent trachea and often is still present after the foreign body has been removed (Fig. 3.170). Such edema, when present, constitutes a contraindication to removal of the foreign body with a Foley catheter (22).

Some foreign bodies may lead to mucosal ulceration (2) and in other instances lead intoxication from ingested lead-containing foreign bodies can occur (15,21,25).

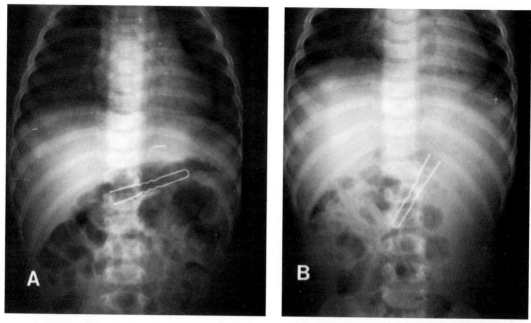

FIGURE 3.168. *Problematic foreign body.* **(A)** Early film showing hairpin in the stomach. **(B)** Later film showing complete change in position of the pin, which thereafter remained lodged at this site. At laparotomy, this turned out to be at the duodenal–jejunal junction.

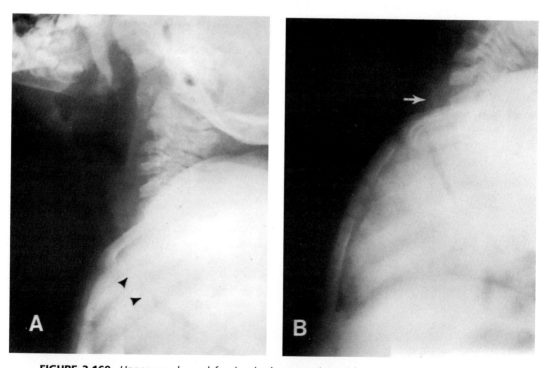

FIGURE 3.169. *Upper esophageal foreign body presenting with stridor.* **(A)** Note the overdistended hypopharynx and upper trachea in this young infant presenting with stridor. Also note that the trachea below the level of the clavicles is narrowed (*arrows*). **(B)** With the neck fully extended, a semiopaque foreign body is demonstrated in the upper esophagus (*arrow*). The site of this foreign body corresponds to the site of tracheal narrowing noted in **(A)**.

(continued on next page)

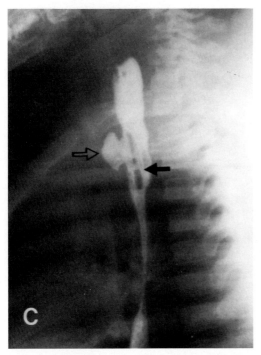

FIGURE 3.169. *(continued)* **(C)** Barium swallow demonstrates the foreign body (*solid arrow*) in the esophagus, and the deep anterior ulcer that it produced (*open arrow*). It is easy to see why this portion of the trachea appeared narrowed on the other studies. (From Smith PC, Swischuk LE, Fagan CJ. An elusive and often unsuspected cause of stridor or pneumonia [the esophageal foreign body]. *AJR* 1974;122:80–89, with permission.)

REFERENCES

1. Alexander AA, Hayden CK, Swischuk LE. Catheter removal of esophageal foreign bodies: Push or pull? *AJR* 1988;151:835.
2. Bonadio WA, Emslander H, Milner D, Johnson L. Esophageal mucosal changes in children with an acutely ingested coin lodged in the esophagus. *Pediatr Emerg Care* 1995;10:333-334.
3. Burrington JD. Aluminum pop-tops: A hazard to child health. *JAMA* 1976;235:2614–2617.
4. Calkins CM, Christians KK, Sell LL. Cost analysis in the management of esophageal coins: Endoscopy versus Bougienage. *J Pediatr Surg* 1999;34:412-414.
5. Campbell DR, Brown SJ, Manchester JA. An evaluation of the radio-opacity of various ingested foreign bodies in the pharynx and esophagus. *Can J Assoc Radiol* 1968;19:183–186.
6. Campbell JB, Quattromani FL, Foley LC. Foley catheter removal of blunt esophageal foreign bodies. Experience with 100 consecutive children. *Pediatr Radiol* 1983;13:116–119.
7. Conners GP, Chamberlain JM, Ochsenschlager DW. Symptoms and spontaneous passage of esophageal coins. *Arch Pediatr Adoles Med* 1995;149:36-39.
8. Eggbli KD, Potter BM, Garcia V, Altman RP, Breckbill DL. Delayed diagnosis of esophageal perforation by aluminum foreign bodies. *Pediatr Radiol* 1986;16:511–513.
9. Harned RK II, Strain JD, Hay TC, Douglas MR. Esophageal foreign bodies: safety and efficacy of Foley catheter extraction of coins. *AJR* 1997;168:443-446.
10. Heller RM, Reichelderfer TE, Dorst JP, Oh KS. The problem with replacement of copper pennies by aluminum pennies. *Pediatrics* 1974;54:684–688.
11. Hodge D III, Techlenburg F, Fleisher G. Coin ingestion: Does every child need a radiograph? *Ann Emerg Med* 1985;14:443–446.

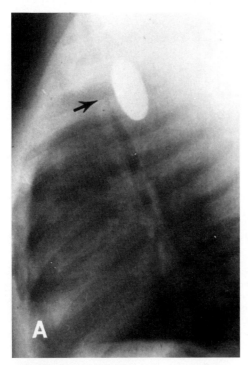
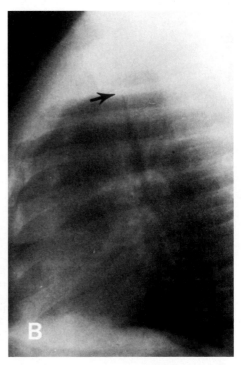

FIGURE 3.170. *Esophageal foreign body with tracheal compression.* **(A)** Note the coin in the esophagus (*arrow*). Also note that the trachea just adjacent to it is narrowed. This is caused by periesophageal edema. **(B)** After removal of the coin, the trachea still is narrowed (*arrow*).

12. Jeffers RG, Weir MR, Wehunt WD, Carter SC. Pull-tab; the foreign body sleeper. *J Pediatr* 1978;92:1023–1024.

13. Kassner EG, Rose JS, Kottmeier PK, Schneider M, Gallow GM. Retention of a small foreign object in the stomach and duodenum: A sign of partial obstruction caused by duodenal anomalies. *Radiology* 1975;114:683–686.

14. Kelley JE, Leech MH, Carr MG. A safe and cost-effective protocol for the management of esophageal coins in children. *J Pediatr Surg* 1993;28:898-900.

15. Lyons JD, Filston HC. Lead intoxication from a pellet entrapped in the appendix of a chld: Treatment considerations. *J Pediatr Surg* 1994;29:1618–1620.

16. Morrow SE, Bickler SW, Kennedy AP, Snyder CL, Sharp RJ, Ashcraft KW. Balloon extraction of esophageal foreign bodies in children. *J Pediatr Surg* 1998;33:266-270.

17. Newman DE. The radiolucent esophageal foreign body: An often forgotten cause of respiratory symptoms. *J Pediatr* 1978;92:60–63.

18. Schidlow DV, Palmer J, Balsara RK, Trutz MG, Williams JL. Chronic stridor and anterior cervical "mass" secondary to an esophageal foreign body. *Am J Dis Child* 1981;135:869–870.

19. Schunk JE, Harrison AM, Corneli HM, Nixon GW. Fluoroscopic Foley catheter removal of esophageal foreign bodies in children: Experience with 415 episodes. *Pediatrics* 1994;94:709-714.

20. Smith PC, Swischuk LE, Fagan CJ. An elusive and often unsuspected cause of stridor or pneumonia (the esophageal foreign body). *AJR* 1974;122:80–89.

21. Sprinkle JD Jr, Hingsbergen EA. Retained foreign body: associations with elevated lead levels, pica, and duodenal anomaly. *Pediatr Radiol* 1995;25:528-529.

22. Tauscher JW. Esophageal foreign body: An uncommon cause of stridor. *Pediatrics* 1978;61:657–658.

23. Towbin R, Lederman HM, Dunbar JS, Ball WS, Strife JL. Esophageal edema as a predictor of unsuccessful balloon extraction of esophageal foreign body. *Pediatr Radiol* 1989;19:359–360.

24. Volle E, Beyer P, Kauffmann HJ. Therapeutic approach to ingested button-type batteries: Magnetic removal of ingested button-type batteries. *Pediatr Radiol* 1989;19:114–118.

25. Wiley JR II, Hearetig FM, Selbst SM. Blood lead levels in children with foreign bodies. *Pediatrics* 1992;89:593-596.

Miscellaneous Ingested Foreign Bodies and Substances

Pills or capsules are usually not identified unless they contain substances such as iron or calcium (3), and in such cases they may be seen, but not always clearly, on abdominal films (Fig. 3.171). This is important, for iron intoxication is not uncommon in children (1) and can result in extensive gastrointestinal damage with bleeding, necrosis, and perforation (2,3). Pica in childhood most often is accounted for by the eating of dirt or clay. In these children, flecks of opaque material can be seen scattered throughout the gastrointestinal tract; in some cases actual pebbles may be noted (Fig. 3.172). Of course, fragments of lead paint also can be seen on roentgenograms, and occasionally such infants present in the emergency room with acute lead intoxication.

Another opaque substance sometimes encountered in the emergency room setting is a bismuth-containing

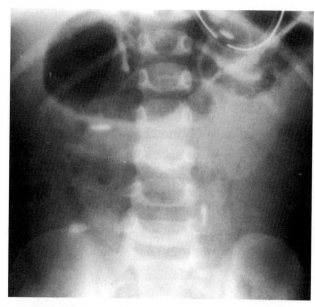

FIGURE 3.171. *Iron-tablet ingestion.* Note numerous, opaque tablets scattered in the abdomen of this toxic infant who has ingested iron tablets.

antacid. Such medications frequently are administered for gastroenteritis and commonly show up as irregular opacities in the intestines of these children (Fig. 3.173). Other foreign materials include dental fillings, teeth, mercury, plaster, erasers, modeling clay, and bubble gum (2).

Finally, an interesting recent study has shown that a significant number of patients who ingest foreign bodies have

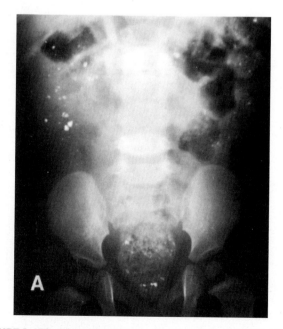

FIGURE 3.172. *Dirt and pebbles in the gastrointestinal tract.* **(A)** Note scattered opacities throughout the tract in this patient. A good many of them are mixed with fecal material in the colon. Similar findings can be seen with lead poisoning, but most often the findings represent dirt eating. *(continued on next page)*

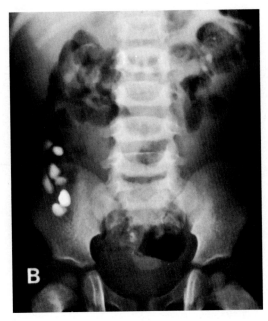

FIGURE 3.172. *(continued)* **(B)** Note pebbles in the cecum of this patient.

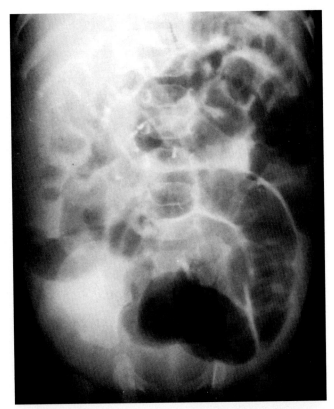

FIGURE 3.173. *Opacities in the gastrointestinal tract in a patient with gastroenteritis.* Note numerous opacities in the distended intestines of this infant with gastroenteritis. Such opacities are common in these patients and represent bismuth in certain antacid preparations.

increased lead levels in the blood (4). This emphasizes the concept that some infants and children simply are chronic ingestors of foreign materials, and that among these materials may be lead.

REFERENCES

1. Everson GW, Oudjhane J, Young LW, Krenzelok EP. Effectiveness of abdominal radiographs in visualizing chewable iron supplements following overdose. *Am J Emerg Med* 1989;7: 459–463.
2. Geller E, Smergel EM. Bubble gum simulating abdominal calcifications. *Pediatr Radiol* 1992;22:298–299.
3. Knott LH, Miller RC. Acute iron intoxication with intestinal infarction. *J Pediatr Surg* 1978;13:720–721.
4. Staple TW, McAlister WH. Roentgenographic visualization of iron preparation in the gastrointestinal tract. *Radiology* 83: 1051.

Genitourinary Foreign Bodies

Genitourinary foreign bodies (1,2) inserted by the patient are more common than generally is appreciated. In girls, these foreign bodies often are inserted into the vagina, and occasionally they are demonstrable on plain films (Fig. 3.174). Urinary bladder foreign bodies also can be encountered in girls, but in boys one more often encounters such foreign bodies in the urethra (Fig. 3.162C). Patients with these foreign bodies can present with hematuria or urinary tract infection.

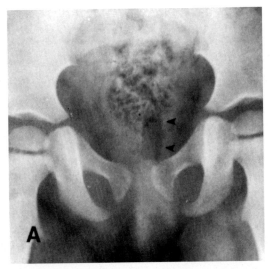

FIGURE 3.174. *Genitourinary foreign bodies.* **(A)** Note the radiolucent (plastic pen cap) foreign body (*arrows*) in the vagina of this girl. *(continued on page 273)*.

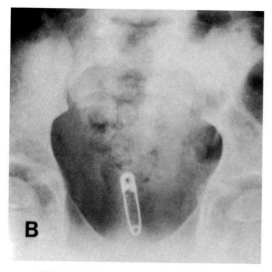
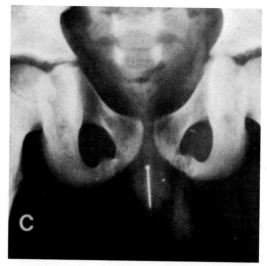

FIGURE 3.174. *(continued)* **(B)** Closed safety pin in the bladder of another girl. **(C)** Straight pin in the urethra of a young boy.

REFERENCES

1. Paradise JE, Willis ED. Probability of vaginal foreign body in girls with genital complaints. *Am J Dis Child* 1985;139:472–478.
2. Swischuk LE. Acute, non-traumatic, genitourinary pediatric problems. *Radiol Clin North Am* 1978;16:147–157.

MISCELLANEOUS ABDOMINAL PROBLEMS

Bezoars

Bezoars most frequently occur in the stomach (1,2,4,5,9) but also may be seen in the small bowel. Most likely, these latter instances represent cases in which portions of the gastric bezoar break off and pass into the small intestine. Once a bezoar enters the small bowel, obstruction with or without intussusception (3,8) may occur (Fig. 3.175).

The most common bezoar in older childhood is a trichobezoar resulting from ingestion of hair, usually from the patient's own head. Although usually considered to be the result of psychiatric difficulties, iron deficiency, much as with clay eating, also has been shown to be a potential contributing factor (7). Next most common is a phytobezoar, (4) but currently in very young infants lactobezoars are more common (1,2,5,6,10). In these instances, a dense milk coagulation results if powdered milk is mixed with inadequate amounts of water. It is especially likely to occur in premature infants. Bezoars secondary to persimmon-seed ingestion are not as common in childhood as in adulthood. In this type of bezoar, the protein material of the persimmon, after being acted upon by gastric acid, is converted to a shellaclike substance.

Plain film findings of a gastric bezoar consist of amorphous, granular, or at times whirlpool-like configurations of solid and gaseous material in the stomach (Fig. 3.175A). In other instances, the bezoar is so compact that a layer of air is seen to surround it (Fig. 3.175B). Barium studies confirm

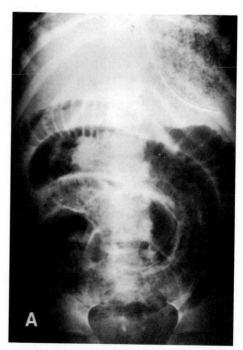

FIGURE 3.175. *Bezoars.* **(A)** Note the granular appearance of a bezoar in the stomach (left upper quadrant). Also note the presence of a classic small-bowel obstruction and numerous granular, linear, and curvilinear densities within the small bowel. This patient had a large bezoar, part of which had become detached, producing a small-bowel obstruction. *(continued on next page)*

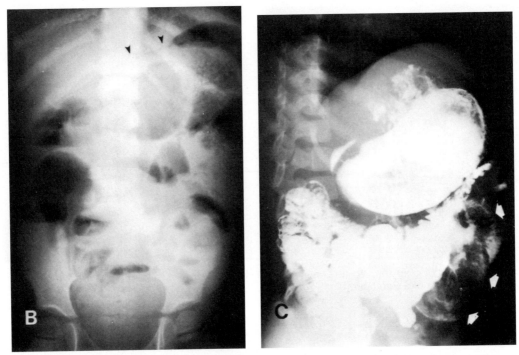

FIGURE 3.175. *(continued)* **(B)** Another bezoar somewhat less well defined. Note, however, the thin rim of air trapped between it and the gastric wall *(arrows)*. **(C)** Subsequent gastrointestinal series demonstrates the large bezoar in the stomach, but in addition, note that a portion of it has become detached and is present in the distal small bowel *(arrows)*. It was causing a moderate degree of obstruction.

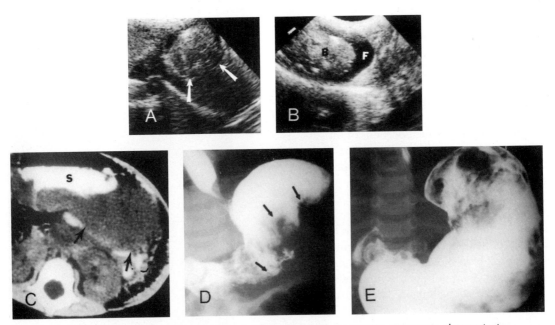

FIGURE 3.176. *Bezoar: ultrasound and CT findings.* **(A)** Transverse sonogram demonstrates echogenic material in the stomach *(arrows)*. **(B)** With a little fluid *(F)* added to the stomach, the echogenic bezoar *(B)* is clearly visualized. **(C)** In this patient, an abdominal mass *(arrows)* displacing the stomach *(S)* was believed to be present. **(D)** Subsequent gastrointestinal series demonstrates large, nodular filling defects in the stomach *(arrows)*. **(E)** With the patient now in prone position, barium coats the entire large nodular bezoar.

the presence of a bezoar and the presence of a gastric ulcer if such a complication is present. On plain films, bezoars must be differentiated from food in the stomach.

On ultrasound, the echogenic arc of air between the bezoar and gastric wall is characteristic (6,9). In addition, an actual mass can be seen if fluid is administered to these patients (Fig. 3.176). CT scanning also can demonstrate these masses very vividly (9) (Fig. 3.176).

REFERENCES

1. Bakken DA, Abramo TJ. Gastric lactobezoar: A rare cause of gastric outlet obstruction.
2. Grosfeld JL, Schreiner RL, Franken EA, Lemons JA, Ballantine TVN, Weber TR, Gresham EL. The changing pattern of gastrointestinal bezoars in infants and children. *Surgery* 1980;88: 425–432.
3. Dalshaug GB, Wainer S, Hollaar GL. The Rapunzel syndrome (Trichobezoar) causing atypical intussusception in a child: A case report. *J Pediatr Surg* 34:479–480.
4. Eshel G, Broide E, Azizi E. Phytobezoar following raisin ingestion in children. *Pediatr Emerg Care* 1988;4:192–193.
5. Majd M, LoPresti JM. Lactobezoar. *AJR* 1972;116:575–576.
6. McCracken S, Jongeward R, Silver TM, Jafri ZH. Gastric trichobezoar: Sonographic findings. *Radiology* 1986;161:123–124.
7. McGehee FT Jr, Buchanan GR. Trichophagia and trichobezoar: Etiologic role of iron deficiency. *J Pediatr* 1980;97: 946–948.
8. Mehta MH, Patel RV. Intussusception and perforations caused by multiple trichobezoars. *J Pediatr Surg* 1992;27:1234–1235.
9. Newman B, Girdany BR. Gastric trichobezoars: Sonographic and computed tomographic appearance. *Pediatr Radiol* 1990;20: 526–527.
10. Singer JI. Lactobezoar causing an abdominal triad of colicky pain, emesis and mass. *Pediatr Emerg Care* 1988;4:194–196.

Abdominal Ascariasis

Ascariasis may be encountered as an incidental finding, but in other cases intestinal obstruction or even intestinal perforation can occur (4,6,7). In addition, during the early phase of the infection, larvae can pass through the lymphatic system or portal system to the right side of the heart and be filtered out in the lungs, causing nonspecific infiltrates. Respiratory distress may be the presenting symptom in these patients.

On abdominal roentgenograms an adult worm of an *Ascaris worm* can be seen as a linear or circular filling defect in a loop of dilated bowel, but more commonly infestation is massive and a whirlpool, bezoarlike mass of linear, opaque, and radiolucent shadows is seen (Fig. 3.177). If

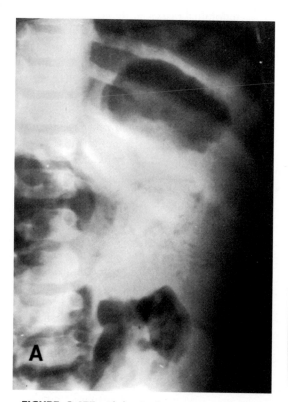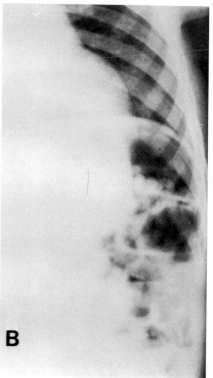

FIGURE 3.177. *Abdominal ascariasis.* **(A)** Note the whirlpool-like effect of worms in the intestines on the left side of the abdomen. **(B)** Another patient demonstrating worms visualized in air-filled loops of intestine.

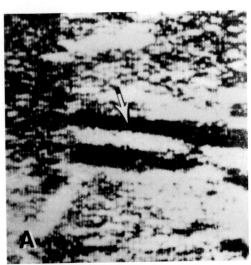 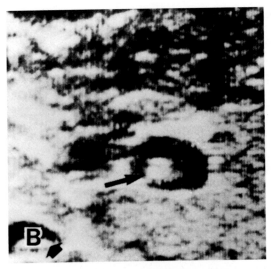

FIGURE 3.178. *Biliary ascaris: ultrasonographic findings.* **(A)** Longitudinal section demonstrating a dilated common bile duct with a worm in the center (*arrow*). **(B)** Cross-sectional view demonstrating the bull's eye sign with the echogenic worms in the center (*arrows*) of the dilated bile duct. (From Cerri GG, Leite GJ, Simoes JB, DaRocha DJC, Albuquerque FP, Machado MCC, Magalhaes A. Ultrasonographic evaluation of ascaris in the biliary tract. *Radiology* 1983;146:753–754, with permission.)

barium is administered, the worms ingest the barium and can be identified by the linear collections of barium in their gastrointestinal tracts. Infection with an ascaris of the biliary system and pancreatic ducts also can occur but is relatively rare. The findings in these cases are readily demonstrable with ultrasound (1–3,5). The worm in the dilated bile ducts is echogenic and produces a bull's-eye configuration (Fig. 3.178).

REFERENCES

1. Cerri GG, Leite GJ, Simoes JB, DaRocha DJC, Albuquerque FP, Machado MCC, Magalhaes A. Ultrasonographic evaluation of ascaris in the biliary tract. *Radiology* 1983;146:753–754.
2. Cremin BJ. Ultrasonographic diagnosis of biliary ascariasis: "A bull's eye in the triple O." *Br J Radiol* 1982;55:683–684.
3. Hoffmann H, Kawooya M, Esterre P, Ravaoalimalala VE, Roth J, Thomas AK, Roux J, Seitz HM, Doehring E. In vivo and in vitro studies on the sonographical detection of Ascaris lumbricoides. *Pediatr Radiol* 1997;27:226–229.
4. Mohta A, Bugga D, Malhotra CJ, et al. Intestinal obstruction due to roundworms. *Pediatr Surg Int* 1993;8:226–228.
5. Price J, Leung JWC. Ultrasound diagnosis of Ascaris lumbricoides in the pancreatic duct: The "four-lines" sign. *Br J Radiol* 1988;61:411–413.
6. Rode H, Cullis S, Millar A. Abdominal complications of Ascaris lumbricoides in children. *Pediatr Surg Int* 1990;5:397–401.
7. Surendran N, Paulose MO. Intestinal complications of round worms in children. *J Pediatr Surg* 1988;23:931–935.

Abdominal Masses, Tumors, and Pseudotumors

Abdominal masses in the emergency room setting are not a particularly common problem. Occasionally, however, with hemorrhage into a tumor, trauma to a hydronephrotic kidney, or so forth, acute abdominal pain may be the presenting problem, and in such cases ultrasonography is the most rewarding screening procedure. Although certain information can be obtained from plain films, ultrasonography usually provides ready information regarding whether the lesion is solid or cystic and its precise location (Fig. 3.179). CT scanning also can be utilized, but ultrasound usually is the first imaging modality employed. If cysts are present, either infected or noninfected, acute rupture of these cysts (e.g., mesenteric cysts, urachal cysts) can lead to acute abdominal problems (1,2).

In the emergency patient, one of the most commonly encountered problems is that of a normal structure presenting as a pseudotumor on abdominal roentgenograms. These so-called pseudotumors are quite common, and among the most common are the distended urinary bladder and the fluid-filled fundus of the stomach. The fluid-filled fundus appears as a soft-tissue "tumor" in the left upper quadrant. In children, another type of pseudotumor occasionally is produced by a peculiar configuration of the stomach on upright view (Fig. 3.180). Pseudotumors anywhere in the abdomen can be seen as a result of fortuitous visualization of fluid-filled

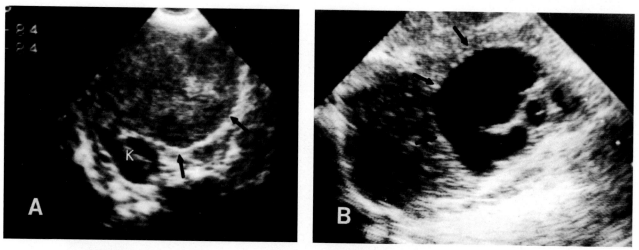

FIGURE 3.179. *Abdominal masses: ultrasound.* **(A)** Solid Wilms' tumor (*arrows*) in patient with abdominal pain and hematuria; compressed kidney (*K*). **(B)** Classic ureteropelvic junction obstruction (*arrows*) in patient with abdominal trauma and hematuria.

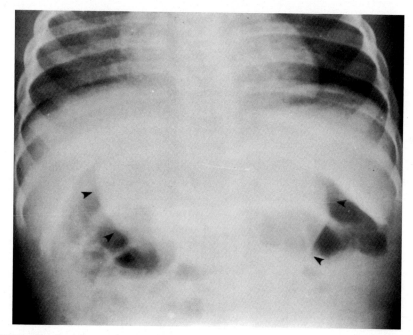

FIGURE 3.180. *Gastric pseudotumor.* Note the fluid-filled stomach presenting as a peculiar mid-abdominal pseudotumor (*arrows*). The *arrows* on the right outline the fluid-filled antrum; those on the left outline the fluid-filled body. This configuration almost always is seen on upright views.

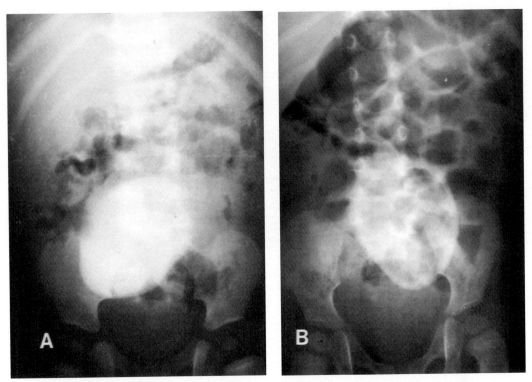

FIGURE 3.181. *Umbilical hernia: pseudotumor.* **(A)** Note a large opaque umbilical hernia producing a pseudotumor in the midabdomen. **(B)** Similar appearance in another patient, but this time the umbilical hernia contains air-filled loops of intestine.

loops of normal intestine. Finally, it should be mentioned that one of the most common pseudotumors in infancy is that produced by an umbilical hernia (Fig. 3.181).

REFERENCES

1. Klein MD. Traumatic rupture of an unsuspected mesenteric cyst: An uncommon cause of an acute surgical abdomen following a minor fall. *Pediatr Emerg Care* 1996;12:40.
2. Ogbevoen JO, Jaffe DM, Langer JC. Intraperitoneal rupture of an infected urachal cyst: A rare cause of peritonitis in children. *Pediatr Emerg Care* 1996;12:41–43.

Rectus Sheath and Psoas Muscle Hematomas

Hematomas of the abdominal wall in the rectus muscle can present with acute abdominal pain and may be mistaken for conditions such as appendicitis or cholecystitis. In other cases, they may be mistaken for abdominal masses. Because the abdomen often is so tense in these patients that physical examination is difficult, ultrasonography has become the best

modality with which to demonstrate these hematomas (1,2). Psoas muscle hematomas are less common but can be seen with trauma and in hemophiliacs. They are demonstrable with ultrasound and CT imaging (Fig. 3.182). Hematomas are echogenic on ultrasound in their early stages, but as they mature and liquefy, they become more anechoic.

REFERENCES

1. Benson M. Rectus sheath haematomas simulating pelvic pathology: The ultrasound appearances. *Clin Radiol* 1982;33:651–655.
2. Kaftori JK, Rosenberger A, Pollack S, Fish JH. Rectus sheath hematoma: Ultrasonographic diagnosis. *AJR* 1977;128: 2.

Psoas Muscle Abscess

Psoas muscle abscesses are not particularly common but do occur. Often they are tuberculous in origin, but idiopathic, pyogenic abscesses also can occur (1,2). The findings are no different from those in any other abscess, except that they are located in the psoas muscles and this is the major clue to proper diagnosis. Ultrasonographically, the abscess may be fluid-filled or show mixed echogenicity; overall, the findings are vividly demonstrable with either ultrasound or CT imaging (Fig. 3.183).

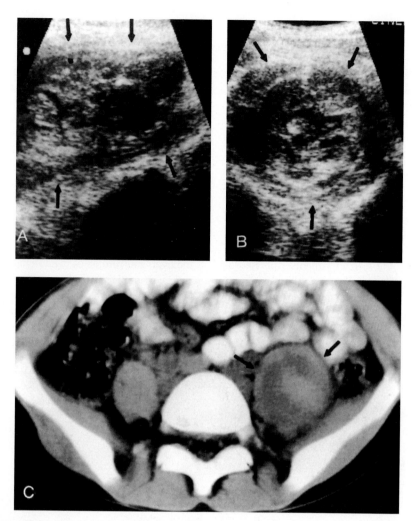

FIGURE 3.182. *Psoas hematoma.* **(A)** Longitudinal ultrasonogram demonstrates a large, heterogeneous mass (*arrows*) in the left psoas muscle. **(B)** Cross-sectional view of the same mass (*arrows*). **(C)** CT study demonstrates the enlarged left psoas muscle (*arrows*) and the hypodense hematoma within it. This patient was a hemophiliac.

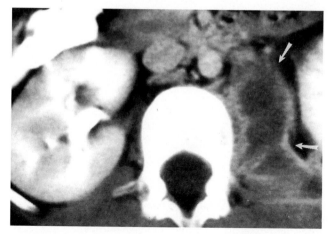

FIGURE 3.183. *Psoas abscess.* Note the abscess on the left (*arrows*). It has a hypodense center and a discrete rim.

REFERENCES

1. Malhotra R, Singh KD, Bhan S, Dave PK. Primary pyogenic abscess of the psoas muscle. *J Bone Joint Surg* 1992;74A: 278–284.
2. Parbhoo A, Govender S. Acute pyogenic psoas abscess in children. *J Pediatr Orthop* 1992;12:663–666.

Abdominal Calcifications

Overall, abdominal calcifications are not particularly common in children, but one must realize the significance of those that are seen from time to time. In this regard, one of the most common *incidental calcifications* found in the abdomen of a child is that *in the adrenal gland.* Such calcifications usually result from a previous, but often undocumented, neonatal adrenal hemorrhage, and if seen in the older child are of no clinical significance. Characteristically, the calcification lies above the kidney and is of triangular or near-triangular shape (Fig. 3.184A). Another innocuous calcification in the abdomen is the so-called mulberry- or popcorn-type calcification of old, inflamed mesenteric or retroperitoneal lymph nodes (Fig. 3.184B). Old healed tuberculosis or histoplasmosis often causes round, punctate, frequently multiple calcifications in the liver or spleen (Fig. 3.184C).

Urinary tract calcifications are not as common in children as in adults, but they do occur (2). Although in the past such calcifications usually were considered secondary to some type of metabolic disease, it is becoming increasingly apparent that most have other causes, including infection, and some are idiopathic. Bladder calculi are seen in patients with neurogenic disease and in other chronically immobilized patients. In the emergency patient, however, the urinary tract calcification of most concern is the calcified renal calculus producing renal colic. Currently one of the best ways to identify such calculi is on noncontrast- enhanced helical CT scanning.

Diffuse calcifications, such as those seen with renal tubular acidosis, oxalosis, and chronic glomerulonephritis and those resulting from renal cortical and medullary necrosis, seldom are encountered other than as incidental findings or in patients presenting with renal failure.

Pancreatic calcifications usually are midabdominal and irregular but on the whole are uncommon in childhood. They can be seen in cystic fibrosis and chronic pancreatitis. They usually are stippled and frequently outline the entire pancreas. Calcification of an appendiceal fecalith is of clear-cut significance and is dealt with in the section of this chapter on appendicitis. Calcification of a stone in a Meckel's diverticulum is uncommon but can mimic an appendiceal fecalith. Other abdominal calcifications may occur in teratomas, hemangiomatous tumors of the liver or other organs, hamartomas of the liver, and tumors of the adrenal glands such as neuroblastomas or adrenal cortical carcinoma. Massive calcification of a large adrenal gland is seen in Wolman's disease (1), and curvilinear or amorphous abdominal calcifications are seen with meconium peritonitis. Calcified phleboliths in the pelvis are not common in the pediatric population.

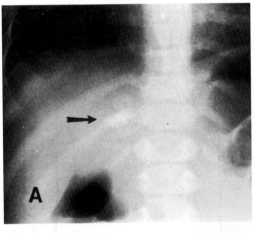
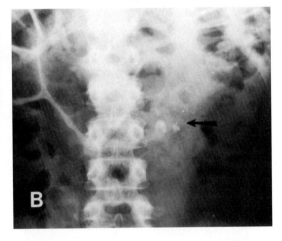
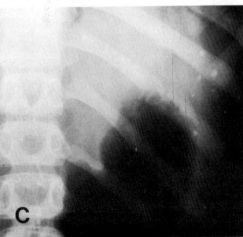

FIGURE 3.184. *Incidental abdominal calcification.* **(A)** Typical incidental calcification in adrenal gland (*arrow*). **(B)** Typical mulberry calcification in retroperitoneal lymph nodes (*arrow*). **(C)** Typical punctate calcification in the spleen. These calcifications often are secondary to healed histoplasmosis or tuberculosis.

REFERENCES

1. Queloz JM, Capitanio MA, Kirkpatrick JA. Wolman's disease: Roentgen observations in 3 siblings. *Radiology* 1972;104:357–359.
2. Walther PC, Lamm D, Kaplan GW. Pediatric urolithiases: A ten-year review. *Pediatrics* 1980;65:1068–1072.

Gastrointestinal Bleeding

Gastrointestinal bleeding is not as common in childhood as in adulthood, but by no means is it rare. Unfortunately, however, as many as 30% of cases remain undiagnosed (1). Arteriography often is helpful in patients suffering from acute bleeding and should be performed on an emergency basis if required. Bleeding must be brisk, however, probably at a rate of 1 mL/min, for the study to be fruitful.

Upper gastrointestinal bleeding, of a massive nature, is usually caused by portal hypertension but also can be seen with esophagitis, peptic-ulcer disease, and hemangiomas of the hypopharynx or gastrointestinal tract. Bleeding from the rectum is very frequently secondary to juvenile polyps of the colon, either single or multiple. In other instances, bleeding may result from colonic tumors and conditions such as ulcerative colitis and the hemolytic uremic syndrome. Indeed, colonic bleeding may be the presenting problem in the hemolytic uremic syndrome.

Bleeding in the form of red currant-jelly stools is a classic feature of intussusception, but in some cases, bright red bleeding or no bleeding may be seen. Meckel's diverticula are notorious for presenting with painless lower gastrointestinal bleeding, as are so-called benign colonic or small intestinal ulcers of unknown cause (2). Bright red rectal bleeding also occasionally is seen in peptic ulcer disease, especially in young infants, in whom gastrointestinal transit times may be rapid.

REFERENCES

1. Grosfeld JL, Schiller M, Weinberger M, Clatworthy HW Jr. Primary nonspecific ileal ulcers in children. *Am J Dis Child* 1970; 120:447–450.
2. Shah MJ. Primary nonspecific ulcer in ileum presenting with massive rectal hemorrhage. *Br Med J* 1968;3:474.

Acute Urinary Retention

Acute urinary retention problems are uncommon in infancy and childhood. Occasionally, however, one encounters a patient with a lower urinary tract obstruction and acute distension of the bladder presenting as an abdominal mass. Acute urinary retention also can be seen in severely injured children and those who might be comatose.

REFERENCE

1. Swischuk LE. Acute, non-traumatic, genitourinary pediatric problems. *Radiol Clin North Am* 1978;16:147–157.

Hematuria

Hematuria can result from renal trauma, calculi, parenchymal disease, infection, or neoplasms. It also may be idiopathic and, as such, is not uncommon. Neoplasms leading to hematuria seldom are encountered in childhood, because most Wilms' tumors do not present with hematuria. Hematuria more often is seen with urinary tract infection where cystitis is the problem. In such cases, ultrasound often demonstrates thickened bladder mucosa. Renal parenchymal disease leading to hematuria, usually glomerulonephritis, may manifest in increased echogenicity and enlargement of the kidneys on ultrasound. With renal trauma, CT with contrast enhancement is much more productive than ultrasonography, and with renal colic, plain films and intravenous pyelography usually were utilized in the past. Ultrasound now also can be employed, but noncontrast helical CT scans are extremely valuable in detecting these calculi. Overall, however, ultrasonography is a good screening examination for hematuria in the pediatric age group (1).

REFERENCE

1. Jequier S, Cramer B, Pititjeanroget T. Ultrasonographic screening of childhood hematuria. *Can J Assoc Radiol* 1987;38:170–176.

Hydrometrocolpos

Although not a common cause of acute abdominal pain in girls, hydrometrocolpos does occur every so often. Classically, it is seen either in the neonatal period or in adolescence. Two types exist, simple imperforate hymen or actual vaginal atresia. The former is more likely to be the problem in the adolescent but is not the exclusive presentation. With the onset of menses, blood accumulates in the obstructed uterus and a painful abdominal mass develops. It can be seen on plain films but is more specifically diagnosed with ultrasonography, where a sonolucent, elongated mass usually is seen behind the bladder (Fig. 3.185). Occasionally the mass is more solid, if uterine and vaginal secretions predominate.

Acute Scrotal Problems

Acute scrotal problems include epididymoorchitis, orchitis, testicular abscess, and testicular torsion. In addition, torsion of the appendix testis can be encountered and actually probably is the most common condition encountered. Additionally, trauma to the testicle also can be a problem.

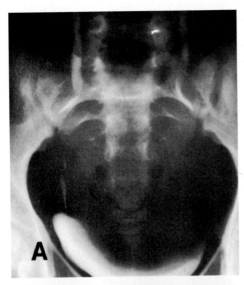

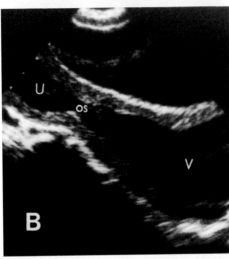

FIGURE 3.185. *Hydrometrocolpos.* **(A)** Note typical central pelvic mass displacing the ureter and bladder. **(B)** Sagittal sonogram demonstrating fluid and debris in an enlarged vagina (*V*) and uterus (*U*). Cervical os (*OS*).

Of course, in such cases a differential diagnosis is not required, but instead the most important job is to determine whether the testicle is intact.

In the past, these problems were best assessed with technetium-99 pertechnetate nuclide imaging (Fig. 3.186), but currently color flow Doppler ultrasonography is preferred (1,9–11,13,16). It also has been demonstrated that power Doppler is most sensitive in detecting intertesticular blood flow (2,3,12).

With testicular torsion, in the early stages one simply sees an enlarged testicle with no blood flow. Later, with hemorrhage into the testicle, a heterogeneous pattern is encountered (Fig. 3.187) and eventually there is reactive

inflammation around the testicle and in the epididymis, resulting in increased blood flow to these structures but no flow to the testicle itself (Fig. 3.187). ***With torsion and detorsion the findings can be confusing.*** Firstly, increased blood flow to the epididymis and surrounding peritesticular tissues can be seen, but in addition there is blood flow to the testicle, although it still may be scant. ***The most important point in these cases is to ask the patient whether the symptoms have resolved.*** Almost invariably the patient is able to say that they have and that pain no longer is a problem. Nonetheless, because torsion could occur again, these patients are best subjected to surgical correction. Bilateral testicular torsion is rare (5).

Other findings associated with testicular torsion include a highly echogenic head of the epididymis, which also may be noted to be displaced from its normal position. In addition, it has been determined that if echogenicity of the testicle is normal, the prognosis usually is good (14). This stands to reason, because this would indicate that the problem has been encountered in its early prenecrotic stages.

Testicular abscesses are rare in childhood and on ultrasound produce variably mixed or hypoechoic collections of fluid. Epididymoorchitis or epididymitis without orchitis are much more common. With epididymoorchitis, blood flow is increased both to the epididymis and the testicle (1,9,15) and is vividly demonstrable with color flow Doppler ultrasonography, especially power Doppler (Fig. 3.188). If epididymitis is without significant orchitis, blood flow to the testicle may be scant or absent; in such cases the findings are difficult to differentiate from missed testicular torsion. In most cases, however, epididymitis and orchitis occur together, and blood flow is clearly visible to both structures.

Torsion of the appendix testis may be the most common acute testicular problem in childhood. The findings may mimic those of testicular torsion but are quite variable (6,8,17). Clinically, visualization of the torsed appendix testis as a blue dot is pathognomonic, and similarly an echogenic dot seen on ultrasound can be highly suggestive of the diagnosis (Fig. 3.189). Other than these, however, the findings are quite variable and often consist of hyperemia of a thickened epididymis and peritesticular tissues. ***If blood flow to the testicle also is present, the findings can be misinterpreted as epididymoorchitis, but if blood flow to the testis is not present (which is a frequent occurrence), the findings cannot be differentiated from those in missed testicular torsion.***

Clearly, the various causes of acute testicular pain and swelling can produce ultrasonographic findings that can overlap. ***Therefore, it is important not so much that one determines exactly what is going on, but rather that one determines whether blood flow to the testicle is present or absent. If it is absent, no matter what the cause, the patient should be explored surgically.*** This may be an oversimplified approach to the problem, but because there

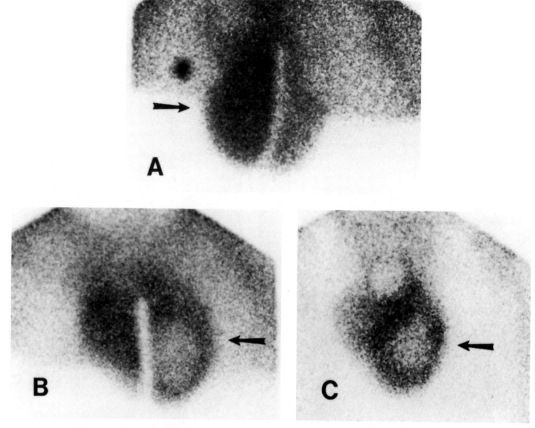

FIGURE 3.186. *Acute testicular problems: scintigraphy.* **(A)** Epididymoorchitis. Note increased isotope activity in the enlarged right testicle (*arrow*). **(B)** Early testicular torsion. Note decreased isotope uptake in the left testicle (*arrow*). A scrotal rim is present, but it is not hyperemic. **(C)** Missed torsion. Characteristically with missed torsion, a similar cold testicular center is seen, but the tissues around it becomes hyperemic (*arrow*).

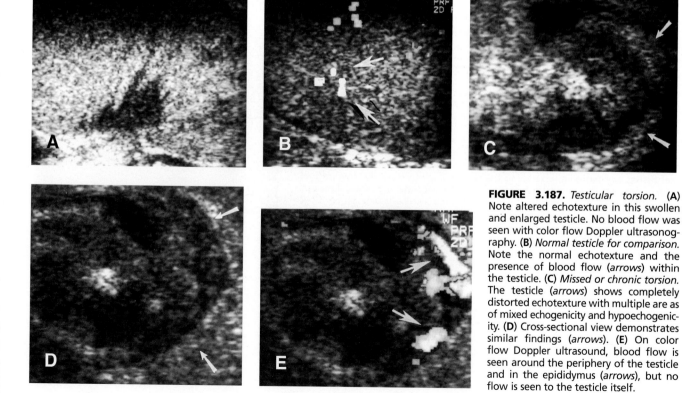

FIGURE 3.187. *Testicular torsion.* **(A)** Note altered echotexture in this swollen and enlarged testicle. No blood flow was seen with color flow Doppler ultrasonography. **(B)** *Normal testicle for comparison.* Note the normal echotexture and the presence of blood flow (*arrows*) within the testicle. **(C)** *Missed or chronic torsion.* The testicle (*arrows*) shows completely distorted echotexture with multiple are as of mixed echogenicity and hypoechogenicity. **(D)** Cross-sectional view demonstrates similar findings (*arrows*). **(E)** On color flow Doppler ultrasound, blood flow is seen around the periphery of the testicle and in the epididymus (*arrows*), but no flow is seen to the testicle itself.

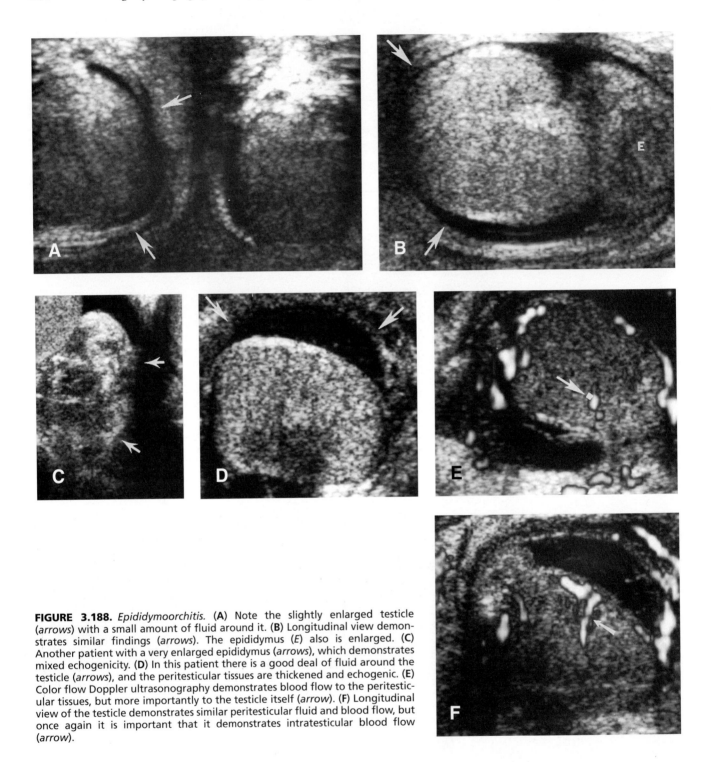

FIGURE 3.188. *Epididymoorchitis.* **(A)** Note the slightly enlarged testicle (*arrows*) with a small amount of fluid around it. **(B)** Longitudinal view demonstrates similar findings (*arrows*). The epididymus (*E*) also is enlarged. **(C)** Another patient with a very enlarged epididymus (*arrows*), which demonstrates mixed echogenicity. **(D)** In this patient there is a good deal of fluid around the testicle (*arrows*), and the peritesticular tissues are thickened and echogenic. **(E)** Color flow Doppler ultrasonography demonstrates blood flow to the peritesticular tissues, but more importantly to the testicle itself (*arrow*). **(F)** Longitudinal view of the testicle demonstrates similar peritesticular fluid and blood flow, but once again it is important that it demonstrates intratesticular blood flow (*arrow*).

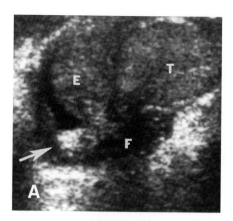
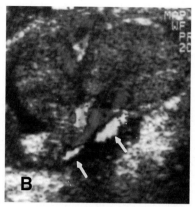
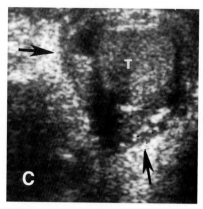

FIGURE 3.189. *Torsion of the appendix testis.* **(A)** Note the testicle (*T*). It appears normal. The epididymus (*E*) is enlarged, and there is an echogenic focus representing the torsed appendix testis (*arrow*). Fluid (*F*) is present in the area. **(B)** On color flow Doppler ultrasound, increased peritesticular blood flow is seen (*arrows*). **(C)** Transverse view of the testicle (*T*) again shows the peritesticular fluid and thickening of the peritesticular tissues (*arrows*).

is little time to waste with torsion of the testicle, in our institution it has become the practice of choice.

With trauma, ultrasound usually demonstrates disorganization of the normally uniform echogenicity of the testicle if testicular fracture is present (7). The ultrasonographic findings are rather straightforward (Fig. 3.190), but in

other cases only enlargement of the testicle may be seen. Thickening of the epididymis and hyperemia of the epididymis are common, as are associated hydroceles (Fig. 3.177). If a hematocele is present, a sonolucent area can be seen, and very often there is associated thickening of the scrotal wall.

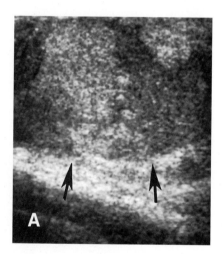
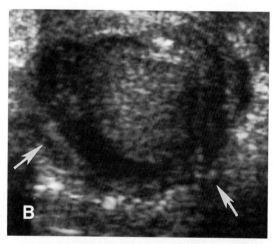
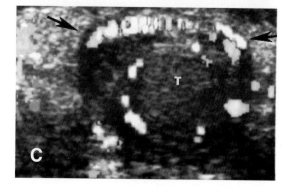

FIGURE 3.190. *Testicular trauma.* **(A)** This testicle demonstrates increase in size and considerable ultrasonographic inhomogenicity. These findings are typical of a "fractured" testicle. **(B)** In this patient the testicle is intact but surrounded by fluid (*arrows*). **(C)** With color flow Doppler ultrasonography, increased peritesticular blood flow is seen (*arrows*). This represents traumatic epididymitis and peritesticular inflammation. *T*, testicle.

Finally, it should be noted that patients with Henoch–Schönlein purpura also can develop an acute scrotum. In such cases, they suffer from hemorrhagic epididymitis (4,18), and the findings are similar to those of infectious epididymitis.

REFERENCES

1. Atkinson GO Jr, Patrick LE, Ball TI Jr, Stephenson CA, Broecker BH, Woodard JR. The normal and abnormal scrotum in children: Evaluation with color Doppler sonography. *AJR* 1992;158:613–617.
2. Bader TR, Kammerhuber F, Herneth AM. Testicular blood flow in boys as assessed at color Doppler and power Doppler sonography. *Radiology* 1997;202:559–564.
3. Barth RA, Shortliffe LD. Normal pediatric testis: Comparison of power Doppler and color Doppler US in the detection of blood flow. *Radiology* 1997;204:389–393.
4. Ben-Chaim J, Korat E, Shenfeld O, Shelhav A, Jonas P, Goldwasser B. Acute scrotum caused by Henoch-Schonlein purpura, with immediate response to short-term steroid therapy. *J Pediatr Surg* 1995;30:1509–1510.
5. Benge BN, Eure GR, Winslow BH. Acute bilateral testicular torsion in the adolescent. *J Urol* 1992;148:134.
6. Cohen HL, Shapiro MA, Haller JO, Glassberg K. Torsion of the testicular appendage. *J Ultrasound Med* 1992;11:81–83.
7. Gordon LM, Stein SM, Ralls PW. Traumatic epididymitis: Evaluation with color Doppler sonography. *AJR* 1996;166:1323–1325.
8. Hesser U, Rosenborg M, Gierup J, Karpe B, Nystrom A, Hedenborg L. Gray-scale sonography in torsion of the testicular appendages. *Pediatr Radiol* 1993;23:529–532.
9. Horstman WG, Middleton WD, Melson GL. Scrotal inflammatory disease: Color Doppler US findings. *Radiology* 1991;179:55–59.
10. Jensen MC, Lee KP, Halls JM, Ralls PW. Color Doppler sonography in testicular torsion. *J Clin Ultrasound* 1990;18:446–448.
11. Kadish HA, Bolte RG. A retrospective review of pediatric patients with epididymitis, testicular torsion, and torsion of testicular appendages. *Pediatrics* 1998;102:73–76.
12. Luker GD, Siegel MJ. Scrotal US in pediatric patients: Comparison of power and standard color Doppler US. *Radiology* 1996;198:381–385.
13. Meza MP, Amundson GM, Aquilina JW, Reitelman C. Color flow imaging in children with clinically suspected testicular torsion. *Pediatr Radiol* 1992;22:370–373.
14. Middleton WD, Middleton MA, Dierks M, Keetch D, Dierks S. Sonographic prediction of viability in testicular torsion: Preliminary observations. *J Ultrasound Med* 1997;16:23–27.
15. Middleton WD, Siegel BA, Melson GL, Yates CK, Andriole GL. Acute scrotal disorders: Prospective comparison of color Doppler US and testicular scintigraphy. *Radiology* 1990;177:177–181.
16. Patriquin HB, Yazbeck S, Trinh B, Jequier S, Burns PN, Crignon A, Filiatrault D, Garel L, Dubois J. Testicular torsion in infants and children: Diagnosis with Doppler sonography. *Radiology* 1993;188:781–785.
17. Strauss S, Faingold R, Manor H. Torsion of the testicular appendages: Sonographic appearance. *J Ultrasound Med* 1997;16:189–192.
18. Sukakoff GS, Burke M, Rifkin MD. Ultrasonographic and color Doppler imaging of hemorrhagic epididymitis in Henoch-Schonlein purpura. *J Ultrasound Med* 1992;11:619–621.

Pregnancy

Of course, it is well known that gastrointestinal upsets are common in pregnancy, but often one does not think of pregnancy in the pediatric age group. Nevertheless, one should be aware of this possibility, for the first indication that a pregnancy is present may come from the abdominal roentgenogram in which a pelvic mass or even a formed fetus is demonstrated. Confirmation now is accomplished readily with ultrasonography (Figs. 3.191 and 3.192) and pregnancy tests.

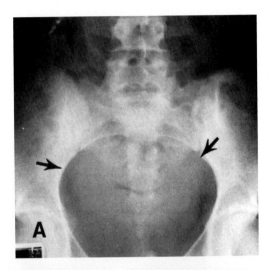

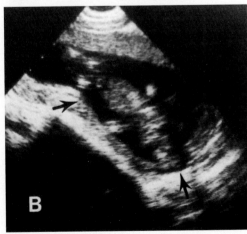

FIGURE 3.191. *Late pregnancy.* **(A)** Note fullness, or a mass in the pelvis (*arrows*). **(B)** Ultrasonogram demonstrating well-developed fetus (*arrows*).

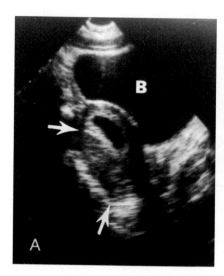
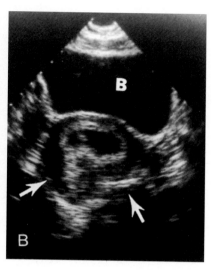

FIGURE 3.192. *Early pregnancy: ultrasound findings.* **(A)** On this sagittal view note the enlarged uterus (*arrows*) with an early decidual sac (sonolucent center) behind the bladder (*B*). **(B)** Transverse sonogram demonstrates the same findings within the enlarged uterus (*arrows*). *B*, Urinary bladder.

NORMAL FINDINGS CAUSING PROBLEMS

Gastric and Colon Contents Mimicking Abscesses and Bezoars

This point seems straightforward, yet in some cases, if gastric or colonic contents are visualized in just the right place, it is most difficult to differentiate them from the findings of an abdominal abscess or gastric bezoar (Fig. 3.193). Contents in the right side of the colon are especially problematic in patients with appendicitis and suspected perforation. Indeed, in some cases it is most difficult to determine whether one is dealing with an appendiceal abscess or fortuitous visualization of feces in the colon. In young infants, milk curds can conglomerate in the stomach to produce a bezoar or even mass-like configuration (Fig. 3.194).

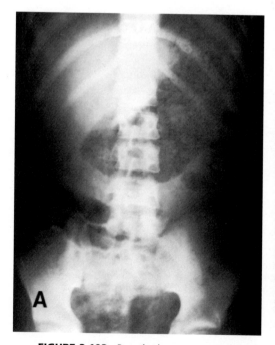
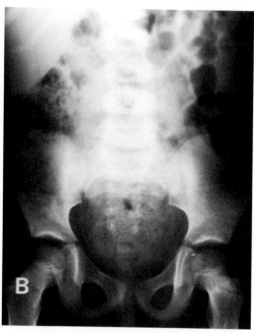

FIGURE 3.193. *Pseudoabscess or pseudobezoar appearance of gastric and colonic contents.* **(A)** Note the granular appearance of food and air mixed within the stomach of this patient. The pattern is similar to that seen with abdominal abscesses or gastric bezoars. **(B)** Another patient with fecal material mixed with air in the rectum and hepatic flexure. Either of these collections alone could be misinterpreted as an abscess.

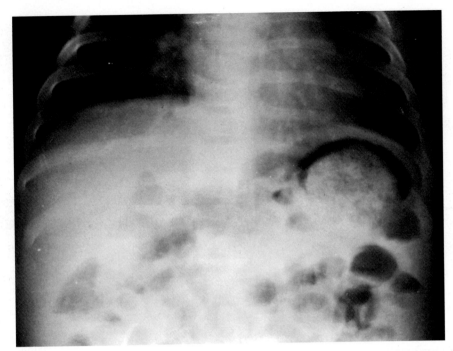

FIGURE 3.194. *Milk curds in stomach of infant.* Note the mass-like collection of milk curds in the fundus of the stomach of this young infant. The findings mimic those of a gastric bezoar, but they are normal and common.

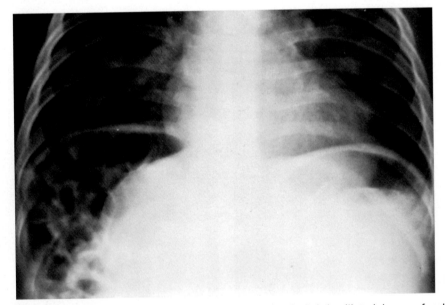

FIGURE 3.195. *Chilaiditi's syndrome.* Note interposition of slightly dilated loops of colon between the liver and the right diaphragmatic leaflet. The findings should not be misinterpreted as free air under the diaphragmatic leaflet, especially on chest films, in which the top of the abdomen only is included on the study.

Abdominal Pseudotumors

These are discussed with abdominal masses elsewhere.

Chilaiditi's Syndrome (Hepatodiaphragmatic Interposition)

This condition usually is considered a normal variation and consists of interposition of the colon between the liver and the diaphragm (1–3). Most often, it is seen on the right, but it can be seen bilaterally. The findings should not be misinterpreted as free peritoneal air (Fig. 3.195).

REFERENCES

1. Behlke FM. Hepatodiaphragmatic interposition in children. *AJR* 1964;91:669.
2. Jackson ADM, Hudson CJ. Interposition of colon between liver and diaphragm (Chilaiditi's syndrome) in children. *Arch Dis Child* 1957;32:151.
3. Vessal K, Borhanmanesh F. Hepatodiaphragmatic interposition of the intestine (Chilaiditi's syndrome). *Clin Radiol* 1976;27:113–116.

Duodenal Air Mimicking Air Under the Liver

In some cases, air trapped in the partially collapsed duodenal bulb is virtually indistinguishable from free air trapped under the liver. Only familiarity with this normal configuration allows the physician to avoid misinterpretation (Fig. 3.196).

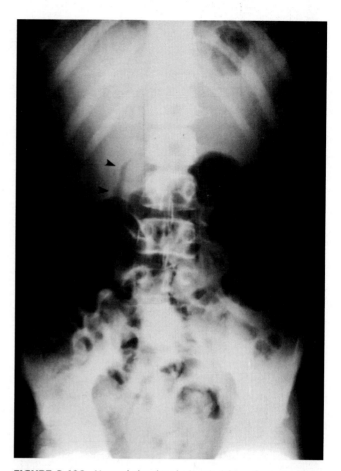

FIGURE 3.196. *Normal duodenal air mimicking free air under the liver.* Note the linear collection of air in the duodenum (*arrows*). Such configurations usually are best visualized on upright views and can mimic the appearance of free air under the liver.

4

THE EXTREMITIES

This chapter primarily addresses the detection of the more subtle and frequently missed fractures and inflammatory lesions of the extremities. There is no attempt to cover all fractures, especially those that require roentgenographic examination merely to confirm their presence or visualize the precise position of the fractured fragments. Although many other injuries represent significant management problems, they offer no real problems for roentgenographic diagnosis. Furthermore, they are dealt with in whole or in part in a number of excellent publications on the subject (2,3).

There also is a greater than usual emphasis on evaluation of the soft tissues and periarticular fat pads. These structures generally are underutilized and underestimated in importance. They are, however, invaluable in yielding data regarding the specific location and nature of a lesion, and their special usefulness in infants and young children is stressed, because in this age group clinical history and physical examination often are less than optimal. Clinical history, however, still is important in determining the nature and possible location of an injury (1), and physical examination is most predictive of a fracture if point tenderness, deformity, and extensive edema are present (4).

REFERENCES

1. Berbaum KS, El-Khoury GY, Franken EA Jr, Kathol M, Montgomery WJ, Hesson W. Impact of clinical history on fracture detection with radiography. *Radiology* 1988;168:507–511.
2. Blount WP. *Fractures in children, 2nd Ed.* Baltimore: Williams and Wilkins, 1980.
3. Rang M. *Children's fractures, 2nd Ed.* Philadelphia: J.B. Lippincott, 1982.
4. Rivara FP, Parish RA, Mueller BA. Extremity injuries in children: Predictive value of clinical findings. *Pediatrics* 1986;78:803–807.

GENERAL CONSIDERATIONS

What Views Should Be Obtained?

At least two views, usually at right angles to each other, are necessary. Most often these views consist of frontal and lateral projections of the involved extremity, and it cannot be stated too forcefully that true frontal and lateral projections are required. One cannot settle for a "sort of" frontal or lateral view, or one will regret it. If these views fail to yield useful information, oblique or other special views should be obtained.

In addition, it is of utmost benefit to obtain **comparative views** of the other (normal) side, especially in cases in which abnormal findings are subtle. These views are extremely useful, because, generally speaking, symmetry from side to side in the normal patient is very consistent and, because of this, any asymmetry, no matter how subtle (2–4), should be treated with the greatest suspicion. Over the years there has been movement towards discouraging the routine use of comparative views (1), but although there is some merit to this posture, *most experienced radiologists, especially those not sustained on a steady diet of pediatric films, still prefer to obtain comparative views. Indeed, even though our institution is a pediatric facility, we obtain comparative views rather liberally, for we do not feel we can detect subtle bony injury or evaluate the soft tissues satisfactorily without them.* It is interesting that, in a summary report, the Committee on Radiology of the American Academy of Pediatrics provided so many loopholes in the premise that comparative views are not required that the loopholes virtually destroyed the original premise. For example, quoting directly from their report (1):

> Injury to the hip joint is a notable exception to the selective approach; at least one view should routinely include the normal hip, with the gonads shielded. Hip injuries in children are most frequently associated with joint effusion, which can be detected only with comparing similar measurements of the opposite joint space.

Other specific areas of the appendicular skeleton may require more comparative views. The elbow, with a relatively large number of ossification centers appearing at widely varying times, may prove confusing even to the experienced radiologist; comparison view of this joint may be requested frequently. Detection of joint effusion in the knee and ankle may necessitate a comparison view, in at least one projection. Comparison views may also be helpful in evaluating the tissue planes and subcutaneous fat in suspected inflammatory conditions of the soft tissues or bones.

Finally, a conclusion from the same communication (1) suggests that no one uniform policy can be expected for all individuals dealing with pediatric trauma:

A number of theoretical and practical considerations will continue to determine the use of comparison views. Personal conviction based on experience and training is the major theoretical consideration. Practical considerations include the availability of radiologic consultation, the expertise of the physician who initially interprets the study and clinical demands. An individual's policy toward the use of comparison images is a balance of these considerations.

The latter paragraph probably is the most important in this ongoing controversy. ***Do what you have to do, but be sure in your mind that you will not miss any fractures when you obtain views of the injured side only. One might ask, "How sure am I that I am not missing a bending fracture, a subtle Salter–Harris type I injury, or a minimal buckle fracture?"***

Recently it has been demonstrated that the cost of obtaining comparative views is negligible, and so is the risk of radiation injury to the patient (5). Indeed, it is difficult to construct a case against comparative views if one wants to be able to detect subtle injuries, peculiar injuries, and otherwise potentially occult and problematic injuries. This is especially true if one does not look at pediatric films on a full-time basis.

REFERENCES

1. Committee on Radiology. Comparison radiographs of extremities in childhood: Recommended usage. *Pediatrics* 1980;65:646–647.
2. John SD, Phillips WA. Imaging evaluation of pediatric extremity trauma, part I: Injury patterns of the immature skeleton and imaging modalities. *Intensive Care Med* 1998;13:124–134.
3. John SD, Phillips WA. Imaging evaluation of pediatric extremity trauma, part II: Upper extremity. *Intensive Care Med* 1998;13:184–194.
4. John SD, Phillips WA. Imaging evaluation of pediatric extremity trauma, part III: Lower extremity and soft tissues. *Intensive Care Med* 1998;13:241–252.
5. Swischuk LE. Comparative views in childhood fractures. *Emerg Radiol* 1997;4:2.

Utilizing the Soft Tissues

Evaluating soft tissue changes in trauma and infection of the extremities in childhood, and even in adulthood (1), is invaluable. The findings one should look for include localized or generalized swelling of the soft tissues, obliteration of the muscle–fat interfaces, and displacement or obliteration of the periarticular fat pads. These structures are displaced if fluid accumulates within the joint and obliterated if edema surrounds the joint. Evaluating the soft tissues in this manner can serve to localize the site of injury or infection, and such an evaluation should be undertaken before the bones themselves are examined (Fig. 4.1). Of course,

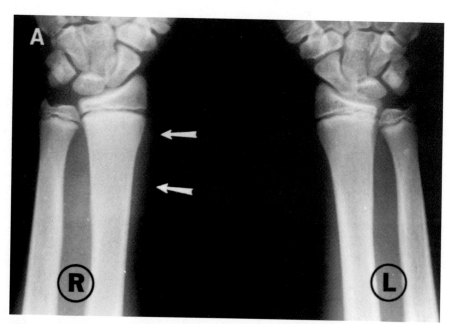

FIGURE 4.1. *Value of soft tissues in localizing an injury.* **(A)** Frontal view of both wrists. Bony abnormality is subtle and consists primarily of a little widening of the distal right radial epiphyseal line. This should signify the presence of a Salter–Harris type I epiphyseal–metaphyseal injury, but the finding is subtle and could be missed. If it is noted that soft-tissue swelling also is present (*arrows*), however, the finding takes on more significance. *(continued on next page)*

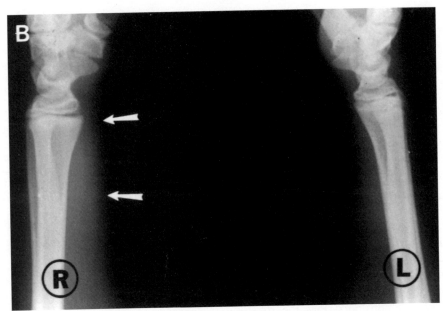

FIGURE 4.1. *(continued)* **(B)** Soft tissue swelling also is noted on the lateral view (*arrows*). Note that not only are the soft tissues thicker, but edema and swelling have obliterated the normal fat–muscle interfaces. Compare with the normal appearance of the left wrist. Note the slightly wider epiphyseal line and mininally displaced (posteriorly) distal, right radial epiphysis.

the changes differ some from joint to joint and bone to bone, but basically abnormality can be placed in one of the three categories just proposed. More detailed discussion of the soft-tissue changes for each joint of the body is presented at subsequent points throughout this chapter.

REFERENCE

1. Curtis DJ, Downey EF Jr, Brower AC, Cruess DF, Herrington WT, Ghaed N. Importance of soft tissue evaluation in hand and wrist trauma: Statistical evaluation. *AJR* 1984;142:781–788.

Significance of Intraarticular Fluid

As a general rule, in children, fluid in the joint in the absence of trauma should be presumed to be pus until proven otherwise. In the elbow and ankle, fluid in the joint is manifested by outward displacement of the anterior and posterior fat pads; in the shoulder and hip, fluid accumulation causes lateral displacement of the humerus or femur and concomitant joint space widening. Knee fluid produces bulging of the suprapatellar bursa, just behind the quadriceps tendon; in the wrist, joint fluid is manifested simply by the presence of swelling around the wrist.

In the presence of trauma, fluid in the joint should cause one to look more diligently at the bones for evidence of a fracture in this area. Not always, however, does one see such a fracture; however, in our study on the subject (2), the incidence of missed fracture was surprisingly low (Table 4.1). This has been corroborated more recently in the elbow (1). It is important to emphasize, however, that in our study liberal use of comparative views was standard. If one does not

TABLE 4.1. OCCULT FRACTURE—PERCENT PROBABILITY[a]

Fracture	Total No. of Cases	Total Cases with No. X-ray Follow-up	Total Cases with X-ray Follow-up	No. of Cases with Fracture Detected	Percent Fracture Probability
Shoulder	0	0	0	0	0
Elbow	46	20	26	4	15.8
Wrist	5	2	3	2	67
Hip	0	0	0	0	0
Knee	16	9	7	0	11
Ankle	61	34	27	3	12.8
Total	128	65	63	8	12.8

[a]Reproduced from: Swischuk, L.E., Hayden, C.K., and Kupfer, M.C.: Significance of intraarticular fluid without visible fracture in children, A.J.R. 142:1261–1262, 1984.

obtain comparative views, one is more likely to miss fractures that become apparent on later studies.

REFERENCES

1. Connelly LF, Klostermeier TT, Klosterman LA. Traumatic elbow effusions in pediatric patients: Are occult fractures the rule? *AJR* 1998;171:243–245.
2. Swischuk LE, Hayden CK, Kupfer MC. Significance of intra-articular fluid without visible fracture in children. *AJR* 1984;142:1261–1262.

What Type of Bony Injuries Are Seen in Children?

The types of fractures most peculiar to childhood are (a) cortical, buckle, or torus fractures; (b) greenstick fractures; (c) bent or bowed bones without a visible fracture line (i.e., acute plastic, bending fractures); and (d) epiphyseal–metaphyseal fractures (Fig. 4.2). Of course, typical midshaft, transverse, spiral, oblique, and comminuted fractures also occur in children, but none are especially peculiar to childhood and most are not difficult to detect. One might make some exception to this statement if these fractures are of the so-called hairline variety, but otherwise these fractures are readily demonstrable roentgenographically and not difficult to diagnose. Hairline fractures occur most commonly in the tibia and small bones of the hands and feet. In the tibia, both transverse (upper metaphysis) and spiral-shaft (toddler's fracture) fractures occur (Fig. 4.3).

Buckle or torus fractures are simple compression fractures that manifest themselves through buckling, kinking, or

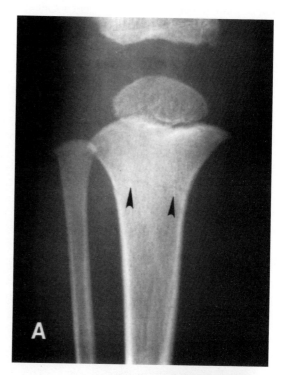

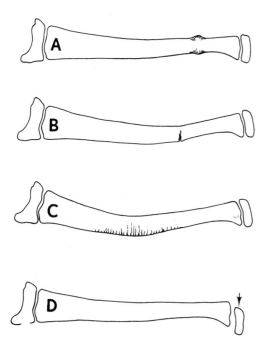

FIGURE 4.2. *Fractures peculiar to children.* **(A)** Typical torus or buckle fracture with buckling of the cortex. **(B)** Greenstick fracture with the fracture visible through one aspect of the cortex only. The fracture is incomplete, and a certain degree of bending coexists. **(C)** Bending or plastic bowing fracture of long bone. No fracture line is visible roentgenographically, but numerous microfractures exist along the outer aspect of the bent bone. **(D)** Epiphyseal–metaphyseal injury with or without displacement of the epiphysis *(arrow)*.

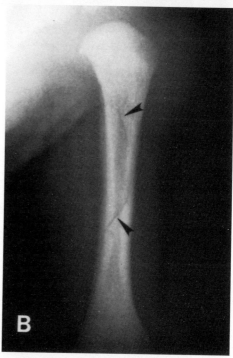

FIGURE 4.3. *Hairline fractures.* **(A)** Note the hairline fracture *(arrows)* traversing the upper right tibia. It is not easy to see. **(B)** Spiral hairline fracture *(arrows)* in a battered infant. The presence of periosteal new bone indicates early healing. Hairline fractures often become more readily visible at this stage.

notching of the cortex. They occur most frequently in the metaphyseal regions of long bones, for this is where the cortex is weakest. They also can be seen, however, in the clavicles, the pubic bones, and even the scapulae. Some of these buckle or torus fractures are quite subtle, but if one follows the rule that the distal ends of the long bones should possess smooth, continuous curves, then one will not accept even the slightest bump, dent, buckle, or cortical irregularity as nor-mal (Fig. 4.4). Nonetheless, some of these fractures do elude initial detection, and if follow-up films are obtained, signs of healing in the form of sclerosis along the fracture line and periosteal new bone deposition can be seen (Fig. 4.5).

Greenstick fractures are bending fractures with a fracture line extending through one cortex of the bone only (Fig. 4.6). The term "greenstick" comes from the comparison of this type of fracture to the manner in which a

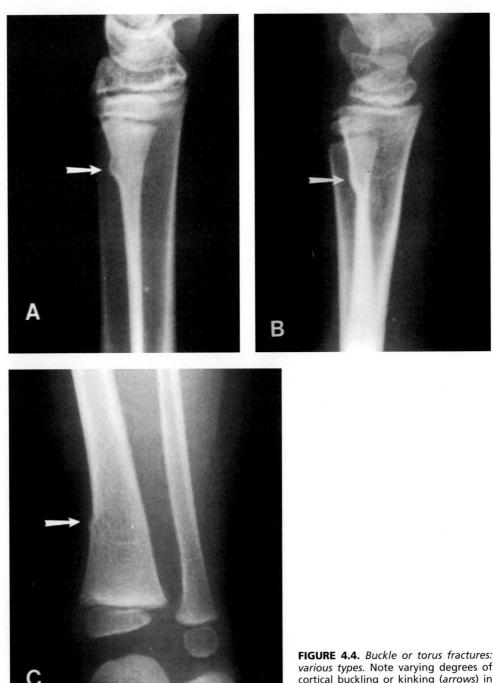

FIGURE 4.4. *Buckle or torus fractures: various types.* Note varying degrees of cortical buckling or kinking (*arrows*) in these typical torus fractures of the wrist (**A** and **B**) and ankle (**C**).

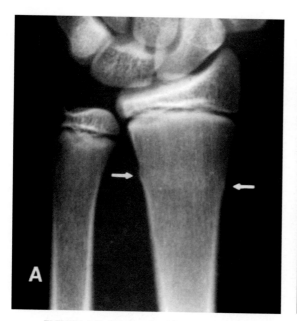
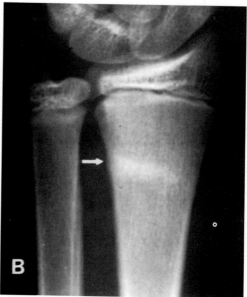

FIGURE 4.5. Healing buckle or torus fracture. (A) Note typical, but subtle, bulging of the cortex (*arrows*). Also note that the trabecular pattern along the fracture line has been disturbed. **(B)** Two weeks later note sclerosis along the fracture line (*arrow*).

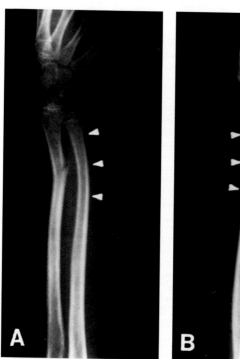
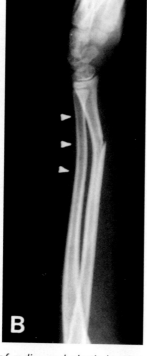

FIGURE 4.6. *Greenstick fracture of radius and plastic bowing fracture of ulna.* Anteroposterior **(A)** and lateral **(B)** views. Note the greenstick fracture of the distal radius. In addition, however, note bending of the ulna (*arrows*). This finding represents an acute plastic bending fracture of the ulna. Some concomitant bending of the fractured radius also is present.

"green," supple tree branch breaks if it is bent. True ***bending or bowing (plastic) fractures,*** without a visible fracture line (2–4,9,13), can be considered the precursor of the classic greenstick fractures (i.e., the greenest of greenstick fractures). These fractures frequently are missed unless comparative views of the normal extremity are obtained, and although a fracture line is not visible roentgenographically, numerous microfractures exist along the outer surface of the bent bone. In these cases, the fracture force is not dissipated at any one site, and thus a single fracture line is not visualized. With enough bending, a single fracture line develops, but until then, only bending is seen (Fig. 4.6). Most often these fractures occur in the forearm (1–4,14), but they also can be seen in the lower extremity (3,14), clavicle, and indeed almost any long bone in the body of the infant or young child. These fractures are discussed in more detail in later sections, but it might be noted at this point that seldom, if ever, do they show classic signs of healing. In other words, whereas with a greenstick fracture one sees sclerosis and periosteal new bone formation, with the usual bending fracture nothing but the deformity persists (Fig. 4.7).

Epiphyseal–metaphyseal fractures are very common in childhood and, of course, occur exclusively in the child. Because the junction between the epiphysis and metaphysis is a weak area, if a shearing force is applied to the end of a long bone, it is quite natural that epiphyseal–metaphyseal slippage or separation results. A variety of injuries can be sustained at this junction, and to facilitate their understanding and categorization, the Salter–Harris classification of five types (12) usually still is employed (Fig. 4.8). More

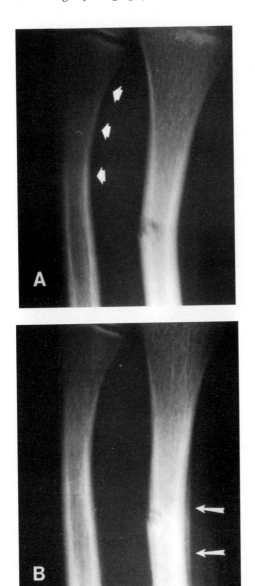

FIGURE 4.7. *Greenstick and plastic bending fracture: healing phase.* **(A)** Note the greenstick fracture of the distal radius. In addition, note bending of the ulna (*arrows*). **(B)** Follow-up films demonstrate classic healing of the radial fracture (*arrows*), but in the ulna, no signs of healing are seen.

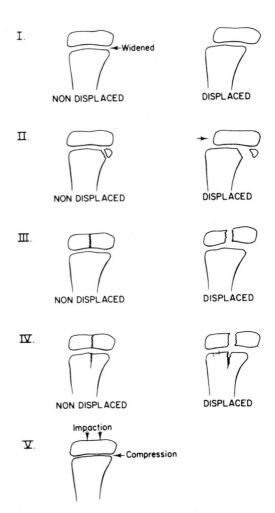

FIGURE 4.8. *Salter–Harris classification of epiphyseal–metaphyseal fractures.* Type I: The epiphyseal line (physis) is widened secondary to some degree of epiphyseal separation. The epiphysis may or may not be displaced. Type II: There is a small or large metaphyseal fracture fragment in association with widening of the epiphyseal line. The epiphysis and fracture fragment may or may not be visibly displaced. Type III: The fracture occurs through the epiphysis and may or may not be displaced. If displacement occurs, usually only part of the fractured epiphysis is displaced. Type IV: Fractures exist through the epiphysis and the metaphysis; displacement of the fragments may or may not be present. Type V: An impaction fracture with compressive injury of the epiphyseal plate only is present. No roentgenographic findings other than swelling around the involved epiphyseal–metaphyseal junction usually are present.

complicated classifications have been suggested, but the Salter–Harris classification is more than adequate and probably will not be replaced.

As far as the radiologist is concerned, the greatest challenge comes from the Salter–Harris type I and II injuries (12). The reason for this is that if in these cases the epiphysis is not displaced, bony changes are subtle, and one must rely more on soft-tissue changes and widening of the epiphyseal line. Salter–Harris type I and II fractures heal in characteristic fashion, and thus, should they not be

detected in their acute phase, repeat roentgenograms 10 days to 2 weeks later show sclerosis and irregularity of the epiphyseal–metaphyseal junction and periosteal new bone deposition along the metaphysis (Fig. 4.9). Salter–Harris type III and IV fractures usually are relatively easy to detect, for often some degree of epiphyseal displacement exists and, in any case, the fracture lines are more readily visible. Type III fractures occur most commonly in the

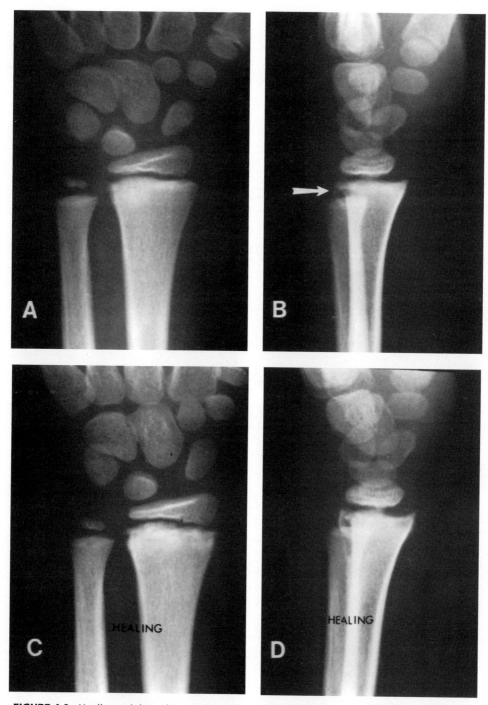

FIGURE 4.9. *Healing epiphyseal–metaphyseal injury.* (**A**) Frontal view demonstrating little if any abnormality of the epiphyseal–metaphyseal junction. (**B**) Lateral view demonstrates posterior displacement of the radial epiphysis and a corner fracture of the posterior metaphysis (*arrow*). These findings are consistent with a Salter–Harris type II injury. (**C**) Two weeks later note how sclerotic and irregular the radial metaphyseal margin has become. This is characteristic of the healing phase of these fractures. (**D**) Lateral view showing similar findings.

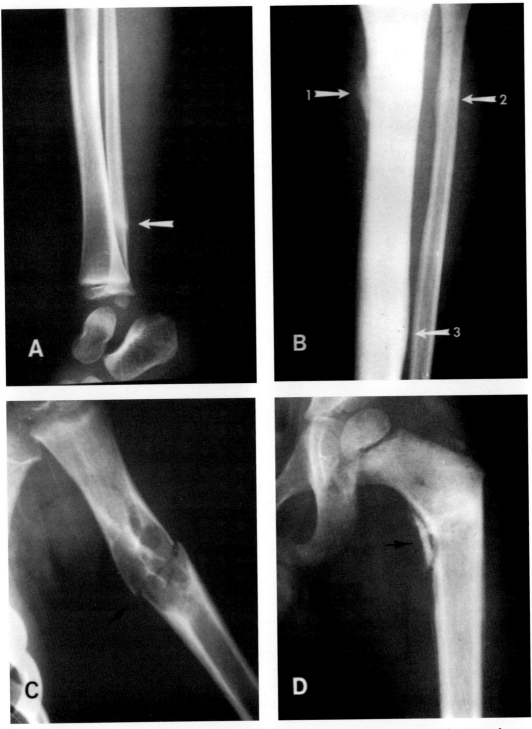

FIGURE 4.10. *Other fractures in childhood.* **(A)** Stress fracture of fibula. Note the area of increased sclerosis and periosteal new bone deposition in the lower fibula (*arrow*). **(B)** Another patient demonstrating multiple stress fractures. First note the large "lump" of periosteal new bone adjacent to the tibial fracture (*1*). Then note a similar, but much less pronounced, finding in the fibula just across from the tibia (*2*); finally, note the old healed stress fracture of the lower tibia (*3*). **(C)** Pathologic fracture through unicameral bone cyst of the humerus (*arrow*). **(D)** Pathologic fracture in Ewing's sarcoma with avulsion of the lesser trochanter (*arrow*). Note that there is destruction of the medullary portion of the bone, and that reactive periosteal new bone is present circumferentially. This patient experienced acute hip pain while running.

distal tibia, followed by the small bones of the hands and feet.

The type V Salter–Harris injury, that is, the one in which only epiphyseal-plate compression occurs (9), is the least common of all. Indeed, a question has been raised as to whether the type V fracture occurs at all (10). It is considered, however, one of the more serious injuries a child can sustain, for epiphyseal-plate damage and subsequent impaired epiphyseal growth are common (7,10,12). Growth abnormalities also are a significant complication of the type IV fracture but are a lesser problem with the other Salter–Harris types of epiphyseal–metaphyseal injuries. Roentgenographically, in the type V fracture the films usually are void of bony abnormality.

Although the fractures outlined here constitute the major portion of childhood fractures, one also can see stress fractures with considerable frequency and, to a lesser extent, pathologic fractures. Stress fractures usually, but not always, occur in perfectly normal individuals, and the most common site for such a fracture in a child is the upper tibia (15). They can occur, however, in almost any bone of the lower extremity (5,13). Stress fractures of the second metatarsal usually are referred to as "march fractures." Shin splints also probably are stress microfractures (1).

It is unusual to detect stress fractures in their initial stages, for unless a fracture line is seen through the involved cortex, one will not even suspect that such an injury is present. Consequently, these fractures frequently go undetected for days or weeks and finally come to the attention of the physician in their healing phase, replete with sclerosis along the fracture line and periosteal new bone deposition over the fracture site (Fig. 4.10A). Indeed, so striking are these changes that very often they are misinterpreted for more serious lesions such as a bone tumor (Fig. 4.10B).

Nuclear scintigraphy also is very useful in the detection of stress fractures. Although the findings are nonspecific, they do localize the site of injury. Stress fractures also now can be detected readily with magnetic resonance (MR) imaging (6,8). However, in most cases plain films and nuclear scintigraphy suffice.

The classic *pathologic fracture* in childhood is the one occurring through a unicameral bone cyst. Unicameral bone cysts are common in children and most often are located in the metaphyses of long bones, especially the upper humerus (Fig. 4.10C). Indeed, in the Spring, when track-and-field and baseball practice begin, many a child has come to the emergency room with such a fracture. Pathologic fractures also occur through tumors (Fig.4.10D).

REFERENCES

1. Anderson MW, Ugalde V, Batt M, et al. Shin splints: MR appearance in a preliminary study. *Radiology* 1997;204:177–180.
2. Borden S. IV. Roentgen recognition of acute plastic bowing of the forearm in children. *AJR* 1975;125:524–530.
3. Cail WS, Keats TE, Sussman MD. Plastic bowing fracture of the femur in a child. *AJR* 1978;130:780–782.
4. Crowe JE, Swischuk LE. Acute bowing fractures of the forearm in children: A frequently missed injury. *AJR* 1977;128:981–984.
5. Haasbeek JF, Green NE. Adolescent stress fractures of the sacrum: Two case reports. *J Pediatr Orthop* 1994;14:336–338.
6. Horev G, Korenreich L, Ziv N, Grunebaum M. The enigma of stress fractures in the pediatric age: Clarification or confusion through the new imaging modalities. *Pediatr Radiol* 1990;20: 469–471.
7. Keret D, Mendez AA, Harcke HT, MacEwen GD. Type V physeal injury: A case report. *J Pediatr Orthop* 1990;10:545–548.
8. Lee JK, Yao L. Stress fractures: MR imaging. *Radiology* 1988;169: 2217–2220.
9. Mabry JD, Fitch RD. Plastic deformation in pediatric fractures: Mechanism and treatment. *J Pediatr Orthop* 1989;9:310–314.
10. Mendez AA, Bartal E, Grillot MB, Lin JJ. Compression (Salter-Harris type V) physeal fracture: An experimental model in the rat. *J Pediatr Orthop* 1992;12:29–37.
11. Peterson HA, Burkhart SS. Compression injury of the epiphyseal growth plate: Fact or fiction? *J Pediatr Orthop* 1981;1: 377–384.
12. Salter RB, Harris WR. Injuries involving the epiphyseal plate. *J Bone Joint Surg* 1963;45A:587–622.
13. St. Pierre P, Staheli LT, Smith JB, Green NE. Femoral neck stress fractures in children and adolescents. *J Pediatr Orthop* 1995;15: 470–473.
14. Strenstrom R, Gripenberg L, Bergius AR. Traumatic bowing of forearm and lower leg in children. *Acta Radiol* 1978;19: 243–249.
15. Walker RN, Green NE, Spindler KP. Stress fractures in skeletally immature patients. *J Pediatr Orthop* 1996;16:578–584.

Occult Fractures and Obscure Extremity Pain

Often a patient presents with obscure skeletal pain and who in fact may have an occult fracture. Nuclear scintigraphy has proved to be the best screening modality for this problem (1,2,6–8). Bone scintigraphy can demonstrate the presence of a bony injury or even infection before plain film roentgenographic findings become apparent. It is especially useful in detecting early osteomyelitis, occult fractures, and stress fractures (Fig. 4.11A–D). Recently MR imaging also has proven useful in detecting occult fractures (4,5). However, it is not in widespread use on an emergent basis and actually probably is not required very often in children. Occult fractures also can be detected with computed tomographic (CT) imaging (3) and even with ultrasound (2,7), with which the cortical break can be imaged.

Finally, it should be remembered that patients with underlying malignancies such as leukemia (5), lymphoma, and metastatic neuroblastoma can present with obscure bone pain. With leukemia, trophic lines may be the only finding (Fig. 4.11E). Bone destruction also may be seen both with metastatic neuroblastoma and leukemia (Figs. 4.11F and G).

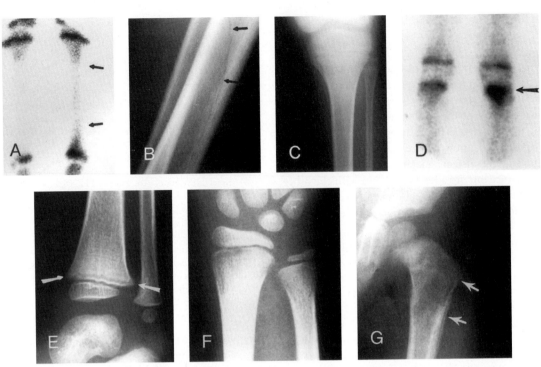

FIGURE 4.11. *Obscure skeletal pain.* **(A)** *Occult fracture.* Nuclear scintigraphy demonstrates an area of increased activity throughout the left tibia (*arrows*). **(B)** Roentgenogram demonstrates a spiral (toddler's) fracture of the tibia (*arrows*). **(C)** Occult osteomyelitis. This patient had acute pain but virtually no swelling in the upper leg on the left. The roentgenographic changes are completely normal and there was little in the way of soft tissue swelling. **(D)** Subsequent bone scan, however, shows marked focal increase in uptake of the isotope in the upper left tibia (*arrow*). **(E)** Patient with leukemia presenting with vague bone pain demonstrates a classic, trophic line in the distal tibia (*arrows*). These trophic lines are nonspecific but highly suggestive of leukemia if bone pain is present. **(F)** Another patient with leukemia demonstrating diffuse bony destruction in the distal radius and ulna. The findings could be mistaken for simple demineralization. **(G)** Metastatic neuroblastoma presenting as hip pain. Note the moth-eaten, permeated bone destruction in the upper femur with some early periosteal new bone (*arrows*).

REFERENCES

1. Aronson J, Garvin K, Seibert J, Glasier C, Tursky EA. Efficiency of the bone scan for occult limping toddlers. *J Pediatr Orthop* 1992;12:38–44.
2. Graif M, Stahl-Kent V, Ben-Ami T, Strauss S, Amit Y, Itzchak Y. Sonographic detection of occult bone fractures. *Pediatr Radiol* 1988;18:383–385.
3. Hindman BW, Kulik WJ, Lee G, Avolio RE. Occult fractures of the carpals and metacarpals demonstration by CT. *AJR* 1989;153: 529–532.
4. Jaramillo D, Hoffer FA, Shapiro F, Rand F. MR imaging of fractures of the growth plate. *AJR* 1990;155:1261–1265.
5. Jonsson OG, Sartain P, Ducore JM, Buchanan GR. Bone pain as an initial symptom of childhood acute lymphoblastic leukemia: Association with nearly normal hematologic indexes. *J Pediatr* 1990;117: 233–237.
6. Park HM, Rothschild PA, Kernek CB. Scintigraphic evaluation of extremity pain in children: Its efficacy and pitfalls. *AJR* 1985;145: 1079–1084.
7. Patten RM, Mack LA, Wang KY, Lingel J. Nondisplaced fractures of the greater tuberosity of the humerus: Sonographic detection. *Radiology* 1992;182:201–204.
8. ter Meulen DC, Majd M. Bone scintigraphy in the evaluation of children with obscure skeletal pain. *Pediatrics* 1987;79:587–592.

Osteomyelitis

Roentgenographic bony changes in osteomyelitis take 10 days to 2 weeks to develop; therefore in the early stages one can only infer the diagnosis from soft tissue changes. Osteomyelitis manifests in deep soft tissue edema; superficial cellulitis demonstrates findings reflecting superficial edema (Fig. 4.12), and thus deep edema should suggest the presence of osteomyelitis until proven otherwise. Soft tissue abscesses also can produce deep edema, but osteomyelitis is more common and is manifest in enlargement of the deep muscle bulk (Fig. 4.12). In addition, at sites such as the distal femur and elbow, displacement of the fat pads overlying the involved metaphyses also can be seen (5).

After 10 to 14 days, bony destruction is seen and can manifest as an acute destructive process or a low-grade

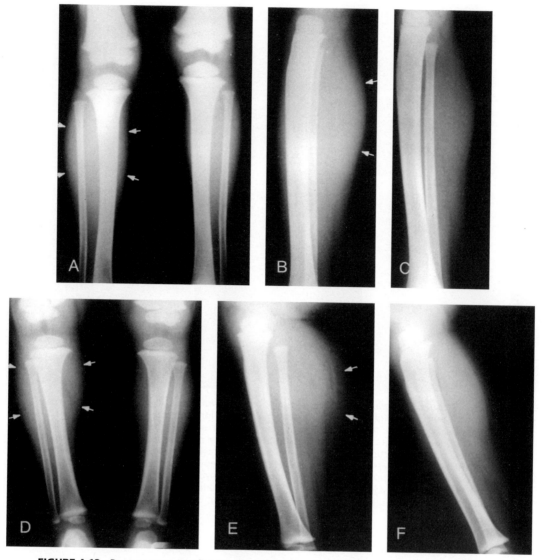

FIGURE 4.12. *Deep versus superficial edema.* **(A)** *Deep edema: osteomyelitis.* Note that the muscle bulk on the right is enlarged (*arrows*), and yet the subcutaneous soft tissues show little in the way of edema. The edge of the muscle is sharp. All of this should point towards a deep inflammatory process (i.e., osteomyelitis or deep abscess). **(B)** Lateral view demonstrating the same phenomenon with marked enlargement of the deep muscle bulk of the calf (*arrows*). The edge of the muscle is sharp. **(C)** Normal side for comparison. Note that the muscle bulk is smaller and less dense. **(D)** Superficial edema: cellulitis. In this patient, note enlargement of the right calf (*arrows*). **(E)** Lateral view shows extensive superficial edema (*arrows*) with thickening and reticulation of the subcutaneous fat. The interface between the muscle and subcutaneous fat is indistinct. **(F)** Normal side for comparison. Compare the muscle bulk with that in **E.** Note that there is no real difference, attesting to the fact that enlargement of the calf on the right results primarily from superficial edema (i.e., cellulitis). The subcutaneous tissues are normal.

smoldering problem. More aggressive permeative and "moth-eaten" changes are seen with the former; with the latter more reactive bony healing or sclerosis is seen (Fig. 4.13). In addition, although osteomyelitis usually is a metaphyseal problem, it can involve the epiphysis (1,3,10) and occasionally the diaphysis only (Fig. 4.13E).

Clinically, in advanced osteomyelitis the extremity is swollen and extremely tender. In the early stages, however, edema may be minimal even though pain is marked, and in such cases an elevated erythrocyte sedimentation rate is a valid positive indicator of underlying infection (11).

If one suspects the presence of osteomyelitis clinically but plain film changes do not support the diagnosis, one should turn to nuclear scintigraphy. Nuclear scintigraphy is the single most effective method with which to detect early underlying bone infection. Although the findings are non-

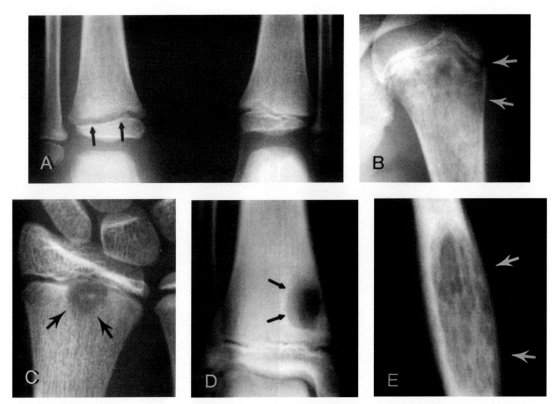

FIGURE 4.13. *Osteomyelitis: various roentgenographic changes.* **(A)** In this patient, only increased lucency and width of the epiphyseal line on the right, resulting from adjacent metaphyseal destruction, are seen (*arrows*). Compare with the normal side. **(B)** Another patient demonstrating more aggressive changes in the upper humeral metaphysis consisting of irregular, permeative bone destruction (*arrows*). **(C)** Low-grade osteomyelitis of the distal radius (*arrows*) with a small central sequestrum. The process has crossed the epiphyseal line and is extending into the epiphysis. **(D)** Low-grade, clean-appearing lytic lesion (*arrows*) with some adjacent sclerosis characteristic of a low-grade Brodie's abscess. **(E)** Unusual middiaphyseal low-grade osteomyelitis (*arrows*). The findings could be mistaken for a Ewing's tumor.

specific, if one utilizes the three-phase technetium-99m pyrophosphate study consisting of the blood flow, blood pool, and static-imaging phases (11), occult osteomyelitis usually is detected and differentiated from cellulitis (Fig. 4.14A–C). It should be remembered, however, that the pyrophosphate bone scan measures reactive (healing) bone activity and not the development of a purulent exudate *per se*. It is for this reason that in some cases imaging with gallium- or indium-labeled white blood cells (9) may be required to determine whether an infection is present. In the pediatric age group, however, osteomyelitis is relatively clean and is a first-time focal event, and thus the technetium-99m pyrophosphate study usually suffices. On the other hand, it should be remembered that in many cases, the technetium bone scan, in the very early stages of the infection, may appear falsely normal (2).

The reason for the bone scan being normal in such early stages is that there is so much congestion of the bone marrow by the developing infection that blood flow, and hence

the delivery of the isotope to the bone, is impaired. Usually within 24 to 48 hr results of the bone scan are positive. Therefore, if one can make the presumptive diagnosis of osteomyelitis on the basis of clinical and plain film roentgenographic (deep edema) findings, then one should assume that such infection is present and begin therapy. The bone scan, primarily for confirmation, then can be delayed for a day or two.

Because of the problem of the falsely negative bone scan, CT and MR imaging also have been utilized in the detection of early osteomyelitis (4,6). In addition, ultrasonography has been utilized for this purpose (7). With ultrasound the findings depend on demonstration of hypoechoic purulent exudate between the periosteum and the cortex of the bone (Fig. 4.15). Of all imaging modalities, however, it is the least useful. On CT scans, bone marrow changes are subtle, with the normally radiolucent bone marrow showing increased density or signal. Bone destruction, however, is very precisely delineated (Fig. 4.15C). With MR imaging

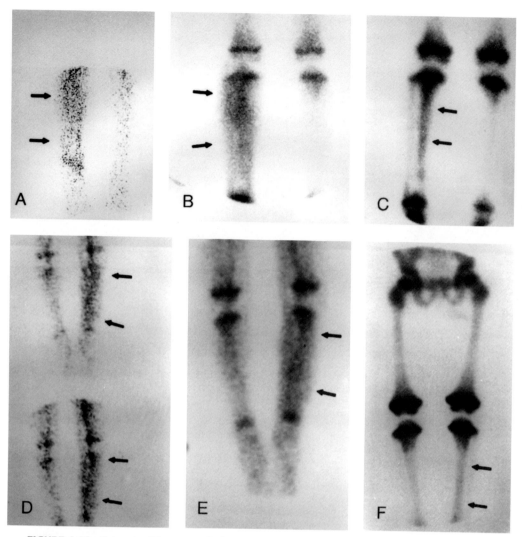

FIGURE 4.14. *Osteomyelitis verus cellulitis: nuclear scintigraphy technetium-99m bone scan.* **(A)** Osteomyelitis. Flow phase demonstrates increased flow to the right lower leg (*arrows*). **(B)** Blood pool phase demonstrates pooling of isotope in the right lower extremity (*arrows*). **(C)** Static scan demonstrates diffusely increased uptake over the entire right tibia (*arrows*). **(D)** Cellulitis. Flow phase demonstrates increased flow to the left lower leg (*arrows*). **(E)** Blood pool phase demonstrates pooling of isotope into the right lower extremity (*arrows*). **(F)** Static scan, however, fails to demonstrate significant accumulation of isotope in the tibial shaft (*arrows*). There is a faint ghost of the shaft suggested. This speaks against osteomyelitis and in favor of cellulitis, for although there always is a minor degree of reactive periosteal activity with adjacent soft-tissue inflammation, for the bone scan to be positive for osteomyelitis, it must show markedly increased uptake of the isotope as seen in **C.**

the normal high signal of fat on the T1-weighted images is lost; on the proton-density or T2-weighted images, increased signal is seen (Fig. 4.15D–F).

Nuclear scintigraphy also can be utilized to differentiate osteomyelitis from cellulitis. Although in these conditions the blood flow and blood pool findings may be identical, with cellulitis there is no significant accumulation of the isotope agent in the bone itself. Only a ghost of the bone may be seen (Fig. 4.14D–F).

Most cases of osteomyelitis in childhood are hematogenous in origin, but some result from puncture wounds, with secondary involvement of the underlying bone. A very small number result from osteomyelitis superimposed on a previous fracture (8). In any event, the bony changes are the same, but it should be noted that osteomyelitis in flat bones (i.e., pelvic bones, clavicle, ribs, scapula) is much more difficult to detect with plain films, and it is in these instances that nuclear scintigraphy has a major role. In addition, CT

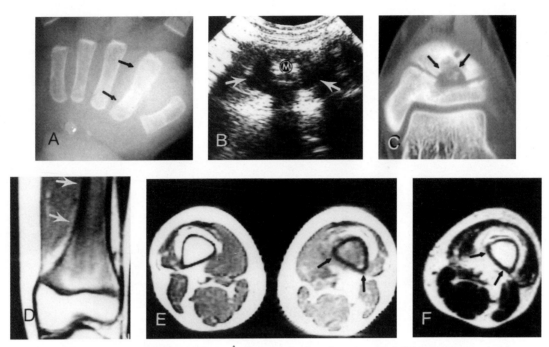

FIGURE 4.15. *Osteomyelitis: Demonstration with various imaging modalities.* **(A)** Note mixed destruction and reactive sclerosis of the second metatarsal (*arrows*) in this infant with osteomyelitis. There is considerable soft tissue swelling. **(B)** Sonogram demonstrates a ring of hypoechoic pus (*arrows*) around the metacarpal (*M*). **(C)** Computed tomographic study in another patient demonstrates a discrete focus of destruction in the distal tibia (*arrows*) with a suggestion of a small bony sequestrum. **(D)** T1-weighted magnetic resonance image in another patient demonstrates decreased signal in the bone marrow of the distal left femur (*arrows*). The plain film changes in this patient were near normal. Only a small focus of suspicious bony destruction was seen on the lateral view. **(E)** T1-weighted axial images demonstrate decreased signal of the marrow of the involved femur (*arrows*). There is surrounding soft tissue edema. **(F)** Proton-density image demonstrates increased signal in the involved marrow (*arrows*) indicating the presence of pus. In addition, surrounding edema now shows increased signal.

and MR imaging can be utilized, but nuclear scintigraphy is less expensive.

REFERENCES

1. Andrew TA, Porter K. Primary subacute epiphyseal osteomyelitis: A report of three cases. *J Pediatr Orthop* 1985;5:155–157.
2. Berkwitz ID, Wenzel W. "Normal" technetium bone scans in patients with acute osteomyelitis. *Am J Dis Child* 1980;134:828–830.
3. Bogoch E, Thompson G, Salter RB. Foci of chronic circumscribed osteomyelitis (Brodie's abscess) that traverse the epiphyseal plate. *J Pediatr Orthop* 1984;4:162–169.
4. Dangman BC, Hoffer FA, Rand FF, O'Rourke EJ. Osteomyelitis in children: Gadolinium enhanced MR imaging. *Radiology* 1992;182:743–747.
5. Hayden CK Jr, Swischuk LE. Para-articular soft tissue changes in infections and trauma of the lower extremity in children. *AJR* 1980;134:307–311.
6. Hernandez RJ, Conway JJ, Poznanski AK, Tachdjian MO, Dias LS, Kelikian AS. The role of computed tomography and radionuclide scintigraphy in the localization of osteomyelitis in flat bones. *J Pediatr Orthop* 1985;5:151–154.
7. Kaiser S, Sosenberg M. Early detection of subperiosteal abscesses by ultrasonography: A means for further successful treatment in pediatric osteomyelitis. *Pediatr Radiol* 1994;24:336–339.
8. Morrissy RT, Haynes DW. Acute hematogenous osteomyelitis: A model with trauma as an etiology. *J Pediatr Orthop* 1989;9:447–456.
9. Raptopoulos V, Dohery PW, Goss TP, King MA, Johnson K, Gantz NM. Acute osteomyelitis: Advantage of white cell scans in early detection. *AJR* 1982;139:1077–1082.
10. Rosenbaum DM, Blumhagen JD. Acute epiphyseal osteomyelitis in children. *Radiology* 1985;156:89–92.
11. Scott RJ, Christofersen MR, Robertson WW Jr, Davidson RS, Rankin L, Drummond DS. Acute osteomyelitis in children: A review of 116 cases. *J Pediatr Orthop* 1990;10:649–652.

Osteomyelitis versus Bone Infarction in Sickle Cell Disease

The problem of differentiating bone infection from bone infarction in patients with sickle-cell disease is difficult. Clinically and roentgenographically the findings may be similar in the early stages, but extremity swelling is usually more marked in osteomyelitis. Nuclear scintigraphy is of value in some of these cases (1), because with a fresh infarct the bone scan shows decreased uptake in the area of infarction. Later, the area becomes positive, for the bone scan records reactive, healing bone activity. In this regard, however, the findings are no different than in osteomyelitis. Therefore, one should proceed to scintigraphy with a bone-marrow imaging agent such as gallium citrate or indium-labeled white blood cells. These studies can yield further data as to whether an infarction or an infection is present. With infarction the gallium- or indium-labeled white blood cell studies are negative (Fig. 4.16A–C).

If a patient has sustained multiple episodes of bone infarction, the findings on nuclear scintigraphy can be more confusing than helpful (Fig. 4.16D–F). Therefore, very often one must make the final determination on the basis of clinical, laboratory, and other imaging findings. If pronounced and extensive swelling of the extremity is present, simple infarction is unlikely. If only focal pain with minimal swelling is present, however, the problem can be caused by either infection or infarction. Furthermore, it is quite likely that infarction precedes infection in many if not most of these cases, and this only adds to the confusion. Even if CT (3) and MR imaging are employed, they may not be helpful, for with both infection and infarction, bone-marrow insult and bone insult occur. If one process affected the bone only and the other the marrow only, then the problem for the most part would be resolved, but because both involve the marrow the problem exists. In the end, there is no simple

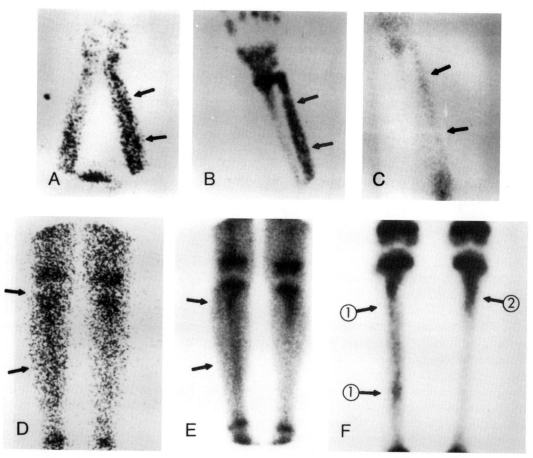

FIGURE 4.16. *Nuclear scintigraphy: bone infarct.* **(A)** Blood flow phase demonstrates increased flow to the right upper extremity (*arrows*). **(B)** Static scans demonstrate markedly increased uptake of isotope throughout the entire ulna (*arrows*) on the right. **(C)** Subsequent gallium bone scan shows vague and very subtle increase in activity in the left ulna. If this patient had osteomyelitis, the signal in the left ulna would be significantly increased. **(D)** Another patient with increased flow to a painful right lower extremity (*arrows*). **(E)** Blood pool phase demonstrates the same findings (*arrows*). Note, however, that the upper left tibial metaphysis also shows increased uptake of isotope. **(F)** Subsequent static scan demonstrates diffuse, but spotty, uptake of isotope throughout the right tibia (*1*). The uptake, however, is irregular. In addition, there is increased uptake in the upper left tibia (*2*). A gallium scan would have been most helpful in this patient; otherwise, it is difficult to interpret the findings, for some result from old healing infarctions. This patient had no signs or symptoms referable to the left leg. Presumably the findings in the upper left tibia result from an old healing infarct. In view of this, how can one be certain that the increased areas of activity in the right tibia are caused by osteomyelitis? One cannot, and that is why these cases are so puzzling and why additional scans are necessary.

answer to the problem, and even ultrasound is helpful only in the later stages (2).

REFERENCES

1. Rao S, Solomon N, Miller S, Dunn E. Scintigraphic differentiation of bone infarction from osteomyelitis in children with sickle cell disease. *J Pediatr* 1985;107:685–688.
2. Sadat-Ali M, Al-Umran K, Al-Habdan I, Al-Mulhim F. Ultrasonography: Can it differentiate between vaso-occlusive crisis and acute osteomyelitis in sickle cell disease? *J Pediatr Orthop* 1998;18: 552–554.
3. Stark JE, Glasier CM, Blasier RD, Aronson J, Seibert JJ. Osteomyelitis in children with sickle cell disease: Early diagnosis with contrast-enhanced CT. *Radiology* 1991;179:731–733.

Septic Arthritis

The roentgenographic assessment of septic arthritis centers around the detection of fluid in the involved joint and periarticular soft tissue edema. For the most part, this is accomplished by noting increased width of the joint space and displacement of fat pads where applicable, and by comparing the suspicious findings on the abnormal side with those on the normal side. Assessment of all of the bony and soft-tissue structures is especially important in the very young infant, in whom little in the way of systemic response to infection often is present. In other words, fever is not high, leukocytosis is not striking, toxicity is not marked, and the only finding may be an inability to move the involved extremity (pseudoparesis). However, with properly positioned roentgenograms and an evaluation of the joint space and soft tissues, one usually detects the problem. In this regard in the absence of trauma fluid in the joint should be considered pus until proven otherwise.

In the past, nuclear scintigraphy has been advocated for the differentiation of septic arthritis from other inflammatory processes around the joint but generally speaking it is not overly productive in this role. Ultimately, one must rely on clinical findings and plain films in most cases, and then, if suspicion is high, arthrocentesis is required. Ultrasonography, however, has become useful, especially in the hip joint, where plain films often are unrewarding. More detailed discussions of the findings of septic arthritis for each joint are undertaken at other points in this chapter.

Pyomyositis

Pyomyositis in children is more common than generally believed (1,2). It can be confused with osteomyelitis, and in some cases frank abscess formation ensues. Plain film findings in pyomyositis simply demonstrate deep soft tissue edema and expansion of the involved muscle compartment. In this regard the findings are not different from those seen with osteomyelitis. On ultrasound, however, if an abscess is present, it becomes clearly visible. Usually one does not require imaging beyond ultrasound to detect these abscesses. If no abscess is present, only swelling of the muscle with increased echogenicity and volume is seen. Nuclear scintigraphy demonstrates accumulation of isotope if gallium or white blood cell examinations are utilized.

REFERENCES

1. Renwick SE, Ritterbusch JF. Pyomyositis in children. *J Pediatr Orthop* 1993;13:769–772.
2. Spiegel DA, Meyer JS, Dormans JP, Flynn JM, Drummond DS. Pyomyositis in children and adolescents: Report of 12 cases and review of the literature. *J Pediatr Orthop* 1999;19:143–150.

UPPER EXTREMITY PROBLEMS
Shoulder
Normal Soft Tissues of the Shoulder

There are no specific fat pads to evaluate around the shoulder, but over the clavicle the companion shadow can be of some use. This shadow represents the edge of the skin and subcutaneous tissues as they pass over the clavicle, and the edge can become obliterated by the edema associated with clavicular fractures (see Fig. 4.18C). Other than this, evaluation of the soft tissues of the shoulder is nonspecific.

Detecting Fluid in the Shoulder Joints

Fluid in the shoulder joints (i.e., pus or blood) causes the humerus to be displaced laterally and the joint space to be widened (Fig. 4.17). Associated swelling, edema, and bulging of the soft tissues around the shoulder may or may not be present and are more likely to occur in young infants.

The shoulder for examination in these cases can be in almost any reasonable anteroposterior position, as long as both the involved and noninvolved extremities are examined in the same position. In other words, one wants to avoid the situation in which one extremity is examined in internal rotation but the other is examined in external rotation. On a practical basis, it often is best to examine the involved extremity in whichever position the patient holds that extremity, and then to match that position in the normal extremity. Furthermore, *it is probably best to obtain views of both shoulders on the same film and not on separate films.*

Clavicular Injuries

Overall, the clavicle is the most commonly injured bone of the shoulder in infants and young children. Injury usually results from falling on an outstretched extremity, falling

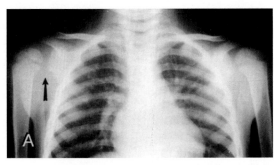
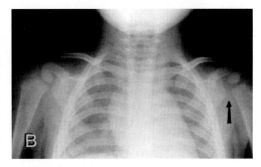

FIGURE 4.17. *Detecting fluid in the shoulder joint.* **(A)** Note widening of the joint space on the right (*arrow*). The upper humerus and humeral head are displaced laterally from the glenoid fossa. This signifies the presence of intraarticular fluid. This child had *Haemophilus influenzae* septic arthritis. **(B)** Another patient with joint widening on the left (*arrow*) resulting from a Salter–Harris type I epiphyseal–metaphyseal fracture. Note that the epiphyseal line between the humeral head and metaphysis is wider than the one on the normal right side.

directly on the shoulder, or a direct blow to the clavicle. By far the most common location for a clavicular fracture is the midshaft, and although many such fractures are easy to identify (Fig. 4.18A), others are more elusive. One reason for this is that many clavicular fractures are greenstick fractures, plastic bowing fractures, or other fractures with a poorly visible fracture line. In all of these cases, one should learn to look first for abnormal angulation or curvature of the injured clavicle. This is best accomplished by comparing one clavicle with the other, and any discrepancy should

be treated with suspicion. In addition, one also should assess the soft tissues for a general increase in density resulting from edema and bleeding, obliteration of the companion shadow of the clavicle, and obliteration of the supraclavicular fat–muscle interfaces (Fig. 4.18B and C).

Complete fractures through the midshaft of the clavicle, with displacement of the fracture fragments, also are common but are not a problem as far as roentgenographic detection is concerned. Even in these cases, however, very often the position of the fracture is such that it is hidden by

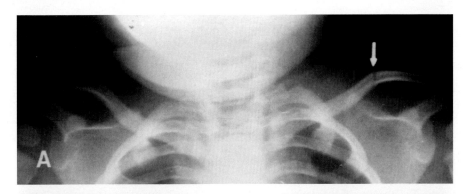
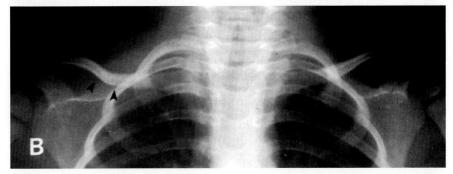

FIGURE 4.18. *Clavicular fractures.* **(A)** *Typical fracture of clavicle.* Note the easily identified fracture (*arrow*) of the bent left clavicle. **(B)** Subtle bending fracture. The only signs of a clavicular injury in this patient are those of unusual downward bending of the right clavicle (*arrows*) and a generalized increase in density (edema) of the soft tissues around it.

(continued on next page)

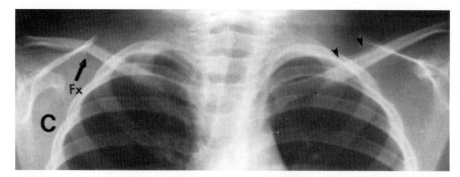

FIGURE 4.18. *(continued)* **(C)** Subtle bending fracture with soft tissue changes. In this patient, there is unusual bending of the right clavicle, but the fracture line (*Fx*) is difficult to see because it is obscured by the overlying scapular tip. Note that there is a generalized increase in soft tissue density of the soft tissues in the right supraclavicular region, however, and that the companion shadow on the right is absent. Compare these findings with the normal findings on the left, including the presence of a normal companion shadow (*arrows*). The companion shadow represents the interface between the air and the skin and subcutaneous tissues overlying the clavicle. With edema and swelling, these soft tissues thicken and the companion shadow is lost.

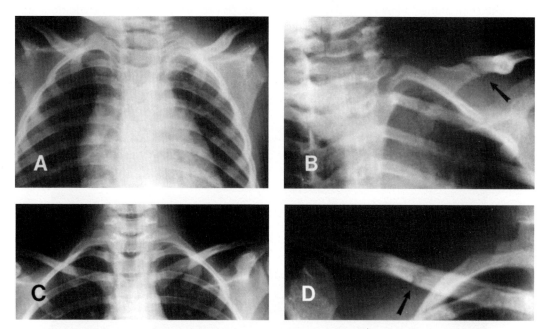

FIGURE 4.19. *Occult clavicular fractures.* **(A)** The clavicles are quite symmetric, but note soft tissue swelling over the left clavicle. Also note that it might be more bent than the right. **(B)** Oblique view demonstrates a clear-cut fracture through the medial portion of the left clavicle (*arrow*). **(C)** Curvature of the clavicles is asymmetric, which is important. This patient had injury to the right shoulder, but one cannot see the fracture behind the second rib. **(D)** Another view, more oblique, demonstrates the fracture (*arrow*).

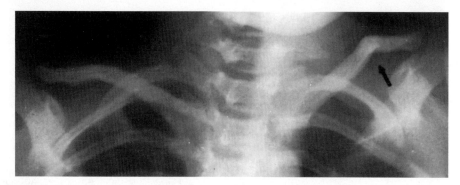

FIGURE 4.20. *Pseudofracture of the clavicle resulting from rotation.* This patient is rotated to the left; this causes the left clavicle to telescope and appear bent (*arrow*).

the first or second ribs. It is only with oblique or lordotic views that one can actually see the fracture (Fig. 4.19).

The most important pitfall in the evaluation of suspected clavicular fractures lies in the misinterpretation of a clavicle distorted by poor positioning or patient rotation, for a fractured clavicle (Fig. 4.20).

Acromioclavicular separations are not particularly common in infancy but do occur in the older child and adolescent. In such cases, one should first look for soft tissue prominence over the acromioclavicular joint and then for separation of the joint itself. Although the acromioclavicular joint is widened, one often also notes widening between the clavicle and the coracoid process of the scapula (Fig. 4.21). Indeed, separation at this site caused by ligamentous sprain often is easier to detect than is acromioclavicular separation. Furthermore, in some of these cases it has been noted that an associated coracoid process fracture can occur (4). In the infant and young child, rather than acromioclavicular separation, an isolated fracture through the lateral end of the clavicle usually is sustained. Even in some of these cases, however, a certain degree of acromioclavicular separation and coracoclavicular ligament sprain exists (Fig. 4.22).

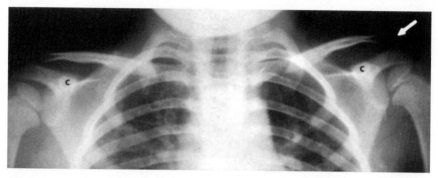

FIGURE 4.21. *Acromioclavicular separation.* First note that the left clavicle is higher than the right, and then note that the acromioclavicular joint on the left is widened (*arrow*). In addition, however, note that the space between the clavicle and the coracoid process (C) also is increased (coracoclavicular ligament sprain).

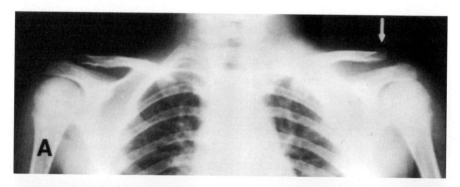

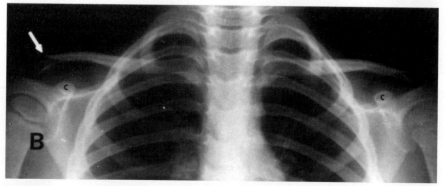

FIGURE 4.22. *Lateral clavicular fracture with varying degrees of acromioclavicular and coracoclavicular separation.* **(A)** Note the fracture of the lateral end of the left clavicle (*arrow*). The space between the fracture fragment and acromial process of the scapula is barely widened. Minimal if any associated acromioclavicular separation exists. **(B)** Note the fracture of the lateral end of the right clavicle (*arrow*). Also note, however, that the space between the clavicle and coracoid process (C) is widened secondary to associated coracoclavicular ligament sprain. Although not visible on this illustration, a mild degree of acromioclavicular separation also was present in this patient.

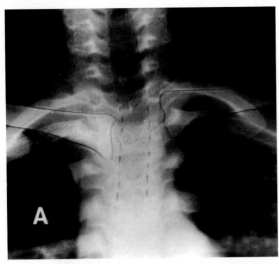
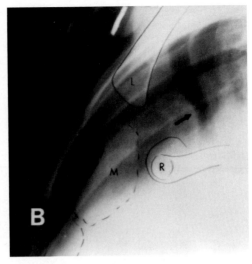

FIGURE 4.23. *Medial clavicular dislocation.* **(A)** Frontal view demonstrating typical downward displacement of the medial end of the right clavicle. This can occur with either posterior or anterior dislocations. **(B)** Oblique view demonstrating the posteriorly displaced right clavicle (*R*) and normally aligned left clavicle (*L*). Note associated anterior indentation of the trachea (*arrow*). *M*, manubrium. (From Lee FA, Gwinn JL. Retrosternal dislocation of the clavicle. *Radiology* 1974;110: 631–634, with permission.)

Medial clavicular injuries usually consist of ***anterior or posterior dislocations,*** for fracturing in this area is relatively uncommon (2). With anterior displacement, a clinically visible and palpable bulge is present over the involved sternoclavicular joint. With posterior displacement, such a bulge is not present, but a more serious problem arises: Tracheal compression occurs (Fig. 4.23). On frontal view, dislocation of the medial end of the clavicle, either anterior or posterior, should be suspected if the medial end of the involved clavicle is lower than the medial end of the normal clavicle (Fig. 4.23). Occasionally the clavicle is displaced upward (Fig. 4.24), but in any case CT scanning should be the next study performed. It can

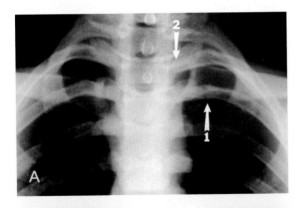

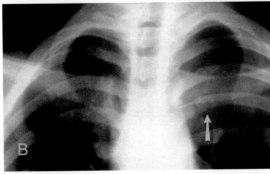

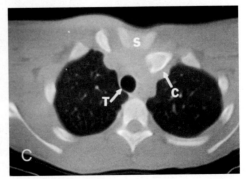

FIGURE 4.24. *Superior medial dislocation of clavicle.* **(A)** Note the elevated medial end of the left clavicle (*1*). The sternoclavicular joint is disrupted and widened (*2*). **(B)** Another patient with an elevated medial end of the left clavicle (*C*). **(C)** Axial computed tomographic study demonstrates the posteriorly displaced left medial clavicle (*arrow*). Note that the trachea is not compressed. Also note the normal position of the medial end of the right clavicle. *C*, clavicle; *T*, trachea.

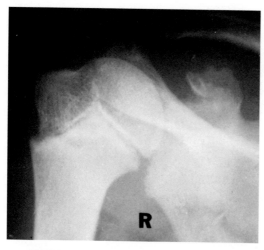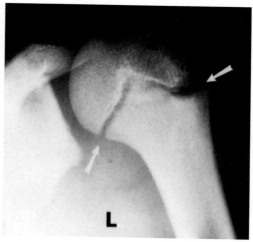

FIGURE 4.25. *Epiphyseal–metaphyseal fracture of the upper left humerus.* Note that the epiphyseal line on the left is wider and more radiolucent (*arrows*) than the one on the right. Such widening of the epiphyseal line denotes the presence of a Salter–Harris type injury, either I or II. The findings above are those of a Salter–Harris type I injury. In addition, note that on the normal side the humeral head along its lateral aspect appears offset or displaced on the metaphysis. This is normal and should not be misinterpreted as a displaced epiphyseal fracture.

very clearly delineate the position of the clavicle and detect any associated avulsion fractures (Fig. 4.24).

Injuries of the Upper Humerus

In childhood, one of the more common injuries of the upper humerus is the Salter–Harris type I or II epiphyseal–metaphyseal injury (Figs. 4.25–4.27). Salter–Harris type III epiphyseal injuries are less common (Fig. 4.27C), and type IV and V injuries are quite uncommon in the shoulder. In those type I and II injuries in which the epiphysis is completely separated, the diagnosis is never in doubt (3), but in the more subtle cases, one should look for widening of the epiphyseal line or the presence of a meta-

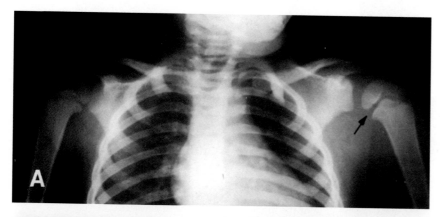

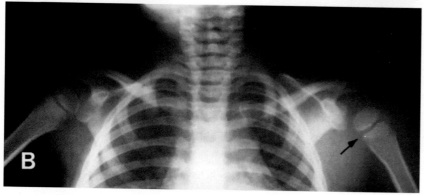

FIGURE 4.26. *Epiphyseal–metaphyseal fracture: shoulder.* (**A**) Note widening of the epiphyseal line of the upper left humerus (*arrow*). Also note that the joint space is widened, suggesting fluid (blood) in the joint. (**B**) Another view demonstrating similar findings. Note especially that the epiphyseal line remains widened (*arrow*). *(continued on next page)*

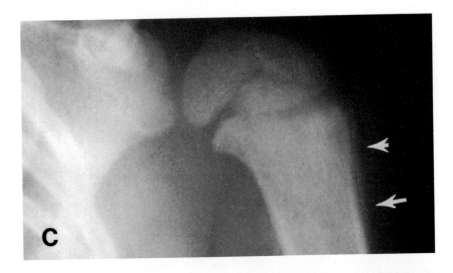

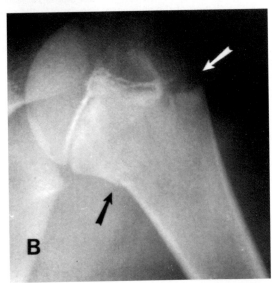

FIGURE 4.26. *(continued)* **(C)** Follow-up film 2 weeks later demonstrates healing of the fracture with periosteal new bone along the upper humeral shaft (*arrows*).

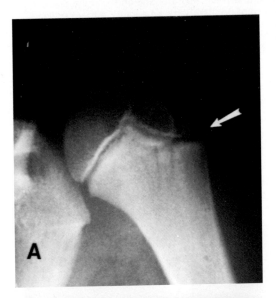

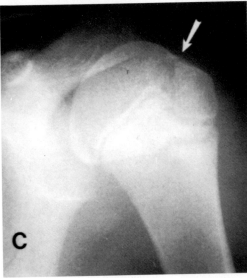

FIGURE 4.27. *Other epiphyseal–metaphyseal fractures of the upper humerus.* **(A)** Salter–Harris type II injury with a widened epiphyseal line laterally (*arrow*) and two poorly defined vertical fracture lines extending into the upper humeral shaft. **(B)** Salter–Harris type II injury with a widened epiphyseal line laterally (*white arrow*) and a cortical break medially (*black arrow*). The metaphyseal fracture fragment is rather large in this patient. **(C)** Salter–Harris type III injury. Note the fracture (*arrow*) through the nondisplaced epiphysis.

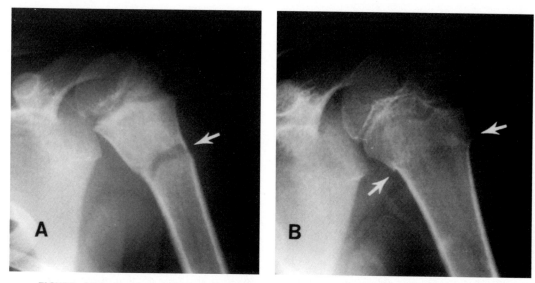

FIGURE 4.28. *Upper humeral shaft fractures.* **(A)** Typical transverse surgical neck fracture (*arrow*). **(B)** Buckle compression-type fracture of the upper humerus (*arrows*). This type of fracture is quite common in infants and young children, because the cortex in this area is still relatively weak.

physeal corner fracture. In chronic form, this same injury is seen in young boys playing baseball and partaking in overexuberant stressful pitching. It is termed **Little Leaguer's shoulder** (1,6).

Other fractures occurring through the upper humerus include the easily identified surgical neck fracture, transverse or oblique upper humeral shaft fractures, and the more subtle buckle or torus fractures (Fig. 4.28). In addition, *it should be noted that pathologic fractures through*

unicameral bone cysts quite commonly occur in the upper humerus (Fig. 4.10C).

A major pitfall in the evaluation of the upper humeral fractures is misinterpretation of the normal epiphyseal line as a fracture. This can occur if the epiphyseal line is open and wide or closing and narrow (Fig. 4.29). Of course, if comparative views of the normal extremity are obtained, almost always the line appears exactly the same, and the problem is solved. This simple solution notwithstanding, it

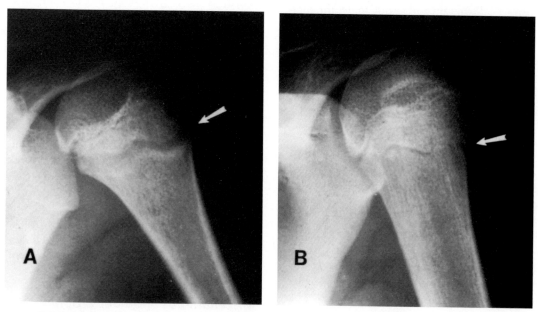

FIGURE 4.29. *Pseudofracture upper humerus: normal epiphyseal line.* **(A)** Normal appearance of a wide epiphyseal line (*arrow*) often misinterpreted as a fracture. **(B)** Older child with narrower epiphyseal line mimicking a fracture (*arrow*).

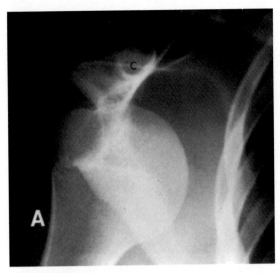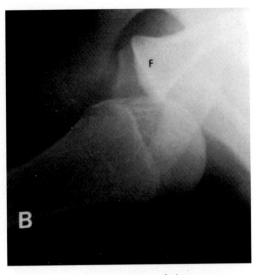

FIGURE 4.30. *Anterior dislocation of the shoulder.* **(A)** Note abnormal position of the upper humerus. It is located below the coracoid process (C). This is a subcoracoid dislocation. **(B)** Transaxillary view showing dislocated humerus anterior to the glenoid fossa (F). With subglenoid dislocations, the humeral head lies under the glenoid fossa; with posterior dislocations it lies posterior to the scapula.

is still very common to mistake this normal finding for a fracture.

Dislocations of the shoulder are not common in the young infant and child, for it is only after the epiphysis closes that it becomes a problem. The dislocations, of course, can be either anterior (i.e., subglenoid or subcoracoid) or posterior. The posterior dislocations are more difficult to detect, for overlapping of the humeral head and the glenoid fossa can be subtle. Anterior dislocations usually have a rather characteristic appearance, with the humeral head being displaced downward and resting under the coracoid process or glenoid fossa (Fig. 4.30). In any case, and especially with posterior dislocations, transaxillary views of the shoulder should be obtained for clearer definition (Fig. 4.30). Of course, CT studies now also can be obtained and are especially useful for locating the humeral head and any associated glenoid avulsions.

Scapular Fractures

These can occur through the body of the scapula or the acromial or coracoid processes of the scapula. Fractures through the body of the scapula usually result from direct blows and can be linear, curvilinear (Fig. 4.31), or stellate. Fractures through the acromial and coracoid processes of the scapula can result from direct blows or falls on the outstretched extremity and may be difficult to detect (Fig. 4.31). Comparative views are of the utmost importance here, especially with the more peculiar fractures (Fig. 4.31E and F), and of course CT studies are invaluable in analyzing fractures of the scapula, especially those of the glenoid fossa (Fig. 4.32).

Septic Arthritis, Osteomyelitis, and Cellulitis of the Shoulder

With septic arthritis, the most important roentgenographic features are joint space widening and lateral displacement of the upper humerus (Fig. 4.33A and B). These findings denote the presence of pus in the shoulder joint (5), and in the very young infant the adjacent soft tissues may appear edematous and cause the whole shoulder to bulge. In the older child, however, joint-space widening usually is the only finding, and in many cases nothing is seen. Ultrasound may be useful for demonstrating occult pus in these cases, for similar to the hip, increase in the width of the joint space may be more difficult to detect in older children.

If osteomyelitis or cellulitis of the shoulder is present, there usually is little in the way of joint space widening, except in the young infant, in whom septic arthritis and osteomyelitis frequently occur together. In such cases, of course, features of both conditions are present (Fig. 4.33C and D). With osteomyelitis alone, however, early findings usually consist of nothing more than soft tissue edema and obliteration of the normal fat–muscle tissue planes. This causes the soft tissues to appear more homogeneously opaque than normal (Fig. 4.34A and B) and, later on, bony destruction can be seen (Fig. 4.34C). Cellulitis around the shoulder is not a particularly common problem in children.

Miscellaneous Shoulder Problems

Occasionally, one can encounter a patient who does not move his or her upper extremity because of scapular or clav-

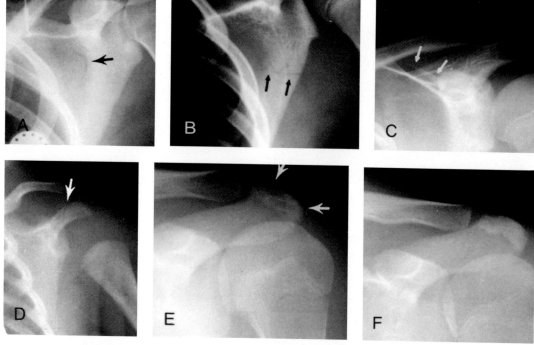

FIGURE 4.31. *Scapular fracture.* **(A)** Typical curvilinear fracture (*arrow*) of the body of the scapula. **(B)** Transverse, linear fracture (*arrows*) of the scapula. **(C)** Avulsion fracture (*arrows*) of the upper scapular edge in an older child. **(D)** Acromial fracture (*arrow*) in a battered infant. **(E)** Bending fracture of acromion. Note peculiar shape of acromial process (*arrows*). This was a bending fracture of the acromion resulting from a direct fall on the tip of the shoulder. **(F)** Normal side for comparison.

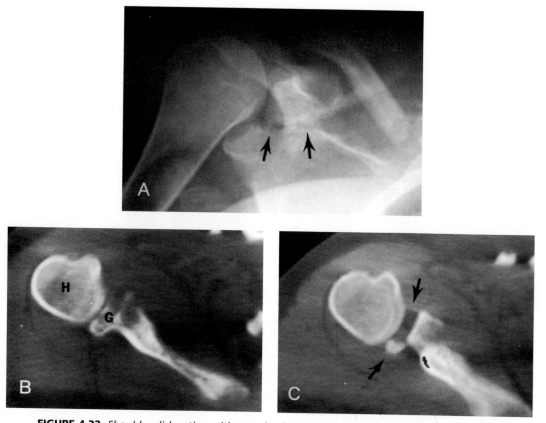

FIGURE 4.32. *Shoulder dislocation with scapular fracture: computed tomographic findings.* **(A)** Note the superiorly dislocated humerus and the associated fracture through the glenoid fossa (*arrows*). The humeral head still is articulating with the superior fragment. **(B)** Upper computed tomographic cut demonstrates the humeral head (*H*) articulating with the superior portion of the glenoid fossa (*G*). **(C)** Lower cut demonstrates widening of the joint space (*upper arrow*) and a small avulsed bony fragment (*lower arrow*).

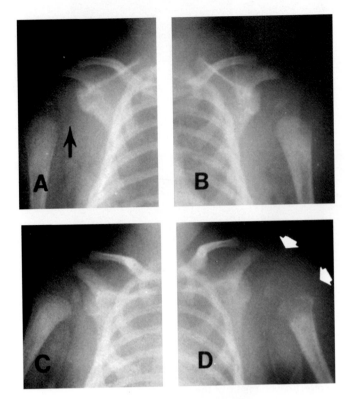

FIGURE 4.33. *Septic arthritis.* **(A)** Note widening of the joint space (*arrow*), resulting from pus in the joint. **(B)** Normal left side for comparison. **(C)** Septic arthritis and osteomyelitis. Normal right shoulder. **(D)** On the left, note bulging of the soft tissues of the left shoulder (*arrows*) and widening of the joint space caused by pus in the joint. Destruction of the upper humerus also is present. If this patient had osteomyelitis alone, little if any joint space widening would occur. Contrarily, if septic arthritis were the only problem, no bone destruction of the metaphysis would be seen, and soft-tissue swelling would be less pronounced.

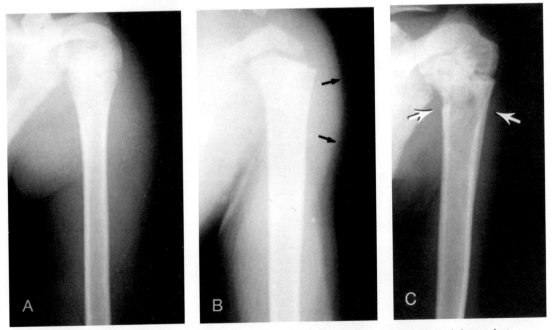

FIGURE 4.34. *Osteomyelitis.* **(A)** *Early changes in older child.* Note that the humerus is intact, but that there is extensive deep and superficial edema of the adjacent soft tissues. No muscle–fat planes are identified, and the soft tissues are of increased, homogeneous density. **(B)** Normal shoulder for comparison, demonstrating the normal interface between the muscle and the subcutaneous fat (*arrows*). Note that the other fat–muscle interfaces also are clearly visible. **(C)** Later, notice destruction of the upper humeral metaphysis and some early periosteal new bone deposition (*arrows*).

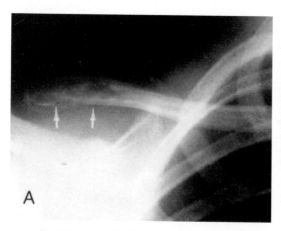

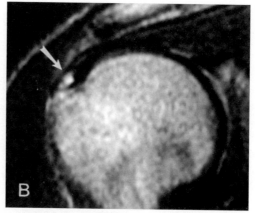

FIGURE 4.35. **(A)** *Histiocytosis X of clavicle.* Note the expanding, lytic, somewhat bubbly lesion of the distal right clavicle (*arrows*). **(B)** Rotator cuff injury. Coronal magnetic resonance image demonstrates a focus of high signal in the supraspinatus tendon (*arrow*).

icular involvement in Caffey's disease (infantile cortical hyperostosis), osteomyelitis of the scapula or clavicle, metastatic disease, or histiocytosis X of the bones of the shoulder (Fig. 4.35A), or a rotator cuff injury. The latter currently is best evaluated with MR imaging but is not a common problem in childhood. With MR imaging, tears of the supraspinatus muscle and tendon produce focal high-signal levels because of the edema and bleeding in the supraspinatus tendon (Fig. 4.35B).

Normal Findings Causing Problems

Misinterpretation of the upper humeral epiphyseal line as a fracture has been dealt with previously and is demonstrated in Figure 4.29. Other normal structures frequently misinterpreted as abnormalities include a bony exostosis along the inferior aspect of the clavicle just at the site of the costoclavicular ligament (Fig. 4.36A) and a normal accessory ossification center at the medial end of the clav-

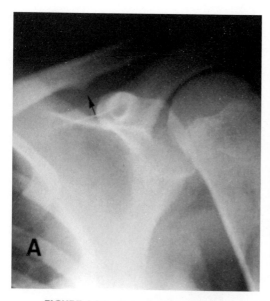

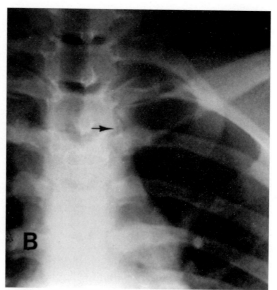

FIGURE 4.36. *Normal variations of the clavicle.* **(A)** Note the bony exostosis (*arrow*) at the site of the insertion of the costoclavicular ligament. **(B)** Normal medial accessory ossification center (*arrow*). The wire loop just below and medial to it is a wire suture in the sternum from a prior thoracotomy.

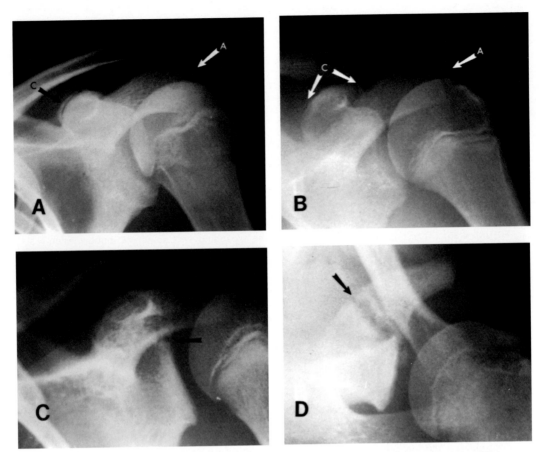

FIGURE 4.37. *Normal findings: scapular ossification centers.* (**A** and **B**) *Usual accessory centers.* Note the variable appearance of the accessory ossification centers of the acromion (*A*) and coracoid (*C*) processes. (**C**) Large coracoid secondary center. Note the junction between the large coracoid secondary center and the scapula (*arrow*), simulating a fracture. (**D**) Special oblique view demonstrating that the fracture fragment actually is a large coracoid secondary center, and that the junction between it and the scapula produces a pseudofracture line (*arrow*). These large secondary centers should not be misinterpreted as fractures. This patient had a similar center in the other scapula.

icle (Fig. 4.36B). Still other normal structures causing problems include the various ossification centers of the scapula (Fig. 4.37); the secondary center for the coracoid process can be very large and surely suggestive of a fracture in some individuals (Fig. 4.37C and D). In addition, the ring apophysis of the glenoid fossa, if caught tangentially, can erroneously suggest a glenoid rim avulsion fracture (Fig. 4.38).

Vascular grooves in the scapula also can create problems and be misinterpreted as fractures (Fig. 4.39). Finally, the normal deltoid notch, a finding frequently misinterpreted as a destructive lesion, and the vacuum-joint phenomenon around the shoulder are examples of other findings causing uncertainties in interpretation (Fig. 4.40).

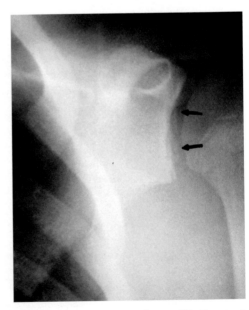

FIGURE 4.38. *Glenoid rim: secondary ossification center.* Note the fracture fragment–like secondary center (*arrows*) of the glenoid fossa.

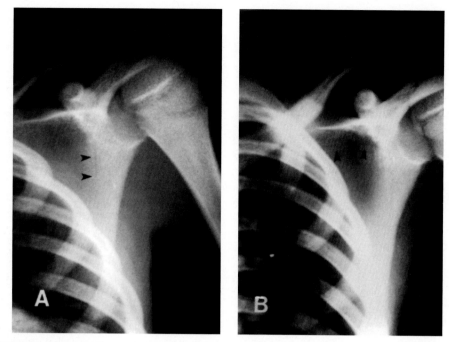

FIGURE 4.39. *Normal vascular grooves of scapula.* (**A** and **B**) Demonstration of vascular grooves of the scapula (*arrows*), frequently misinterpreted as fractures.

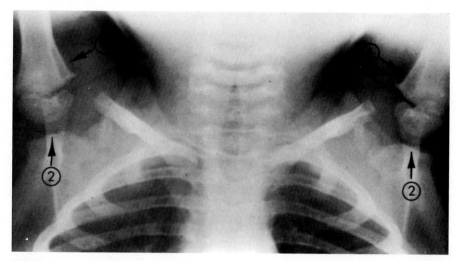

FIGURE 4.40. *Normal humeral notch and vacuum-joint phenomenon.* Note bilateral humeral notches (*1*), often misinterpreted as destructive lesions of the proximal humerus. These notches represent a normal depression of the bone in the region of insertion of the deltoid muscle. The notch characteristically is visualized if the extremity is upwardly extended. Also note the normal vacuum-joint phenomenon in both shoulders (*2*). This phenomenon occurs when the upper extremities are stretched and is normal. Although the term "vacuum joint" is used to describe this finding, there is debate as to whether the radiolucent area actually represents a vacuum, or a space filled with nitrogen or water vapor.

REFERENCES

1. Bowerman JW, McDonnell EJ. Radiology of athletic injuries: Baseball. *Radiology* 1975;116:611–615.
2. Lee FA, Gwinn JL. Retrosternal dislocation of the clavicle. *Radiology* 1974;110:631–634.
3. Nicastro JF, Adair DM. Fracture-dislocation of the shoulder in a 32-month-old child. *J Pediatr Orthop* 1982;2:427–429.
4. Protass JJ, Stampfli FV, Osmer JC. Coracoid process fracture diagnosis in acromioclavicular separation. *Radiology* 1975;116:61–64.
5. Schmidt D, Mubarak S, Gelberman R. Septic shoulders in children. *J Pediatr Orthop* 1981;1:67–72.
6. Torg JS, Pollack H, Sweterlitsch P. The effect of competitive pitching on the shoulders and elbows of preadolescent baseball players. *Pediatrics* 1972;49:267–272.

Humeral Shaft

Midshaft fractures of the humerus commonly occur in infancy and childhood. The most common is the spiral or oblique fracture, but transverse fractures also are seen. Usually these fractures are so obvious that there is no problem in their roentgenographic detection, but occasionally they are hairline and undisplaced and more difficult to detect. Cortical buckling or torus fractures do not usually occur in the midshaft of the humerus, for the cortex is thick in this area, and the only normal finding that can be misinterpreted as a fracture is a normal vascular groove (Fig. 4.41).

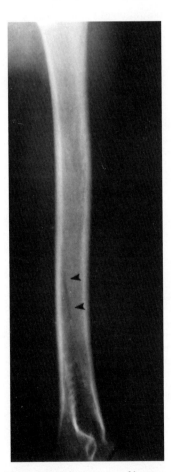

FIGURE 4.41. *Normal vascular groove of humerus.* Note the vascular groove (*arrows*) in the distal humerus. These vascular grooves can be confused with linear or spiral fractures. If one notes that the radiolucent line is rather wide and that there is slight sclerosis along either edge, however, one should make the diagnosis of normal vascular groove.

Elbow

Normal Soft Tissues and Fat Pads

In the elbow, the most important fat pads to assess are the anterior and posterior pads (3). The anterior fat pad is located in the coronoid fossa; the posterior fat pad is located in the olecranon fossa. These fat pads must be evaluated on true lateral, flexed views of the elbow, for with any degree of rotation, their usefulness diminishes or is totally invalidated. Normally, on the true lateral flexed view of the elbow, the anterior fat pad is visible, but the posterior fat pad is not (Fig. 4.42A). The reason for the lack of visualization of the posterior fat pad is that it lies deep in the olecranon fossa. It becomes visible only if fluid in the joint displaces it posteriorly. On extension it may be visible normally, but never on a flexed view. These fat pad configurations are very consistent, and consequently, any deviation from the configurations illustrated in Fig. 4.42 should be considered abnormal.

The supinator fat pad (16) is another normal fat pad around the elbow. It also is seen on true lateral views and overlies the anterior aspect of the supinator muscle (Fig. 4.42B). Overall, however, this fat pad is less useful than the other elbow fat pads, for it is less consistently visualized, especially in infants and young children. Nonetheless, it can be obliterated or displaced with fractures of the proximal radius. It also can be obliterated with generalized edema around the elbow.

Evaluation of the soft tissues around the elbow, other than the fat pads, is nonspecific. Basically, it consists of noting whether the fat–muscle interfaces are distinct or indistinct. If they are indistinct, edema is present.

Detecting Fluid in the Elbow Joint–Displaced Fat Pads

Fluid in the elbow joint usually produces upward and outward displacement of the anterior and posterior fat pads (Fig. 4.43A). These fat pads overlie the capsule of the elbow joint, and their displacement is very accurate in reflecting the presence of intraarticular fluid. It should be noted, however, that if edema also surrounds the elbow, the displaced fat pads are obliterated or just faintly visible (Fig. 4.43D and E).

Ultrasonography also can be used to detect fluid in the elbow joint (11) but seldom is needed, because the findings on lateral elbow films are very sensitive. Nonetheless, the anatomy as visualized on plain films is exactly the same on ultrasound (Fig. 4.44).

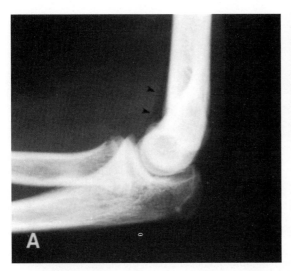
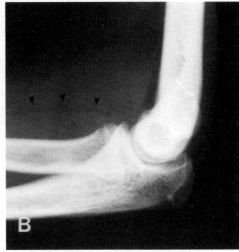

FIGURE 4.42. *Normal elbow fat pads.* **(A)** The anterior fat pad (*arrows*) normally is visible as a thin, triangular radiolucency anterior to the humerus. The posterior fat pad, on true lateral flexed views of the elbow, is not visible under normal circumstances. **(B)** The supinator fat pad (*arrows*) is thin and more often visible in older children.

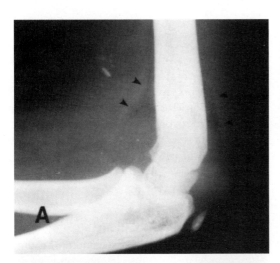
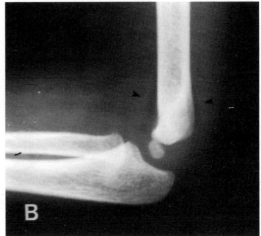

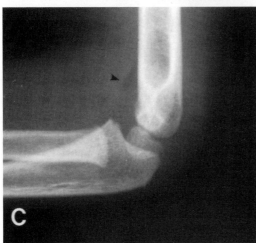

FIGURE 4.43. *Abnormal fat pad configurations.* Elevation and displacement denote the presence of fluid in the joint; obliteration denotes periarticular edema and swelling. Both can occur together. **(A)** Elevation and displacement only. Note that both the anterior and posterior fat pads are visible and displaced upward and outward (*arrows*). This patient had an occult supracondylar fracture of the humerus. **(B)** Less pronounced displacement of the fat pads (*arrows*). The fact that the posterior fat pad is even visible is abnormal in itself, for if it is visible, it is displaced. **(C)** Anterior fat pad displacement only. The anterior fat pad is displaced and elevated (*arrow*); the posterior fat pad is not displaced and not visible. This patient had a minimal fracture of the lateral condyle. *(continued on next page)*

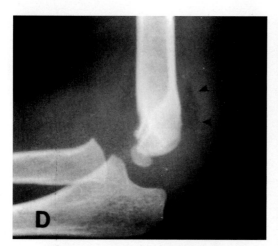 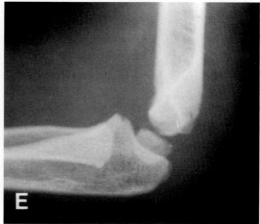

FIGURE 4.43. *(continued)* **(D)** Displacement and obliteration. The posterior fat pad is markedly displaced (*arrows*) and a little hazy (obliterated) because of edema around the elbow. The anterior fat pad also is displaced, but because of edema it also is obliterated. Only a subtle suggestion of its presence, in its abnormally elevated position, is noted. **(E)** Displacement and marked obliteration. Both fat pads are displaced and elevated, but both are barely visible because of extensive edema around the elbow. Both this patient and the patient in **D** had subtle distal humerus fractures.

Injuries around the Elbow

Injuries, including fractures, of the three bones around the elbow are perhaps the most commonly encountered fractures in infancy and childhood. Each of these bones, however, because of their configurations and articulations with each other, tend to fracture in different ways. It is most important to appreciate the mechanisms of injury in these patients (9), because this enables one to detect the more subtle injuries. For the most part, elbow injuries are sustained by falling on the outside extremity ("foosh" injury). In the hyperextended arm, axial forces act on all three bones, hyperextension forces act on the distal humerus, and rotatory forces along with varus and valgus forces act on the radius and ulna (9). These force patterns are reviewed as the individual fractures are dealt with as they occur in this chapter.

In our recent study of over 400 infants and children with elbow fractures (9) the most commonly injured bone, by far, was the distal humerus (81%). Supracondylar fractures were most common and overall constituted approximately 60% of injuries encountered. Radial head and proximal ulnar fractures constituted approximately 9 to 10% of the total fractures each; medial epicondylar fractures constituted 7% and lateral condylar fractures 19% of the total injuries (9).

Injuries of the Distal Humerus

Common injuries of the distal end of the humerus include supracondylar fractures, lateral condylar fractures, and medial epicondylar fractures. The most common of these,

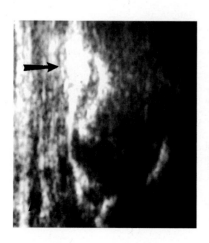 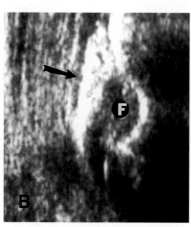

FIGURE 4.44. *Elbow fluid: ultrasound findings.* **(A)** *Normal side.* Note the echogenic anterior fat pad (*arrow*) in its normal location. **(B)** With joint fluid (*F*) on the other side, the echogenic anterior fat pad (*arrow*) has been anteriorly displaced. Compare these findings with the plain-film findings in Figure 4.43.

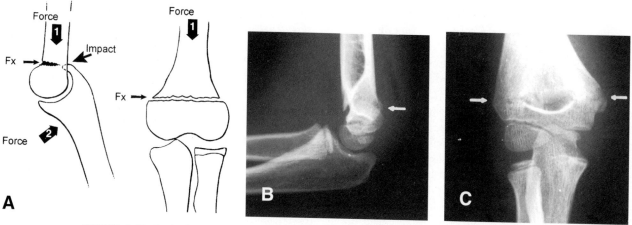

FIGURE 4.45. *Typical supracondylar fracture.* (**A**) *Diagrammatic representation.* Two forces are at play, axial loading (*1*) and hyperextension (*2*). Note the point of impact (*impact*) resulting in the fracture (*FX*). (**B**) Lateral view demonstrating typical supracondylar fracture (*arrow*) with posterior tilting of the distal fracture fragment. (**C**) Frontal view demonstrates the barely visible transverse fracture line (*arrows*) (Part A with permission from reference 9).

however, is the supracondylar fracture; generally this fracture results from a fall on the outstretched upper extremity. With the olecranon locking into the olecranon fossa a hyperextension force is applied to the distal humerus, and because this is the weakest part of the humerus, a fracture occurs (Fig. 4.45A). ***The problem can be equated to opening a soda pop bottle with a bottle opener.*** The

result is posterior tilting of the distal fracture fragment (Fig. 4.45B).

The classic, clearly visible supracondylar fracture with angulation and posterior displacement of the distal fragment is not difficult to recognize (Fig. 4.45B and C). Very often, however, even though a fracture is visible on lateral view it is not seen on frontal view (Fig. 4.46). In addition,

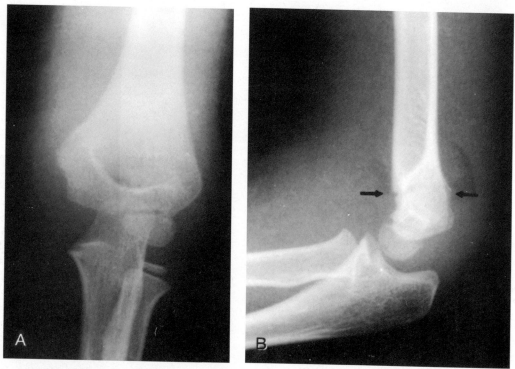

FIGURE 4.46. *Supracondylar fracture not visible on anteroposterior view.* (**A**) On the anteroposterior view there is considerable soft-tissue swelling, but the fracture through the supracondylar region is not visible. (**B**) Lateral view demonstrates the typical fracture (*arrows*), with obliteration and elevation of the anterior fat pad and elevation of the posterior fat pad.

if the fracture is hairline or merely a plastic, bending fracture, little angulation occurs. In such cases, one must rely more on fat-pad abnormalities and an abnormal anterior humeral line (Fig. 4.47). The anterior humeral line is a line drawn along the anterior aspect of the distal humerus and should be applied on true lateral views. Under normal circumstances, it intersects the ossified capitellum somewhere through its middle third (17). If it intersects the capitellum through the anterior third, or if it misses it entirely, a supracondylar fracture probably is present (Fig. 4.47). The anterior humeral line is a little more difficult to apply in the young infant, in whom the capitellum is incompletely ossified, but even in these cases, if the findings are compared with those on the normal side, posterior displacement can be detected. In addition, in almost every instance, the fat pads are elevated or obliterated in these patients, and if they are, one should assume that an elbow injury has occurred. ***This is not always a supracondylar fracture, but because***

such a fracture is so common, in the absence of other visible fractures one should assume that it is present. In many of these cases, on follow-up healing-phase films, one's original suspicions are confirmed (Fig. 4.48). There are, of course, cases in which no such evidence of healing is present, and in such cases one assumes that only a traumatic joint effusion was present. It is better, however, to have a few of these cases than to miss those with occult supracondylar fractures.

Although most fractures through the supracondylar region are of the type demonstrated in Figures 4.45 through 4.48, in the young infant in whom the cortex is relatively thin and weak one can encounter a variety of often extremely subtle buckle fractures in this region (Fig. 4.49). Of course, as with any fracture, one view may be better than another for fracture visualization and, indeed, one often requires oblique views for full demonstration of these fractures. Most often these buckle fractures are caused by hyperextension and varus

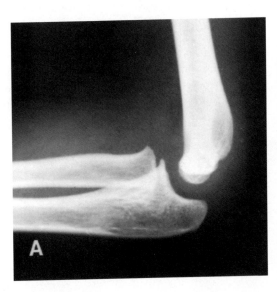

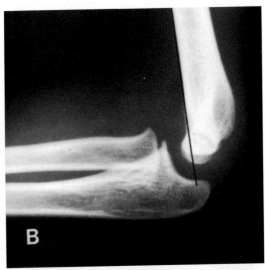

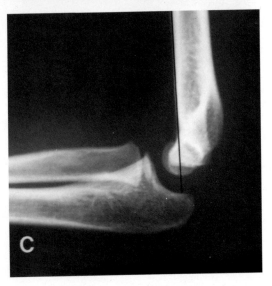

FIGURE 4.47. *Subtle supracondylar fractures: value of soft tissues and anterior humeral line.* **(A)** Young child with elbow injury. Note soft-tissue swelling around the elbow and a partially obliterated and elevated anterior fat pad. **(B)** Same elbow. The anterior humeral line intersects the capitellum through its anterior third. An occult, greenstick, or bending fracture should be suspected. **(C)** Normal elbow for comparison. Note the position of the normal anterior fat pad and the normal position of the anterior humeral line. It intersects the capitellum through its middle third.

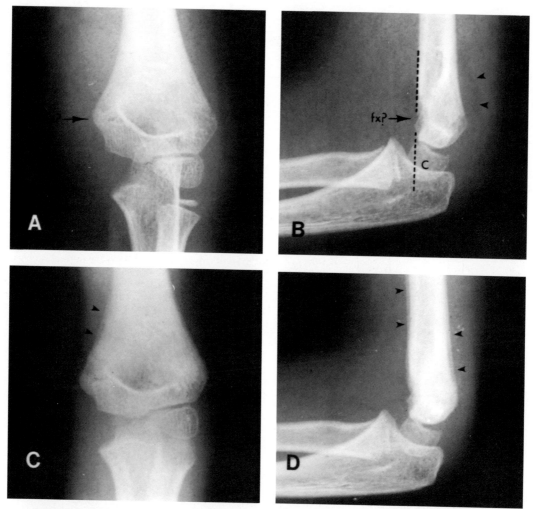

FIGURE 4.48. *Subtle supracondylar fracture with healing.* **(A)** Frontal view demonstrating little or no abnormality. A subtle fracture line (*fx*) is suggested medially. **(B)** Lateral view demonstrating abnormal fat pads and an anterior humeral line that intersects the capitellum (*C*) through its anterior third. This should suggest posterior displacement of the capitellum, and an underlying supracondylar fracture. A fracture line (*arrow*) also is suggested, but it is questionably visible. **(C)** Two weeks later, note periosteal new-bone deposition along both sides of the distal humerus (*arrows*). The fracture line is more clearly visible. **(D)** Lateral view demonstrating periosteal new-bone deposition along the shaft of the humerus (*arrows*). Also note that the fat pads have returned to normal, but that the capitellum still is displaced posteriorly.

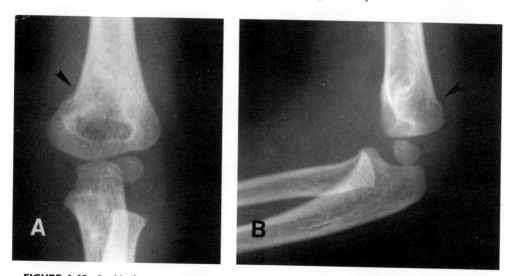

FIGURE 4.49. *Buckle fracture of the distal humerus.* **(A)** Note buckling of the cortex along the medial aspect of the distal humerus (*arrowhead*). **(B)** Lateral view demonstrating buckling of the cortex posteriorly (*arrowhead*), and posterior displacement of the capitellum. Also note the faintly visible but definitely elevated posterior fat pad. The anterior fat pad is, for the most part, obliterated.

325

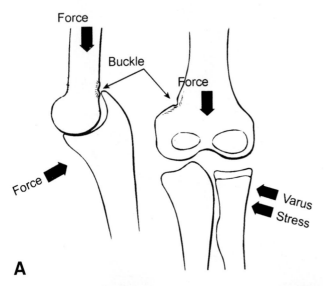

A

FIGURE 4.50. *Minimal buckle, plastic bending supracondylar fracture.* (**A**) *Diagrammatic representation.* In addition to axial loading and hyperextension forces, varus stress forces (*varus stress*) are present and cause buckling of the medial and posterior cortices of the distal humerus (*buckle*). A discrete fracture line is not visible on either view. (**B**) There is a minimal buckle through the distal humerus (*arrow*). (**C**) Normal side for comparison. Note smooth curving contour of the cortex (*arrow*). (**D**) Lateral view. Note slight buckle posteriorly (*arrow*) and that the anterior humeral line intersects the anterior third of the capitellum. (**E**) On the normal side no buckle is seen. The anterior fat pad is normal, and the anterior humeral line intersects the capitellum through its posterior third. All of these findings indicate the presence of a subtle plastic bending fracture of the distal humerus. (Part A reproduced with permission from reference 9.)

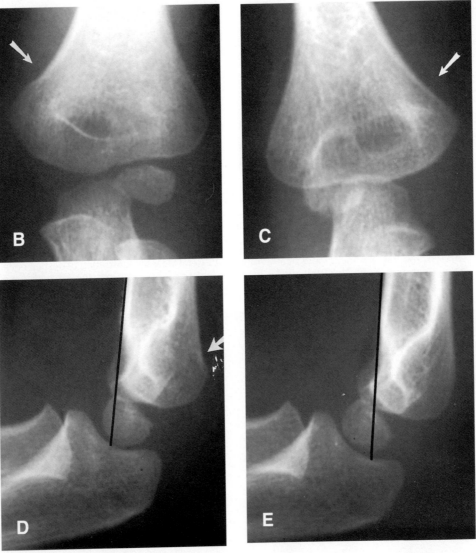

forces, and on anteroposterior views they can be very subtle (Fig. 4.50). Another fracture occurring through the distal humerus in conjunction with the supracondylar hyperextension fracture is the "T" fracture. In these cases not only are hyperextension forces applied to the distal humerus but axial loading on both the lateral and medial condyles also results in splitting of the distal humerus and the resultant T fracture (Fig. 4.51). Pseudodislocation of the elbow occurs with complete transverse fractures through the supracondylar region. In these cases (4) the distal fragment is so displaced that clinically dislocation is erroneously suggested (Fig. 4.52). Finally, it should be noted that in some cases a supracondylar fracture with faulty alignment results in a cubitus varus (gun-stock) deformity of the elbow (10), which may need surgical correction.

In condylar and epicondylar injuries of the distal humerus, it is the medial epicondyle and lateral condyle that most commonly are injured. Medial condylar (13) and lateral epicondylar fractures are rare. Lateral condylar fractures tend to occur in young infants and children; medial epicondylar fractures more often occur in older children. Many of these fractures are subtle and, once again, examination of the soft tissues becomes important. In this regard, an abnormality of the fat pads of the elbow usually is present, but not always. More importantly, however, there usually is telltale unilateral swelling and edema of the soft tissues. With medial epicondylar fractures, such swelling occurs medially; with lateral condylar fractures, it occurs laterally. The pres-

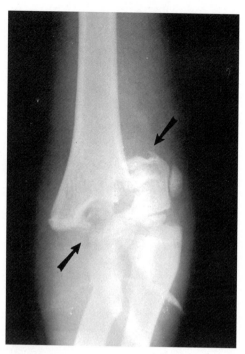

FIGURE 4.52. *Complete fracture distal elbow: clinical pseudo-dislocation.* Note the completely displaced fracture of the distal humerus (*arrows*). Clinically, this type of injury can cause the elbow to appear dislocated, but in actual fact no dislocation is present. Note that the displaced distal humeral fracture fragment is in normal alignment with both the radius and ulna. Compare with true dislocation of the elbow in Fig. 4.57.

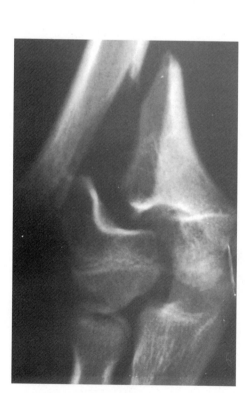

FIGURE 4.51. *Supracondylar "T" fracture.* Note the typical comminuted T fracture. Clinically the elbow may appear dislocated.

ence of such unilateral soft-tissue edema is especially important in the assessment of those medial epicondylar injuries in which minimal or no displacement of the epicondyle occurs (Fig. 4.53), or in children younger than 7 years of age, in whom the epicondyle is not yet ossified.

A wide range of medial epicondylar injuries occurs, and injuries seen range from those with simple separation of the epicondyle to those with complete dislocation or intraarticular entrapment of the epicondyle (Fig. 4.54). These injuries result from rotation applied to the bones distal to the elbow, resulting in avulsion of the medial epicondyle by the pull of the flexor pronator tendon. In some cases minimal or no displacement of the medial epicondyle is seen (Fig. 4.55A); in others not only is displacement present, but the medial epicondyle also is rotated (Fig. 4.55B). If entrapment of the medial epicondyle occurs, the medial epicondyle is not visible in its normal position (Fig. 4.56). In addition to these injuries of the medial epicondyle, it should be noted that avulsion of this secondary center frequently accompanies true dislocations of the elbow. In these cases, the fact that the medial epicondyle is displaced can elude detection until postreduction films are obtained (Fig. 4.57).

Lateral condylar fractures result if varus stresses are placed upon the elbow, on the bones distal to the joint (i.e.,

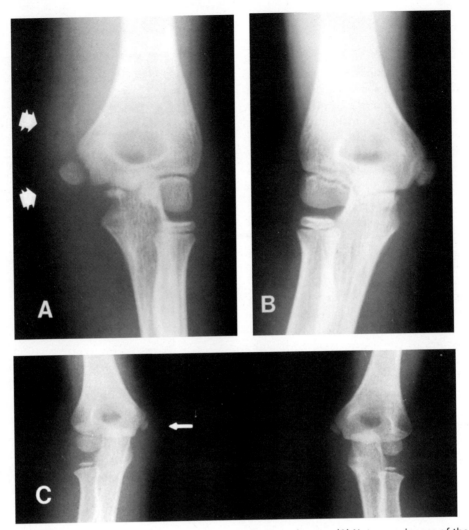

FIGURE 4.53. *Medial epicondyle injury: value of soft tissue changes.* **(A)** Note prominence of the soft tissues over the medial epicondyle (*arrows*), and that the medial epicondyle appears displaced. **(B)** Comparative view of the other side demonstrates normal position of medial epicondyle and lack of soft-tissue swelling. **(C)** More subtle case. Note swelling over the right medial epicondyle (*arrow*). The epicondyle itself, however, does not appear particularly displaced. On the normal side, note that there is no soft-tissue swelling over the medial epicondyle.

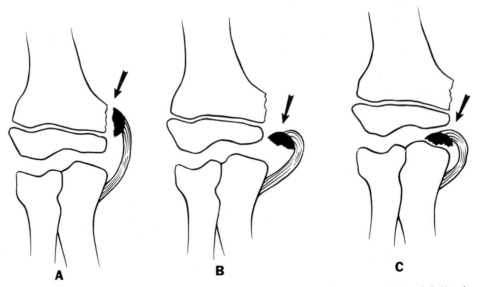

FIGURE 4.54. *Range of medial epicondylar injuries: diagrammatic representation.* **(A)** Simple separation of fracture fragment (*arrow*). **(B)** Separation with rotation of fragment (*arrow*). **(C)** Separation with entrapment of fragment (*arrow*) in joint space.

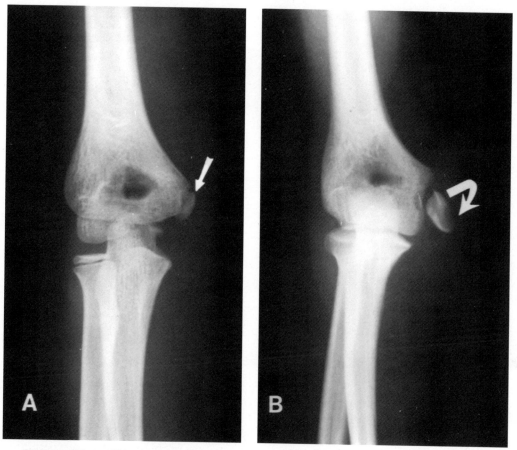

FIGURE 4.55. *Medial epicondylar avulsions: varying degrees.* (**A**) Minimal separation of the medial epicondyle with slight downward displacement (*arrow*). Note that the soft tissues over the area are a little thickened. (**B**) Markedly displaced and completely rotated medial epicondyle (*arrow*).

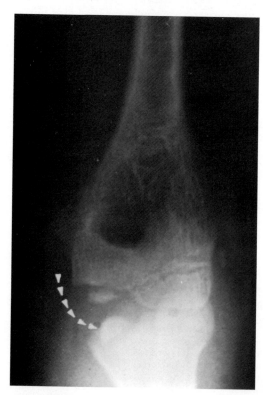

FIGURE 4.56. *Medial epicondylar entrapment.* Note the abnormal position of the entrapped medial epicondyle. It has been displaced from its normal position and now lies in the intraarticular space (*arrows*). (Courtesy of Lee Rogers, M.D., and Harvey White, M.D.)

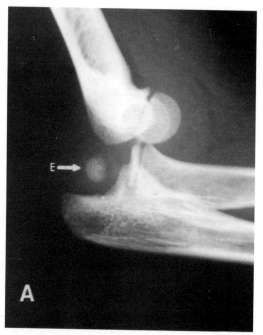

FIGURE 4.57. *Medial epicondyle separation secondary to elbow dislocation.* (**A**) Lateral view: total dislocation of the elbow. Note position of the medial epicondyle (*E*).

(continued on next page)

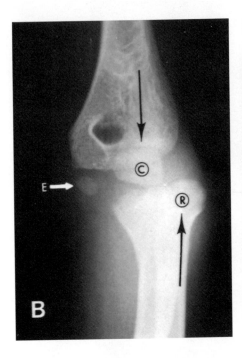

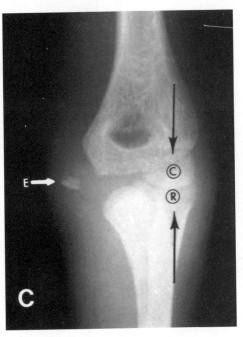

FIGURE 4.57. *(continued)* **(B)** Frontal view demonstrating complete dislocation of the elbow. Note that the capitellum (*C*) does not line up with the proximal radial head (*R*). Also note, however, the position of the displaced medial epicondyle (*E*). Just beneath it is a small, avulsed, sliverlike metaphyseal bony fragment. **(C)** Postreduction film demonstrates extensive edema of the elbow and persistent separation of the medial epicondyle (*E*). Note that the capitellum (*C*) is now in a straight-line relationship with the head of the radius (*R*).

radius and ulna) (Fig. 4.58). The resultant distracting forces cause avulsion of the underlying subcondylar metaphysis. Many times a transverse fracture of the ulna also occurs, and it is most important to determine whether the condylar fracture is displaced or undisplaced.

Displacement and/or rotation occur if the fracture extends through the articular cartilage of the distal humerus. In these cases, the stabilizing, hingelike function of the nondisplaced fracture fragment is lost, and the injury becomes unstable (Fig. 4.58). Such fractures require inter-

nal fixation, and thus it is most important to identify them accurately. Examples of displaced and nondisplaced lateral condylar fractures are presented in Fig. 4.59. Another variation of the lateral condylar fracture occurs in young infants in whom only a small sliver of the metaphysis is avulsed. In these cases, which are very common, close inspection of roentgenograms and assessment of the fat pads and adjacent soft tissues are most worthwhile (Fig. 4.60), but in other cases oblique views become more important (Fig. 4.61). These fractures can occur alone or can be seen with other

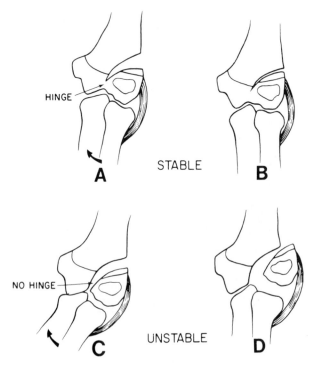

FIGURE 4.58. *Lateral condyle fractures: mechanics of stability and instability.* **(A)** Stable fracture. Twisting forces (*arrow*) cause separation of the lateral condyle from the humeral metaphysis. The articular cartilage, however, is incompletely broken, and a stabilizing hinge remains. **(B)** If the fracture-causing forces are removed, the fracture fragment returns to a nearly normal position; it is stable. **(C)** Unstable fracture. Same twisting forces (*arrow*) causing complete fracture through the articular cartilage, with no residual hinge. **(D)** With removal of the forces, the totally separated lateral condyle rotates upward and outward. Because there is no hinge remaining, the fracture is unstable. (Adapted from Rang M.: *Children's fractures.* Philadelphia: J.B. Lippincott, Philadelphia, 1974.)

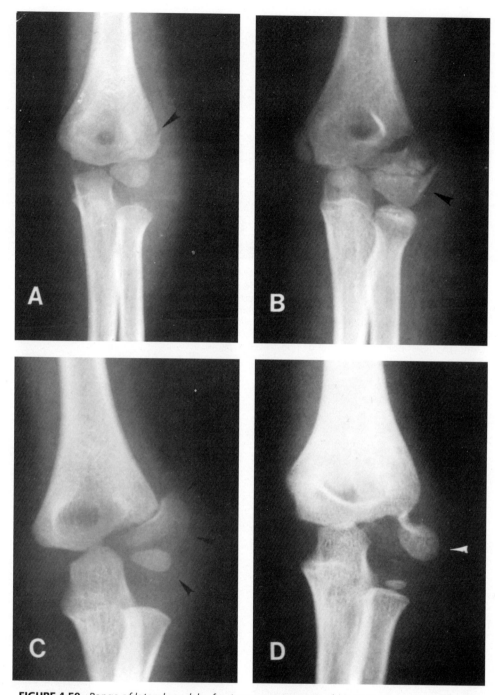

FIGURE 4.59. *Range of lateral condylar fractures: roentgenographic appearance.* (**A**) Stable fracture, hinge intact. Note the undisplaced lateral condylar fracture (*arrow*). Also note the presence of adjacent unilateral edema of the soft tissues. (**B**) Unstable fracture, hinge not intact. There is more downward displacement of the fractured fragment (*arrow*). (**C**) Unstable fracture, hinge not intact. Note pronounced lateral and upward displacement of the fractured lateral condyle (*arrows*). (**D**) Unstable fracture, hinge not intact. Note complete rotation and marked upward displacement of the lateral condyle (*arrow*).

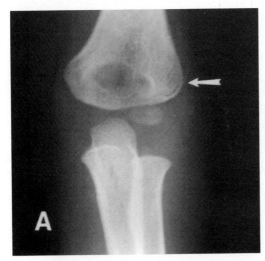
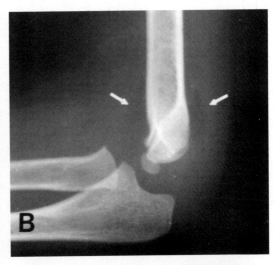

FIGURE 4.60. *Subtle lateral condylar fracture.* **(A)** Frontal view demonstrating a subtle fracture line through the lateral condyle (*arrow*). A sliverlike piece of bone has been avulsed. **(B)** Lateral view demonstrating abnormal displacement of both the anterior and posterior fat pads (*arrows*). This is a stable and very common fracture. In addition, note the slight buckle of the medial humeral cortex on the anteroposterior view and slight posterior tilting of the distal humerus on lateral view. These signify the presence of an associated plastic bending supracondylar fracture. Compare these findings with those demonstrated in Figure 4.50.

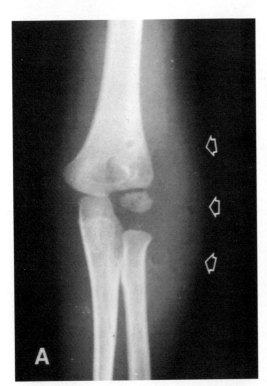
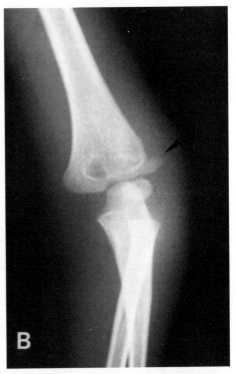

FIGURE 4.61. *Lateral condylar fracture: value of oblique film.* **(A)** Frontal view demonstrating no significant abnormality in the bones. Note, however, prominent unilateral swelling of the soft tissues over the lateral aspect of the elbow (*arrows*). This should signify the presence of an injury to the lateral condyle. **(B)** Oblique view demonstrates the displaced fracture fragment with greater clarity (*arrow*).

fractures to the other bones resulting from the same varus forces. For example, minimal buckle fractures of the distal humerus on the medial side can be seen (Fig. 4.60). In addition, transverse and buckle fractures along the medial aspect of the upper ulna can be seen (Fig 4.62). In a few cases impaction fractures of the radial head also occur.

Lateral epicondylar and medial condylar fractures (13), as noted previously, are much less common than the fractures just discussed. Not so rare, however, are avulsion fractures of the capitellum itself. These fractures can be confused with avulsion fractures of the lateral epicondyle (Fig. 4.63).

Little Leaguer's elbow usually is devoid of significant soft tissue or bony abnormalities on the roentgenograms. It is a traumatic lesion resulting from too much pitching at too young an age, and if long-term bony changes occur, they consist of fragmentation and enlargement of the medial epicondyle. In other cases, if such stress on the elbow continues, the following can occur: overgrowth and fragmentation of various other epiphyses and secondary centers around the elbow (6), chronic anterior angulation of the radial head (5,6), and nonunion of the olecranon apophysis (14).

Injuries of the Radial Head

Radial head fractures are impaction fractures and result if valgus forces are placed on the elbow distal to the joint itself (Fig. 4.64). The radial head becomes impacted, and a Salter–Harris type II fracture results with variable displacement of the proximal fracture fragment. This fracture can be associated with transverse, medially diastatic fractures of the ulna, and of course avulsion of the medial epicondyle.

Gross, fragmented, or displaced fractures of the radial head are not difficult to detect (Fig. 4.64B), but the more subtle corner buckle fracture frequently is missed (Fig. 4.65). Of course, in most cases, abnormalities of the soft tissues and fat pads around the elbow alert one to the presence of this fracture, but still the fracture remains elusive. As important as not missing the fracture, however, is not misinterpreting a normal notch in the radial head of many

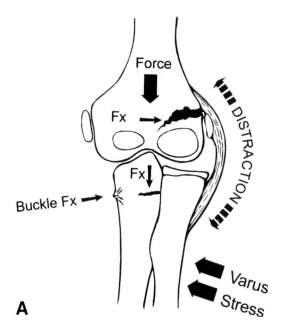

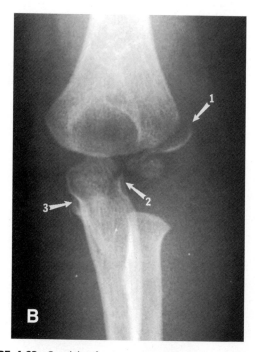

FIGURE 4.62. *Condylar fracture, associated ulnar fracture.* **(A)** Diagrammatic representation. Lateral distracting forces (*varus stress*) lead to a lateral condylar fracture (*upper FX*). In addition, a transverse fracture (*lower FX*) of the ulna along with a buckle fracture of the ulna can occur. **(B)** Note the lateral condylar avulsion fracture (*1*), the transverse fracture of the ulna (*2*), and the buckle fracture of the ulna (*3*), Part A reproduced with permission from reference 9.

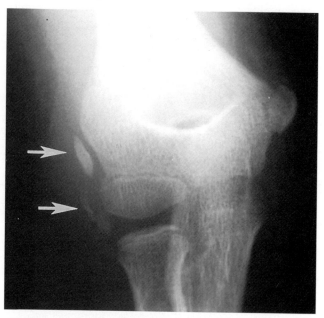

FIGURE 4.63. *Capitellar avulsion fracture.* Note the avulsion fracture of the capitellum (*lower arrow*); the upper arrow designates the normal lateral epicondyle.

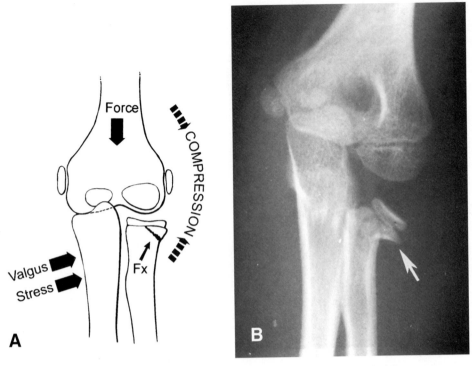

FIGURE 4.64. *Radial head compression fracture.* **(A)** Axial loading forces along with valgus stress forces applied to the elbow result in compression laterally. This results in an impaction fracture of the radial head (*FX*). **(B)** Note the impacted, displaced radial head fracture (*arrow*). Part A reproduced with permission from reference 9.

young infants as an actual fracture (Fig. 4.66). The notch defect in question usually is seen in infants and young children in whom the radial head epiphysis is not ossified. In the older child, it usually is not a problem.

Most radial head fractures are impaction fractures, with the capitellum hammering the radial head. Again, many of these are subtle, and in such cases it is of the utmost importance to obtain comparative views of the normal extremity and then to look for any subtle evidence of cortical buck-ling, radial head tilting, or cortical fracturing (Fig. 4.67). Even then, the most subtle of these fractures can elude one's initial detection, and only if follow-up films are obtained does it come to one's attention that such a fracture existed in the first place (Fig. 4.68).

Dislocation of the radius (radial head) obviously occurs if the entire elbow is dislocated, but dislocation of the radius alone usually occurs in association with a fracture of the ulna (i.e., Monteggia's fracture). The ulnar fracture can

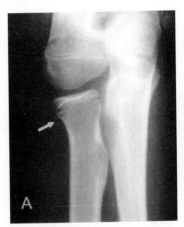
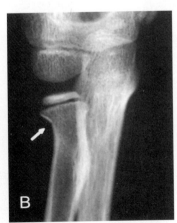
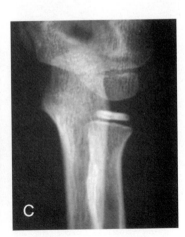

FIGURE 4.65. *Radial head corner: impaction fracture.* **(A)** Note the minimally impacted corner fracture of the radial head (*arrow*). **(B)** Another patient with a more pronounced impaction (*arrow*). **(C)** Normal side for comparison.

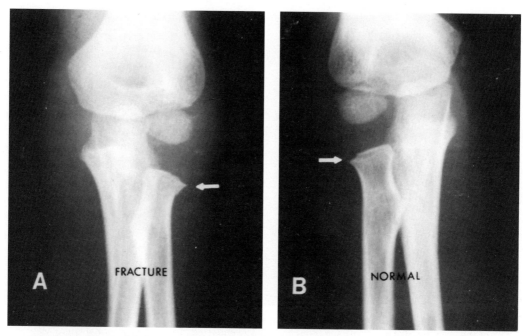

FIGURE 4.66. *Radial head corner fracture versus normal notch.* **(A)** Note typical, slightly impacted corner fracture of the proximal radial head (*arrow*). **(B)** Normal side for comparison. Note normal notch in radial head (*arrow*), frequently misinterpreted as a fracture. Also note that the soft tissues in **A** (fracture side) are fatter and more opaque because of edema and swelling.

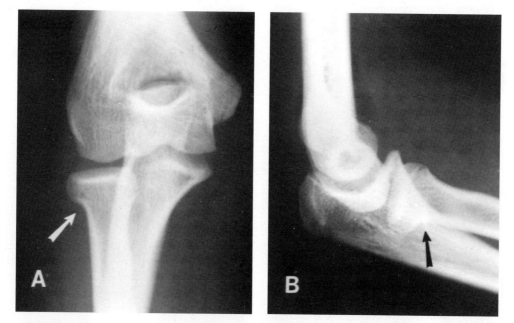

FIGURE 4.67. *Impacted radial head fracture.* **(A)** Note the minimal cortical buckle in the radial head (*arrow*). **(B)** Lateral view demonstrating displaced fat pads and subtle suggestion of the same fracture in the radial head (*arrow*). The findings on both views might be overlooked unless compared with the same area on the normal side. *(continued on next page)*

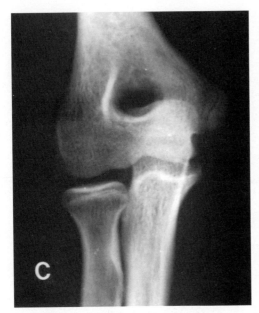

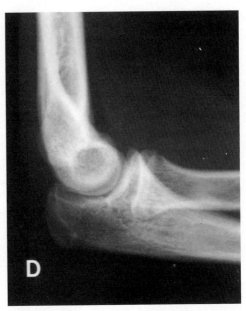

FIGURE 4.67. *(continued)* **(C)** Normal frontal view for comparison. Compare the configuration of the normal radial head with the tilted and slightly impacted head in **A**. **(D)** Normal lateral view for comparison. Compare again this normal radial head with the slightly impacted and tilted head in **B**.

occur through the proximal end of the ulna (Fig. 4.69) or the midshaft of the ulna. In assessing the radius for dislocation, one should determine whether the radial head and capitellum line up in a straight line. If they do not, the radius is dislocated (Fig. 4.69). This rule is valid on both lateral and anteroposterior views (15). These dislocations result if the annular ligament ruptures as a result of varus forces

being applied to the elbow distal to the joint (Fig. 4.70A). In most such cases a fracture of the ulna also occurs, but in other cases no such fracture is seen (Fig. 4.70B and C).

Dislocation of the radial head from the annular ligament without fracture, or the so-called *pulled, curbstone, or nursemaid's elbow,* is not true dislocation (7). Rather, there is subluxation of the radial head from the annular lig-

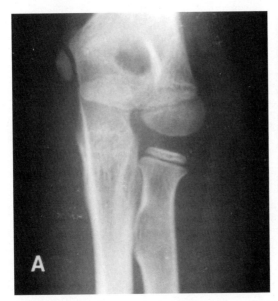

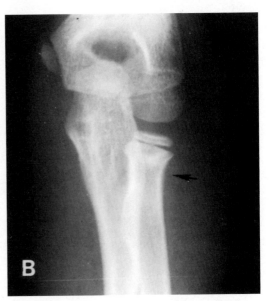

FIGURE 4.68. *Subtle radial head fracture with healing.* **(A)** The radial head appears normal, but the elbow in this patient was painful. **(B)** Two weeks later, note periosteal new-bone deposition *(arrow)* and sclerosis of the metaphysis, indicating the presence of a healing, impacted radial head fracture.

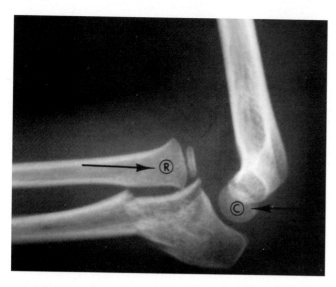

FIGURE 4.69. *Dislocated radial head.* Note that the radial head (*R*) is displaced upward. It does not line up in a straight-line relationship with the capitellum (*C*). Also note the angulated fracture of the proximal ulna. The ulna is not dislocated.

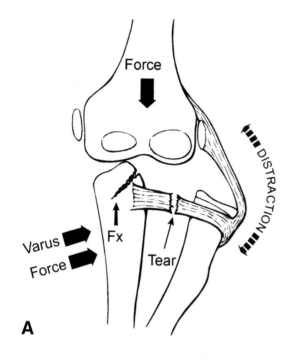

FIGURE 4.70. *Radial head dislocation.* **(A)** With varus forces, distracting forces exist laterally, and if the ligament between the radius and ulna tears, the radial head can dislocate. In addition, transverse fractures of the ulna can occur (*FX*). **(B)** Simple radial-head dislocation (*arrow*). **(C)** In this patient, in addition to the radial head dislocation, a fracture through the ulna (*arrow*) has occurred. This latter fracture constitutes a form of Monteggia's fracture. Part A reproduced with permission from reference 9.

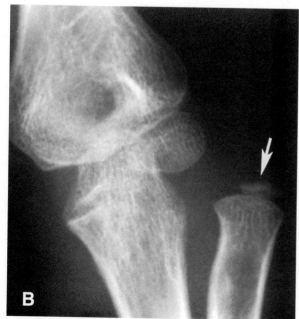
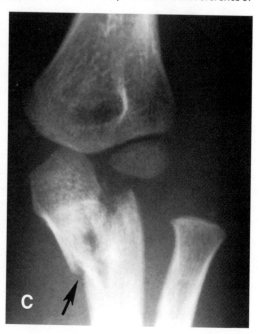

337

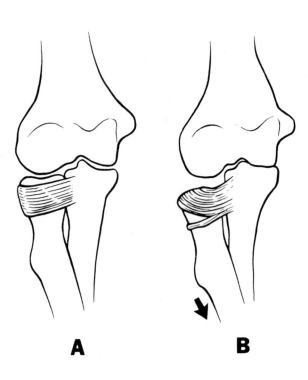

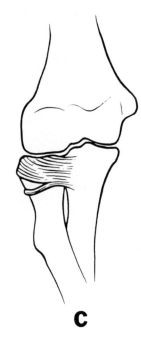

A   **B**   **C**

FIGURE 4.71. *Pulled-elbow mechanics.* **(A)** Note the position of the normal annular ligament. It is wrapped around the radial head. **(B)** With pulling on the elbow, the annular ligament is torn, and some of the fibers roll over the radial head. **(C)** After pulling stops, the fibers that rolled over the radial head remain in that position and the elbow becomes painful. (Adapted from Rang, M.: *Children's fractures.* Philadelphia: J.B. Lippincott, 1974.)

ament, incomplete tearing of the ligament, and subsequent entrapment of a portion of the ligament in the joint space (Fig. 4.71). This is a very common elbow injury in infancy and early childhood and results from a brisk pull on the elbow such as occurs in lifting the child by one arm. The condition produces exquisite pain and a most unhappy child. The clinical picture is absolutely characteristic: A previously well child suddenly refuses to move the involved extremity. Clinical examination is not productive, because no matter which way one moves or, indeed, even touches the arm, the child reacts violently. The arm is held in slight flexion and pronation, and supination is impossible without great pain. Occasionally the problem can be bilateral (12).

The roentgenographic findings in "pulled" elbow usually are negative, in terms of both bony and soft tissue abnormality. Usually, however, the views obtained are suboptimal, for it is very difficult to position these patients for adequate roentgenograms. On the other hand, many times trying to position the arm properly leads to reduction. Indeed, almost as if by magic, there is an immediate full return to normal movement of the extremity, and a previously crying, tormented child is all smiles. In other cases, mild discomfort may persist for 30 min to 1 or 2 hr. Actually, if one is cognizant of this injury, it can be reduced before roentgenograms are ever obtained, for with the thumb over the radial head, supination and slight flexion of the elbow result in a palpable click and reduction of the radial head. After reduction, one can encounter, in some cases, evidence of edema and fat pad displacement suggesting minimal fluid accumulation in the joint.

Fractures of the Proximal Ulna

Fractures of the proximal ulna are varied. One of the reasons for this is that the ulna, more than the other two bones around the elbow, is subject to all of the forces applied to the elbow during "foosh" injuries. The ulna in the outstretched extremity injury is locked into the olecranon fossa and cannot move freely. The radius, of course, can rotate easily around the capitella, but the ulna is rigidly fixed and prone to a number of leverage- and twisting-induced fractures.

Transverse fractures, through the proximal ulna, visualized on frontal view can occur both with varus and valgus forces applied to the bones distal to the elbow joint (Fig. 4.72). They seldom occur alone; there usually is an associated radial fracture. With valgus forces in action, compression fractures of the radial head occur, and the transverse fracture through the ulna is diastatic on the medial aspect. With varus forces, distraction of the structures along the lateral aspect of the elbow can lead to radial-head dislocation or capitellar fractures. In these cases, the transverse fracture through the upper ulna tends to be somewhat oblique and diastatic on the lateral side. In addition, buckle fractures along the medial aspect of the ulna are common.

On lateral view, transverse fractures of the ulna often are hairline and occur from posteriorly applied forces. With broad-surface injuries, impact usually results in a linear fracture, and pull by the brachialis and triceps muscles causes variable separation of the fracture fragments (Fig. 4.73). If the fall is on a sharp or wedge-like object, a ful-

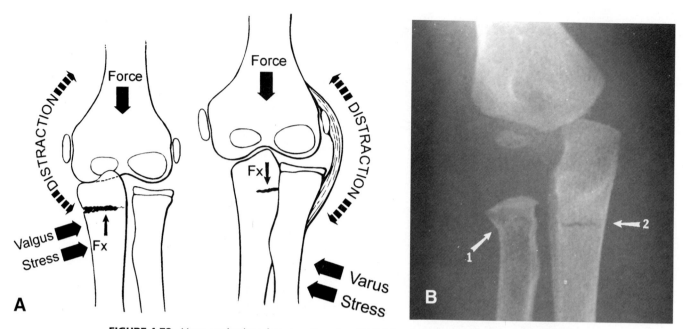

FIGURE 4.72. *Varus and valgus forces on the ulna.* (**A**) With valgus stress, distracting forces cause a transverse fracture (*FX*) through the ulna. With varus forces, similar lateral distracting forces produce a similar fracture (*FX*). (**B**) Valgus stress produces a buckle fracture of the radial head (*1*) and a transverse fracture of the ulna (*2*). Part A reproduced with permission from reference 9.

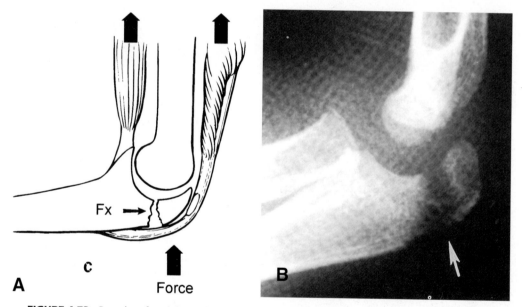

FIGURE 4.73. *Broad-surface injury of the olecranon.* (**A**) With broad-surface injuries, forces (*force*) on the olecranon produce a fracture (*FX*). Often the fracture fragments are separated (diastatic) because of pull of the triceps and biceps muscles. (**B**) Typical separated fracture fragments (*arrow*). Reproduced with permission from reference 9.

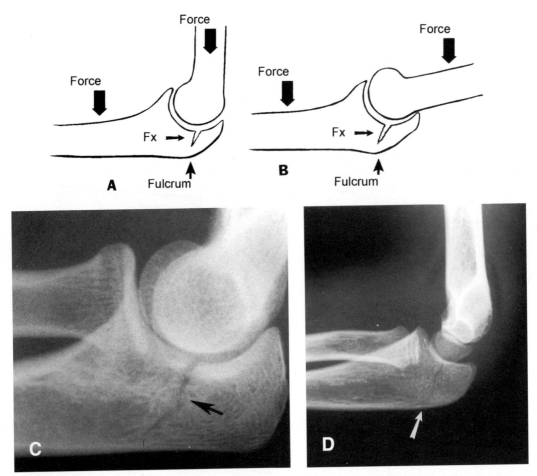

FIGURE 4.74. *Broad-surface injury of olecranon with fulcrum.* **(A and B)** If the point of impact is focal, a fulcrum exists and a V-shaped fracture (*FX*) occurs at the site. This can occur with flexion or extension of the elbow. **(C)** Note the readily visible, slightly V-shaped fracture (*arrow*). **(D)** A very subtle hairline fracture (*arrow*). Parts A and B reproduced with permission from reference 9.

crum results and the fracture is then V-shaped, being diastatic at the articular surface (Fig. 4.74).

Still another fracture peculiar to the proximal ulna is the longitudinal linear, often hairline, fracture (19). This fracture results from a shearing force applied to the proximal ulna with rotation through the elbow (Fig. 4.75). Because the ulna is locked into the olecranon fossa, twisting forces result in longitudinal, often slightly spiral, fractures (Fig. 4.76). The problem is similar to that which occurs with the mechanism that results in the typical toddler's fracture of the tibia, in which rotational forces cause hairline, spiral fractures. In the ulna the resulting linear fractures also can be extremely subtle and commonly missed unless comparative views of the normal side are obtained (Figs. 4.77 and 4.78).

Finally, one should be aware of the fact that avulsion fractures of the proximal ulna also occur. The most common is that which involves the coronoid process (Fig. 4.79A). This fracture occurs with elbow dislocations or hyperextension–rotation injuries in which forceful contraction of the brachial muscle causes avulsion of the coronoid process (2,9). The avulsed fragment is usually relatively small and can be overlooked. Its characteristic location, however, allows its identification with confidence (Fig. 4.79B). Less commonly, avulsion of the olecranon apophysis occurs. This results from forceful contraction of the triceps muscle, but because the muscle tends to insert more distally on the ulna, the apophysis seldom is avulsed. Occasionally, however, such avulsion fractures occur (Fig. 4.80). Avulsion of the apophysis of

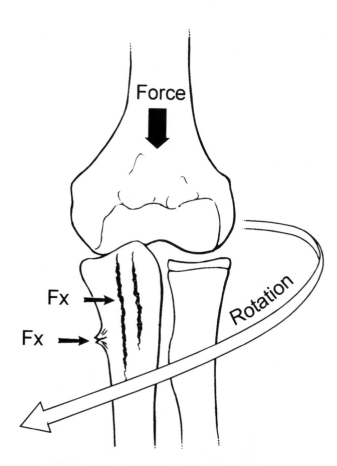

FIGURE 4.75. *Longitudinal spiral and linear hairline fractures of the proximal ulna: diagrammatic representation.* With axial loading (*force*) and rotation (*rotation*), linear shredding and buckle fractures can occur in the proximal ulna (*FX*). Reproduced with permission from reference 9.

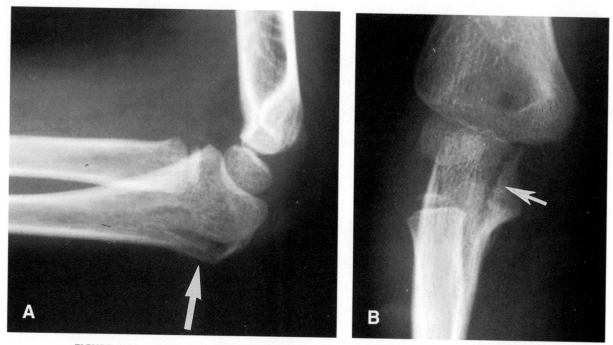

FIGURE 4.76. *Longitudinal spiral fractures of the proximal ulna.* (**A**) Readily apparent longitudinal buckle fracture (*arrow*). (**B**) Another readily apparent vertical fracture (*arrow*) through the proximal ulna.

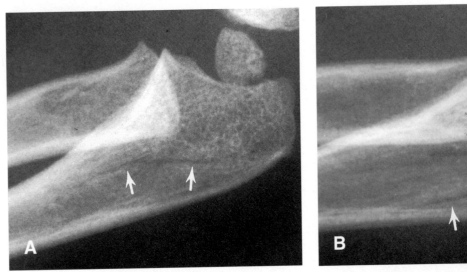

FIGURE 4.77. *Subtle linear hairline fractures of the proximal ulna.* (**A**) A hairline longitudinal fracture (*arrows*). (**B**) More subtle linear longitudinal fracture (*arrow*).

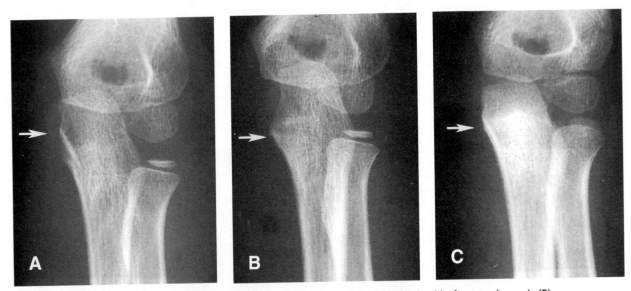

FIGURE 4.78. *Subtle proximal ulnar buckle fracture.* (**A**) Note the buckle fracture (*arrow*). (**B**) Normal side for comparison. Note the smooth cortex (*arrow*). (**C**) With healing, diffuse sclerosis is present (*arrow*).

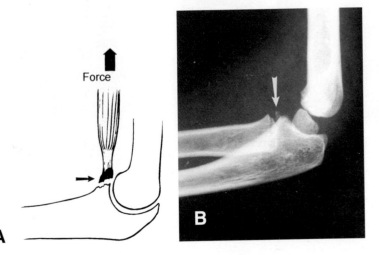

FIGURE 4.79. *Avulsion of coronoid process.* (**A**) Diagrammatic representation of the fracture fragment (*arrow*) secondary to avulsion by the brachialis muscle. (**B**) Typical appearance of the avulsed bony fragment (*arrow*). Part A reproduced with permission from reference 9.

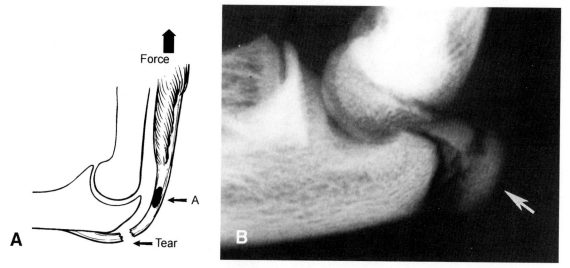

FIGURE 4.80. *Avulsion of the olecranon apophysis.* **(A)** Diagrammatic representation demonstrates rupture (*Tear*) of the tendinous insertion of the triceps muscle. The apophysis (*arrow*) then becomes avulsed. **(B)** Note separation of the ulnar apophysis (*arrow*). Part A reproduced with permission from reference 9.

the olecranon also can result from direct blows to the elbow.

Dislocation of the Elbow

Total dislocation of the elbow is not particularly common in infancy but can occur in the older child. In these cases it frequently is associated with avulsion of the medial epicondyle and entrapment of the epicondyle in the joint (Fig. 4.57). More often what occurs is that a complete fracture through the transcondylar region is sustained and the entire fracture fragment is so displaced that, clinically, dislocation of the elbow is mimicked (Fig. 4.52). There is, however, no true dislocation of the elbow in these cases.

Osteochondritis of the Elbow

Although not a common problem, osteochondritis of the elbow can involve the capitellum, trochlear epiphysis (8,18), or radial head. Involvement of the capitellum perhaps is most common and produces a bony defect with subtle adjacent sclerosis (Fig. 4.81). MR imaging is useful in determining the exact position of the fragment, if required.

Septic Arthritis, Osteomyelitis, and Cellulitis of the Elbow

Septic arthritis of the elbow is not as common as is septic arthritis of the shoulder and hip. If it occurs, however, it

produces marked swelling around the elbow and displacement or obliteration of the elbow fat pads (Fig. 4.82A). Although it is not necessary for diagnosis, joint fluid in the elbow also can be demonstrated with ultrasound (Fig. 4.44). Usually, however, there is little in the way of joint space widening.

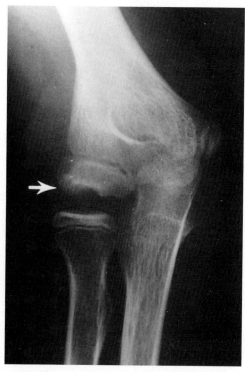

FIGURE 4.81. *Osteochondritis of capitellum.* Note lytic defect with sclerotic border in the capitellum (*arrow*).

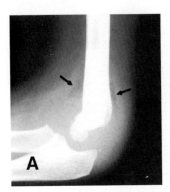
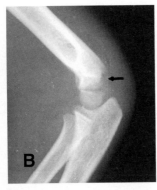

FIGURE 4.82. *Septic arthritis and osteomyelitis.* **(A)** Note elevation of both fat pads (*arrows*), attesting to fluid in the joint in this patient with septic arthritis. **(B)** This patient demonstrates edema around the elbow, partial obliteration of the elevated fat pads, and a destructive focus in the distal humerus (*arrow*), signifying the presence of osteomyelitis. Septic arthritis is also present.

Osteomyelitis of the bones around the elbow usually produces extensive deep soft tissue swelling and obliteration of the normal soft tissues and fat pads (Fig. 4.82B). In the early stages, there is little in the way of bony destruction, but after 10 to 14 days or so bone destruction and periosteal new-bone deposition appear.

With cellulitis of the elbow, if edema is circumferential, the findings are difficult to differentiate from those of early osteomyelitis (Fig. 4.83A) In many cases one actually is dealing with an acute epitrochlear adenitis, which frequently results from cat-scratch disease. These findings also can be detected with ultrasound (1) in the form of epitrochlear adenitis (Fig. 4.83B).

Normal Variations Causing Problems

The most common normal variations misinterpreted as fractures are the various secondary ossifications centers

around the elbow. Of these, the sliverlike lateral epicondyle and the frequently irregularly ossified medial condyle are the two most problematic bones (Fig. 4.84). They are followed, however, in short order by the accessory center of the olecranon (Fig. 4.84B). Another normal finding misinterpreted as abnormality is a circular radiolucency in the distal humerus representing an area of normal thinning of the floor of the olecranon fossa (Fig. 4.84A). In young infants, this radiolucency can erroneously suggest osteomyelitis. Finally, it should be reiterated that the normal radial head notch demonstrated in Figure 4.66 should not be misinterpreted as a radial head corner fracture.

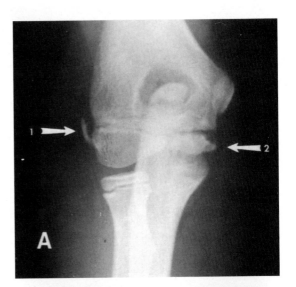
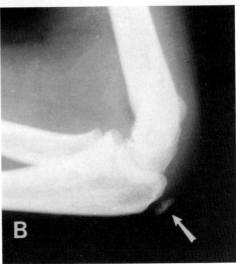

FIGURE 4.84. *Normal secondary ossification centers of the elbow.* **(A)** The accessory centers most commonly misinterpreted as fractures are the lateral epicondyle (*1*) and the irregularly ossified medial condyle (*2*). The central radiolucency in the humerus results from normal thinning of the base of the olecranon fossa. **(B)** The accessory ossification center of the olecranon (*arrow*) also often is misinterpreted as a fracture.

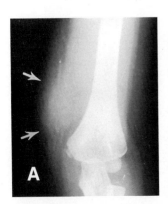
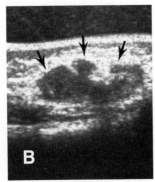

FIGURE 4.83. *Epitrochlear adenitis.* **(A)** Note extensive soft-tissue edema manifested by reticulation of the soft tissues (*arrows*). A central soft tissue density also is present. **(B)** Ultrasound demonstrates an enlarged inflamed, partially liquefied lymph node (*arrows*).

REFERENCES

1. Barr LL, Kirks DR. Ultrasonography of acute epitrochlear lymphadenitis. *Pediatr Radiol* 1993;23:72–73.
2. Blamoutier A, Klaue K, Damsin JP, Carlioz H. Osteochondral fractures of the glenoid fossa of the ulna in children: Review of four cases. *J Pediatr Orthop* 1991;11:638–640.
3. Bohrer SP. The fat pad sign following elbow trauma. Its usefulness and reliability in suspecting "invisible" fractures. *Clin Radiol* 1970;21:90–94.
4. DeLee JC, Wilkins KE, Rogers LF, et al. Fracture-separation of the distal humeral epiphysis. *J Bone Joint Surg* 1980;62A: 46–51.
5. Ellman H. Anterior angulation deformity of the radial head: an unusual lesion occurring in juvenile baseball players. *J Bone Joint Surg* 1976;11:281.
6. Gore RM, Rogers LF, Bowerman J, Suker J, Compere CL. Osseous manifestations of elbow stress associated with sports activities. *AJR* 1980;134:971–977.
7. Illingworth CM. Pulled elbow: Study of 100 patients. *Br Med J* 1975;2:672–674.
8. Jawish R, Rigault P, Padovani JP. Osteochondritis dissecans of the humeral capitellum in children. *Eur J Pediatr Surg* 1993;3: 97–100.
9. John SD, Wherry K, Swischuk LE, Phillips WA. Improving detection of elbow fractures by understanding their mechanics. *Radiograph* 1996;16:1443–1460.
10. Labelle H, Bunnell WP, Duhaime M, Poitras B. Cubtius varus deformity following supracondylar fracture of the humerus in children. *J Pediatr Orthop* 1982;2:539–546.
11. Markowitz RI, Davidson RS, Harty MP, Bellah RD, Hubbard AM, Rosenberg HK. Pictorial essay. Sonography of the elbow in infants and children. *AJR* 1992;159:829–833.
12. Michaels MG. A case of bilateral nursemaid's elbow. *Pediatr Emerg Care* 1989;5:226–227.
13. Papavasiliou V, Nenopoulos S, Venturis T. Fractures of the medial condyle of the humerus in childhood. *J Pediatr Orthop* 1987;7: 421–423.
14. Pavlov H, Torg JS, Jacobs B, Vigorita V. Non-union of olecranon epiphysis: Two cases in adolescent baseball pitchers. *AJR* 1981; 136:819–829.
15. Quan L, Marcuse EK. The epidemiology and treatment of radial head subluxation. *Am J Dis Child* 1985;139:1194–1197.
16. Rogers SL, MacEwan DW. Changes due to trauma in the fat plane overlying the supinator muscle: A radiologic sign. *Radiology* 1969;92:954–958.
17. Rogers LF, Malave S Jr, White H, Tachdjian MO. Plastic bowing, torus and greenstick supracondylar fractures of the humerus: Radiographic clues to obscure fractures of the elbow in children. *Radiology* 1978;128:145–150.
18. Vanthournout I, Rudelli A, Valenti P, Montagne J. Osteochondritis dissecans of the trochlea of the humerus. *Pediatr Radiol* 1991;21:600–601.
19. Wherry K, John SD, Swischuk LE, Phillips W. Linear fractures in the proximal ulna (A frequently missed injury). *Emerg Radiol* 1995;2:197–201.

Forearm

Injuries of the Forearm

Fractures through the midshaft of the radius and ulna are common, and either both bones or one bone only can be fractured. If a midshaft fracture is encountered in one bone, it is worthwhile to look for a fracture in the other bone, not only in its midshaft but at either end (Fig. 4.85). The types of fractures that can occur through the midshaft of the bones of the forearm include clearly visible transverse, spiral, and oblique fractures and the more subtle hairline, greenstick, and plastic bending or bowing fractures. Buckle or torus fractures are uncommon in the midshaft of these bones, because compared with the metaphyseal regions, the cortex of the midshaft is rather sturdy and not prone to buckling. Many overt midshaft fractures result from direct blows, but many also result from falls on the outstretched extremity.

Acute plastic or bowing fractures of the forearm are commonly missed, despite of the fact that pain and deformity are present clinically (1–4). In these patients, there often is loss of supination–pronation function, but if roentgenograms are obtained, a classic fracture with a visible fracture line is not detected. Rather, one notes only a variable degree of bowing of one or another, or both, of the bones of the forearm (Figs. 4.86 and 4.87). In this regard, one should note that the entire bone or just one part of it can be bent. These fractures can be considered the "green-

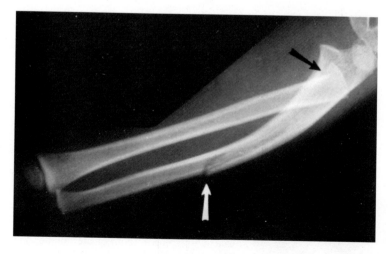

FIGURE 4.85. *Ulnar fracture with occult radial-head fracture.* Note the clearly visible fracture through the midshaft of the ulna (*white arrow*). It is a greenstick fracture with considerable bending of the ulna. In addition, note that there has been a metaphyseal fracture of the proximal radius (*black arrow*). The radial head is not dislocated in this patient, but the fracture could be overlooked because of the potentially distracting ulnar fracture.

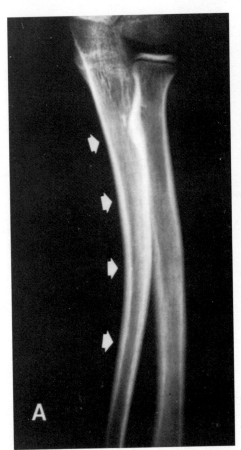
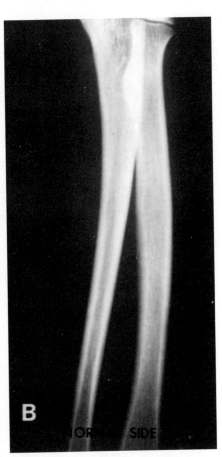

FIGURE 4.86. *Plastic bending fracture of the ulna.* (A) Note the marked degree of bending of the entire ulna (*arrows*). No fracture line is visible, but unless a comparative view of the normal side is examined, the bony deformity could be missed. (B) Normal side for comparison. Note the configuration of the normal ulna and compare it with the bent ulna in (A).

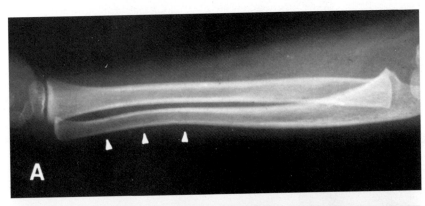
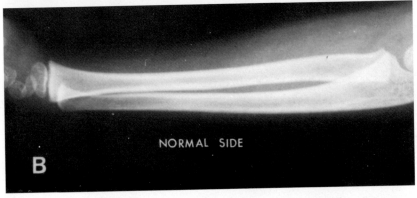

FIGURE 4.87. *Acute plastic bending fracture of the distal ulna and radius.* (A) Note bending of the distal ulna (*arrows*) and, to a lesser extent, of the distal radius. (B) Normal side for comparison. Although the views are not exactly the same in terms of positioning, one still can see that the normal ulna and radius are not bent.

est of greenstick" fractures, and although numerous microfractures may exist along the outer surface of the bones, none are large enough to be visualized as a single fracture roentgenographically. Because of this, the entire injury may go undetected unless comparative views of the other arm are obtained, and when they are the curvature of the involved bone should be compared inch-for-inch with the normal contralateral bone (Fig. 4.88). This is most important, for if only one extremity is examined, normal bowing can be misinterpreted as a plastic bending fracture (Fig. 4.89).

Overall, acute plastic bowing or bending fractures of the forearm are more common than generally believed and are quite variable. In some cases, both bones are involved in the bending process; in others only one is involved. In still other cases, one bone may be bent and the other frankly fractured. Another interesting feature of these fractures is that, unlike other fractures of the forearm, when they heal they usually produce little in the way of periosteal bone reaction. Bone scans are positive, but usually they are not required. Clinically there is no attempt to reduce these frac-

tures, and thus residual bowing with supination–pronation motion impairment can persist well after healing is complete.

The other noteworthy fracture of the bones of the forearm is Monteggia's fracture. This fracture consists of a fracture of the ulna and a dislocation of the radial head (Fig. 4.90). Both anterior and posterior Monteggia's fractures occur, and in either case it is the associated dislocation of the radial head that is the missed portion of this injury. *It cannot be stated often enough that one should always line up the radial head and capitellum to determine whether they are in a straight-line relationship.* If they are not, dislocation of the radial head is present.

Normal Variations Causing Problems

The only normal finding in the midshaft of the radius and ulna that can be misinterpreted as a fracture is a vascular groove in either bone. These vascular grooves are diaphyseal and appear no different from those in other long bones.

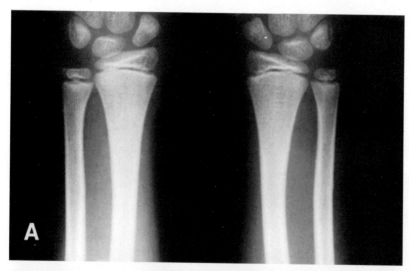

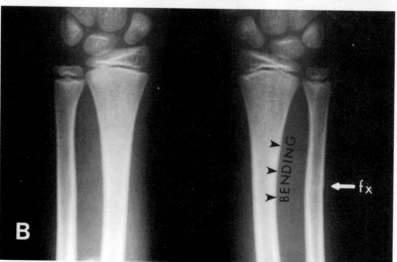

FIGURE 4.88. *Subtle bending fracture.* **(A)** Note slight bending of the left radius. There also is a subtle greenstick fracture of the distal ulna. **(B)** Fractures are labeled. Bending fracture of radius (*black arrows*). Fracture of ulna (*fx*).

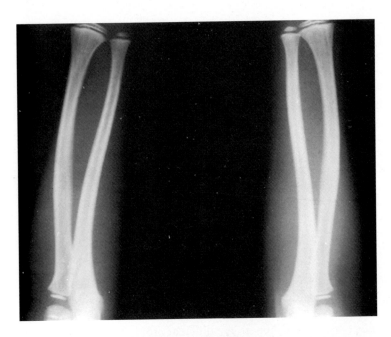

FIGURE 4.89. *Normal bowing of bones of the forearm.* Note the normal degree of bowing of the bones of the forearm on both sides. This is the reason why comparative views should always be obtained if a bending fracture is suspected. Only with comparative views can one be certain that such a fracture exists. If only one of these extremities were examined, the degree of bending could be misconstrued as being abnormal.

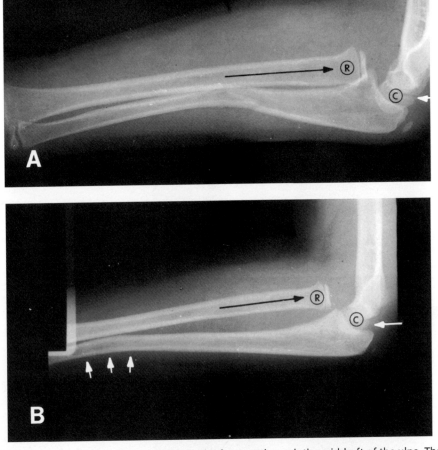

FIGURE 4.90. *Monteggia fracture.* **(A)** Note the fracture through the midshaft of the ulna. There is considerable associated bending of the ulna. Also note that the radial head (*R*) is dislocated and does not line up in a straight line with the capitellum (*C*). **(B)** Another patient with a dislocated radial head (*R*). This time, however, the only other fracture is a subtle bending fracture of the ulna (*arrows*). C, capitellum.

REFERENCES

1. Attia MW, Glasstetter DS. Plastic bowing type fracture of the forearm in two children. *Pediatr Emerg Care* 1997;13:392–393.
2. Borden S. Roentgen recognition of acute plastic bowing of the forearm in children. *AJR* 1975;125:524–530.
3. Crowe JE, Swischuk LE. Acute bowing fractures of the forearm in children: A frequently missed injury. *AJR* 1977;128:981–984.
4. Stenstrom R, Gripenberg L, Bergius AR. Traumatic bowing of forearm and lower leg in children. *Acta Radiol* 1978;19:243–249.

Wringer Injuries

For the most part, washing machine wringer arm injuries are uncommon in this day and age, but some still do occur (1). Bone injury is very uncommon, however, and although an occasional epiphyseal dislocation may be encountered, these injuries are mainly soft tissue injuries.

REFERENCE

1. Stone HH, Cantwell DV, Fullenwider JT. Wringer arm injuries. *J Pediatr Surg* 1976;11:375–379.

Wrist

Normal Fat Pads

There are two fat pads around the wrist that can be utilized in the assessment of wrist injuries. The first is the pronator

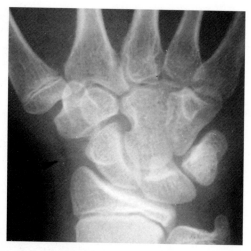

FIGURE 4.92. *Normal navicular fat pad.* The navicular fat pad (*arrow*) is best visualized in older children. It can be obliterated or displaced with navicular bone injuries.

quadratus fat pad (9), and the second is the navicular fat pad (4,15). The pronator quadratus fat pad is seen on lateral views of the wrist and lies along the pronator quadratus muscle (Fig. 4.91). The navicular fat pad lies just medial to the navicular bone and is seen on posteroanterior views of the wrist (Fig. 4.92). In young infants, this latter fat pad is not visualized with as much consistency as it is in older children. This is not so unfortunate, however, because obliteration of the navicular fat pad is utilized primarily for the detection of navicular fractures, and these fractures are not particularly common in infants and young children. Distal, radial, and ulnar fractures, on the other hand, are quite common, and it is in this regard that viewing displacement and obliteration of the pronator quadratus fat pad becomes most useful.

Determining the Presence of Fluid in the Wrist Joint

Determining the presence of fluid in the wrist joint simply amounts to noting whether the soft tissues around the wrist are swollen. Apart from this, there is little else to look for, for the joint space seldom becomes widened, and except for the navicular fat pad, no other useful fat pads are present. With wrist joint fluid, most of the swelling occurs distal to the radial and ulnar epiphyseal lines (Fig. 4.93A). If edematous swelling results from a distal radioulnar fracture, such swelling is located primarily proximal to the epiphyseal lines (Fig. 4.93B).

Injuries of the Distal Radius and Ulna

Although a variety of overt ***transverse and oblique fractures*** commonly occur through the distal third of the radius

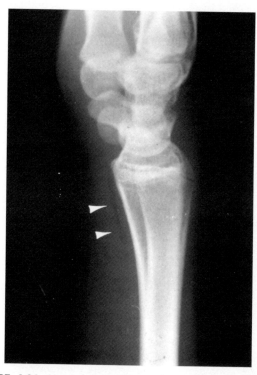

FIGURE 4.91. *Normal pronator quadratus fat pad.* Note the normal appearance and location of the pronator quadratus fat pad (*arrows*).

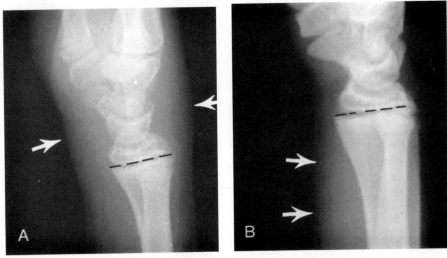

FIGURE 4.93. *Joint fluid in the wrist.* **(A)** *Navicular fracture.* In this patient with joint fluid secondary to a navicular fracture, note that most of the swelling (*arrows*) is located above the epiphyseal line of the distal radius (*dotted line*). **(B)** *Distal radial fracture.* Wrist swelling is again present, but most of the swelling (*arrows*) is located below the epiphyseal line of the distal radius (*dotted line*). This speaks against the presence of any significant wrist joint fluid.

and ulna, with or without angulation or displacement, these fractures usually are not difficult to detect (Fig. 4.94). On the other hand, if they are hairline or subtle greenstick fractures, they may elude early diagnosis unless one studies the soft tissues first (Fig. 4.95). The same can be said for subtle bending fractures (Fig. 4.88).

Cortical buckle or torus fractures also are common in this area and most often are sustained from falls on the outstretched

extremity. The cortical buckles and kinks are of an almost endless variety of configurations, and usually are more clearly visible on one view than another (Fig. 4.96). This is especially true of posterior buckle fractures of the distal radius, in which the fracture and associated posterior tilting of the articular surface frequently are seen on the lateral view only (Fig. 4.97A and B) A similar problem occurs with Smith's fractures. If these fractures are overt there is no problem in diagnosis, but if they are

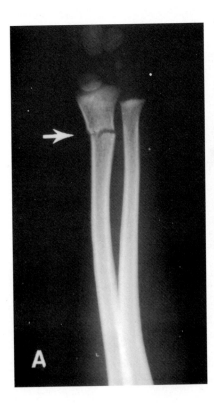

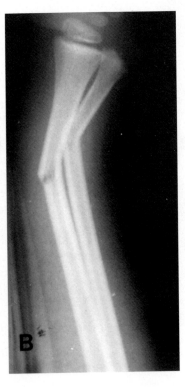

FIGURE 4.94. *Distal radial and ulnar fractures: varying configurations.* **(A)** Note the transverse, slightly angulated fracture through the distal radius (*arrow*). **(B)** Markedly angulated fractures through both bones of the forearm.

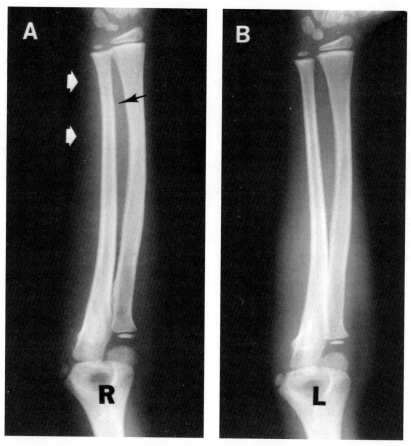

FIGURE 4.95. *Subtle ulnar fracture: value of soft tissues.* **(A)** First, note thickening and prominence of the soft tissues along the distal ulna (*white arrows*). A greenstick fracture through the distal ulna basically is invisible (*black arrow*), and slight generalized bending of the ulna is a subtle finding. **(B)** Normal side for comparison. Note the normal appearance of the soft tissues. Also note that the normal ulna is straighter than the fractured ulna, further attesting to the presence of the ulnar fractures on the right.

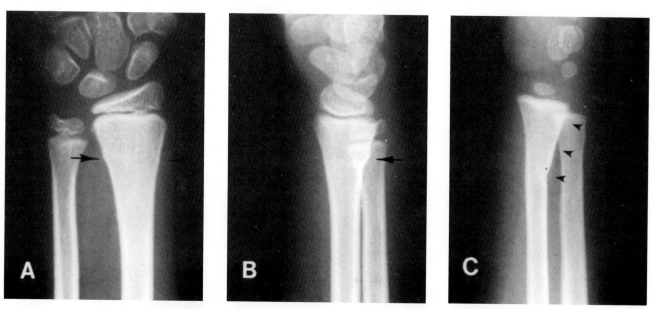

FIGURE 4.96. *Buckle (torus) fractures of the distal forearm.* **(A)** Subtle buckling of the cortex is seen in the distal radius (*arrows*). **(B)** Lateral view more clearly demonstrates the buckling (*arrow*). Note that the soft tissues are swollen and that the pronator quadratus fat pad has been obliterated **(C)** Another infant with a buckle fracture of the distal radius (*arrows*).

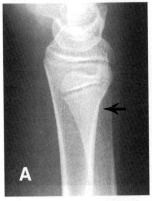
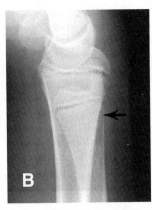
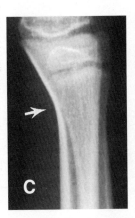
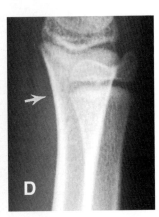

FIGURE 4.97. *Buckle fractures of distal radius: value of lateral film.* **(A)** Childhood equivalent of Colles' fracture. Note posterior buckle (*arrow*). **(B)** Normal side for comparison. Note that the cortex is smooth (*arrow*). **(C)** Childhood equivalent of Smith's fracture. Note the anterior cortical buckle (*arrow*). **(D)** Normal side for comparison. Note the smooth cortex (*arrow*).

subtle, the buckling of the cortex over the anterior aspect of the distal radius can be missed (Fig. 4.97C and D).

The most common epiphyseal–metaphyseal injuries are Salter–Harris type I and II injuries. Types III, IV, and V injuries are relatively uncommon. Most often the Salter–Harris type I or II fracture involves the epiphyseal–metaphyseal junction of the radius, but occasionally the ulna also is involved. In most instances the injury results from falling on the outstretched extremity, and if there is

displacement of the distal radial epiphysis it is posterior. In this regard this type of fracture is the childhood equivalent of a Colles' fracture. In detecting these injuries, one should look for one or more of the following changes: soft tissue edema, obliteration or displacement of the pronator quadratus fat pad, widening of the involved epiphyseal line, an associated metaphyseal corner fracture, or displacement of the epiphysis (Figs. 4.98–4.100). Widening of the epiphyseal line, however, is most important.

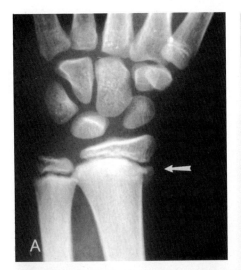
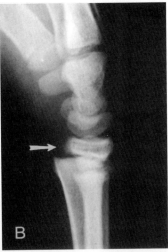

FIGURE 4.98. *Displaced Salter–Harris type II epiphyseal–metaphyseal fracture of the radius.* **(A)** Note that the distal radial epiphysis is displaced laterally, and that there is a small metaphyseal corner fracture (*arrow*). **(B)** Lateral view demonstrates the marked degree of posterior displacement of the distal radial epiphysis (*arrow*). There is slight impaction of the posterior corner of the distal radial metaphysis. **(C)** Subtle Salter–Harris type I fracture of radius (*arrows*) in older child with epiphysis almost closed. **(D)** Normal side for comparison.

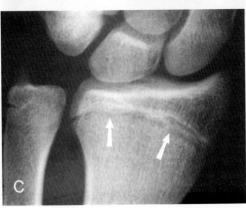
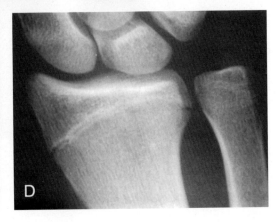

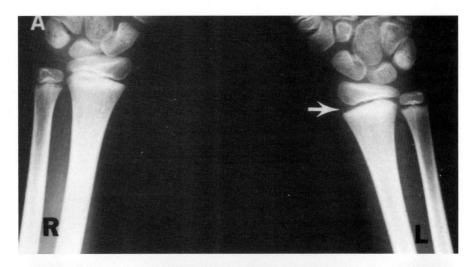

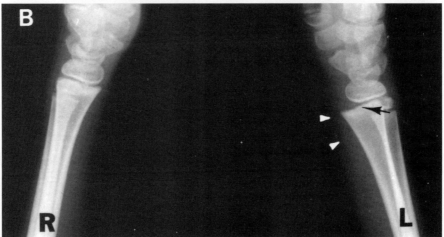

FIGURE 4.99. *Epiphyseal–metaphyseal fracture of the wrist with small avulsed fragment (Salter–Harris type II injury).* **(A)** On frontal view, note that the left distal radial epiphysis is slightly displaced, and that the epiphyseal line is a little wider than the normal epiphyseal line on the right. Also note the thin sliverlike avulsed metaphyseal fragment (*arrow*). **(B)** Lateral view demonstrating swelling of the soft tissues around the left wrist, anterior displacement of the pronator quadratus fat pad (*white arrows*), posterior displacement of the distal radial epiphysis, and the sliverlike avulsed metaphyseal fragment (*black arrow*).

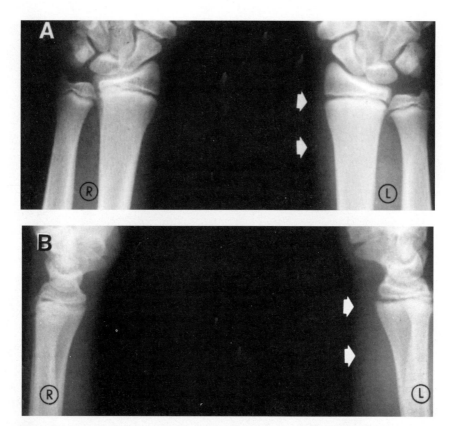

FIGURE 4.100. *Salter–Harris type I epiphyseal–metaphyseal fracture of the wrist: value of soft tissues.* **(A)** On frontal view, one might suspect that the epiphyseal line through the distal left radius is a little wider than the one on the right, but if one first notes that soft tissue swelling in the area also is present (*arrows*), then the finding becomes even more suspicious. **(B)** Confirmation is present on the lateral view, in which one can see marked swelling of the soft tissues anterior to the wrist (*arrows*) and complete obliteration of the pronator quadratus fat pad. In addition, the distal radial epiphysis is slightly displaced posteriorly.

An interesting manifestation of wrist injuries in childhood is the presence of an ulnar styloid tip avulsion fracture. This is an important fracture because virtually always if it is present a radial fracture also is present (14). The reason for this is that the ligaments surrounding the two bones are strong and do not allow for isolated ulnar styloid injuries. Therefore, if there is enough force to fracture the ulnar styloid tip, a radial fracture occurs also. If the fracture is overt, there is no problem with its recognition, and the ulnar styloid process fracture is incidental (Fig. 4.101). If the radial fracture is subtle, however, it can be overlooked and the entire problem misinterpreted as a rather innocuous ulnar styloid tip fracture (Fig. 4.102). Most often the radical fractures are dorsal buckle fractures of the radius or Salter–Harris type I or II injuries with minimal displacement of the epiphysis. Isolated ulnar styloid fractures can be seen if direct blows to the styloid process are sustained (14).

Old, ununited styloid avulsion fractures may erreoneously suggest the presence of a secondary ossification

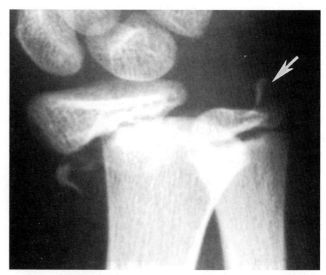

FIGURE 4.101. *Overt radial fracture with ulnar styloid fracture.* Note the overt displaced epiphyseal–metaphyseal fracture of the radius. Also note the subtle ulnar styloid tip fracture (*arrow*).

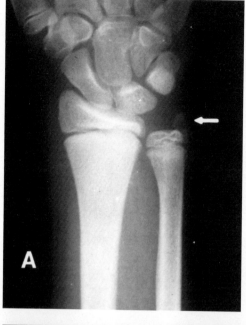

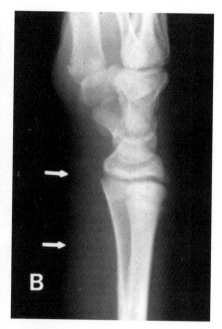

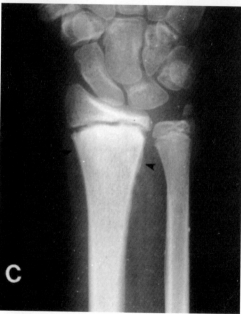

FIGURE 4.102. *Epiphyseal–metaphyseal fracture of the wrist with distracting ulnar styloid fracture.* (**A**) Note swelling around the wrist and a fractured ulnar styloid process (*arrow*). At first one might think this is the only injury present. (**B**) On lateral view, however, one can see that there is considerable swelling anterior to the wrist (*arrows*), and that the pronator quadratus fat pad is totally obliterated. Under these circumstances, one should suspect an underlying epiphyseal–metaphyseal injury of the radius, for an isolated ulnar styloid process fracture would not result in this much swelling. (**C**) Two weeks later, note evidence of healing of the occult epiphyseal–metaphyseal fracture of the distal radius. Some periosteal new bone is seen along the distal radial shaft (*arrow*), and sclerosis along the epiphyseal–metaphyseal junction is clearly evident. The ununited ulnar styloid process fracture is noted again.

center (Fig. 4.103A). In these cases the ossicle is located at the tip of the styloid process. If the styloid process itself forms as a separate center, the ulnar epiphysis is hypoplastic and the entire styloid process is seen as a separate ossicle (Fig. 4.103B and C). The ulnar epiphysis also can be bipartite through its midportion. In these cases there usually is no confusion with an ulnar styloid tip fracture (Fig. 4.103D).

Finally it should be noted that chronic stress–induced epiphyseal–metaphyseal fractures of the distal radius and ulna can be seen in gymnasts and other young athletes who overuse the wrist (1,2,4,8). These fractures appear no different than healing, classic epiphyseal–metaphyseal injuries (Fig. 4.104). They often are discovered somewhat incidentally, however, because acute presentation of these injuries is not the rule. The problem is one of chronic repetitive subclinical stress.

Galeazzi's fracture, which often is associated with radioulnar disassociation, is rare in childhood (7). The radioulnar disassociation is best evaluated on lateral views and usually is finally delineated with CT scanning (12).

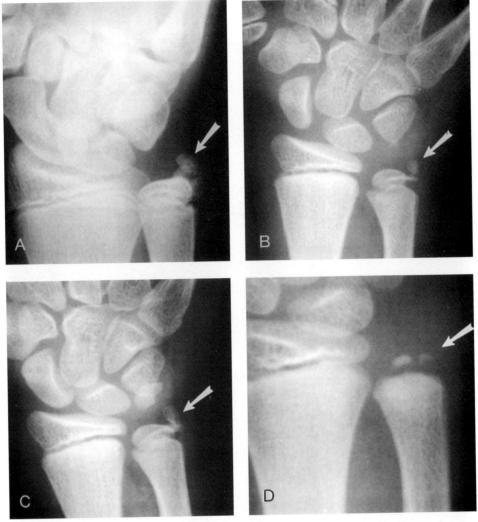

FIGURE 4.103. (A) *Ununited styloid fracture.* Note the smooth, ununited styloid tip fracture (*arrow*), and note that the ulnar epiphysis is normal in configuration. **(B)** Separate ulnar styloid ossification center. Note the accessory ossification center (*arrow*). The underlying epiphysis is dysplastic and flat. **(C)** As the child grows older, the accessory epiphysis begins to unite (*arrow*). The ulnar epiphysis itself remains thin and dysplastic. (A-C are from Stansberry SD, Swischuk LE, Swischuk JL, Midgett WT. Signficance of ulnar styloid fractures in childhood. *Pediatr Emerg Care* 1990;6:99-103, With permission.) **(D)** Bipartite normal ulnar epiphysis (*arrow*).

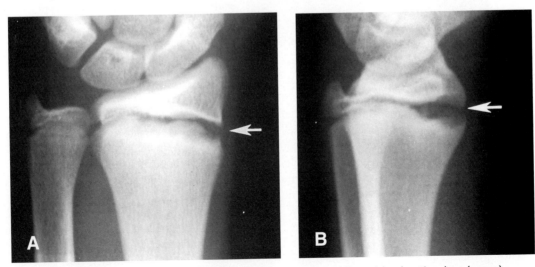

FIGURE 4.104. *Gymnast's wrist.* **(A)** Note widened epiphyseal line with sclerotic edges (*arrow*). **(B)** Lateral view demonstrating similar findings (*arrow*). These findings represent a chronic Salter–Harris type 1 injury.

Injuries of the Carpal Bones

Fractures or dislocations of the carpal bones in infants and young children are uncommon. They are more common in the older child; of these, ***fractures of the navicular bone*** are most common (16). The clinical findings in these fractures are similar to those seen in adults (i.e., acute tenderness in the anatomic snuff box). These fractures result from falls on the outstretched extremity.

Roentgenographically, this fracture can be suspected if there is localized soft tissue swelling or obliteration of the navicular fat pad (4,9,15), shortening or telescoping of the navicular bone, rotation and resultant increase in density of one of the fracture fragments, or a visible fracture line (Fig. 4.105). In some cases, oblique (navicular) views may be necessary for clearer visualization of the suspected fracture, and in those cases in which the presence of a fracture is in doubt, nuclear scintigraphy (10) or MRI (3,6) can be of

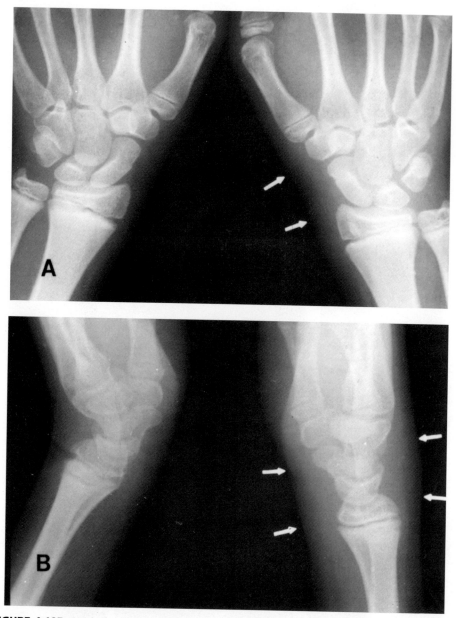

FIGURE 4.105. *Navicular fracture.* **(A)** First note that the soft tissues adjacent to the navicular bone are thickened and edematous (*arrows*). In addition, note that the navicular bone on the left is shorter (impacted) than the normal one on the right. A subtle fracture line through its upper third also is suggested. **(B)** Lateral view demonstrating extensive swelling around the wrist. Swelling extends both anteriorly and posteriorly (*arrows*). Note that the site of the swelling is located primarily around the carpal bones. With distal radial injuries, it usually is located more proximally.

value. Overall, navicular fractures are quite variable and often subtle (Fig. 4.106). The reason for this is that not only can one encounter typical hairline fractures such as seen in adults, but in addition, because the bones of the child are soft, a number of buckle-impaction fractures occur (Fig.

4.106). Comparative views are essential in these cases. In addition, oblique views of the wrist are mandatory.

Aseptic necrosis as a complication of scaphoid (navicular) fractures is not as common in children as in adults (13), but it does occur. Usually it is the proximal fragment that

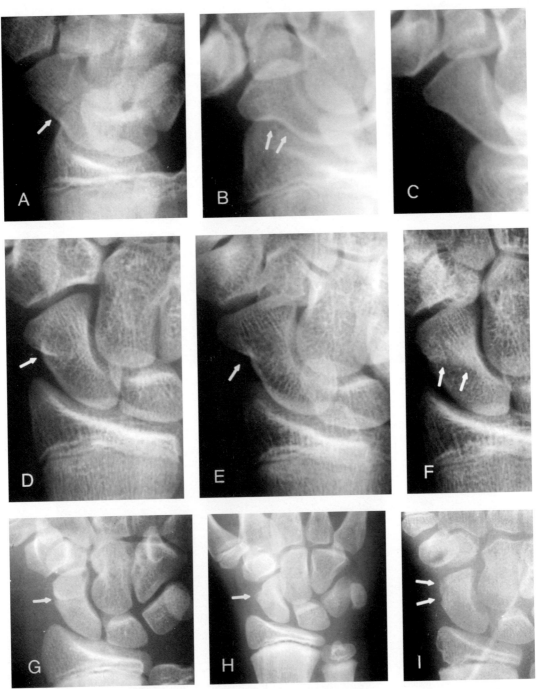

FIGURE 4.106. *Navicular fractures.* **(A)** Subtle, barely visible hairline fracture (*arrow*). **(B)** Subtle bending fracture (*arrows*). **(C)** Normal side for comparison. **(D)** Another patient with a buckle fracture (*arrow*). **(E)** Oblique view in the patient in **D** demonstrates the same fracture (*arrow*). **(F)** Later, with healing, note the area of sclerosis (*arrows*). **(G)** Transverse fracture (*arrow*) with slight tilting of the upper fragment in another patient. **(H)** Markedly angulated fracture with a small avulsed fragment (*arrow*). **(I)** Another fracture with multiple fragments.

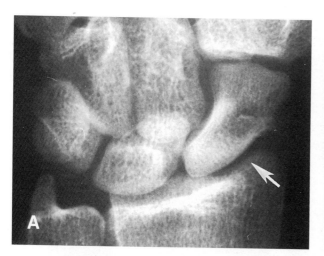
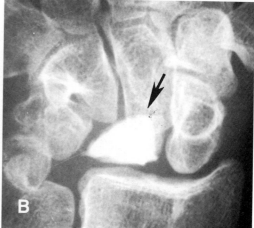

FIGURE 4.107. *Aseptic necrosis: carpal navicular.* (**A**) Note the sclerotic proximal fracture fragment (*arrow*). (**B**) Note sclerotic lunate bone (*arrow*).

becomes necrotic, and the radiographic findings consist of nonunion of the fracture and increasing sclerosis of the necrotic fragment (Fig. 4.107). Aseptic necrosis of the other carpal bones is uncommon but occasionally is encountered (Fig. 4.107B).

The only other bones in the wrist to fracture with any frequency in childhood are the pisiform and triquetrum. The pisiform fracture can result from a direct blow, but the triquetral fracture usually results from falling on the outstretched extremity. These fractures can be subtle (Fig. 4.108).

In terms of carpal bone dislocations, the occasional case of lunate or perilunate dislocation of the wrist in the older child occurs. These injuries present with malalignment of the proximal row of carpal bones and associated discrepancy in the width of the perilunate joint spaces. In other words, the joint spaces are narrower or completely obliterated on one side, and wider on the other (Fig. 4.109A). Obliteration of the joint space results from overlap of the dislocated carpal bones, and widening, of course, is caused by distraction of the involved bones. On lateral view, the normal vertical, sequential arrangement of the capitate, lunate, and distal radial epiphysis is lost in these cases (Fig. 4.109B). This latter point is most important, for any deviation from this arrangement of the carpal bones should indicate an underlying dislocation. Of course, with a lunate dislocation, the lunate lies anterior to the capitate and distal radial epiphysis, but with a perilunate dislocation both the lunate and distal radius and its epiphysis move forward and lie anterior to the other bones of the wrist.

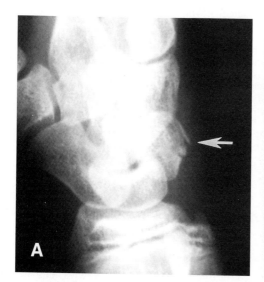
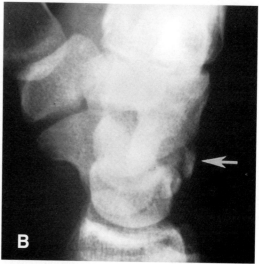

FIGURE 4.108. *Fracture of triquetrum.* (**A**) Note the comminuted fracture (*arrow*) of the triquetral bone. (**B**) Another patient with similar fragmentation (*arrow*).

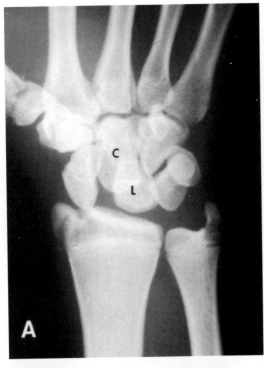

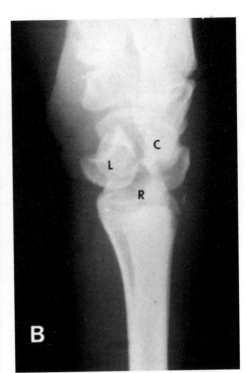

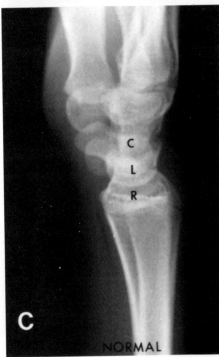

FIGURE 4.109. *Dislocation of the lunate.* **(A)** Note that the joint spaces to either side of the lunate bone (*L*) are unequal. This should alert one to the dislocation. In addition, note that the lunate bone overlies the capitate (*C*), and that the wrist is foreshortened. Also note fractures of the ulnar styloid process, distal radial epiphysis, proximal thumb, and navicular bone (foreshortening and rotation). **(B)** Lateral view demonstrating abnormal anterior location of the lunate bone (*L*). The capitate (*C*) and distal radial epiphysis (*R*) lie behind the lunate bone. **(C)** Normal view for comparison showing the normal vertical, sequential arrangement of the capitate (*C*), lunate (*L*), and distal radial epiphysis (*R*).

Other dislocations in the wrist are quite uncommon. These include isolated rotatory subluxation of the navicular bone (5) (Fig. 4.110) and dislocation of the carpal–metacarpal joints. In assessing the wrist for a suspected underlying dislocation of any of the bones one should follow two rules. First, one should identify each of the carpal bones with clarity, and second, one should note whether the individual joint spaces are uniform and delineated by parallel lines. In other words, one should try to determine whether any bony overlap or joint widening is present. If any of the individual bones are not clearly visualized and if any of the joint spaces appear suspiciously narrow or wide, one should turn to oblique and lateral views for further delineation and verification. Finally, a form of Galeazzi's injury is a fracture dislocation (7) of the wrist. The ulna is dislocated, and in addition the pisiform also can be dislocated. The ulna also can dislocate alone (Fig. 4.111).

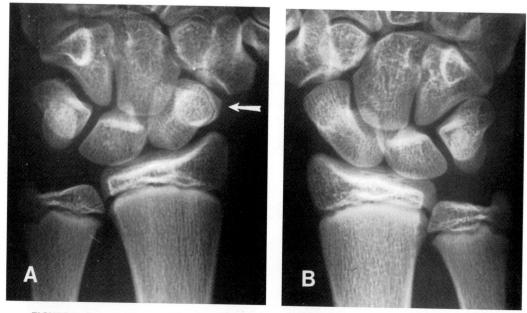

FIGURE 4.110. *Rotatory subluxation of navicular bone.* **(A)** Note slight increase in the navicular–lunate joint space and also telescoping of the navicular bone (caused by rotation) resulting in the circle sign (*arrow*). **(B)** Normal side for comparison.

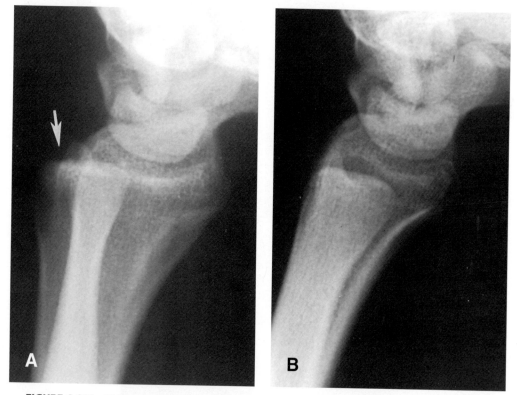

FIGURE 4.111. *Dislocation of ulna.* **(A)** Note posterior displacement of the ulna (*arrow*). **(B)** Normal side for comparison. Note the normal position of the ulna. Both of these are true lateral views of the wrist.

Sprained Wrist

There is a good rule to follow with wrist injuries: "A sprained wrist is a fractured wrist until proven otherwise." This rule, taught to me by a colleague, has proven most trustworthy. This is not to say that simple sprains of the wrist do not occur, but rather that many so-called sprains actually turn out to be epiphyseal–metaphyseal or cortical buckle injuries. Even in those cases in which the radiographic findings are confined to soft tissue swelling and obliteration of the pronator quadratus fat pad, clinical tenderness along the epiphyseal line or distal radius indicates the presence of an epiphyseal–metaphyseal injury. It is quite a different problem from the one encountered in the ankle, in which a sprained ankle more often than not turns out to be just a sprained ankle.

Septic Arthritis, Osteomyelitis, and Cellulitis of the Wrist

Generally speaking, septic arthritis, osteomyelitis, and cellulitis of the wrist all lead to pronounced swelling in and around the wrist joint. The various normal soft tissue struc-

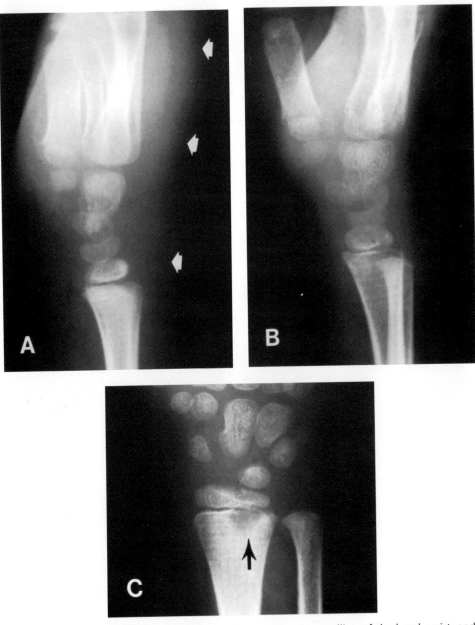

FIGURE 4.112. *Osteomyelitis: distal radius.* **(A)** Note extensive swelling of the hand, wrist, and distal forearm (*arrows*). **(B)** Normal side for comparison. **(C)** Frontal view demonstrating metaphyseal defect due to osteomyelitis (*arrow*).

tures are obliterated, and early on, soft tissue swelling is most pronounced around the area of primary involvement (Fig. 4.112). In less advanced cases, less bone destruction is seen, and nuclear scintigraphy often is required (10).

Normal Findings Causing Problems

For the most part, the carpal bones ossify as single smooth foci, but occasionally irregular ossification of one or another of the carpal bones can be misinterpreted as a fracture. This occurs with the pisiform bone more than any other (Fig. 4.113A). Another problem in the wrist, although far less common, is that of misinterpreting a bipartite navicular bone as a fractured navicular bone (Fig. 4.113B). In the distal radius and ulna, an incompletely obliterated but nor-

mally closing epiphyseal line (14) can be misinterpreted as a fracture (Fig. 4.113C), and occasionally normal bony spicules extending into the epiphyseal line suggest an epiphyseal–metaphyseal injury (Fig. 4.113D).

REFERENCES

1. Caine D, Roy S, Singer KM, Broekhoff J. Stress changes of the distal radial growth plate. *Am J Sports Med* 1992;20:290–298.
2. Carter SR, Aldridge MJ, Fitzgerald R, Davies AM. Stress changes of the wrist in adolescent gymnasts. *Br J Radiol* 1988;61:109–112.
3. Breitenseher MJ, Metz VM, Gilula LA, Gaebler C, Kukla C, Fleischmann D, Imhof H, Trattnig S. Radiographically occult scaphoid fractures: Value of MR imaging in detection. *Radiology* 1997;203:245–250.

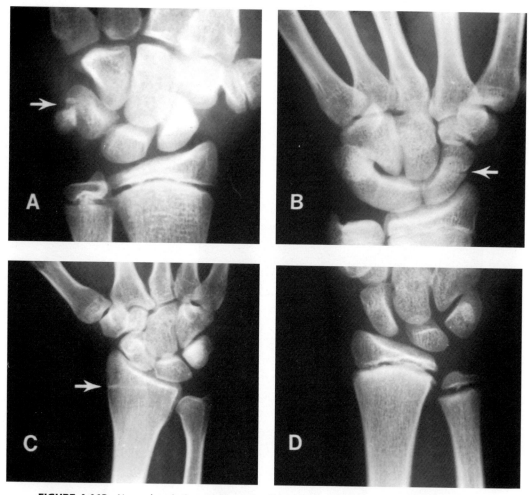

FIGURE 4.113. *Normal variations in the wrist.* **(A)** Irregular ossification of the pisiform (*arrow*). This should not be misinterpreted as a fracture of the pisiform. **(B)** Bipartite navicular. Note the bipartite navicular (*arrow*). Also note that the lunate and triquetral bones are fused. The bipartite navicular should not be misinterpreted as a fracture. **(C)** Incompletely obliterated radial epiphysis. Note the incompletely obliterated epiphysis of the distal radius (*arrow*), often misinterpreted as a fracture. **(D)** Epiphyseal–metaphyseal spicules. Note normal spicules extending from the ulnar epiphysis, and normal metaphyseal spicules and irregularity along the inner aspect of the distal radial metaphysis.

4. Haverling M, Sylven M. Soft tissue abnormalities at fracture of the scaphoid. *Acta Radiol* 1978;19:497–501.
5. Hudson TM, Caragol WJ, Kaye JJ. Isolated rotatory subluxation of the carpal navicular. *AJR* 1976;126:601–611.
6. Hunter JD, Escobedo EM, Wilson AJ, Hanel DP, Zink-Brody GC, Mann FA. MR imaging of clinically suspected scaphoid fractures. *AJR* 1997;168:1287–1293.
7. Landfried MJ, Stenclik M, Susi JG. Variant of Galeazzi fracture-dislocation in children. *J Pediatr Orthop* 1991;11:332–335.
8. Liebling MS, Berdon WE, Ruzal-Shapiro C, Levin TL, Roye D Jr, Wilkinson R. Case report. Gymnast's wrist (pseudorickets growth plate abnormality) in adolescent athletes: Findings on plain films and MR imaging. *AJR* 1995;164:157–159.
9. MacEwan DW. Changes due to trauma in the fat plane overlying the pronator quadratus muscle: A radiologic sign. *Radiology* 1964;82: 879–886.
10. Rolfe EB, Garvie NW, Khan MA, Ackery DM. Isotope bone imaging in suspected scaphoid trauma. *Br J Radiol* 1981;54: 762–767.
11. Roy S, Caine D, Singer KM. Stress changes of the distal radial epiphysis in young gymnasts: A report of twenty-one cases and a review of the literature. *Am J Sports Med* 1985;13:301–308.
12. Scheffler R, Armstrong D, Hutton L. Computed tomographic diagnosis of distal radio-ulnar joint disruption. *J Can Assoc Radiol* 1984;35:212–213.
13. Southcott R, Rosman MA. Nonunion of carpal scaphoid fractures in children. *J Bone Joint Surg* 1977;59B:20–23.
14. Stansberry SD, Swischuk LE, Swischuk JL, Midgett TA. Significance of ulnar styloid fractures in childhood. *Pediatr Emerg Care* 1990;6:99–103.
15. Terry DW Jr, Ramin JE. The navicular fat stripe: A useful roentgen feature for evaluating wrist trauma. *AJR* 1975;124:25–28.
16. Wulff RN, Schmidt TL. Carpal fractures in children. *J Pediatr Orthop* 1998;18:462–465.

Hand

Evaluation of the Fat Pads and Soft Tissues

There are no specific fat pads to evaluate in the hand, and evaluation of the soft tissues consists primarily of noting whether localized soft tissue edema and swelling are present. This latter finding, however, as nonspecific as it is, is very helpful in localizing the site of injury in the fingers (Fig. 4.114).

Detecting Fluid in the Small Joints of the Hand

Detection of fluid in the small joints of the hand depends primarily on noting the presence of swelling around the joint. In some cases, the joint space may be widened (5), but this finding often is subtle. There are no specific fat pads to evaluate, and thus, in most cases, one is left only with generalized swelling around a knuckle (Figs. 4.114 and 4.115).

Injuries of the Metacarpals and Phalanges

Crush injuries to the terminal phalanges are hardly worth obtaining roentgenograms, because unless the fracture is a compound fracture, little needs to be done for these

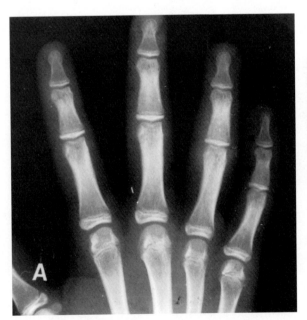
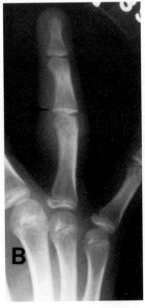

FIGURE 4.114. *Phalangeal fracture: value of soft tissues.* **(A)** Note soft tissue swelling localizing the site of injury to the proximal interphalangeal joint of the ring finger (*arrows*). **(B)** Oblique view demonstrates the swelling again but in addition also demonstrates the presence of a small chip fracture of the epiphysis (*arrow*). This is a Salter–Harris type III injury with bleeding into the joint and associated periarticular soft tissue swelling.

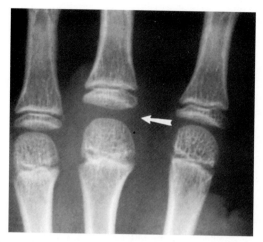

FIGURE 4.115. *Joint fluid.* Note the widened joint space (*arrow*) at the metacarpal joint. This resulted from traumatic hemarthrosis.

injuries. The typically comminuted terminal phalangeal tuft is not difficult to detect roentgenographically, and even if it is missed, no dire sequelae develop. Other injuries to the fingers and thumb result from hyperextension, twisting, or direct blows to the digits. *The types of fractures sustained include buckle (torus) fractures, epiphyseal–metaphyseal injuries, fracture dislocations, and linear, transverse, or spiral fractures.* They come in an almost endless assortment of configurations, and some are illustrated in Fig. 4.116. In addition, although rare, plastic bending fractures can occur (Fig. 4.117).

An important point regarding cortical buckle (torus) fractures occurring at the proximal end of the phalanges or distal ends of the metacarpals is that if one sees one such fracture, then one should look at the neighboring digits for other similar fractures. In addition, usually all of these frac-

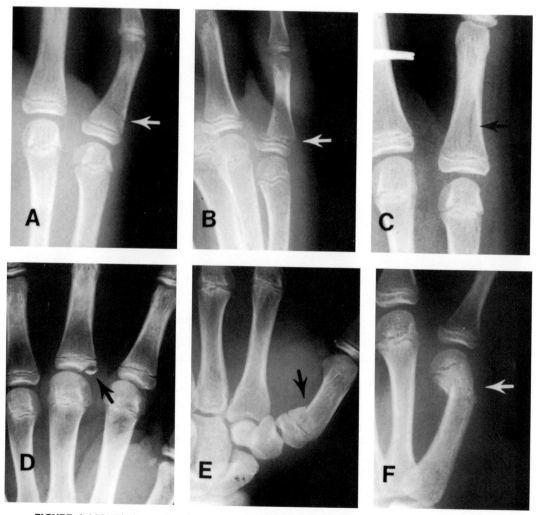

FIGURE 4.116. *Phalangeal and metacarpal fractures: various types.* **(A)** Typical transverse fracture (*arrow*). **(B)** Epiphyseal–metaphyseal fracture with displacement (*arrow*). Clinically, this type of fracture can be mistaken for a true dislocation. **(C)** Longitudinal fracture through phalanx (*arrow*). **(D)** Epiphyseal chip fracture (*arrow*). **(E)** Epiphyseal–metaphyseal fracture (Salter–Harris type II injury) of the base of the first metacarpal (*arrow*). **(F)** Typical angulated fracture (*arrow*) through the head of the fifth metacarpal. This fracture usually is sustained by punching someone or something and often is termed the "boxer's fracture."

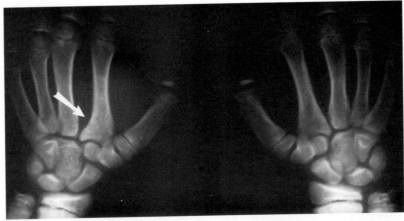

FIGURE 4.117. *Plastic bending fracture: metacarpal.* Note swelling over the left hand and a wavy, bent appearance of the first metacarpal (*arrow*). Compare with its normal, straight appearance on the other side.

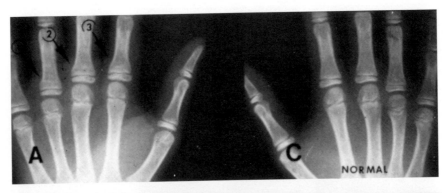

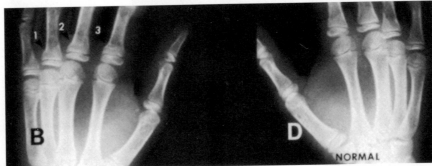

FIGURE 4.118. *Buckle (torus) fractures of the base of the phalanges.* **(A)** Frontal view demonstrating a buckle fracture through the base of the proximal phalanx of the fourth digit (*1*). A more subtle but similar fracture is present through the base of the proximal phalanx of the third digit (*2*). An even more subtle fracture is present through the base of the proximal phalanx of the second digit (*3*). This last fracture is so subtle that it might not be appreciated on this view alone. **(B)** Oblique view more clearly demonstrates all three fractures. **(C and D)** Normal frontal and oblique views for comparison. Specifically, compare the contour of the cortices of the involved bones.

tures are more clearly defined on oblique views (Fig. 4.118). Direct blows to the dorsum of the hand can result in transverse fractures through the metacarpal bones that often elude initial observation. The reason for this is that many times the fracture line is barely visible, and little or no displacement of the fracture fragments occurs. In such cases, it is of great benefit to examine the soft tissues first, and then, if edema and swelling are noted, to focus one's attention on the underlying bones (Fig. 4.119).

Dislocations of the fingers and thumb (Fig. 4.120) are not particularly common in childhood, for rather than a dislocation an epiphyseal–metaphyseal separation occurs (Fig. 4.116B). Clinically, however, these separations often appear to be true dislocations. The classic fracture dislocation of the base of the first metacarpal bone (Bennett's

fracture) occurs only after the epiphysis of the thumb has fused. Until this time, this fracture is the equivalent of a Salter–Harris type I or II injury (Fig. 4.116E). This, however, is not to say that the thumb never dislocates in childhood, for indeed it does, but usually this occurs at the metacarpal–phalangeal joint. Frequently, this dislocation is associated with an epiphyseal–metaphyseal fracture (Fig. 4.120), and in the older child in whom the epiphysis has fused or is near fusion, the same injury can result in the so-called gamekeeper's thumb. In this injury, the avulsion fracture indicates the presence of a severe collateral ligament injury, leading to instability and an inability to grasp objects with the thumb. In chronic cases, the injury can be quite disabling, and thus surgical intervention usually is required. Roentgenographically, the presence of this

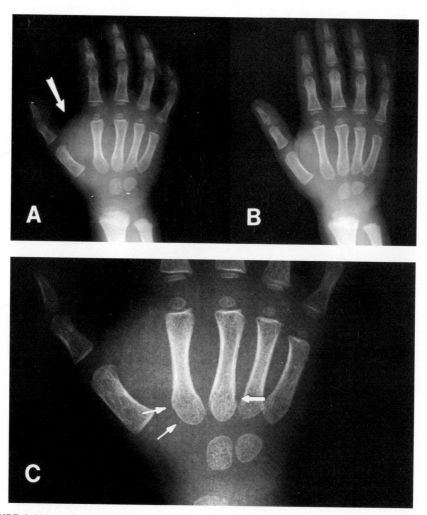

FIGURE 4.119. *Subtle metacarpal cortical fractures: value of soft tissues.* **(A)** First, note soft tissue swelling (increased thickness and density of the soft tissues between thumb and index finger; *arrow*). **(B)** Normal side for comparison. Look back at the right hand in **A** and note that there is a subtle bending buckle fracture through the base of the second metatarsal and a transverse fracture through the base of the third metatarsal. **(C)** Close-up view demonstrating the buckle bending fracture of the second metacarpal and the transverse fracture through the base of the third metacarpal (*arrows*).

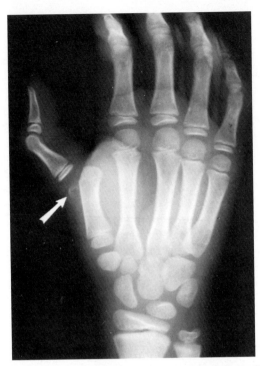

FIGURE 4.120. *Fracture dislocation of the thumb.* Note the dislocated metacarpal–phalangeal joint of the first digit, and the avulsed bony fragment (*arrow*).

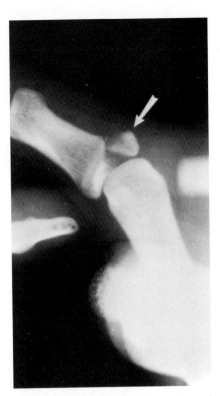

FIGURE 4.121. *Gamekeeper's thumb.* Note the avulsed epiphyseal–metaphyseal fragment (*arrow*). In this condition, there is an associated injury of the medial joint capsule and ligament, and the injury is unstable. The patient is unable to grasp anything with the thumb.

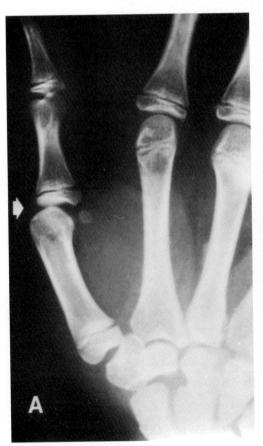

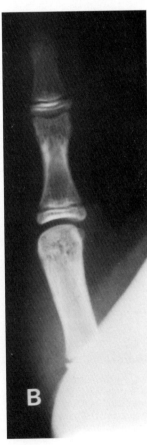

FIGURE 4.122. *Pseudodislocation of the thumb: pitfall.* **(A)** Note that the first metacarpal–phalangeal joint appears dislocated (*arrow*). The small bony ossicle along the inner aspect of the joint is a normal sesamoid bone. **(B)** With proper anteroposterior positioning, one can see that the joint is not dislocated.

injury can be detected if the avulsed fragment is noted (Fig. 4.121).

In assessing the thumb for the presence of a dislocation, it is important to note that if the thumb is examined in oblique position, it can erroneously appear dislocated. This pseudodislocated appearance of the thumb is a common finding, for almost always the thumb is in oblique position as the remainder of the hand is being examined in true frontal projection. Under such circumstances, the first metacarpal joint appears dislocated, but with proper positioning one soon sees that the joint is normal (Fig. 4.122).

Septic Arthritis, Osteomyelitis, and Cellulitis of the Hand

Cellulitis of the fingers is very common and produces generalized soft tissue swelling without joint or bone abnormalities. Osteomyelitis of the small bones of the hands also produces soft tissue swelling, virtually indistinguishable from that seen with cellulitis. If bone destruction is present, of course, the diagnosis becomes relatively easy. With septic arthritis, pronounced swelling around the involved joint is noted, and if enough pus has accumulated in the joint space, one may see some widening of the joint space.

A note regarding the **hand–foot syndrome in sickle cell disease** is in order at this point. In these cases, edema and swelling of the soft tissues of the hand can be extensive, and in some cases one may note the presence of healing changes from similar episodes in the past (Fig. 4.123). The bony changes result from infarction and are indistinguishable from those of osteomyelitis, in which the organism often is a *Salmonella* sp (1).

Frostbite

Frostbite injuries, on an acute basis, produce nothing more than soft tissue swelling. Later on, however, resorption of the involved bones and eventual autoamputation and deformity can be seen (2–4).

Normal Findings Causing Problems

The small bones of the hand have numerous epiphyses and pseudoepiphyses (apophyses), which commonly are misinterpreted as fractures (Fig. 4.124). Bipartite epiphyses also can be misinterpreted as epiphyseal fractures but are not particularly common in the hand. A number of sesamoid bones also can be seen in the hand, but seldom are they misinterpreted as fractures. Only if they are bipartite is there a tendency to make such a misinterpretation, and this problem is more common in the foot. The most common sesamoids of the hand are those located just over the heads of the first and second metacarpals (Fig. 4.122).

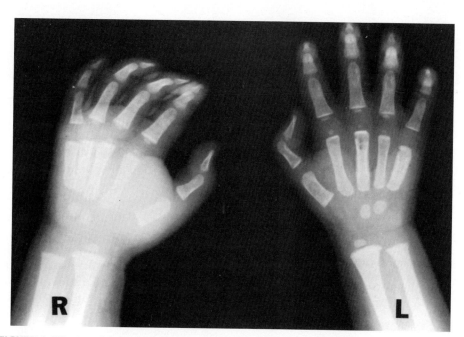

FIGURE 4.123. *Hand–foot syndrome.* Note extensive swelling of the entire right hand. These are acute soft tissue changes of the hand–foot syndrome. The bones are intact. On the left, however, note periosteal new-bone deposition along the third and fifth metatarsals, providing evidence of previous infarcts. In addition, lytic lesions are noted through the distal ends of these bones. The findings are similar to those of osteomyelitis.

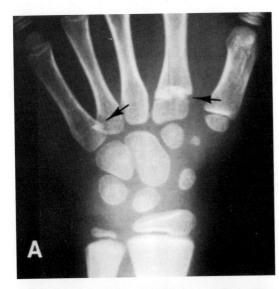

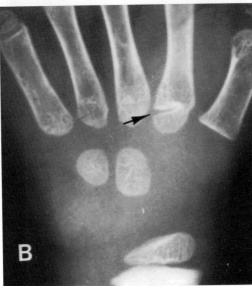

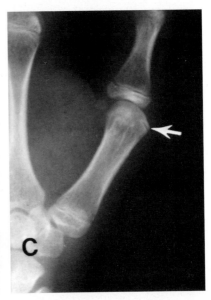

FIGURE 4.124. *Normal secondary ossification centers: pseudofractures.* **(A)** Note pseudofractures through the base of the fifth and second metacarpals (*arrows*). **(B)** Another infant with an incompletely fused secondary center at the base of the second metacarpal (*arrow*). **(C)** Incompletely fused accessory center producing fracturelike appearance through the distal end of the first metacarpal (*arrow*).

REFERENCES

1. Bennett OM. Salmonella osteomyelitis and the hand-foot syndrome in sickle cell disease. *J Pediatr Orthop* 1992;12:534–538.
2. Brown FE, Spiegel PK, Boyle WE Jr. Digital deformity: An effect of frostbite in children. *Pediatrics* 1983;71:955–959.
3. Mooney WR, Reed MH. Growth disturbances in the hands following thermal injuries in children. *Can J Assoc Radiol* 1988;39:91–94.
4. Reed MH. Growth disturbances in the hands following thermal injuries in children: 2. Frostbite *Can J Assoc Radiol* 1988;39: 95–99.
5. Weston WJ. Joint space widening with intracapsular fractures in joint of the fingers and toes of children. *Australas Radiol* 1971;15:367–371.

LOWER EXTREMITY PROBLEMS

Pelvis and Sacrum

Injuries of the Pelvis

Pelvic fractures frequently are multiple and can range from simple buckle or torus cortical fractures to extensive fracture dislocations associated with internal organ or vascular injury (11,12). Most often these latter fractures are sustained in automobile accidents. Pelvic fractures resulting in separation of the symphysis pubis, fractures through the acetabulum, and so-called diametric fractures of the pelvis are considered unstable; other fractures are not. With ring fractures, it is important to note whether the fracture forces resulted from lateral compression, anteroposterior compression, or vertical shearing (16). With lateral compression, diastasis of the symphysis pubis is rare, but on the other hand, vertical fractures through the sacral ala are common, as are vertical fractures through the iliac wing and horizontal fractures of the pubic bones. Sacroiliac diastasis is not as common as if anteroposterior compressive forces are at work. With the latter, however, separation of the symphysis pubis is more common. With vertical shearing forces, vertical fractures through the ischium and pubis are seen along with vertical disassociation of the sacroiliac joints.

Separation of the Symphysis Pubis

Gross separation of the symphysis pubis leading to pelvic instability often is associated with dislocation at the sacroiliac joints and is not difficult to detect. As just mentioned, the problem usually stems from anteroposterior compressive forces. With lesser degrees of diastasis, it may be more difficult to appreciate the problem initially, especially in young infants in whom underossification of the pubic bones leads to a normally wide space between them and a picture suggestive of separation (see Fig. 4.143). If looking

for true separation, however, one should look for asymmetric alignment (offsetting) and associated fractures of the pubic bones (Fig. 4.125).

Diametric Fractures

In this type of injury, fractures exist both anteriorly and posteriorly (ring fracture), and they may be on the same or opposite sides of the pelvis. The more severe diametric fractures tend to be unstable (16), and oblique views of the pelvis may be required for demonstration of all the individ-

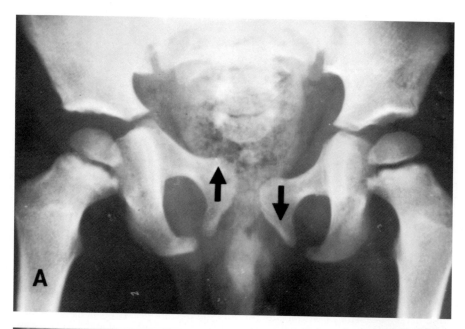

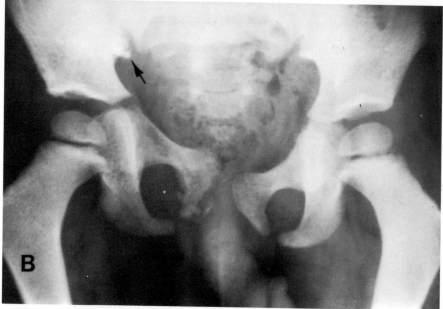

FIGURE 4.125. *Pubic separation.* **(A)** Note on this well-positioned pelvic film that the right pubic bone rides higher than the left (*arrows*). This boy was run over by a farm wagon and complained of right-hip pain. **(B)** One month later, note persistent malalignment of pubic bones and signs of healing around the inferior right pubic ramus. Also note development of an osteophyte along the inferior aspect of the right sacroiliac joint (*arrow*), indicating a previously suspected injury at this site. Most likely there was a mild degree of sacroiliac joint separation sustained at the time of initial injury.

ual fractures present. Posteriorly, these can occur through the iliac bone, sacrum, or sacroiliac joint; anteriorly they occur through the pubic bone or anterior portion of the ischium (Fig. 4.126). These fractures usually result from lateral compressive forces (16).

Isolated Pelvic Fractures

Most often isolated fractures of the pelvis occur through the pubic bone or iliac wing (Fig. 4.127), but occasionally they can occur through the ischium or even the ischiopubic synchondrosis (Fig. 4.128). Isolated torus or buckle fractures of

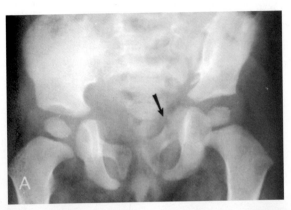

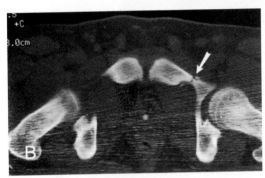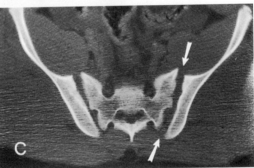

FIGURE 4.126. *Diametric pelvic fracture.* **(A)** Note the fracture of the left pubic bone (*arrow*). Also note separation of the left sacroiliac joint and a small chip fracture along the inferior aspect of the joint. The left iliac wing is abnormally rotated and appears smaller than the right. **(B)** Another patient demonstrating a similar fracture on computed tomographic scan. Note the superior ramus fracture on the right. **(C)** A lower slice demonstrates diastasis of the right sacroiliac joint (*arrows*).

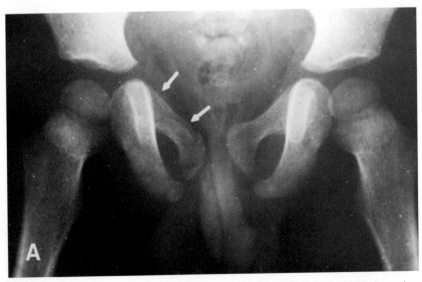

FIGURE 4.127. *Isolated pelvic fractures.* **(A)** Note the fracture of the right pubic bone (*arrows*).

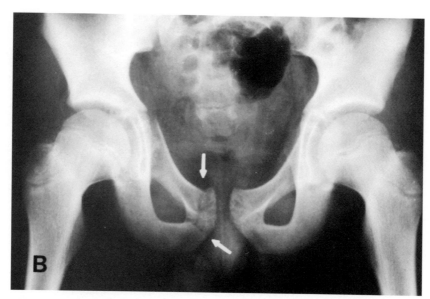

FIGURE 4.127. *(continued)* **(B)** Note the buckle fracture through the left pubic bone (*upper arrow*). Also note soft tissue swelling causing obliteration of the obturator fat pad along the inner margin of the bony pelvis, and a nondisplaced fracture through the ischiopubic synchondrosis (*lower arrow*).

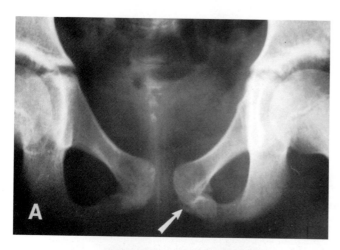

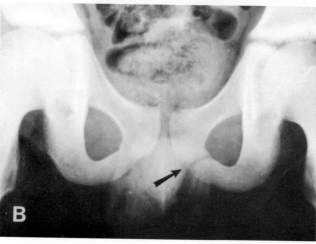

FIGURE 4.128. *Ischiopubic synchondrosis fractures.* **(A)** Note the fracture through the ischiopubic synchondrosis on the left (*arrow*). It is most important to differentiate this fracture from the normal ischiopubic synchondrosis (Fig. 4.143). **(B)** Another, more subtle fracture through the ischiopubic synchondrosis (*arrow*). A similar fracture is seen in Figure 4.127B. **(C)** A displaced fracture through the ischiopubic synchondrosis (*arrow*). Separation of the symphysis also is present.

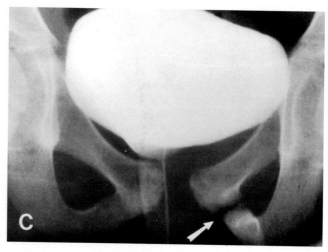

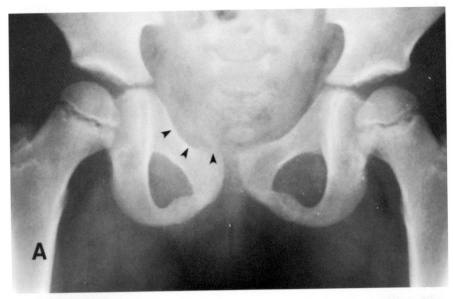

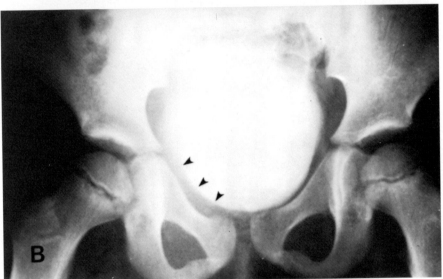

FIGURE 4.129. *Cortical bending (plastic) fracture of superior pubic ramus.* **(A)** Note the abnormal curvature of the superior aspect of the right pubic ramus (*arrows*), compared with the normal left pubic ramus. Also note the increase in soft tissue density over the right pubic ramus and obliteration of the fat pads and soft tissues in the area. **(B)** Follow-up cystogram demonstrates increased soft tissue thickness between the right pubic ramus and contrast-filled bladder (*arrows*). This is caused by bleeding and edema secondary to the cortical bending fracture of the right pubic ramus.

the cortex of the pubic bone also can be seen in childhood, and one can avoid missing them if one looks for subtle bends or kinks in the cortex and adjacent soft tissue edema (Fig. 4.129).

Acetabular Fractures

Acetabular rim fractures are not particularly common in childhood but can be seen in association with posterior hip dislocations (Fig. 4.130). Fractures through the center of the acetabulum usually occur in older children and result from the femoral head being impacted into the acetabulum (Fig. 4.130A). Often they are difficult to detect on plain films (7). Indeed, the findings may consist of nothing more than widening of the joint space (hemarthrosis) and obliteration of the soft tissues along the obturator internus fat pad (edema and bleeding). In the infant and young child, these fractures tend to occur through the triradiate cartilage (Fig. 4.131), but generally speaking they are not very common. Furthermore, care

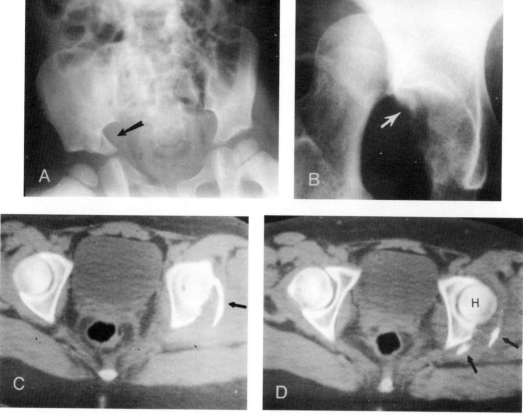

FIGURE 4.130. *Acetabular fracture.* **(A)** Note the fracture through the acetabular roof (*arrow*). The fracture fragment is rotated, and there is associated soft tissue thickening medially. The joint space also is widened by blood in the joint. **(B)** Another patient with a hip dislocation and a barely visible acetabular fracture (*arrow*). **(C)** Computed tomographic scan, however, clearly demonstrates the avulsed acetabular fragment (*arrow*). **(D)** A slightly lower cut demonstrates the femoral head (*H*) and the acetabular fracture (*arrows*). Study obtained after reduction.

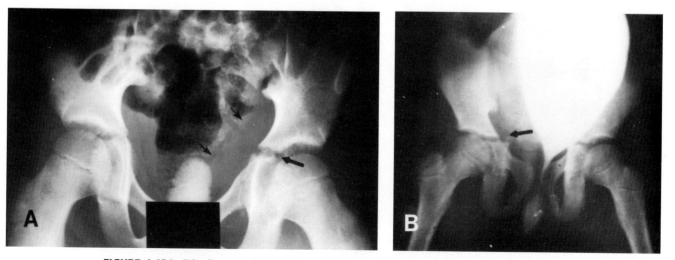

FIGURE 4.131. *Triradiate cartilage fractures.* **(A)** Note soft-tissue swelling along the left inner pelvic margin (*multiple arrows*). Also note that the triradiate cartilage is wider (*single arrow*) than the one on the right. **(B)** Note the dislocation through the triradiate cartilage on the right (*arrow*). Also note that on this well-positioned anteroposterior view the joint space on the right is distorted and narrower than that on the left. Furthermore, the bladder has been displaced and elevated by a large intrapelvic hematoma. (Courtesy of Charles J. Fagan, M.D.)

375

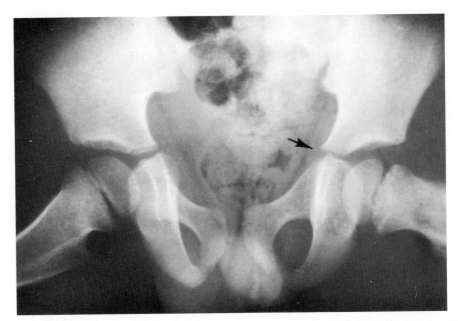

FIGURE 4.132. *Pseudotriradiate cartilage fracture–dislocation.* Note that the pelvis is rotated in this patient (i.e., compare the size of the foramina outlined by the pubic and ischial bones on either side; they are unequal, indicating that rotation is present). Rotation causes apparent off-setting or pseudodislocation of the bones about the triradiate cartilage on the left (*arrow*).

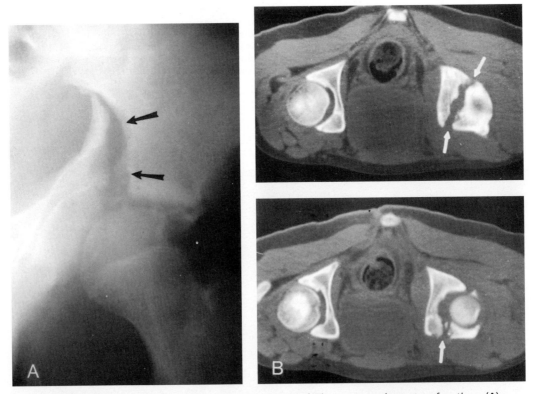

FIGURE 4.133. *Plain films and computed tomographic (CT) scans: complementary functions.* (**A**) Note the gross fracture through the acetabulum (*arrows*). (**B**) High CT cut (*top scan*) demonstrates the fracture through the iliac bone, above the acetabulum (*arrows*). Lower CT cut (*bottom scan*) demonstrates the fracture (*arrow*) and, even more clearly, its relationship to the femoral head. Overall, the two studies provide a very accurate three-dimensional picture of the fracture.

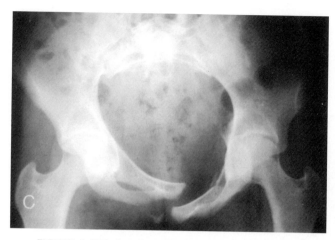
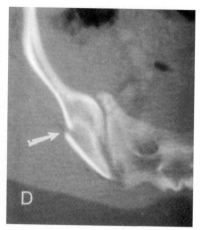

FIGURE 4.133. *(continued)* **(C)** Another patient with extensive displaced fractures of the pubic bones, overriding of the symphysis pubis, disruption of the right sacroiliac joint, and a vaguely apparent fracture through the right iliac wing. **(D)** CT study clearly demonstrates the iliac wing fracture *(arrow)*. Again, the two studies together provide a complete picture of the fractured pelvis.

should be taken not to confuse the normal triradiate cartilage distorted by faulty positioning of the pelvis (15) with one rendered abnormal by a fracture (Fig. 4.132). Most often, such faulty positioning results from rotation, but it also can result from a combination of rotation and utilization of the angled inlet view.

Many times, the first clue to the presence of an otherwise occult triradiate cartilage fracture is the presence of edema and soft-tissue thickening along the inner aspect of the pelvis (Fig. 4.131). If one notes this finding, one may also note that the triradiate cartilage is wider than normal, or that the bones on either side are displaced (Fig. 4.131).

CT scanning, of course, is invaluable in the assessment of pelvic fractures. This is especially true of acetabular injuries (7) (Figs. 4.130 and 4.133). Because CT images of the pelvis are in the axial plane, however, many fractures

still are more clearly visualized with plain films (11). Therefore, one cannot rely on CT scanning alone. It should be used in combination with plain films, so that all fractures are visualized adequately. Of course, with coronal or sagittal reconstruction one may obtain CT data in other than the axial plane, but in any case a combination of CT scanning and plain films is invaluable in the assessment of pelvic injury.

With extensive pelvic fractures, internal visceral and vascular injury is quite common. Indeed, as mentioned previously, exsanguination and other catastrophic complications can result. Once again, CT scanning is invaluable in the assessment of many of these injuries, and if the urinary tract is involved, positive contrast cystography, usually retrograde, is in order (Fig. 4.134). Arteriography can be utilized in certain cases if time permits.

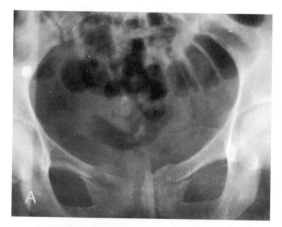
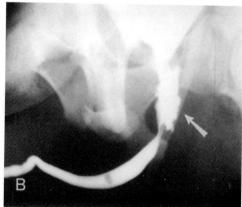

FIGURE 4.134. *Pelvic fractures with bladder and urethral trauma.* **(A)** Note numerous bilateral pubic bone fractures. **(B)** Retrograde cystogram showing numerous sites of extravasation of contrast material *(arrow)*.

(continued on next page)

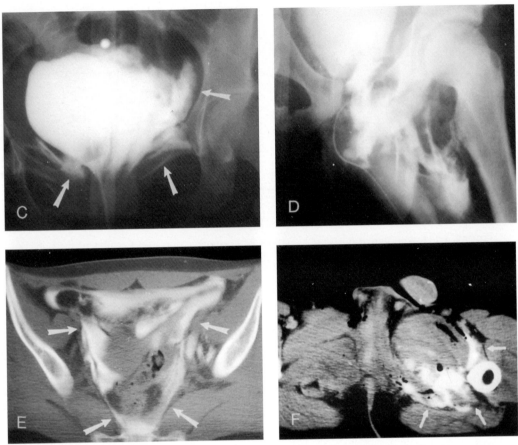

FIGURE 4.134. *(continued)* **(C)** Computed tomographic (CT) study through the upper pelvis demonstrates extensive contrast and urine extravasation throughout the peritoneal cavity (*arrows*). **(D)** Another patient with a posterior urethral tear whose retrograde urethrogram demonstrates early extravasation of contrast material. **(E)** CT scan demonstrates extensive extravasation of contrast material into the pelvic soft tissues (*arrows*). **(F)** A lower CT cut demonstrates contrast material extravasated into the left groin (*arrows*). Air bubbles are seen scattered in the soft tissues.

Avulsion Fractures

Avulsion fractures of the pelvic bones commonly occur in children, and most often they are seen along the outer aspect of the iliac wing, the anterior–inferior iliac spine (8), and the inferior aspect of the ischium (Figs. 4.135–4.137). Less commonly they occur over the upper portion of the superior pubic ramus (Fig. 4.135D), at the top of the iliac wing. In the femur, they occur over the greater and lesser trochanters (see Fig. 4.151). CT scanning can be used to identify the more obscure of these fractures (6), but most often plain films suffice.

With most pelvic avulsion fractures, actual fracture fragments are seen, but in some cases not enough bone is avulsed for this to occur. This is especially common over the ischium, where often only bone resorption, causing a cortical defect, is seen in the early stages (Fig. 4.137A). Later, as this fracture heals, considerable intermixed bony resorption and

osteoblastic reparative change occurs, and bizarre roentgenographic configurations result (Figs. 4.137 and 4.138). These healing avulsion fractures also can occur at other sites (Fig. 4.138), and it always has been cautioned, rightly, that these bizarre configurations not be misinterpreted as those of a more serious lesion such as a bone tumor or osteomyelitis (1,2,6,8,14,16). *The key is to keep in mind just where these very predictable avulsions occur.*

Before leaving the topic of pelvic avulsion fractures, it should be noted that the normal apophyses, along the inferior aspect of the ischium and superior aspect of the iliac wing, can mimic nondisplaced avulsion fractures (see Fig. 4.144). Of course, this does not mean that the apophyses themselves are never avulsed, for this would be untrue, but it does mean that one sees many more normal apophyses than avulsed ones.

Stress fractures of the pelvic bones are quite uncommon in children and are more likely to occur in adolescents

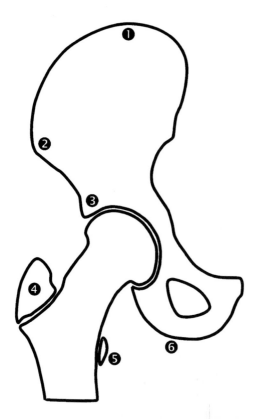

FIGURE 4.135. *Sites of avulsion fractures around the hip.* Superior iliac crest (*1*). Anterior, superior iliac spine (*2*). Anterior, inferior iliac spine (*3*). Greater trochanter (*4*). Lesser trochanter (*5*). Inferior aspect of ischium (*6*).

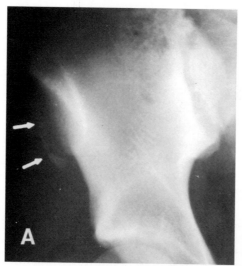
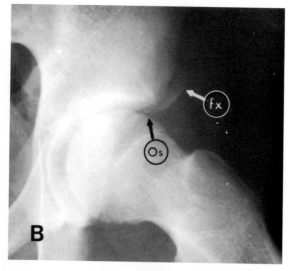
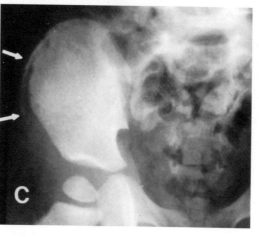
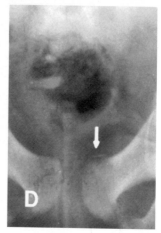

FIGURE 4.136. *Acute pelvic avulsion injuries.* (**A**) Note typical iliac wing avulsion (*arrows*) of anterior superior iliac spine. (**B**) Another iliac bone avulsion fracture (*fx*), this time involving the anterior, inferior iliac spine. The normal os acetabulum (*Os*) should not be confused with these fractures (Fig. 4.145). The os acetabulum lies under the acetabular roof; the fractures occur lateral to the acetabulum. (**C**) Long, linear avulsion of iliac wing (*arrows*). (**D**) Small pubic bone avulsion (*arrow*).

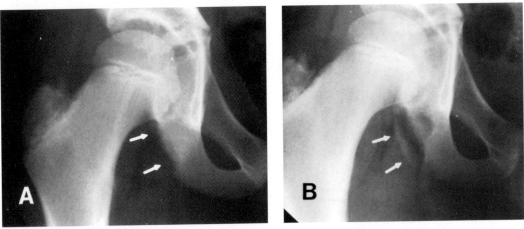

FIGURE 4.137. *Ischial avulsion with healing.* **(A)** Early phase shows nothing more than bone resorption (*arrows*). **(B)** Later, with healing, the avulsed fracture fragment is visible (*arrows*), as hypertrophic bone is beginning to form.

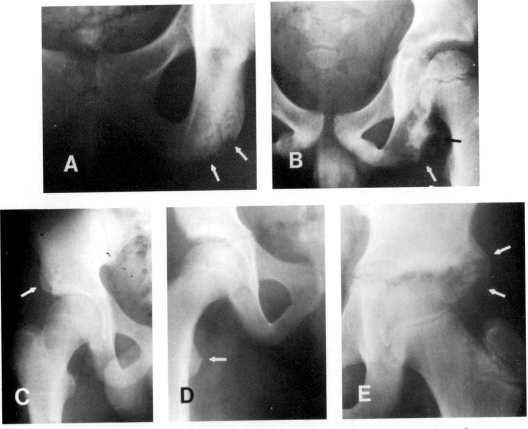

FIGURE 4.138. *Chronic avulsion injuries.* **(A)** Expanded ischium with irregular new-bone formation (*arrows*). **(B)** Tumorlike appearance of a healing ischial avulsion fracture (*arrows*). **(C)** Chronic avulsion of the anterior, inferior iliac spine (*arrow*). **(D)** Chronic avulsion of lesser trochanter (*arrow*). **(E)** Marked hyperostosis resulting from chronic avulsion of the anterior, inferior iliac spine (*arrows*).

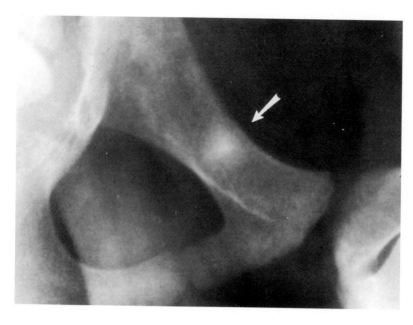

FIGURE 4.139. *Stress fracture: pubic bone.* Note area of sclerosis in pubic bone (*arrow*). Later, periosteal new bone was seen, and the bone scan was positive in this patient. (Courtesy of Jack Riley, M.D.)

and adults (9). The key findings include an area of sclerosis and associated periosteal new bone (Fig. 4.139). They are positive on isotope bone scans, and the main differential diagnosis is osteoid osteoma, which unfortunately also is positive on regular technetium-99m pyrophosphate bone scans. On indium or gallium bone scans, however, osteoid osteoma usually is not positive.

Fractures of the Sacrum

Sacral fractures commonly are associated with pelvic injuries and overall may be difficult to detect. If one sys- tematically compares the cortical margins of the sacral foramina on one side to those on the other, however, disruption of their margins (arcuate lines) (3) provides a clue to the presence of a fracture (Fig. 4.140A). In addition to sacral fractures, many of these patients demonstrate associated sacroiliac joint separations. Once again, CT scanning is useful in confirming or initially detecting these sacral injuries (Fig. 4.140). Other injuries associated with pelvic fractures include fractures of the femur or injuries to the bladder, urethra, or pelvic blood vessels. Indeed, rapid death secondary to exsanguination associated with vascular injury is not uncommon at all.

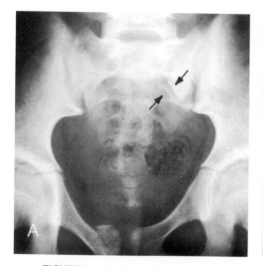
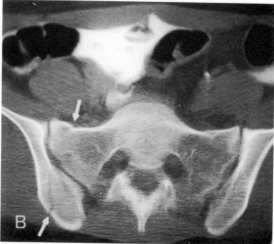

FIGURE 4.140. *Sacral fractures.* **(A)** Note the disrupted ala of the intervertebral foramina on the left. Two disrupted cortices are seen on edge (*arrows*). In addition, note the pubic bone fracture on the right. **(B)** Computed tomographic study in another patient demonstrates a sacral fracture on the right (*upper arrow*). In addition, note the fracture through the iliac bone (*lower arrow*). Contrast material in the peritoneal cavity was secondary to a urinary bladder tear.

Osteomyelitis of the Pelvic Bones and Sacroiliac Joints

Osteomyelitis of the pelvic bones is more common than generally appreciated, but very often its diagnosis is delayed. In the early stages, one may see nothing more than nonspecific, but often extensive, soft tissue swelling around the area of bone involvement. Bone scans are invaluable in such cases and should be utilized whenever the osteomyelitis is suspected even remotely (Fig. 4.141). This is particularly important because destruction of the bones of the pelvis may be very subtle in the early stages (Fig. 4.142).

Osteomyelitis of the sacroiliac joint also can be very elusive and, once again, is diagnosed more readily in its early stages with bone scans (Fig. 4.142C–D). Patients with sacroiliac joint infection can present with acute back pain, referred pain down the leg, a limp, or symptoms suggestive of an intraabdominal problem. As with osteomyelitis of the flat bones of the pelvis, initial roentgenographic findings often are very subtle or nonexistent. Later, destruction along the sacroiliac joint becomes apparent, but in the meantime it is the isotope bone scan that delivers the most useful information. CT and MR imaging (10) also are useful in detecting early bone destruction around the sacroiliac joints and in fact are much more sensitive than plain films (Fig. 4.142F and G).

In addition to osteomyelitis of the pelvis and sacrum, one occasionally encounters deep soft tissue abscesses not associated with bone infection. These lesions usually are best demonstrated with CT scanning, MR imaging, ultrasonography, or indium or gallium nuclear scintigraphy.

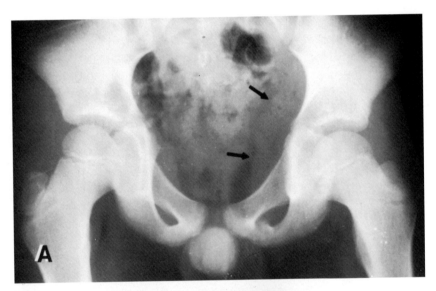

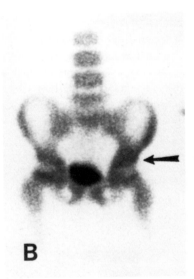

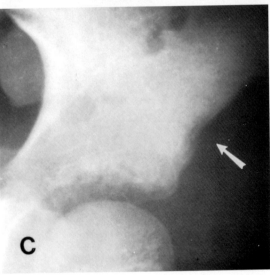

FIGURE 4.141. *Pelvic bone osteomyelitis with bone scan.* **(A)** Note soft tissue thickening along the inner left pelvic margin (*arrows*). Bone changes are virtually nonexistent. **(B)** Anterior bone scan, however, demonstrates increased uptake in the left iliac bone (*arrow*). **(C)** Film of the iliac wing obtained 2 weeks later shows bone destruction (*arrow*).

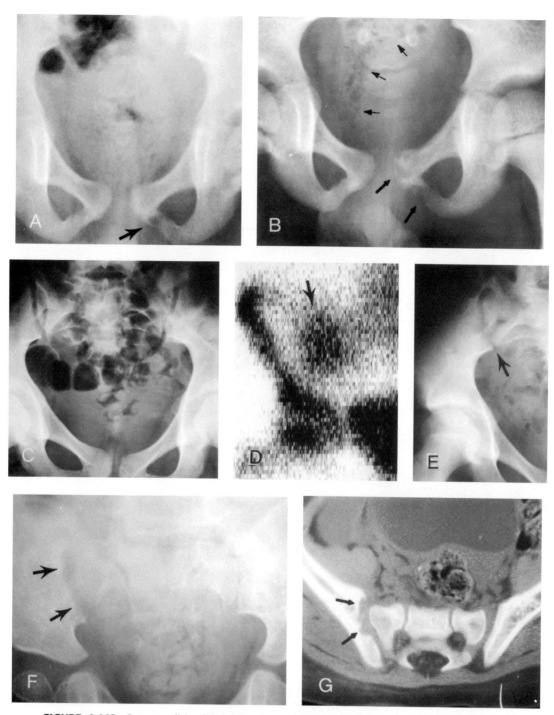

FIGURE 4.142. *Osteomyelitis:.* (**A**) Ischiopubic synchondrosis. Note faint radiolucency in the region of the left ischiopubic synchondroses (*arrow*). This finding could be normal but was the early lesion in this case. Also note that the obturator fat pad on the left is a little less distinct than the one on the right. This patient presented with acute left-hip pain. (**B**) A few weeks later, note extensive destruction of the pubic bones on the left (*lower arrows*), consistent with extensive osteomyelitis. Also note the large, soft tissue mass (abscess) in the pelvis causing displacement of the gas and feces-filled rectum to the right (*upper arrows*). (**C**) Osteomyelitis of sacroiliac joint. This patient presented with back pain and a right limp. No abnormalities are noted, especially in the right sacroiliac joint. (**D**) Bone scan, however, demonstrates increased activity over the right sacroiliac joint (*arrow*). (**E**) Two weeks later, note complete destruction of the right sacroiliac joint (*arrow*). (**F**) Another patient with visible destruction of the right sacroiliac joint (*arrows*). (**G**) Computed tomographic study demonstrates destruction of the iliac bone around the sacroiliac joint (*arrows*).

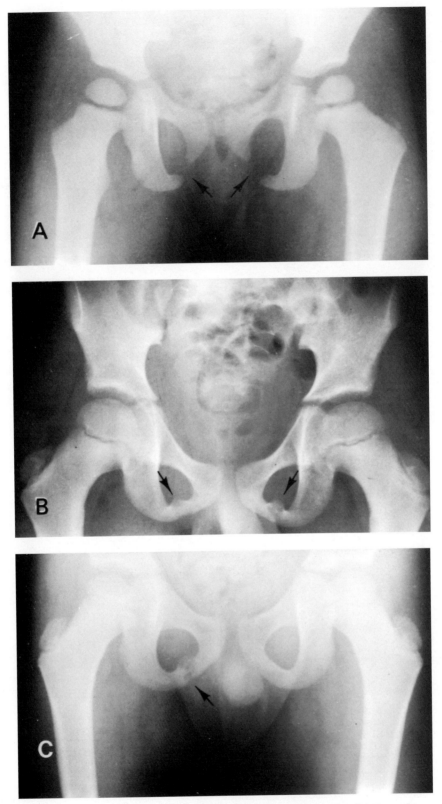

FIGURE 4.143. *Normal pubic symphysis: and ischiopubic synchondroses.* (**A**) Note the normal width between the pubic bones in this young infant. Also note the normal width of the ischiopubic synchondroses (*arrows*). (**B**) Older patient showing normal appearance of the ischiopubic synchondroses (*arrows*). Also note that the space between the pubic bones still is wider than in adults. (**C**) Unilateral ischiopubic synchondrosis on the right (*arrow*).

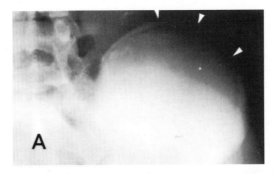

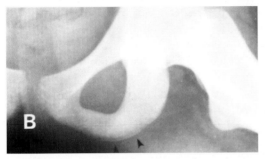

FIGURE 4.144. *Normal iliac and ischial apophyses.* **(A)** Note the normal iliac wing apophysis (*arrows*). **(B)** Normal ischial apophysis (*arrows*).

Normal Findings Causing Problems

There are a number of normal findings in the pelvis that frequently are misinterpreted as pathology. First of all, the normally wide space between the pubic bones in the infant and young child frequently is mistaken for a pubic bone separation (Fig. 4.143); second, the exceedingly variable and pathology-suggestive appearance of the ischiopubic synchondrosis is misinterpreted as a lesion (Fig. 4.143). The normal ischiopubic synchondrosis is positive on nuclear scintigraphy (5), but if osteomyelitis involves the synchondrosis, the activity over the area is more marked. This is important to appreciate, for osteomyelitis of the ischiopubic synchondrosis is not uncommon (4) (Fig. 4.142A).

The apophyses along the superior aspect of the iliac bone and inferior aspect of the ischial bone are another source of erroneous interpretation (Fig. 4.144), as are the numerous normal fragments of the lateral aspect of the normally ossifying acetabulum (Fig. 4.145). These normal bony fragments (os acetabulae) and apophyses can be misinterpreted as fractures, especially avulsion-type fractures. Finally, the nearly obliterated triradiate cartilage remnant must not be misinterpreted as a central acetabular fracture (Fig. 4.145).

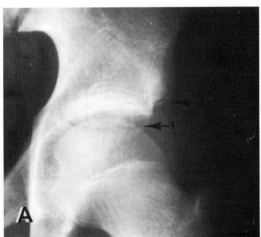

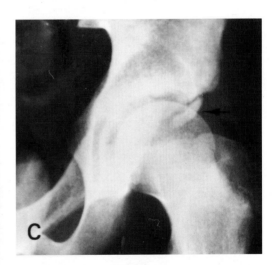

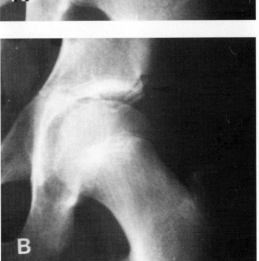

FIGURE 4.145. *Normal triradiate cartilage remnant and acetabular ossicles (os acetabulae).* **(A)** Note the incompletely obliterated triradiate cartilage remnant (*1*), which might be misinterpreted as a central acetabular fracture. Also note the normal, small acetabular ossicle (os acetabulum) or accessory ossification center (*2*). **(B)** Multiple acetabular ossicles (*arrow*). **(C)** Large acetabular ossicle (*arrow*), which might be misinterpreted as an acetabular rim fracture. Note, however, its classic location under the lateral acetabular margin. Fractures occur laterally, outside the acetabular roof.

REFERENCES

1. Brandser EA, El-Khoury GY, Kathol MH. Adolescent hamstring avulsions that stimulate tumors. *Emerg Radiol* 1995;2:273–278.
2. Goergen TG, Resnick D, Riley RR. Post-traumatic abnormalities of the pubic bone simulating malignancy. *Radiology* 1978;126:85–87.
3. Jackson H, Kam J, Harris JH Jr, Harle TS. The sacral arcuate lines in upper sacral fractures. *Radiology* 1982;145:35–39.
4. Jarvis J, McIntyre W, Udjus K, Kloiber R. Osteomyelitis of the ischiopubic synchondrosis. *J Pediatr Orthop* 1985;5:163–166.
5. Kloiber R, Udjus K, McIntyre W, Jarvis J. The scintigraphic and radiographic appearance of the ischiopubic synchondroses in normal children and in osteomyelitis. *Pediatr Radiol* 1988;18:57–61.
6. Kozlowski K, Campbell JB, Azouz EM. Traumatized ischial apophysis: Report of six cases. *Australas Radiol* 1989;33:140–143.
7. Mack LA, Harley JD, Winquist RA. CT of acetabular fractures: Analysis of fracture patterns. *AJR* 1982;138: 407–412.
8. Mader TJ. Avulsion of the rectus femoris tendon: An unusual type of pelvic fracture. *Pediatr Emerg Care* 1990;6:198–199.
9. Meurman KOA. Stress fracture of the pubic arch in military recruits. *Br J Radiol* 1980;53:521–524.
10. Murphey MD, Wetzel LH, Bramble JM, Levine E, Simpson KM, Lindsley HB. Sacroiliitis: MR imaging findings. *Radiology* 1991;180:239–244.
11. Resnik CS, Stackhouse DJ, Shanmuganathan K, Young JWR. Diagnosis of pelvic fractures in patients with acute pelvic trauma: Efficacy of plain radiographs. *AJR* 1992;158:109–112.
12. Sauser DD, Billimoria PE, Rouse GA, Mudge K. CT evaluation of hip trauma. *AJR* 1980;135:269–274.
13. Schaad UB, McCracken GH Jr, Nelson JD. Pyogenic arthritis of the sacroiliac joint in pediatric patients. *Pediatrics* 1980;66:375–379.
14. Schneider R, Kay JJ, Ghelman B. Abductor avulsive injuries near the symphysis pubis. *Radiology* 1976;120:567–569.
15. Shipley RT, Griscom NT, Kirkpatrick JA, Gross G. Artifact of projection simulating a pelvic fracture. *AJR* 1983;141:479–480.
16. Young JWR, Resnik CS. Fracture of the pelvis: Current concepts of classification. *AJR* 1990;155:1169–1175.

Hip

Normal Fat Pads and Joint Space

The two views generally obtained for evaluating the hip are the straight anteroposterior and anteroposterior frog-leg views. The fat pads surrounding the hip and the joint space are best assessed on the straight anteroposterior view (Fig. 4.146). The fat pads around the hip include the obturator internus, iliopsoas, and gluteus (Fig. 4.146). These fat pads do not lie against the joint capsule directly and thus are not displaced outwardly if fluid accumulates within the joint. The only exception occurs with the gluteus fat pad, which can be displaced outwardly with the femur, if it is displaced by joint fluid. With soft tissue edema, of course, the fat pads become obliterated.

Detecting Fluid in the Hip Joint

If fluid (blood, pus, serous fluid) accumulates in the hip joint, the femoral head is displaced laterally (Fig. 4.147). This is a natural and easily accomplished decompressive phenomenon, for outward displacement of the femur is the avenue of least resistance in the hip joint. If such decom-

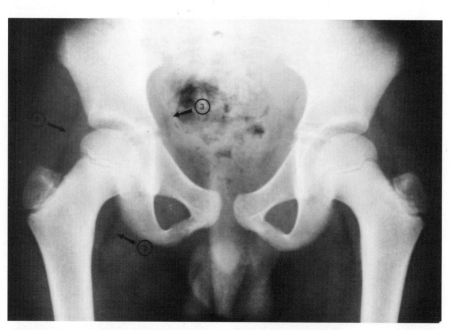

FIGURE 4.146. *Normal hip joint: soft tissues and fat pads.* Note that the joint space both superiorly and medially is of equal width on each side. The visible fat pads include the gluteus (*1*), iliopsoas (*2*), and obturator internus (*3*).

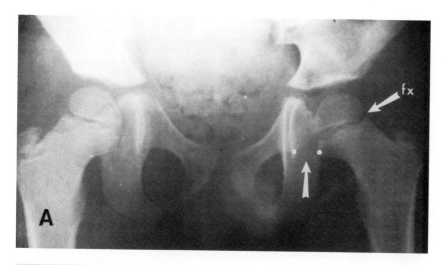

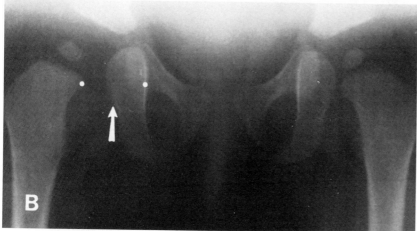

FIGURE 4.147. *Detecting fluid in the hip joint.* **(A)** Note that the left joint space is wider (*arrows*) than the right. Such lateral displacement of the femoral head with widening of the joint space is indicative of fluid in the joint. This patient sustained a mild Salter–Harris type I epiphyseal–metaphyseal injury; note subtle widening of the epiphyseal line on the left (*fx*). The fluid, of course, was blood. **(B)** Young infant with septic arthritis on the right. Note marked widening of the joint space (*arrow*). *Dots* mark the best place to make one's measurements.

pression occurs, it causes the joint space to become widened medially; this is the most important roentgenographic finding in the detection of fluid in the hip joint. In addition, one may note displacement or bulging of the gluteus fat pad, but this finding is less consistent and dependable.

Proper positioning of the hips is mandatory for the evaluation of joint-space widening, for any deviation from normal positioning can lead to erroneous interpretations. In this regard, optimal positioning of the hips is accomplished if the legs are rotated internally (i.e., the toes point toward each other and the kneecaps point upward). If pelvic rotation occurs or if one leg is out of position, erroneous measurements result.

With regard to joint space widening, it has been demonstrated that widening of the joint space secondary to the accumulation of joint fluid is less likely to occur in older children (25). This also has been our experience, and most likely this occurs because the ligaments are tighter in older children. In young children and infants, however, the femur is readily displaced laterally if joint fluid accumulation occurs, and thus joint-space widening in this age group is a

reliable finding for the presence of fluid in the hip joint (25).

Currently, detecting fluid in the hip joint is accomplished best with ultrasonography (25,26). By means of imaging in the sagittal plane through the hip joint, one easily can determine whether joint fluid is present. If joint fluid is present, the overlying iliopsoas muscle is displaced outwardly from the underlying femur (Fig. 4.148). To detect minimal displacement, it is always wise to compare the findings with the normal side. Blood and pus can produce echogenic debris in the joint fluid.

Injuries of the Upper Femur

Fractures through the femoral neck and intertrochanteric region of the femur are distinctly less common in children than in adults. Epiphyseal–metaphyseal injuries, on the other hand, are more common and most often are Salter–Harris type I or II injuries. In assessing the upper femur for the presence of these fractures, one first should look for an increase in the width and radiolucency of the

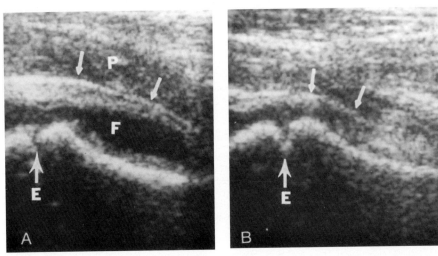

FIGURE 4.148. *Fluid in the hip joint: ultrasound findings.* **(A)** There is distension of the joint capsule (*arrows*) caused by fluid (*F*) in the joint. The femoral neck and femoral head produce the echogenic curved line below. The break in the curved line represents the epiphyseal plate (*E*). Psoas muscle (*P*). **(B)** Normal side for comparison. Compare the width of the joint space. The joint capsule (*arrows*) is not bulging. *E,* epiphyseal plate.

involved epiphyseal line, and then for widening of the medial joint space (Fig. 4.149A). The first finding indicates the presence of an epiphyseal–metaphyseal separation; the second indicates the presence of associated bleeding into the joint. Of course, if dislocation of the femoral capital epiphysis also is present, the injury is not difficult to detect (Fig. 4.149B). With Salter–Harris type II injuries, an associated metaphyseal corner fracture also is present.

Anterior or posterior dislocation of the hip is not particularly common in childhood (18). The reason for this is that, because the epiphysis is still open, it represents the weakest point of the bone, and thus Salter–Harris type I or II injuries are more likely to result. Of course, in the older child, with epiphyseal closure a dislocation is more likely and, as in adults, posterior dislocations are much more common (Fig. 4.150). Acetabular rim fractures are fre-

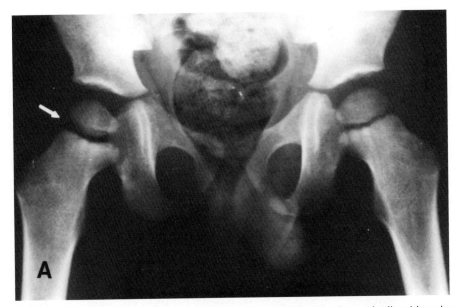

FIGURE 4.149. *Epiphyseal–metaphyseal injuries of the hip.* **(A)** Note the markedly widened epiphyseal line on the right (*arrow*). The joint space is widened minimally because of associated hemarthrosis. This is a Salter–Harris type I injury, undisplaced. Also see Figure 4.17B for a more subtle fracture. Note the clearly detached epiphysis on the right (*arrow*).

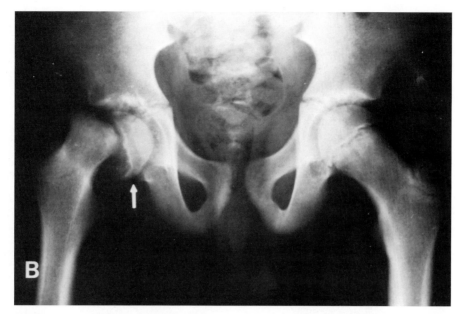

FIGURE 4.149. *(continued)* **(B)** This is a displaced Salter–Harris type I epiphyseal–metaphyseal injury. In this patient, a previously present subclinical slipped capital epiphysis probably was present. Such acute slips can occur under such circumstances.

quently associated injuries, and indeed a fragment of the acetabulum can become trapped in the joint space. Roentgenographically, this complication can be suspected if the joint space fails to return to its normal width after reduction. This can be a most important observation, for the fragment frequently is cartilaginous and not visible, and thus only a high index of suspicion leads to subsequent CT or MR scanning for definitive diagnosis.

Trochanteric Avulsion Fractures

Avulsion fractures of the trochanteric apophyses, especially of the lesser trochanter, are not particularly common (Fig. 4.151A). These latter avulsions, however, often are difficult to diagnose or differentiate from the normal lesser trochanter apophysis, which is not avulsed. In this regard, an important point to remember is that if the lesser trochanter apophysis is visible and appears avulsed on the normal anteroposterior view of the hips (i.e., with the hips in internal rotation), then an avulsion probably is present. If the femur is externally rotated, however, or held in the frog-leg position, the apophysis of the lesser trochanter normally is visualized on edge and then erroneously "appears" avulsed (Fig. 4.151B).

Stress fractures are not particularly common in the femur but most often occur in the femoral neck (4). The character-

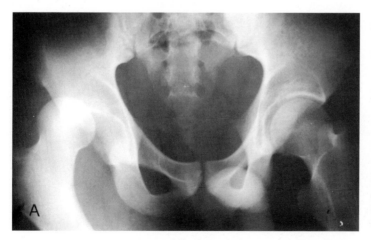
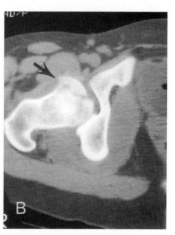

FIGURE 4.150. *Posterior dislocation of the hip.* **(A)** Note the typical position of a posteriorly dislocated femur in this teenager. The injury was sustained in an automobile accident. **(B)** Another patient who sustained a dislocated hip, which then was relocated. A computed tomographic scan demonstrates an underlying femoral head fracture (*arrow*).

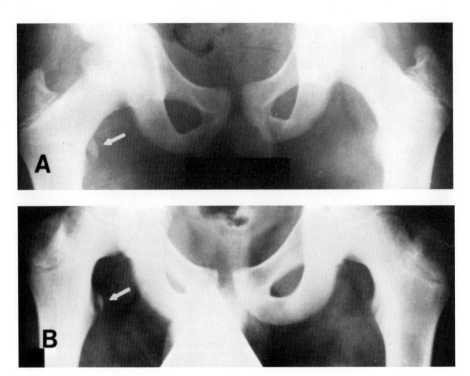

FIGURE 4.151. *True versus pseudoavulsion of the lesser trochanter.* **(A)** True avulsion. Note the avulsed lesser trochanter on the right (*arrow*). Compare the position of both hips. Both are held in internal rotation. In this position, the lesser trochanter should not be visualized on edge; it should appear as it does on the left. **(B)** Pseudoavulsion. Note the avulsed appearance of the lesser trochanter on the right (*arrow*). Note, however, that the position of the right hip is different from that on the left. The left is internal rotation; the right is an external rotation. External rotation causes the hip to assume a coxa valga configuration, and under such circumstances the lesser trochanter is seen on edge and can appear avulsed.

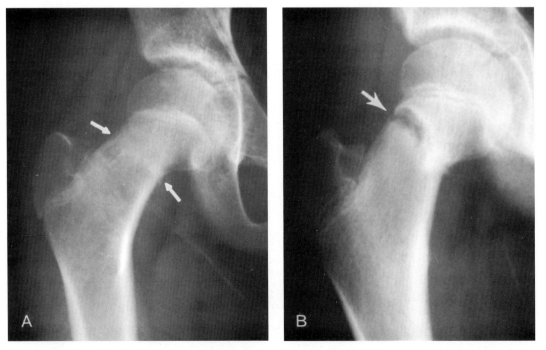

FIGURE 4.152. *Stress fracture.* **(A)** Note the subtle sclerotic line (*arrows*) through the right femoral neck in this patient with a stress fracture. **(B)** Another patient with a healing and refractured stress fracture (*arrow*).

istic findings on plain films consist of sclerosis along the fracture line or, more often, nonspecific sclerosis (Fig. 4.152).

Septic Arthritis, Toxic Synovitis, Osteomyelitis, and Cellulitis of the Hip

The differentiation of these conditions often is a difficult task, for the clinical and roentgenographic findings can be very similar. In most cases plain films and ultrasonography lead to the correct diagnosis, but these two studies can be augmented by the three-phase bone scan (2). Plain films can provide information regarding the presence of joint fluid and, of course, bony destruction with osteomyelitis, but it is ultrasound that is most effective in demonstrating the presence of joint fluid (5,25). With transient synovitis the fluid usually is clear, but with bacterial infection debris in the fluid and, in some cases, thickening of the joint capsule can be seen. Ultrasonographically the findings depend on demonstrating an increase in the distance between the femoral neck and the overlying iliopsoas muscle (see Fig. 4.155).

With toxic or transient synovitis, systemic symptoms usually are less pronounced than with septic arthritis. Indeed, infants with toxic or transient synovitis often smile as they limp and hobble along, but with septic arthritis, well-established pain rules. The precise cause of toxic synovitis is unknown, but it probably is a viral joint infection that afflicts older infants and children. It seldom occurs before the age of 2 years. Roentgenographically, the findings are normal in many cases, but in some more pronounced cases, there is widening of the joint space, bulging of the gluteus fat pad, and obliteration of the obturator fat pad (Fig. 4.153). These latter findings are very similar, if not identical, to those of septic arthritis, and similarly, the ultrasonographic findings demonstrating the presence of fluid are the same.

Transient synovitis is usually a one-time affair. Recurrences do occur, however, and then one should consider the possibility of a more indolent disease process. In this regard, Legg–Perthes disease is the problem in some of these patients, but the incidence is low, probably no more than 10%. Another possible cause for apparent recurrence of the condition may be the presence of a problem such as rheumatoid arthritis. This is quite rare, however, and most often once one diagnoses transient synovitis, it is treated conservatively and never recurs.

In the classic case of **septic arthritis of the hip,** there is considerable pain secondary to capsular distension and marked diminution in the range of motion of the hip; there

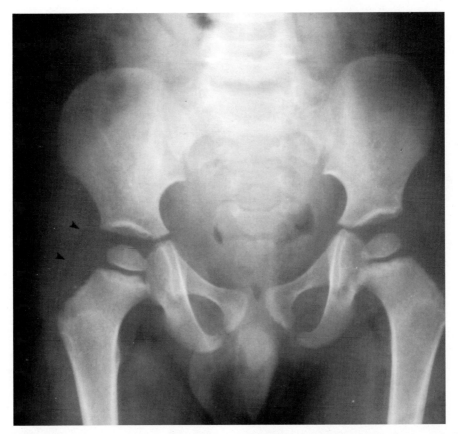

FIGURE 4.153. *Toxic synovitis: right hip.* First note that the joint space on the right is a little wider than that on the left (resulting from fluid). Then note that the right gluteus fat pad shows slight bulging (*arrows*). In addition, there is complete obliteration of the obturator internus fat pad (edema). Compare these findings with those on the normal left side.

also may be swelling and redness over the hip. The systemic reaction usually is pronounced, and both fever and a marked leukocytosis are common (25). An exception to this occurs in the newborn and very young infant, in whom the lesion may be surprisingly silent. Indeed, in these patients the systemic reaction may be very mild, a leukocytosis may not be present, and the only problem may be a loss of motion of the hip. It is in these cases that the roentgenographic and ultrasonographic examination of the hip becomes of paramount importance.

Roentgenographically, the hallmark of septic arthritis of the hip is widening of the joint space resulting from lateral displacement of the femoral head and upper femur (Fig. 4.154). This occurs sooner and more often in infants and young children. In older children joint pus may be present, but because of tighter ligaments the joint is not widened

(27). With larger collections of pus in the hip joint, the obturator fat pad often is obliterated, and in infants and younger children there also is a generalized increase in the density of the soft tissues around the hip secondary to associated edema (Fig. 4.154). On ultrasonography, distension of the joint space is seen (Fig. 4.155).

Acute, fulminant osteomyelitis of the upper femur is common in children, and in very young infants it often is accompanied by septic arthritis. This occurs because in the young infant the blood supply to the femoral metaphysis and epiphysis is contiguous, and thus spread of infection from one side of the epiphyseal cartilage to the other is accomplished readily. This is not unique to the hip joint, of course, but it definitely is unique to the young infant. In such cases, roentgenographic changes of both conditions are present, but in the older child, in whom osteomyelitis

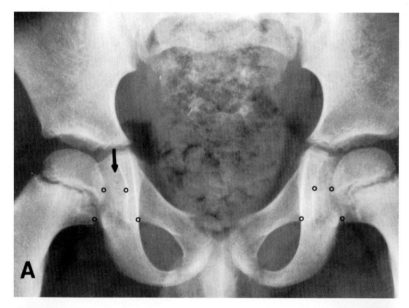

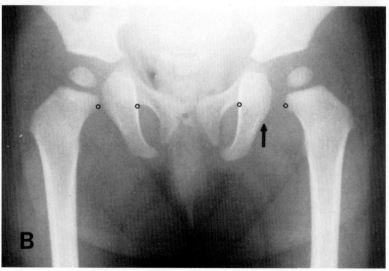

FIGURE 4.154. *Septic arthritis.* **(A)** Note widening of the joint space on the right (*arrow*). In this older child, widening is more apparent through the upper dots. **(B)** Infant with more pronounced widening of the left joint (*arrow*). The distance between the dots is more easily assessed. Also note that there is increased density of the soft tissues along the inner aspect of the acetabulum, causing obliteration of the obturator internus fat pad. This is characteristic of more advanced cases of septic arthritis.

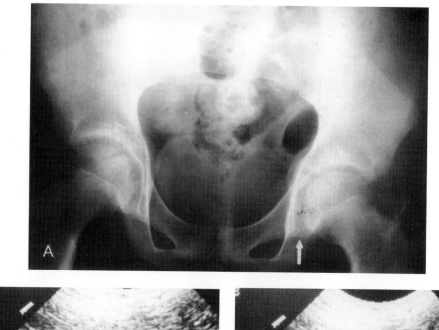

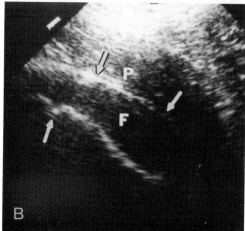
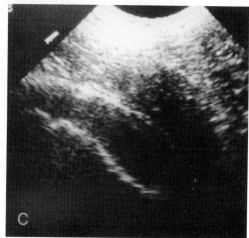

FIGURE 4.155. *Septic hip: value of ultrasound.* **(A)** In this older child the left hip was very tender. The joint space (*arrow*) may be slightly widened. **(B)** Ultrasound, however, clearly demonstrates a markedly bulging joint capsule (*arrows*) resulting from fluid (*F*) in the joint. The psoas muscle (*P*) lies above the capsule. The lower, curved echogenic line represents the femoral neck. The break in the line represents the epiphyseal line (*E*). Compare this with normal findings in Fig. 4.148. **(C)** Unlabeled scan for comparison.

alone exists, there usually are no signs of joint involvement. Absence of joint space widening, plus obliteration of the iliopsoas fat pad, serve to differentiate septic arthritis from osteomyelitis, even in those cases of osteomyelitis in which a small sympathetic joint effusion occurs. In such cases, periarticular soft tissue changes so outweigh the slight degree of joint space widening that one is forced to conclude that septic arthritis could not be the primary problem. If it were, and were causing so much soft tissue change, joint space widening would be pronounced. Later on, of course, bony destruction of the metaphysis occurs, and the diagnosis of osteomyelitis is established more readily (Fig. 4.156). Low-grade osteomyelitis also can occur in the upper femur, and in some cases it can appear as a frank Brodie's

abscess, but in the area of the greater trochanter it often has a less specific and more subtle appearance (Fig. 4.157). Indeed, because the infection often is so low in grade, it may elude initial detection (6,25). It is in such cases, and in early cases, that nuclear scintigraphy is most valuable and should be employed promptly.

Cellulitis of the soft tissues around the hip, in the absence of underlying bone infection also can occur. Most often, such infection results from inflammation of the inguinal lymph nodes, and the findings may be difficult to differentiate from those of osteomyelitis or septic arthritis. However, ultrasound now can be of assistance, for it can clearly identify joint fluid with septic arthritis, and enlarged lymph nodes with increased blood flow with inflammatory adenopathy.

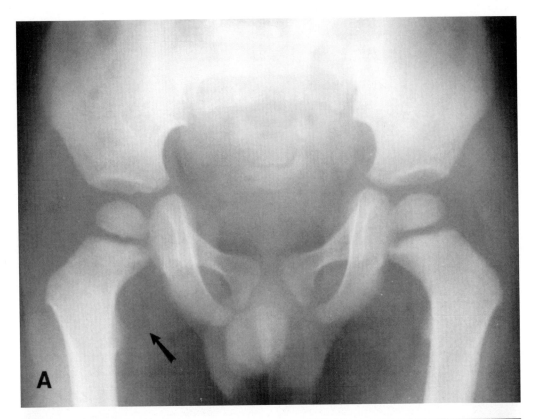

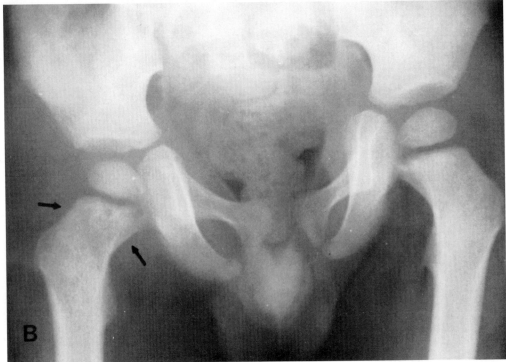

FIGURE 4.156. *Osteomyelitis, upper femur.* (**A**) First, note that the iliopsoas fat pad on the right is obliterated (*arrow*). Compare with the normal fat pad on the left. The joint space is only minimally widened, resulting from a small sympathetic effusion. The fact that septic arthritis (i.e., joint-space widening) is not the primary problem can be deduced from the roentgenographic findings. It would be most unusual for septic arthritis to cause enough edema to obliterate the iliopsoas fat pad and yet not cause any more widening of the joint space. (**B**) Follow-up films demonstrate irregular lytic lesions in the upper femur (*arrows*), consistent with osteomyelitis (surgically confirmed).

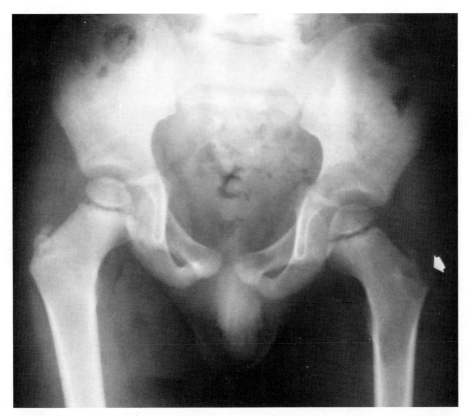

FIGURE 4.157. *Low-grade osteomyelitis of the femur.* This patient presented with a limp on the left. Roentgenograms demonstrated a large lytic lesion just under the greater trochanter (*arrow*). (Surgically proven low-grade osteomyelitis.)

Miscellaneous Hip Problems

Occasionally, on an acute basis, one can be presented with see a painful hip resulting from monoarticular rheumatoid arthritis, nonspecific synovitis, or early Legg–Perthes disease. Any of these conditions can present with findings resembling toxic synovitis or early septic arthritis, and indeed it is generally held that as many as 10% of patients with so-called toxic synovitis eventually are determined to have Legg–Perthes disease. This is not to say that the two are related, nor that one is necessarily a precursor of the other, but only to indicate that their initial presentations may be very similar (Fig. 4.158). Early on in Legg–Perthes disease, demineralization and smallness of the involved femoral head occur (24). These are the earliest bony findings of the disease, and although subchondral fractures (Fig. 4.159) also occur relatively early (17), they are not nearly as common as are the other early findings.

Other early findings include lateral displacement of the femoral head, widening of the joint space and atrophy of the muscles (24). This results in widening of the so-called teardrop sign (9) (Fig. 4.159A). Muscle atrophy and cartilage hypertrophy also are demonstrable with ultrasound (22).

Intraepiphyseal gas also occasionally can be encountered, and in all cases the femoral head eventually shows increasing sclerosis and then fragmentation as the necrotic bone disintegrates and is absorbed (Fig. 4.158C). In many cases associated irregularities of the metaphyses occur (23). These changes are secondary and consist of reactive fibrous tissue extensions into the metaphysis, with resultant irregular bone resorption. Generally they are considered a poor prognostic sign.

If the plain film findings are equivocal, or they are normal and one still suspects Legg–Perthes disease, one can turn to nuclear scintigraphy (1,3) or MR imaging (16,19). There are those who believe that MR imaging is more sensitive, but nuclear scintigraphy is less expensive. With nuclear scintigraphy, one looks for photon-deficient areas in the femoral head, usually laterally (Fig. 4.158D). With MR imaging, there is loss of the normal high signal of fatty marrow in the femoral head. Once again, the changes in the early stages tend to be more lateral than medial.

Aseptic necrosis also can occur with sickle cell disease and in patients on steroid therapy. Often the problem is bilateral in these patients; with idiopathic Legg–Perthes dis-

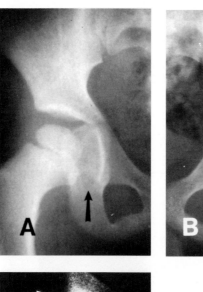
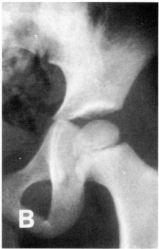
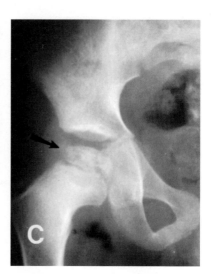

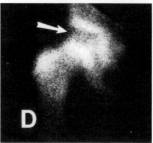

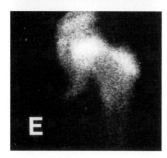

FIGURE 4.158. *Legg–Perthes disease mimicking acute arthritis.* **(A)** This patient presented with an acute limp and hip pain on the right. The roentgenographic findings suggest slight widening of the joint space on the right (*arrow*), and a general increase in soft-tissue density resulting from edema. The findings would be impossible to differentiate from toxic synovitis or early septic arthritis. **(B)** Normal side for comparison. **(C)** Months later, note typical changes of advanced Legg–Perthes disease, consisting of a small sclerotic femoral head and metaphyseal irregularity (*arrow*). **(D)** Isotope study in another patient shows characteristic photon-deficient area (*arrow*) in the epiphysis. **(E)** Normal side for comparison.

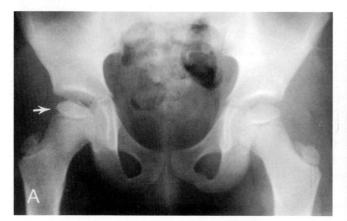
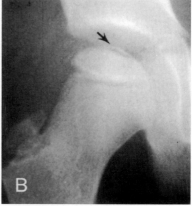

FIGURE 4.159. *Early findings in Legg–Perthes disease.* **(A)** Note the slightly smaller and slightly more sclerotic femoral head (*arrow*). A subchondral fracture also is present. **(B)** Magnified view of the right hip demonstrates the subchondral fracture (*arrow*). These are all early findings in Legg–Perthes disease, but smallness and sclerosis of the head are more common than the subchondral fracture.

ease, only about 10% of cases demonstrate bilateral involvement. Roentgenographically the changes are no different than in the idiopathic form, but they may be more acute in onset. In idiopathic Legg–Perthes disease, a delay in bone age has been noted (10).

The so-called *slipped capital femoral epiphysis* of childhood is another lesion that occasionally presents on an acute basis. This occurs if a superimposed acute slip occurs (Fig. 4.160A and B). More often, however, these patients have a history of chronic hip pain or limp for a number of months (25). The symptoms tend to be low grade and in some cases very minimal, with virtually no pain (11). The classic early roentgenographic findings consist of smoothing of the curve of the epiphyseal line, increased sclerosis on the epiphyseal side, widening and increased lucency of the epiphyseal line, and slight slipping of the epiphysis (2,25) (Fig. 4.160A). Later these changes become more profound and are associated with more pronounced medial and posterior tilting of the epiphysis. The latter often is best seen on the frog-leg view (Fig. 4.160B).

On frontal view, a line drawn along the outer aspect of the femoral neck can aid in determining whether the epiphysis has slipped medially, for in those cases in which such slippage has occurred, the line does not intersect the femoral capital epiphysis (Fig. 4.160A). Posterior slippage of the femoral head usually accompanies medial slippage and, actually, often predominates. It is best detected, as noted previously, on frog-leg views of the hips (Fig. 4.160B).

The precise cause of the slipped capital femoral epiphysis in childhood is unknown, but it probably represents a subclinical Salter–Harris type I injury. In this regard, it has been suggested that in many of these patients the epiphyseal–metaphyseal junction is more vertical than normal (15,20), and because of this the epiphysis is more prone to slippage. Lack of normal anteversion also has been noted to predispose to slippage (7,8) and, of course, so has obesity (7). Slippage is slightly more common in males and occurs primarily in early adolescence (12). In addition, the following predisposing hormonal factors have been identified: decreased growth hormone (21,29), hypothyroidism (13, 28,29), and decreased testosterone (29). Bilaterality is more common in these later cases. In idiopathic slips, bilateral disease usually is asymmetric and occurs in up to 30% of cases. Contralateral slips usually occur within 2 or 3 years of the primary slip (12).

Osteochondritis dessicans of the femoral head is rare (30).

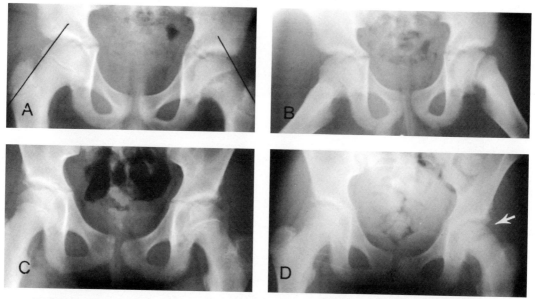

FIGURE 4.160. *Slipped capital femoral epiphysis.* **(A)** Note that on the left the epiphyseal line between the femoral capital epiphysis and femoral neck is wider than that on the right. In addition, note that the line applied along the outer aspect of the femoral neck fails to intersect the femoral capital epiphysis. On the normal right side, it intersects the epiphysis. **(B)** Frog-leg view demonstrating posterior slippage of the left femoral head. In addition, note how much wider the epiphyseal line is compared with the normal one on the right. **(C)** This patient had pain on the left. The findings are very subtle. There is some generalized demineralization of the bones secondary to disuse, and the epiphyseal line is just slightly more rounded and sclerotic than the one on the right. **(D)** Two weeks later, a frank slip on the left (*arrow*) has occurred. The findings in **C** represent the so-called preslip stage.

Normal Variations
Causing Problems

In and around the hip, irregularity of the acetabulum and femoral head are the normal variations most commonly misinterpreted as fractures or other abnormalities. Irregularity of femoral head ossification can be pronounced in children; the normal femoral head can appear quite fragmented (Fig. 4.161). These findings often are misinterpreted as those of Legg–Perthes disease and have been referred to as *Meyer's dysplasia* (14).

The possibility of the normal apophysis of the lesser trochanter being mistaken for an avulsion fracture has been dealt with earlier (Fig. 4.151), but it also should be noted that the normal greater trochanter, because of its frequently very irregular appearance, also can be subject to misinterpretation as a chronic avulsion injury (Fig. 4.162B). Similarly, the cartilage remnant between the greater trochanter and femur, as visualized on frog-leg views, can be mistaken for a fracture (Fig. 4.162). The vacuum-joint phenomenon demonstrated in the shoulder also is common in the hip. It is especially prone to occur with stretching of the hips for the frog-leg views.

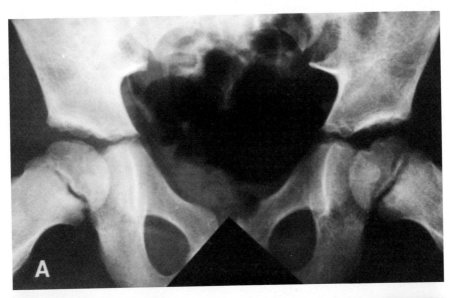

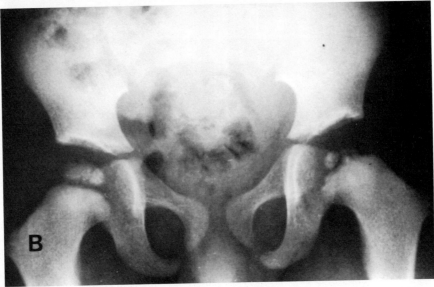

FIGURE 4.161. *Normal femoral head and acetabular-roof irregularities.* **(A)** The irregularities of both acetabular roofs and of the femoral head on the left are normal. **(B)** Normal irregular and asymmetric ossification of the femoral heads.

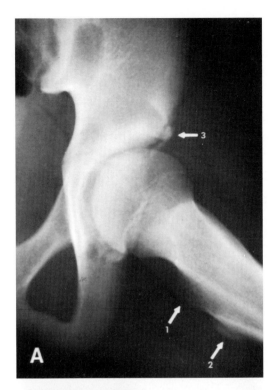

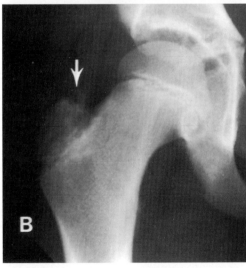

FIGURE 4.162. *Other normal upper femoral findings causing problems.* **(A)** Note the fracturelike cartilaginous remnant between the greater trochanter and femur (*1*), normal lesser trochanter apophysis (*2*), and normal acetabular ossicles (*3*). **(B)** Normal irregular greater trochanter (*arrow*).

REFERENCES

1. Bensahel H, Bok B, Cavailloles F, Csukonyi Z. Bone scintigraphy in Perthes disease. *J Pediatr Orthop* 1983;3:302–305.
2. Boles CA, El-Khoury GY. Slipped capital femoral epiphysis. *RadioGraphics* 1997;17:809–823.
3. Canale ST, Bourland WL. Fracture of the neck and intertro-chanteric region of the femur in children. *J Bone Joint Surg* 1977;59A:431–443.
4. Coldwell D, Gross GW, Boal DK. Stress fracture of the femoral neck in a child (stress fracture). *Pediatr Radiol* 1984;14:174–176.
5. Erken EHW, Katz K. Irritable hip and Perthes' disease. *J Pediatr Orthop* 1990;10:322–326.
6. Frazier JK, Anzel SH. Osteomyelitis of the greater trochanter in children. *J Bone Joint Surg* 1981;63A:833–836.
7. Galbraith RT, Gelberman RH, Hajek PC, Baker LA, Sartoris DJ, Rab GT, Cohen MS, Griffin PP. Obesity and decreased femoral anteversion in adolescence. *J Orthop Res* 1987;5:523–528.
8. Gelberman RH, Cohen MS, Shaw BA, Kasser JR, Griffin TT, Wilkinson RH. The association of femoral retroversion with slipped capital femoral epiphysis. *J Bone Joint Surg* 1986;68A:100–107.
9. Kahle WK, Coleman SS. The value of the acetabular teardrop figure in assessing pediatric hip disorders. *J Pediatr Orthop* 1992;12:586–591.
10. Keenan WNW, Clegg J. Perthes' disease after "irritable hip:" delayed bone age shows the hip is a "marked man." *J Pediatr Orthop* 1996;16:20–23.
11. Ledwith CA, Fleisher GR. Slipped capital femoral epiphysis without hip pain. *Pediatrics* 1992;89:660–662.
12. Loder RT, Farley FA, Herzenberg JE, Hensinger RN, Kuhn JL. Narrow window of bone age in children with slipped capital femoral epiphyses. *J Pediatr Orthop* 1993;13:290–293.
13. Loder RT, Wittenberg B, DeSilva G. Slipped capital femoral epiphysis associated with endocrine disorders. *J Pediatr Orthop* 1995;15:349–356.
14. Meyer J. Dysplasia epiphysealis capitis femoris. *Acta Orthop Scand* 1964;34:183–197.
15. Mirkopulos N, Weiner DS, Askew M. The evolving slope of the proximal femoral growth plate relationship to slipped capital femoral epiphysis. *J Pediatr Orthop* 1988;8:268–273.
16. Mitchell MD, Kundel HL, Steinberg ME, Kressel HY, Alavi A, Axel L. Avascular necrosis of the hip: Comparison of MR, CT and scintigraphy. *AJR* 1986;147:67–71.
17. Norman A, Bullough P. The radiolucent crescent line: An early diagnostic sign of avascular necrosis of the femoral head. *Bull Hosp Joint Dis* 1963;24:99–104.
18. Offerski CM. Traumatic dislocation of the hip in children. *J Bone Joint Surg* 1981;63B:194–197.
19. Pinto MR, Peterson HA, Berquist TH. Magnetic resonance imaging in early diagnosis of Legg-Calve-Perthes disease. *J Pediatr Orthop* 1989;9:19–22.
20. Pritchett JW, Perdue KD. Mechanical factors in slipped capital femoral epiphysis. *J Pediatr Orthop* 1988;8:385–388.
21. Rappaport EB, Fife D. Slipped capital femoral epiphysis in growth hormone-deficient patients. *Am J Dis Child* 1985;139:396–399.
22. Robben SGF, Meradji M, Diepstraten AFM, Hop WCJ. US of the painful hip in childhood: Diagnostic value of cartilage thickening and muscle atrophy in the detection of Perthes disease. *Radiology* 1998;208:35–42.
23. Smith SR, Ions GK, Gregg PJ. The radiological features of the metaphysis in Perthes disease. *J Pediatr Orthop* 1982;2:401–404.
24. Stansberry SD, Swischuk LE, Barr LL. Legg-Perthes disease: Incidence of the subchondral fracture. *Appl Radiol* 1990;19:30–33.
25. Swischuk LE. Childhood limp: Early diagnosis of this problem. In: Margulis AR, Gooding CA (eds.): *Diagnostic Radiology.* San Francisco: University of California Press, 1975, pp. 61–80.
26. Terjesen T, Osthus P. Ultrasound in the diagnosis and follow-up of transient synovitis of the hip. *J Pediatr Orthop* 1991;11:608–613.
27. Volberg FM, Sumner TE, Abramson JS, Winchester PH. Unreli-

ability of radiographic diagnosis of septic hip in children. *Pediatrics* 1984;74:118–120.

28. Wells D, King JD, Roe TF, Kaufman FR. Review of slipped capital femoral epiphysis associated with endocrine disease. *J Pediatr Orthop* 1993;13:610–614.

29. Wilcox PG, Weiner DS, Leighley B. Maturation factors in slipped capital femoral epiphysis. *J Pediatr Orthop* 1988;8:196–200.

30. Wood JB, Klassen RA, Peterson HA. Osteochondritis dissecans of the femoral head in children and adolescents: A report of 17 cases. *J Pediatr Orthop* 1995;15:313–316.

Femoral Shaft

Fractures of the femoral shaft are common in childhood but generally not difficult to detect. Usually they result from serious, known injuries and are of the transverse, spiral, or oblique variety. It is important to note that with femoral shaft fractures a small degree of overriding of the fracture fragments is desirable (Fig. 4.163). Furthermore, healing with abundant callus formation is the rule. The reason overriding is desirable is that the hyperemia associated with the fracture leads to accelerated growth of the femur. The fact that the femur is the fastest-growing long bone in the body, especially at its distal end, causes this combination of factors to lead to overgrowth and excessive length of the femur. Initial overriding protects against this.

Greenstick, buckle (torus), and plastic bending fractures are distinctly uncommon in the femur in any age group. They can occur, however (3). Stress fractures of the mid-shaft of the femur occasionally can be encountered in children (2), but more often they occur in the femoral neck (Fig. 4.152).

Recently, some note has been made of the fact that many times what appears to be an ordinary fractured femur in an infant is actually part of the battered child syndrome (1,4). The main theme of these reports is that in young infants, in whom one might not expect to see femoral-shaft fractures with any degree of frequency, if any suspicion regarding the fracture arises, the possibility of the infant having been battered should be entertained and; the yield, indeed, is relatively high. This problem is discussed in more detail later in the section dealing with infant abuse.

REFERENCES

1. Beals RK, Tufts E. Fractured femur in infancy: The role of child abuse. *J Pediatr Orthop* 1983;3:583–586.
2. Burks RT, Sutherland DH. Stress fracture of the femoral shaft in children: Report of two cases and discussion. *J Pediatr Orthop* 1984;4:614–616.
3. Cail SS, Keats TE, Sussman MD. Plastic bowing fracture of the femur in a child. *AJR* 1978;130:780–782.
4. Gross RH, Stranger M. Causative factors responsible for femoral fractures in infants and young children. *J Pediatr Orthop* 1983;3:341–343.

Knee

Normal Fat Pads and Soft Tissues

There are numerous normal fat pads around the knee, and all can be useful. Those demonstrable on lateral view, however, are the most beneficial (Fig. 4.164). Indeed, one of the best ways to determine whether fluid is present in the knee joint is to assess the soft tissues and fat pads on the lateral view of the knee (as described in the next section).

Detection of Fluid in the Knee Joint

The knee joint does not widen significantly with accumulations of fluid, and thus one must depend on soft tissue and fat pad changes for the detection of fluid in the knee joint (17,18). In this regard, it is the lateral view of the knee that is most useful. On this view, fluid almost always first accumulates in the suprapatellar bursa, which lies behind the quadriceps tendon and in front of the prefemoral fat pad. If this occurs, the quadriceps tendon is displaced anteriorly and the fat pad posteriorly. Early on, just the neck of the suprapatellar bursa may be distended (Fig. 4.165A), but this finding, almost always, is seen in older children and not in infants.

With greater fluid accumulations, the bursa itself can be identified as a discrete structure (Fig. 4.165B), and once again, this most often occurs in older children after trauma. In infants and young children, especially if the fluid is pus, the discrete nature of the distended suprapatellar bursa may be lost, and the confluent soft tissue density of the quadriceps tendon and distended bursa erroneously suggests that

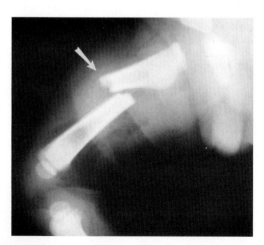

FIGURE 4.163. *Femoral-shaft fracture with overriding fragments.* Note the overriding femoral fracture *(arrow)*. This is desirable to prevent overgrowth of the femur during the healing phase. This infant was a battered child.

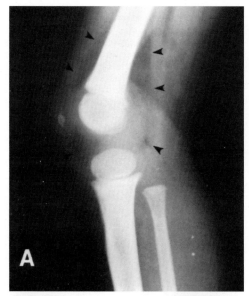

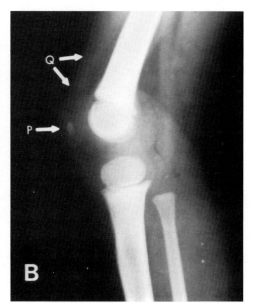

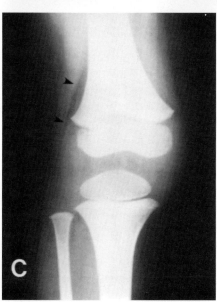

FIGURE 4.164. *Normal soft tissues and fat pads of the knee.* **(A)** Lateral view: the most useful view for evaluation of the joint space and fat pads. The *anterior upper arrows* delineate the prefemoral fat pad; the fat pad posterior to the distal femur is outlined by the *posterior upper arrows*. The *lower anterior arrow* delineates the infrapatellar fat pad; the fat pad over the cartilaginous tibial epiphysis is outlined by the *posterior lower arrow*. **(B)** Same knee, other findings. Note the small ossification center of the basically cartilaginous patella (*P*) and the easily visualized quadriceps tendon (*Q*), just anterior to the prefemoral fat pad. **(C)** Frontal view demonstrating the most frequently visible fat pad (*arrows*).

the entire tendon is thickened (Fig. 4.165C and D). In addition to these findings, it should be noted that fluid eventually begins to accumulate in the posterior popliteal bursa (Fig. 4.165E), but one always should look at the suprapatellar bursa first, becase fluid accumulates here before it does in the posterior popliteal bursa. Seldom, then, does one look at the posterior popliteal bursa for fluid detection.

Fluid in the knee also is detectable on ultrasound, CT, and MR images. Ultrasound, of course, is noninvasive and easily demonstrates the presence of knee joint fluid, and MR imaging is exquisite in demonstrating such fluid (Fig. 4.166). Because plain films are so dependable, however, seldom is there need for these studies to be performed solely for the detection of fluid in the knee joint.

Injuries of the Distal Femur and Proximal Tibia

Cortical buckle (torus) fractures around the knee are uncommon, especially in older children, because the cortices of both the distal femur and proximal tibia are sturdy. They still can occur, however, especially in infants and young children with hyperextension injuries of the knee (38). In such cases there often is a history of someone or some object falling on the infant's knee, and in overt cases the findings are not difficult to detect (Fig. 4.167). In other cases, however, in which the findings are more subtle, they are more difficult to detect (see Figs. 4.178–4.180).

Other fractures and injuries of the knee include epiphyseal–metaphyseal fractures, patellar fractures, cruciate liga-

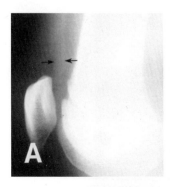

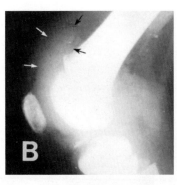

FIGURE 4.165. *Detecting fluid in the knee joint.* **(A)** Lateral view. Early findings consisting of distension of the neck (*arrows*) of the suprapatellar bursa. **(B)** Another patient with discrete distension of the suprapatellar bursa (*arrows*). **(C)** In this case, fluid in the suprapatellar bursa blends in with the quadriceps tendon and causes subtle pseudothickening of the tendon (*arrows*). **(D)** Normal side for comparison. Note normal quadriceps tendon (*arrows*). **(E)** More extensive fluid collection in the suprapatellar bursa leads to marked pseudothickening of the quadriceps tendon. Also note that the prefemoral fat pad is compressed against the femur (*upper arrows*), and that there is early accumulation of fluid in the posterior popliteal bursa (*posterior arrows*).

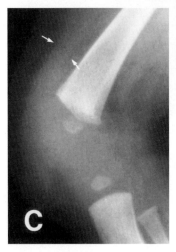

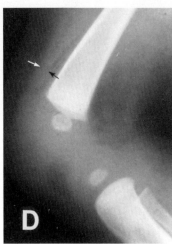

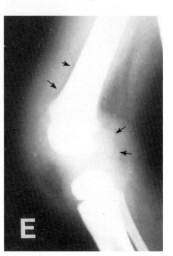

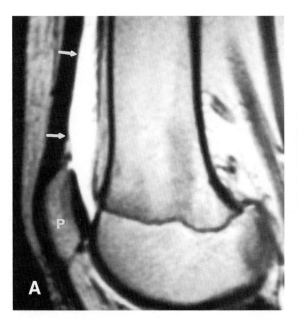

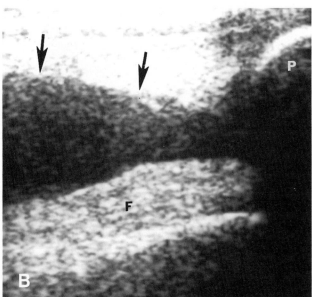

FIGURE 4.166. *Fluid in knee joint: ultrasound and magnetic resonance findings.* **(A)** T2-weighted image demonstrates fluid in the suprapatellar bursa (*arrows*). Just between the fluid collection and the femur is the prefemoral fat pad. *P*, patella. **(B)** Ultrasound study demonstrates fluid (*arrows*) in the suprapatellar bursa. Beneath it lies the prefemoral fat pad (*F*). *P*, patella.

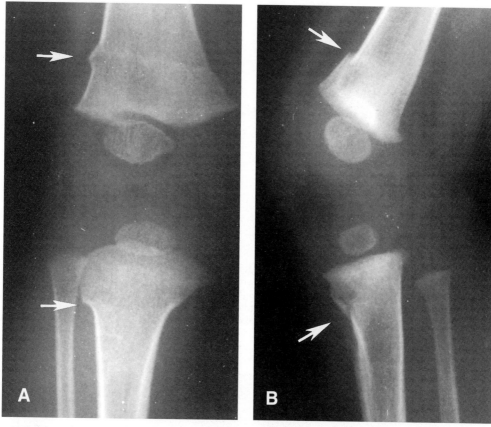

FIGURE 4.167. *Hyperextension fractures of knee and tibia.* (**A** and **B**) Note overt hyperextension buckle-compression fractures of the distal femur and proximal tibia (*arrows*).

ment avulsions with tibial spine fractures, and meniscal injuries. In addition chronic tibial tubercle and inferior patellar tendon avulsion injuries are common.

Epiphyseal–metaphyseal injuries are common about the knee and in gross form are not difficult to detect (Fig. 4.168). The more subtle, nondisplaced Salter–Harris type I or II injuries, on the other hand, frequently elude initial observation. In these cases, one once again must learn to study the soft tissues first and then to be suspicious of the slightest degree of widening of the epiphyseal line (Fig.

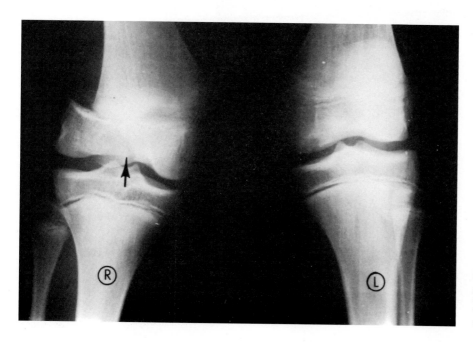

FIGURE 4.168. *Salter–Harris type III epiphyseal–metaphyseal injury.* Note the grossly displaced epiphysis and the fracture through the middle of the epiphysis (*arrow*) of the distal right femur.

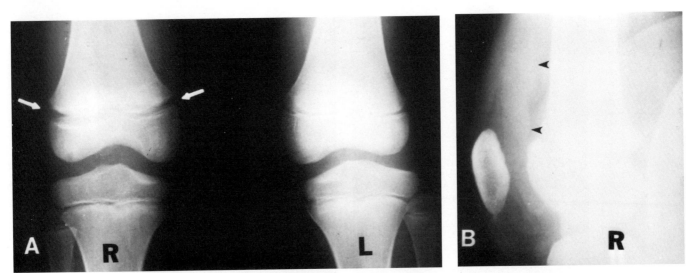

FIGURE 4.169. *Subtle Salter–Harris type I epiphyseal–metaphyseal injury.* (**A**) First, note that the soft tissues are more opaque around the right knee. This indicates the presence of edema. In addition, however, note that the epiphyseal line of the distal right femur is wider (*arrows*) than its counterpart on the normal left side. The findings represent a nondisplaced epiphyseal–meta-physeal separation. (**B**) Lateral view showing associated hemarthrosis manifesting in distension of the suprapatellar bursa (*arrows*).

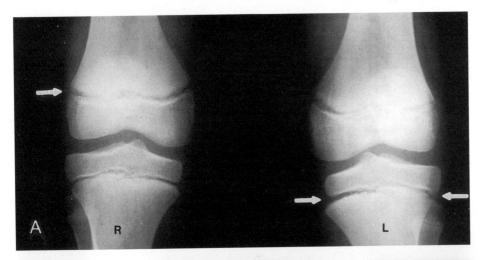

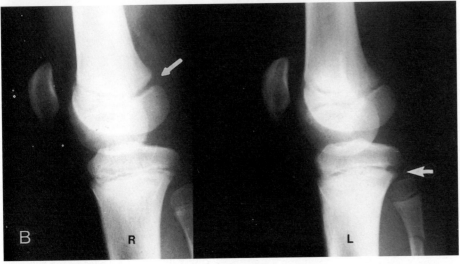

FIGURE 4.170. *Multiple, subtle, Salter–Harris type I epiphyseal–meta-physeal injuries.* (**A**) Note widening of the epiphyseal line of the distal right femur and proximal left tibia (*arrows*). Compare these epiphyseal lines with their normal counterparts on the other side. Also note a frac-ture in the upper left fibula. (**B**) Oblique view demonstrating widen-ing of the right distal femoral and left proximal tibial epiphyseal lines (*arrows*). The left fibular fracture is noted again.

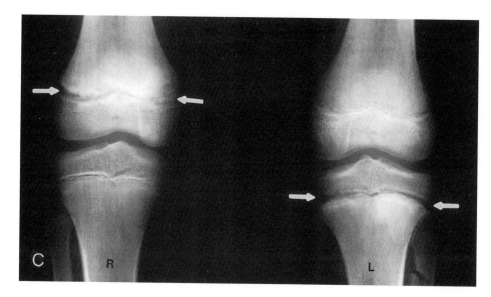

FIGURE 4.170. *(continued)* (C) Two weeks later note evidence of healing of the previously noted epiphyseal–metaphyseal fractures. There is irregular sclerosis along the distal right femoral epiphyseal–metaphyseal junction (*arrows*) and along the upper left tibial epiphyseal–metaphyseal line (*arrows*). The fibular fracture is noted again.

4.169). In other cases, additional oblique (Fig. 4.170) or stress views may be required to confirm or further delineate the injury. Epiphyseal–metaphyseal injuries of the knee can be sustained in a number of ways, but usually trauma is not minor (automobile accidents, athletic injuries [32,33], and so forth), and most often the stresses applied to the knee are dissipated through the epiphyseal–metaphyseal junctions. In some cases, however, rather than the forces being dissipated through this area, collateral ligament strains cause small, marginal avulsions of either the epiphysis or metaphysis (Fig. 4.171A). MR imaging is especially useful in detecting these injuries if no fracture fragment is visible on plain films (Fig. 4.171B).

Cruciate ligament avulsions most often involve the anterior cruciate ligament at its bony insertion into the anterior tibial spine of the tibial epiphysis (16). With large fragment avulsions, the findings are straightforward, and it is difficult to miss the fragment (Fig. 4.172). With smaller avulsions, however, it is easy to miss the fragment on initial studies (Fig. 4.173A). A similar problem can arise, although

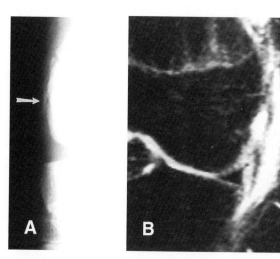

FIGURE 4.171. *Collateral ligament injuries.* (A) Note the barely visible avulsed bony epiphyseal fragment (*arrow*). This patient sustained a lateral knee sprain injury. (B) Another patient with a medial collateral ligament sprain demonstrated on a magnetic resonance image. On this fat-supressed image the injured ligament has a bright signal (*arrows*).

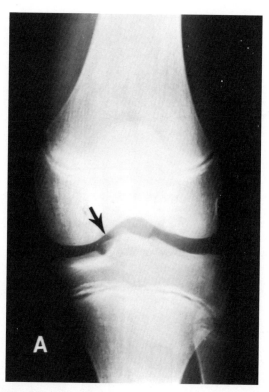

FIGURE 4.172. *Anterior cruciate ligament avulsion: large fragment.* (A) Frontal view demonstrating large avulsed bony fragment (*arrow*).
(continued on next page)

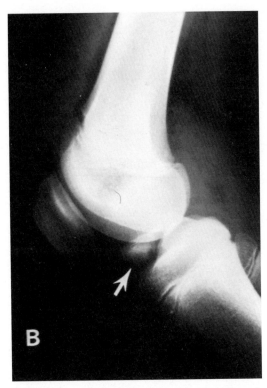

FIGURE 4.172. *(continued)* (B) Lateral view demonstrating the same avulsed bony fragment *(arrow)*. Also note distension of the suprapatellar bursa (hemarthrosis).

less commonly, with cruciate ligament avulsions involving the femoral condyle (Fig. 4.173B). In either case, tunnel views of the knee usually more clearly delineate the avulsed fragment (Fig. 4.173C).

Cruciate ligament injuries currently are best assessed with MR imaging. Occult associated subclinical bone bruises also can be detected with MR imaging, on which they show focal decrease in the normal high signal level of fatty bone marrow on T1-weighted images. More importantly, however, one should look for distortion and indistinctness of the anterior cruciate ligament and buckling of the posterior cruciate ligament (Fig. 4.174). Anterior translocation of the tibia also occurs (40) but is an ancillary finding.

Supracondylar fractures of the distal femur are not difficult to identify if they are gross. Seldom do these fractures occur in healthy bones, however, for in such bones the weakest area is the epiphyseal–metaphyseal junction, and thus fracture through this area is more likely to occur. On the other hand, if the femur is severely demineralized or otherwise weakened, such fractures can occur. In addition it should be noted that buckle, supracondylar fractures can occur in normal bones with hyperextension injuries in infants and young children (Fig. 4.167).

In the proximal tibia one commonly sees transverse metaphyseal fractures, and if these fractures are hairline, they are difficult to detect (Fig. 4.175). These fractures can

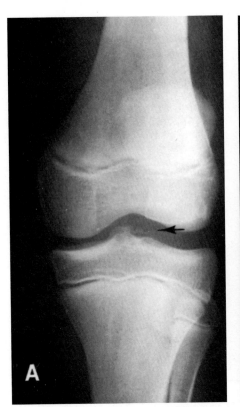
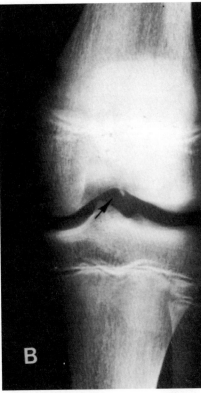
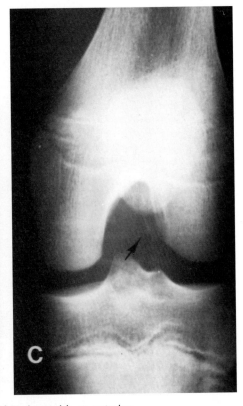

FIGURE 4.173. *Cruciate ligament avulsions: more subtle changes.* **(A)** Patient with an anterior cruciate ligament avulsion. **(B)** Another patient with a small avulsed bony fragment *(arrow)* from the lateral femoral condyle. **(C)** Tunnel view in same patient demonstrating the avulsed bony fragment *(arrow)* to greater advantage.

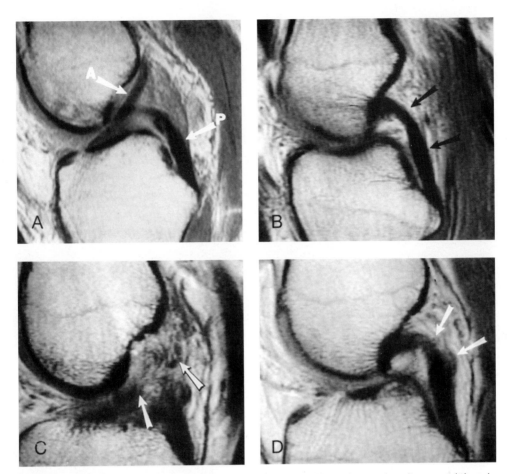

FIGURE 4.174. *Anterior cruciate ligament tear.* **(A)** Normal anterior cruciate ligament (*A*) and partially visible, normal posterior cruciate ligament (*P*). **(B)** Another patient with a normal posterior cruciate ligament (*arrows*). **(C)** Anterior cruciate ligament tear completely disrupts the normal architecture of the anterior cruciate ligament (*arrows*). **(D)** Concomitantly, there is laxity and buckling of the posterior cruciate ligament (*arrows*).

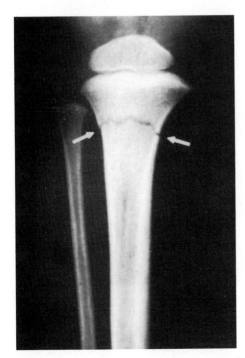

FIGURE 4.175. *Transverse fracture, upper tibia.* Note the clearly visible transverse fracture through the upper left tibia (*arrows*).

occur with forces applied to the lateral or anterior aspect of the knee, and fractures resulting from the latter force often are subtle (38,39). A problematic feature of fractures that occur after lateral forces are applied to the knee is resultant valgus deformity of the tibia (6,21). This deformity, often initially minimally present, can become more pronounced and persistent as time goes by (Fig. 4.176). For the most part, this is believed to result from the fact that there is overgrowth of the tibia, during healing, through the medial portion of the epiphyseal–metaphyseal junction (14,21,32,41). This probably is related to hyperemia associated with the fracture, which in the end causes accelerated growth of the medial aspect of the proximal tibia. It has been noted that normally there is a greater blood supply to the upper medial tibia, and that with trauma this is exaggerated (21).

In subtle form, fractures resulting from purely anterior forces applied to the knee can be difficult to detect. There is, however, a constellation of findings, although not all are always present in any given patient, that aid in their detection and diagnosis (38). In such cases there is anterior buckling of the upper tibial cortex, increased scooping of the notch for the tibial tubercle, a diastatic posterior fracture, and anterior tilting of the epiphyseal–metaphyseal plate

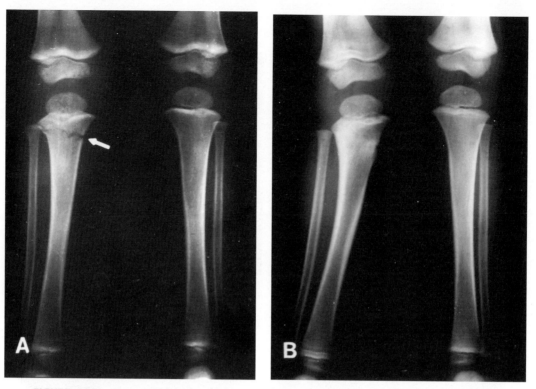

FIGURE 4.176. *Upper tibial fracture with inward bending.* **(A)** Note the clearly visible fracture through the upper right tibia (*arrow*). Also note that the fracture line is wider medially and that there is slight inward angulation of the tibia. **(B)** Late healing phase, demonstrating pronounced knock-knee deformity.

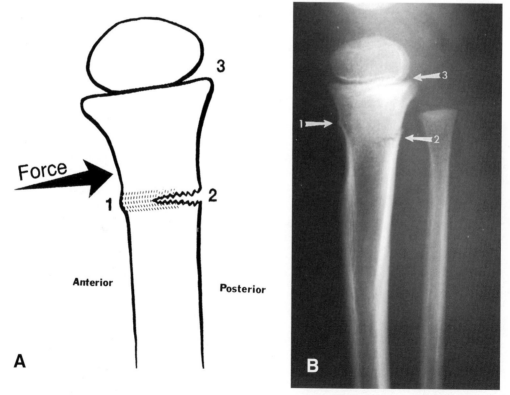

FIGURE 4.177. *Hyperextension injury of upper tibia.* **(A)** Forces (*force*) producing hyperextension result in anterior buckling (*1*), posterior fracturing with diastasis (*2*), and anterior tilting of the epiphyseal plate (*3*). **(B)** Anterior buckle fracture (*1*), posterior diastatic fracture (*2*), and anteriorly tilted epiphyseal plate (*3*). (From Swischuk LE, John SD, Tschoepe EJ. Upper tibial hyperextension fractures in infants: another occult toddler's fracture. *Pediatr Radiol* 1999;29:6–9, with permission.)

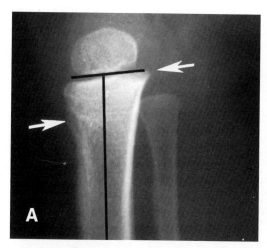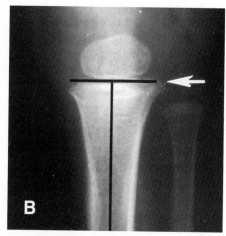

FIGURE 4.178. *Hyperextension injury with tilting of epiphyseal plate.* **(A)** Note the anterior buckle fracture (*anterior arrow*) and the tilted epiphyseal plate (*posterior arrow*). **(B)** Normal side for comparison. The epiphyseal plate is basically horizontal (*arrow*). Note that there is no buckling of the anterior cortex of the tibia. (From Swischuk LE, John SD, Tschoepe EJ. Upper tibial hyperextension fractures in infants: another occult toddler's fracture. *Pediatr Radiol* 1999;29:6–9, with permission.)

(Fig. 4.177). These fractures usually are sustained from some object or some person falling on the infant's knee, but this is not always the case. They also are common trampoline-induced injuries (4), but in any case they can be quite subtle. It is important to appreciate the possibility that such a fracture exists in a patient who is limping, and it is only if one appreciates all of these relatively subtle radiographic findings that one can make the diagnosis with certainty (Figs. 4.178–4.180). *Comparative views are extremely helpful with these fractures, because the findings frequently are very subtle.* Of course, nuclear scintigraphy can reveal the presence of such fractures, but once again the study has no specificity.

Compression fractures of the tibial plateau are less common in children than in adults, but upper fibular fractures occur rather frequently, both with knee injuries (Fig. 4.170) and ankle injuries. Compression fractures of the proximal tibia also occur with trampoline injuries and may be related to chronic stress factors (4).

Stress fractures around the knee most commonly occur in the upper tibia. Although some can be seen in the distal femur, most occur in the proximal tibia. In the acute phase, the fracture line usually is not visible, and it is only after healing begins that the fracture and typical sclerosis and periosteal new bone deposition are seen (Fig. 4.181). In the early stages, these changes can be quite subtle, but later

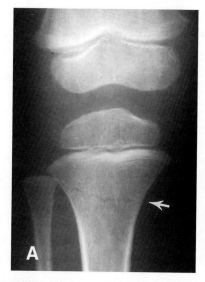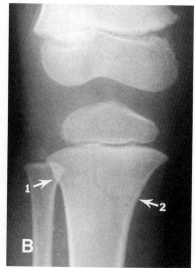

FIGURE 4.179. *Hyperextension injury of upper tibia: hairline and buckle fractures.* **(A)** Note the transverse hairline fracture (*arrow*). **(B)** A subtle buckle fracture (*1*) along with a subtle hairline fracture (*2*) are present. (From Swischuk LE, John SD, Tschoepe EJ. Upper tibial hyperextension fractures in infants: another occult toddler's fracture. *Pediatr Radiol* 1999;29:6–9, with permission.)

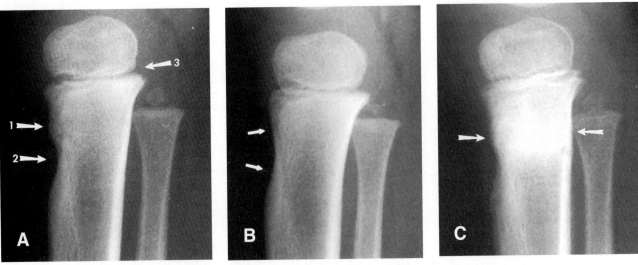

FIGURE 4.180. *Hyperextension injury, upper tibia: scooping of anterior tibial tubercle notch.* **(A)** Note the buckle fracture (*1*) and increased scooping of the tibial tubercle notch (*2*). The epiphyseal plate also is tilted (*3*). **(B)** Normal side for comparison. Note normal appearance of the anterior tibia including the more shallow notch for the tibial tubercle. **(C)** Healing phase of injury in **A**. Note sclerosis in the upper tibia (*arrows*). (From Swischuk LE, John SD, Tschoepe EJ. Upper tibial hyperextension fractures in infants: another occult toddler's fracture. *Pediatr Radiol* 1999;29:6–9, with permission.)

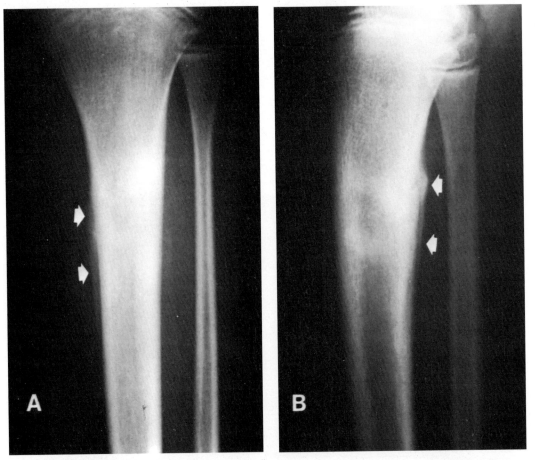

FIGURE 4.181. *Stress fracture of upper tibia.* **(A)** Frontal view demonstrating periosteal deposition along the upper inner aspect of the tibia (*arrows*). **(B)** Lateral view demonstrating typical posterior deposition of periosteal new bone around the fracture site (*arrows*). In addition, note sclerosis through the medullary cavity, indicating the location of the healing stress fracture.

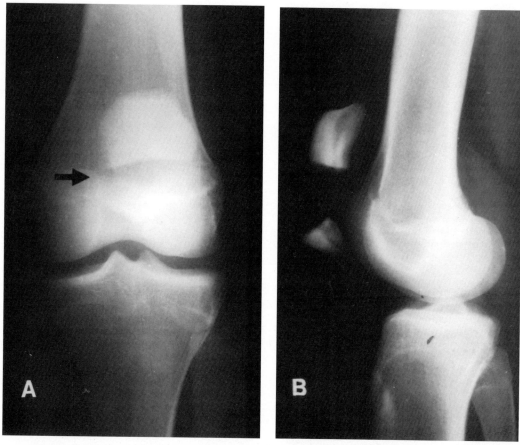

FIGURE 4.182. *Overt patellar fracture.* **(A)** Note the clear-cut patellar fracture (*arrow*). **(B)** Lateral view demonstrating marked separation of the bony fragments.

periosteal new bone deposition is profound, and often a more serious lesion such as a bone tumor is erroneously suggested (7). Periosteal new bone typically is deposited most abundantly posteriorly. The findings also can be demonstrated on CT scanning and are especially well seen in the early stages with MR imaging. In these cases, the occult fracture line becomes visible as a line of decreased signal on T1-weighted images. ***MR imaging is not usually required, however, if plain films are assessed adequately.***

Patellar Fractures and Dislocations

Fractures of the patella usually occur with direct blows to the patella or with injuries producing quadriceps tendon stresses. If these fractures are gross, they are not difficult to detect (Fig. 4.182), but lesser injuries may be difficult to visualize, and one may be left with soft tissue and joint-effusion changes only (Fig. 4.183). This is especially true of

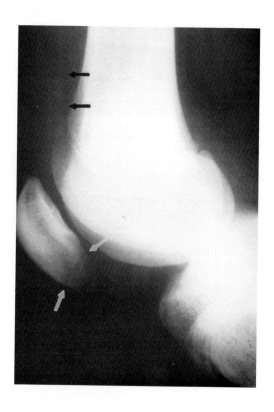

FIGURE 4.183. *Subtle patellar fracture.* First note the presence of fluid in the suprapatellar bursa (*upper arrows*). Then note the barely detectable transverse fracture through the inferior aspect of the patella (*lower arrows*).

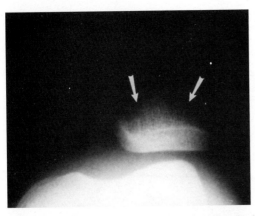

FIGURE 4.184. *Acute dislocation of the patella.* Note the lateral displacement of the patella (*arrows*); it has been dislocated out of the patellofemoral groove.

small avulsion injuries of the patella (see Fig. 4.185). In interpreting these chip fractures, the greatest pitfall lies in the misinterpretation of the so-called bipartite or tripartite patella, or a normal irregularly ossified patella, as a fracture (see Fig. 4.209). Avulsion fractures can involve the superior pole (quadriceps tendon), inferior pole (infrapatellar tendon), or medial edge (13,15). The latter is associated with acute patellar dislocation (see Fig. 4.186).

Both acute and chronic, recurrent dislocation of the patella are reasonably common in childhood (Fig. 4.184), but in most cases the patella relocates before roentgenograms are obtained. In some cases, a residual telltale sign consisting of a medial avulsion fracture of the patella can be seen (13,15) (Fig. 4.185), but most often bony changes are

absent. If the fracture is present, it is best demonstrated on tangential or so-called skyline views of the patella. Patients with chronic recurrent dislocation often have associated patella alta, a condition in which the patella is higher in position than normal (20,23). Abnormal tracking of the patella results, and the patellofemoral groove becomes shallow (26). Patella alta is best seen on lateral view; the shallow groove and associated flattening of the lateral condyle are best seen on skyline views (with 30% flexion) of the patella. Most dislocations, whether acute or chronic, are lateral dislocations.

Avulsion fractures of the lateral condyle are less well appreciated but are not uncommon with injuries to the knee in which dislocation of the patella also occurs. In many cases the only telltale sign of this injury is an avulsed bony fragment seen in the knee joint, frequently floating in the suprapatellar bursa. The fragment can be large or small, but its presence should signify the presence of this underlying injury (Figs. 4.186 and 4.187).

Chondromalacia of the patella is a difficult diagnosis to make with certainty. It is not particularly common in children and currently is evaluated best with MR imaging (27). In these cases there are abnormal levels of signal and variable degrees of deficiency of the cartilage on the posterior aspect of the patella. Stress fractures of the patella are uncommon, but linear, lateral stress fractures have been identified (26).

Miscellaneous Knee Problems

Miscellaneous knee problems include acute and chronic tibial tubercle and inferior patellar avulsions, osteochondritis dissecans, and meniscus injuries. ***Acute total tibial tubercle***

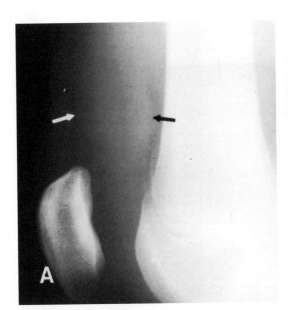
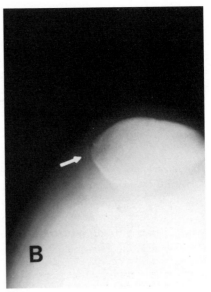

FIGURE 4.185. *Acute dislocation of patella with fracture fragments.* **(A)** Note only fluid in the suprapatellar bursa (*arrows*). **(B)** Two weeks later, note small fracture fragment (*arrow*) attesting to the previous dislocation.

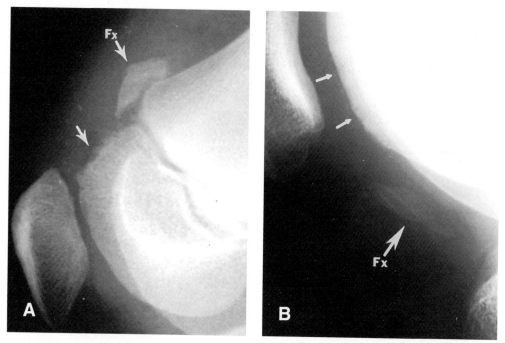

FIGURE 4.186. *Avulsion fracture, lateral femoral condyle.* (**A**) Note the avulsed fracture fragment (*FX*). The defect (*arrow*) of the donor site along the anterior aspect of the lateral femoral condyle is seen. Fluid is present in the suprapatellar bursa. (**B**) Another patient with a displaced fracture fragment (*FX*) and irregularity over the lateral condyle indicating the donor site (*arrows*).

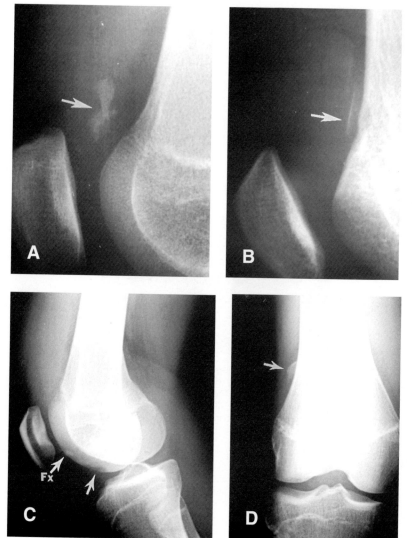

FIGURE 4.187. *Avulsion, lateral femoral condyle: floating fracture fragment.* (**A**) Note the large fracture fragment (*arrow*) in the suprapatellar bursa, which is full of fluid. (**B**) In this patient, with initial patellar dislocation, a small avulsed lateral condylar fragment (*arrow*) is seen in the fluid-distended suprapatellar bursa. (**C**) The fracture fragment (*FX*) in this patient is somewhat obscure. Note the defect, however, in the lateral femoral condyle (*arrow*), indicating the donor site. (**D**) Anteroposterior view demonstrates that the fracture fragment (*arrow*) has now moved upward into the suprapatellar bursa.

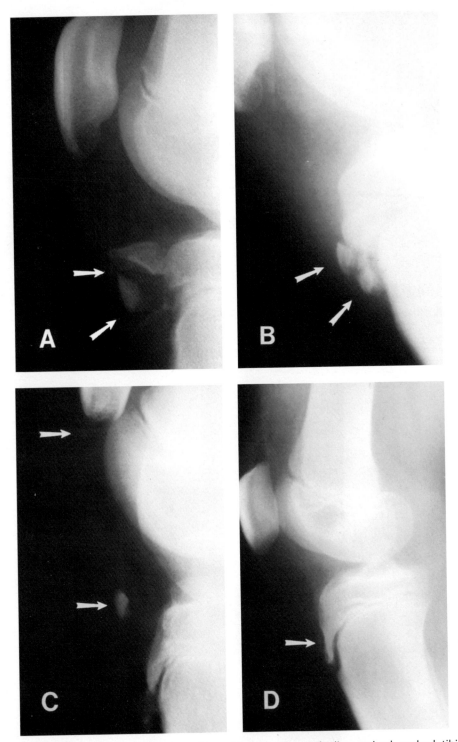

FIGURE 4.188. *Acute tibial tubercle avulsions.* **(A)** Note the grossly disorganized, avulsed, tibial tubercle: basketball injury. **(B)** Another patient with a more subtle tibial tubercle avulsion (*arrows*). Also note soft tissue edema extending into and obliterating the infrapatellar fat pad. **(C)** Note the avulsed tibial tubercle fragment (*lower arrow*) and the small sliver of avulsed bone from the patella (*upper arrow*). **(D)** Very subtle tibial tubercle avulsion consisting of a small sliver of bone (*arrow*). Note again that the infrapatellar fat pad is obliterated.

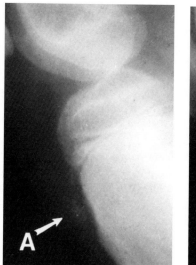
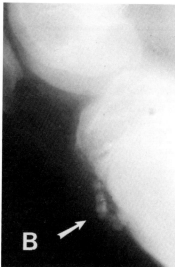
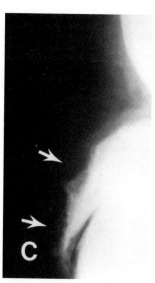

FIGURE 4.189. *Osgood–Schlatter disease.* **(A)** Minimal changes consisting of slight irregularity of the tibial tubercle and a little overlying edema (*arrow*). **(B)** More pronounced changes in the same patient, in the other knee (*arrow*). **(C)** Another patient with very gross irregularity of the tibial tubercle (*arrows*).

avulsions are relatively uncommon but tend to occur in athletes. Clinically and roentgenographically, these fractures are not difficult to detect (Fig. 4.188A–C), but the more subtle minimal avulsion can pose a greater problem (Fig. 4.188D). ***Osgood–Schlatter disease*** results from repeated, subclinical avulsions of the tibial tubercle (2,12,24), and the findings consist of pretubercular swelling and tubercular fragmentation (Fig. 4.189). With healing, a considerable amount of hypertrophic bone can be seen at the site of avulsion (Fig.

4.189C). All of these configurations are virtually pathognomonic of the condition, but occasionally Osgood–Schlatter disease can be mimicked by the very rare periosteal chondroma of the tibial tubercle (22). This lesion is more bulky, mostly lytic, and is associated with destruction of the upper tibia under the tibial tubercle. Rarely, tibia recurvation can result from Osgood-Schlatter disease (25).

A lesion similar to Osgood–Schlatter disease occurring along the inferior aspect of the patella (Fig. 4.190) is termed

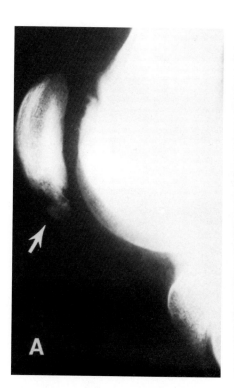
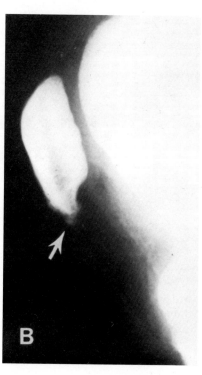

FIGURE 4.190. *Sinding–Larsen–Johansson disease of the patella.* **(A)** Note the large bony fragment just below the inferior aspect of the patella (*arrow*). **(B)** Less pronounced changes in another patient (*arrow*).

Sinding–Larsen–Johansson disease (37). It should be noted that both Osgood–Schlatter disease and Sinding–Larsen–Johansson disease are chronic manifestations of acute avulsion injuries at these sites. They are more tendinous than bony in nature, and both can now be demonstrated with ultrasound, CT, and MR imaging (24,34). ***Plain films, however, usually suffice.*** Finally, it should be noted that both conditions tend to be self-limiting, although they may leave a residual lump in the area. This is especially likely to occur with Osgood–Schlatter disease. Only rarely do significant complications result. Tibia recurvatum has been noted to develop (29), but this is quite uncommon.

Another cause of knee pain in childhood is osteochondritis dissecans of the distal femoral epiphysis and, less often, the patella. Most often, these lesions occur in older children and adolescents, and although many patients are symptomatic, other individuals are asymptomatic. Roentgenographically, typical findings are those of a bony defect along the anteromedial aspect of the medial femoral condyle (Fig. 4.191). This should be differentiated from normal irregularity, which often occurs along the posterior aspect of the lateral femoral condyle. In the patella, osteochondritis dissecans produces an irregular defect on the posterior aspect of the patella (Fig. 4.192). All of these lesions probably represent subchondral fractures and now are assessed with MR imaging if there is question of instability (9,28). MR imaging clearly demonstrates whether the fragment is displaced and extends beyond the articular surface of the involved bone (Fig. 4.191D).

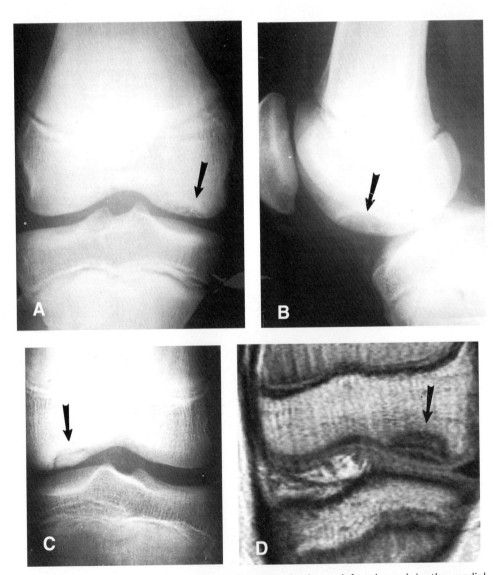

FIGURE 4.191. *Osteochondritis dissecans.* **(A)** Note the bony defect (*arrow*) in the medial condyle. **(B)** Lateral view demonstrates the same defect (*arrow*). **(C)** Another patient with a defect and a sequestrated piece of bone (*arrow*). **(D)** Magnetic resonance study in another patient demonstrates a similar fragment of bone (*arrow*).

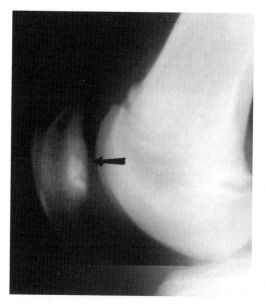

FIGURE 4.192. *Osteochondritis dissecans of patella.* Note irregularity with surrounding sclerosis along the posterior aspect of the patella (*arrow*). Also note distension of the suprapatellar bursa and its neck, caused by an associated effusion.

Meniscus injuries are not as common in childhood as in the adolescent and young adult, but they do occur. Plain film findings usually are absent, and most cases subsequently are diagnosed by MR imaging. In terms of meniscal injuries in childhood, a note about the lateral meniscus in children is in order. Often this meniscus is very large and, rather than being disk-shaped, assumes a semicircular shape. Consequently, the medial aspect extends almost to the intercondylar notch (8,24); because of this, the cartilage

is very prone to tearing. This is termed the ***discoid lateral meniscus*** and is best demonstrated with MR imaging.

A detailed dissertation of all of the findings associated with meniscal tears and other meniscal abnormalities is beyond the scope of this book. Of importance in evaluating these tears, however, is determining whether the suspected tear reaches the articular surface (1,10). In addition, with bucket-handle tears the usual bowtie configuration of the meniscus is lost (19). Joint effusions are common, as are bone bruises. Some of these findings are demonstrated in Fig. 4.193.

An uncommon problem related to trauma around the knee is rupture of the synovium of the knee joint (36). In such cases, chronic extrasynovial fluid collections can extend deep into the calf, and the clinical findings can be confused with deep vein thrombosis (36). Ultrasonography is invaluable in these cases, because it demonstrates the fluid collection resulting from synovial rupture. By the same token, it is also useful in the detection of deep vein thrombosis.

Septic Arthritis, Osteomyelitis, and Cellulitis of the Knee

In the knee, one of the more common clinical problems is that of differentiating septic arthritis from simple cellulitis. Indeed, this comes up far more often than does the differentiation of septic arthritis from osteomyelitis, for soft tissue infections (cellulitis) are especially likely to develop over the patella, and many times it is difficult to clinically determine whether the joint space is involved. This is especially true in the young child and infant. The problem must be resolved, however, for with septic arthritis arthrocentesis is required, but with cellulitis it is con-

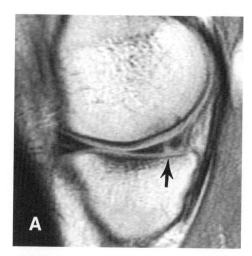
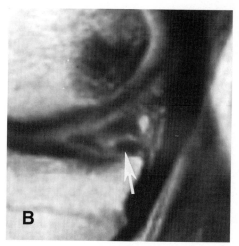

FIGURE 4.193. *Meniscal injuries.* **(A)** Meniscal tear (*arrow*) in the posterior limb of the medial meniscus. **(B)** Another patient with a tear (*arrow*) extending to the articular surface.

(continued on next page)

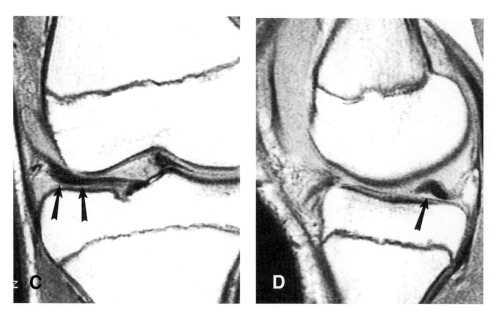

FIGURE 4.193. *(continued)* **(C)** *Bucket-handle tear.* Note the displaced lateral meniscus *(arrows)*. **(D)** Sagittal view demonstrates the posterior limb of the meniscus *(arrow)*. It has a crumpled appearance.

traindicated. Although it is not well appreciated, the lateral view of the knee can solve this dilemma in almost every instance.

With septic arthritis, fluid (pus) accumulates in the various bursae, but it first always accumulates in the suprapatellar bursa (Fig. 4.194A). If it does so, it displaces the quadriceps tendon anteriorly and the prefemoral fat pad posteriorly. As a result, the soft-tissue space between the quadriceps tendon and the prefemoral fat pad becomes thickened (Fig. 4.194B). At first the findings might suggest that the entire quadriceps tendon is thickened, but actually they represent the confluent images of the normal quadri-

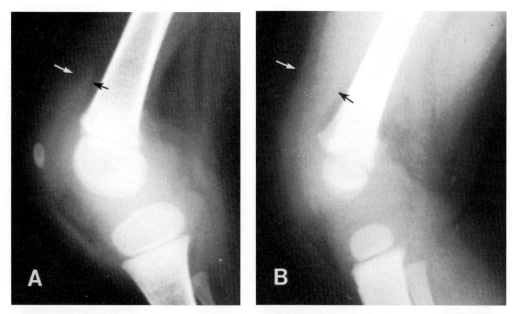

FIGURE 4.194. *Septic arthritis of the knee.* **(A)** Note discrete suprapatellar bursal distension *(arrows)*. **(B)** Another patient. The distended suprapatellar bursa blends with the quadriceps tendon to produce subtle pseudothickening of the tendon *(arrows)*. Associated soft-tissue swelling (fat pad obliteration) also has extended behind the knee.

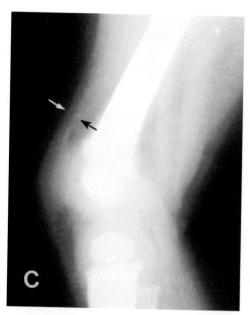

FIGURE 4.194. *(continued)* (C) Normal side for comparison. Note normal thickness of quadriceps tendon *(arrows)*.

ceps tendon and abnormal, pus-filled suprapatellar bursa. In addition to these findings, sooner or later there is bulging of the posterior popliteal bursa: The greater the accumulation of pus, the greater is the bulging (Fig. 4.194). With more extensive collections, the suprapatellar and posterior

popliteal bursae can show enormous bulging, and even the infrapatellar fat pad can become obliterated. No matter how extensive the accumulation of pus in the joint, however, the soft tissues anterior to the patella usually remain normal and distinct. They do not become edematous; this is most important in differentiating septic arthritis from prepatellar cellulitis. In advanced cases of septic arthritis, the deep soft tissues around the knee may become edematous, but distension of the suprapatellar bursa should identify the problem as septic arthritis or septic arthritis with osteomyelitis (Fig. 4.194B).

With prepatellar cellulitis or hematoma, as opposed to septic arthritis, the suprapatellar bursa does not become distended, but rather the soft tissues anterior to the quadriceps tendon and patella become thickened and edematous (Fig. 4.195). Of course, if soft-tissue edema is extensive, the suprapatellar and infrapatellar fat pads may become hazy, and the soft tissues behind the femur also may become indistinct (Fig. 4.195B). Such extensive edema also can be seen with severe septic arthritis or osteomyelitis, but with septic arthritis suprapatellar bursal distention occurs (Fig. 4.194B). Prepatellar edema generally is not seen with either septic arthritis or osteomyelitis (Figs. 4.194B and 4.196B).

With osteomyelitis of the distal femur, early findings consist only of soft tissue edema and obliteration or displacement of the fat pads (18) around the distal femur

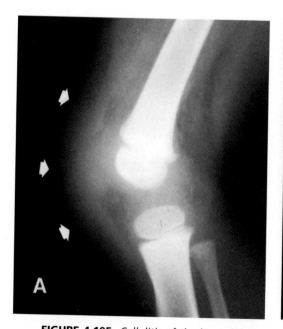

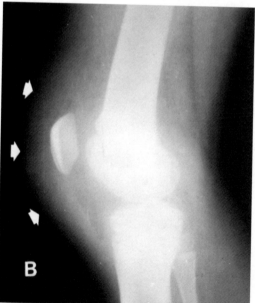

FIGURE 4.195. *Cellulitis of the knee.* (A) First, note that swelling is present in the soft tissues anterior to the quadriceps tendon and unossified cartilaginous patella only *(arrows)*. The quadriceps tendon is still clearly visible, and there is no evidence of accumulation of fluid in the suprapatellar bursa. **(B)** Another patient demonstrating extensive swelling of the soft tissues anterior to the patella and quadriceps tendon *(arrows)*. In this case, soft-tissue swelling is so pronounced that there is associated obliteration of the quadriceps tendon and suprapatellar fat pad. The findings, however, are not those of septic arthritis, for edema of the soft tissues anterior to the patella and quadriceps tendon generally does not occur with septic arthritis. Also note edema posterior to the femur.

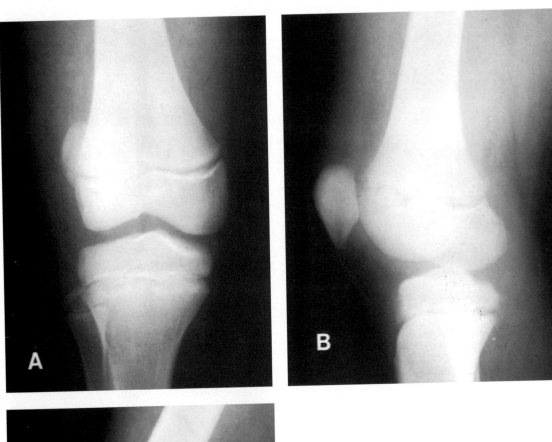

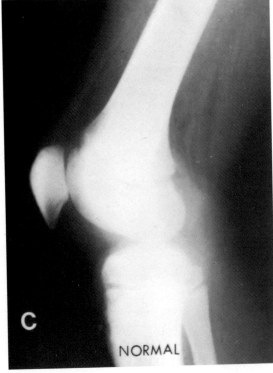

FIGURE 4.196. *Osteomyelitis: deep soft-tissue changes.*
(A) Note extensive swelling of all the soft tissues around
the distal femur. No normal fat–muscle interfaces
remain. **(B)** Lateral view demonstrating similar findings.
Note that the suprapatellar fat pads and the fat pads
posterior to the distal femur have been totally obliterated. Obliteration of these fat pads, especially the ones
posterior to the distal femur, is a most important finding,
for it is not seen with septic arthritis. **(C)** Normal knee of
the same patient for comparison. Note the clearly identified fat–muscle interfaces and the various normal fat
pads, both anterior and posterior to the distal femur.

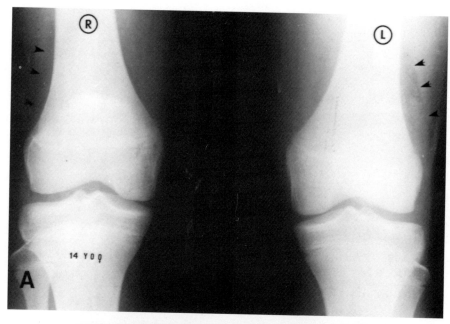

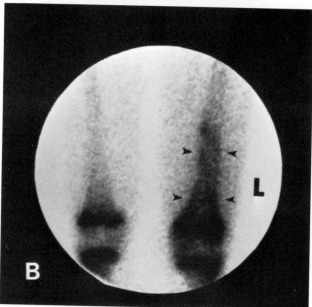

FIGURE 4.197. *Osteomyelitis: early displacement of the fat pads.* **(A)** First note the generalized increase in soft-tissue density and thickness around the distal left femur. Then note displacement of the lateral fat pad outwardly (*arrows*). Compare this with the same fat pad on the normal right side (*arrows*). **(B)** Bone scan demonstrating increased uptake of isotope in the distal left femur (*arrows*), characteristic of osteomyelitis. (Courtesy of M. Capitanio, M.D.)

(Figs. 4.196 and 4.197). Unlike with septic arthritis, there is no filling of the suprapatellar bursa with pus, and unlike with prepatellar cellulitis, prepatellar edema is absent (Fig. 4.196). Of course, once again one must make an exception in the young child or infant, for in this age group osteomyelitis and septic arthritis often occur together and present features of both conditions.

In more advanced cases of osteomyelitis, frank bony destruction and periosteal new-bone deposition are seen, and the diagnosis is no problem. In early cases, however, the area of bone destruction may be small and subtle and may cause confusion with a benign cortical defect (Fig. 4.198). Of course, as with osteomyelitis anywhere, one should turn to nuclear scintigraphy or MR imaging for

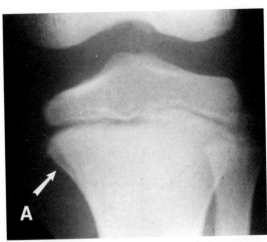
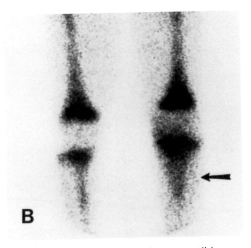

FIGURE 4.198. *Osteomyelitis: subtle findings.* **(A)** Note the subtle lytic lesion in the upper tibia (*arrow*). This could be confused with a benign cortical defect. **(B)** Bone scan, however, demonstrates increased isotope activity in the upper tibia (*arrow*). This does not occur with benign cortical defects. The patient had surgically proven osteomyelitis.

further delineation if there is doubt on the basis of the plain films.

Tendonitis

Tendonitis, either inflammatory or traumatic, can occur anywhere in the body, but it most commonly occurs around the shoulder and knee. Even then, it is more common around the knee than around the shoulder in children. Both the infra- and suprapatellar tendons can be involved, and the findings on plain films are simply those of thickening and indistinctness of the tendon (Fig. 4.199A). These findings also can be demonstrated with ultrasound and with MR imaging (8). With each of these modalities, the findings are those of a thickened, swollen, edematous tendon, but MR imaging also can show focal areas of high signal representing foci of inflammation or bleeding (Fig. 4.199C). In addition, actual tears of the tendons can be demonstrated with ultrasound (3).

Normal Findings Causing Problems

One of the more common normal findings around the knee is *irregularity of the distal femur,* just along the *medial supracondylar ridge.* It occurs most commonly in older children and adolescents and should not be misinterpreted

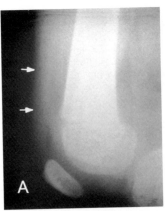
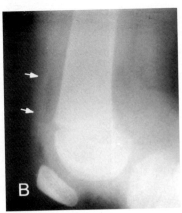
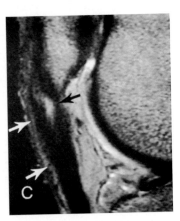

FIGURE 4.199. *Tendonitis.* **(A)** Lateral view demonstrates a thickened, edematous quadriceps tendon (*arrows*). **(B)** Contralateral normal side for comparison. Note the normal width of the quadriceps tendon (*arrows*). **(C)** Magnetic resonance evaluation of tendonitis. Note the thickened infrapatellar tendon (*white arrows*) and the area of high signal at the patellar insertion (*black arrow*) caused by bleeding.

as an area of osteomyelitis or a bone tumor. The irregularity occurs along the line of muscle insertion, recently suggested to be that of the adductor magnus (31). There is histologic support for the concept that this lesion results from chronic avulsion (11) and, depending on the degree of healing, the lesion can appear quite ragged or somewhat scalloped (Fig. 4.200). Unfortunately, however, benign cortical defects also occur here and can appear somewhat similar. Technetium-99 pyrophosphate bone scanning shows no increased isotope activity in most of these lesions (5). This attests to the low-grade activity of these lesions. They are not a serious finding, but it is very tempting to assign a more causative, often serious, role to them in patients with nonspecific knee pain. These irregularities also are seen on CT and MR scanning, and the findings are dependent on the degree of posttraumatic inflammatory activity present (Fig. 4.201).

Benign cortical (fibrous) defects can be found in any of the long bones and frequently are multiple. However, they most commonly occur in the distal femur and proximal tibia and characteristically are eccentric and very peripheral (cortical) in location. They seldom extend beyond a half centimeter or so into the medullary cavity of the bone (Fig. 4.202). When seen *en face*, they can resemble a lytic lesion of the bone and should not be mistaken for low-grade osteomyelitis (i.e., Brodie's abscess) or a bone tumor (Fig. 4.203). Benign cortical defects are related to the somewhat larger benign nonossifying fibroma. This lesion also is eccentric but often more definitely corticated and larger than a benign cortical defect (Fig. 4.202B). Benign cortical defects proper have variably sclerotic margins. In a few cases, ***benign cortical defects appear very cystic and possess a thin cortex.*** In such cases, normal muscle pull on the cortex can cause acute

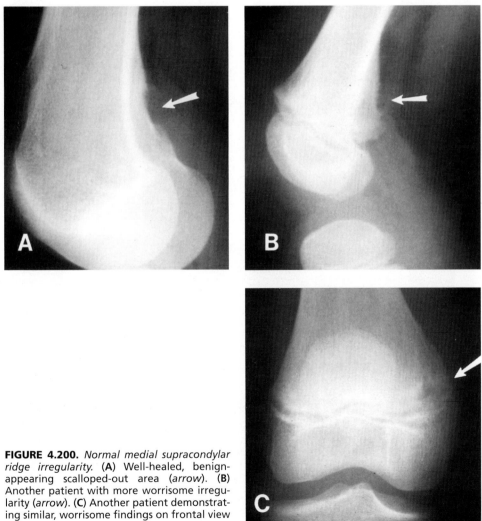

FIGURE 4.200. *Normal medial supracondylar ridge irregularity.* **(A)** Well-healed, benign-appearing scalloped-out area *(arrow)*. **(B)** Another patient with more worrisome irregularity *(arrow)*. **(C)** Another patient demonstrating similar, worrisome findings on frontal view *(arrow)*.

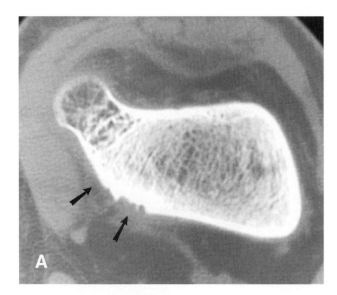

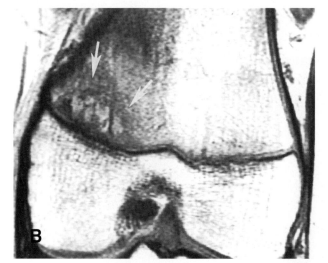

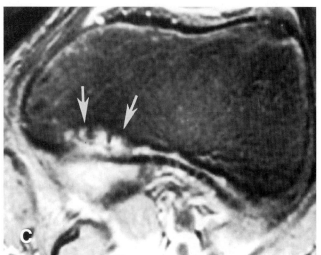

FIGURE 4.201. *Supracondylar ridge irregularity: computed tomographic and magnetic resonance findings.* **(A)** Computed tomographic scan in this patient demonstrates irregularity of the cortex (*arrows*). **(B)** Coronal-view magnetic resonance image in another patient demonstrates the area of irregularity (*arrow*). **(C)** On axial view, high-signal fluid (edema) is seen in the area (*arrows*). This supports the concept of a subclinical avulsion injury.

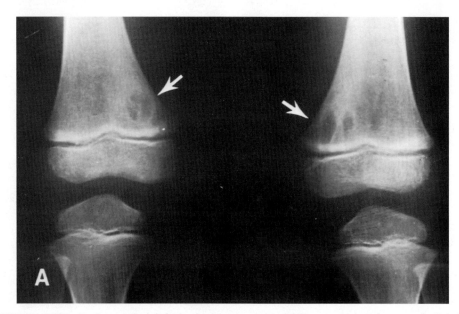

FIGURE 4.202. *Benign cortical defects, classic appearance.* **(A)** Note typical oval or round, slightly sclerotic, benign cortical defects in both distal femurs (*arrows*).

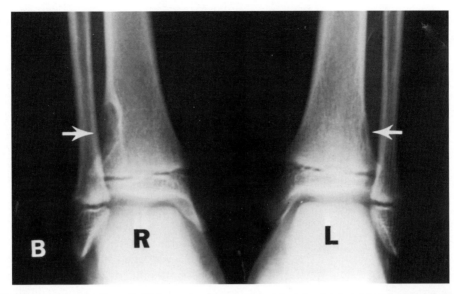

FIGURE 4.202. *(continued)* **(B)** Large benign cortical defect in distal right tibia *(arrow)*. This lesion is large enough to be considered a small nonossifying fibroma. The two lesions probably are related. On the left, a very small benign cortical defect is noted in the distal tibia *(arrow)*.

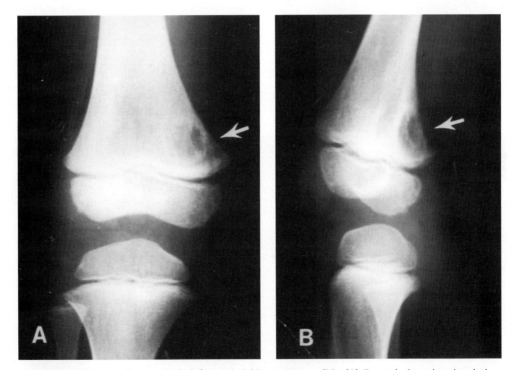

FIGURE 4.203. *Benign cortical defect mimicking osteomyelitis.* **(A)** Frontal view showing lytic lesion in the distal femur *(arrow)*. This patient presented with a swollen, hot knee. **(B)** Oblique view demonstrates the "pseudolytic," destructive appearance of this lesion *(arrow)*.

(continued on next page)

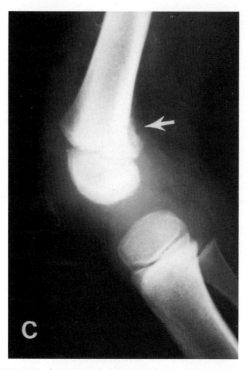

FIGURE 4.203. *(continued)* (C) Lateral view demonstrating the irregular lesion (*arrow*). This was misinterpreted as osteomyelitis, although in fact it was a benign cortical defect. The knee was swollen because of cellulitis of the soft tissues anterior to the patella.

avulsion and fragmentation. In these patients, the roentgenographic findings often first suggest malignancy (Fig. 4.204).

In older children, the ***tibial tubercle has a normal defect along its inferior aspect.*** On lateral view, this defect is not difficult to interpret, but on frontal view, it can be taken for a lytic lesion of the knee (Fig. 4.205). In young infants, the tibial tubercle is not ossified at all, and a scoop-like bony defect in the area can present a problem (Fig. 4.206).

The patella is very prone to irregular ossification (Fig. 4.207). Furthermore, if it finally does ossify, a number of peculiar irregularities and deformities can persist. Some of these are so fracturelike in appearance that it is almost impossible to differentiate them from true fractures (Fig. 4.208). Very often, however, the same configuration is present on the other side, and this solves the problem. Another common normal ossification anomaly of the patella is the bipartite or tripartite patella. In these cases, the extra portion of the patella usually lies in the upper outer quadrant (Fig. 4.209), and very often the anomaly is bilateral. There has been a suggestion that occasionally the bipartite patella can be painful (30). In such cases it has been suggested that the bipartite patella actually represents an incompletely united stress fracture, and that it is positive on isotope bone scanning. Most bipartite patellae, however, are asympto-

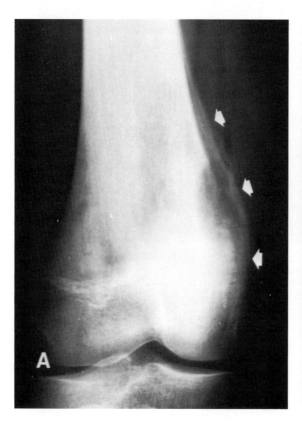

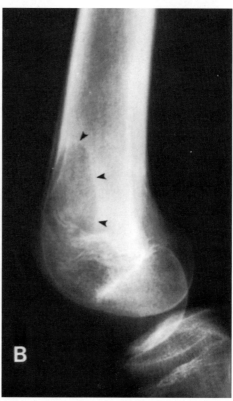

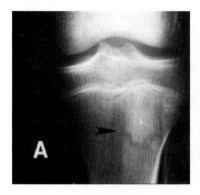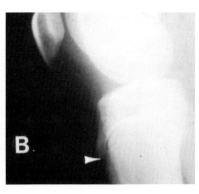

FIGURE 4.205. *Normal tibial tubercle defect.* (**A**) On frontal view, note the radiolucent line (*arrow*) just beneath an area of sclerosis. The area of sclerosis represents the inferior aspect of the tibial tubercle; the radiolucent line is the normal defect just beneath it. (**B**) Lateral view demonstrating the site of the radiolucent defect (*arrow*) under the normal tibial tubercle.

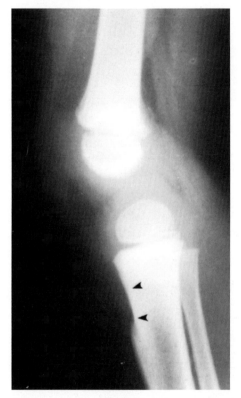

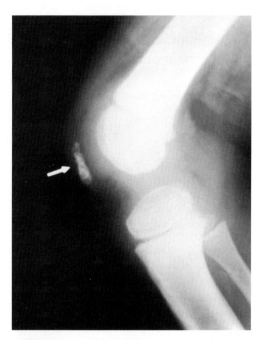

FIGURE 4.206. *Normal upper tibial notch.* In young infants, the tibial tubercle does not ossify and a normal notch is noted at its site (*arrows*). This notch should not be misinterpreted as a destructive lesion.

FIGURE 4.207. *Normal irregular patellar ossification.* Note the normal, irregularly ossified patella (*arrow*). The patella usually begins to ossify at about 5 years of age.

FIGURE 4.204. *Cystic benign cortical defect with periosteal new bone.* (**A**) Note the layered periosteal new bone over the cystic lesion of the distal femur (*arrows*). This young boy presented with recent onset of knee pain. (**B**) Lateral view demonstrating the lytic nature of the lesion and periosteal new bone anterior to it. The findings represent avulsion of the thin cortex of this benign cortical defect with subsequent periosteal new bone formation (histologically proven). (Reprinted with permission from Kumar R, Swischuk LE, Madewell JE. Benign cortical defect: Site for an avulsion injury. *Skeletal Radiol* 1986;15:553–555.)

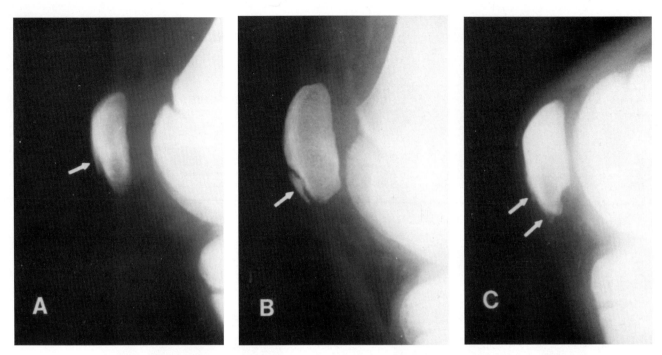

FIGURE 4.208. *Various normal patellar ossification patterns.* (**A**) Sliverlike normal ossicle (*arrow*). In some cases, this thin sliverlike piece of bone can appear completely detached from the patella. (**B**) Larger accessory ossification center of the patella (*arrow*). (**C**) Normal irregular ossification of the anterior–inferior aspect of the patella (*arrows*). This should not be confused with Sinding–Larsen–Johansson disease, in which similar fragmentation associated with pain and local swelling can be seen.

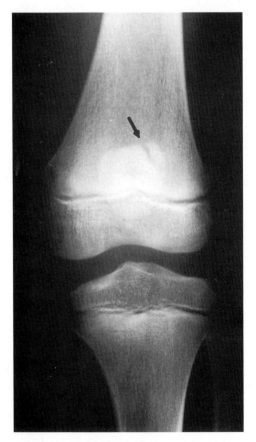

FIGURE 4.209. *Bipartite patella.* Note typical appearance and location of a bipartite patella (*arrow*).

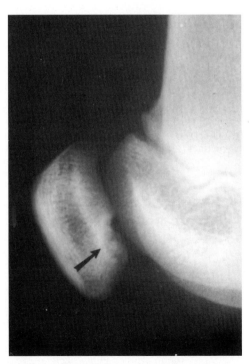

FIGURE 4.210. *Dorsal defect of patella.* Note the irregular dorsal defect (*arrow*). This patient was entirely asymptomatic. The finding can be confused with osteochondritis dessicans.

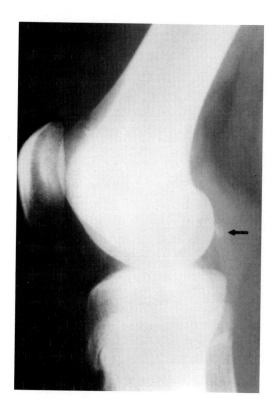

FIGURE 4.211. *Fabella.* The fabella is a normal sesamoid bone occurring in the gastrocnemius tendon (*arrow*).

matic. Finally, a normal dorsal fibrous defect of the patella (1,35) should not be confused with a lesion such as osteomyelitis or osteochondritis dessicans (Fig. 4.210).

The fabella is a normal ossicle occurring in the lateral limb of the gastrocnemius tendon and is best visualized on lateral view (Fig. 4.211). The distal femoral epiphysis fre-

quently ossifies irregularly and can appear very disturbing to the uninitiated (Fig. 4.212). These irregularities are common, however, especially in infants and young children, in whom the epiphysis may appear irregular all around its periphery. In older children, normal irregularities tend to occur in the lateral condyle, posteriorly (Fig. 4.213).

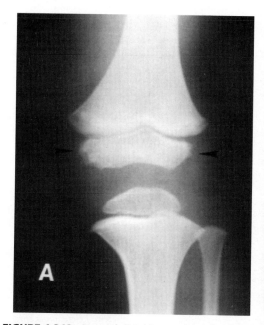
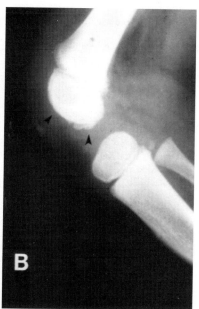

FIGURE 4.212. *Normal distal femoral epiphyseal irregularities.* **(A)** Frontal view showing normal irregularity of the distal femoral epiphysis (*arrows*). Radiolucencies in the metaphyseal corners also are normal. **(B)** Lateral view showing normal irregular ossification pattern of distal femoral epiphysis (*arrows*).

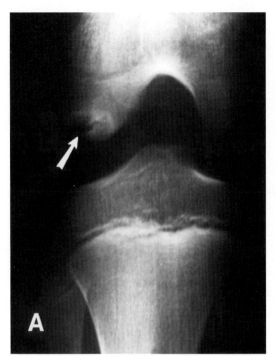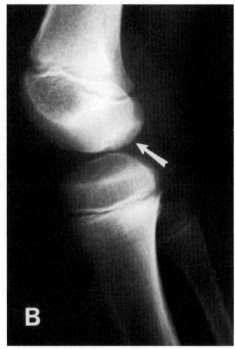

FIGURE 4.213. *Normal distal femoral epiphyseal irregularities.* **(A)** Note deep, focal irregularity of lateral condyle (*arrow*). **(B)** Lateral view demonstrating the irregularity to be posterior (*arrow*). This patient was asymptomatic. (Courtesy of Virgil Graves, M.D.)

REFERENCES

1. Alexander JE, Seibert JJ, Aronson J. Dorsal defect of the patella and infection. *Pediatr Radiol* 1987;17:325–327.
2. Aparicio G, Abril JC, Calvo E, Alvarez L. Radiologic study of patellar height in Osgood-Schlatter disease. *J Pediatr Orthop* 1997;17:63–66.
3. Bianchi S, Swass A, Abdelwahab IF, Banderali A. Diagnosis of tears of the quadriceps tendon of the knee: Value of sonography. *AJR* 1994;162:1137–1140.
4. Boyer RS, Jaffe RB, Nixon GW, Condon VR. Trampoline fracture of the proximal tibia in children. *AJR* 1986;1467:83–85.
5. Burrows PE, Greenberg ID, Reed MH. The distal femoral defect: Technetium-99m pyrophosphate bone scan results. *Can J Assoc Radiol* 1982;33:91–93.
6. Currarino G, Pinckney LE. Genu valgum after proximal tibial fractures in children. *AJR* 1981;136:915–918.
7. Davies AM, Evans N, Grimer RJ. Fatigue fractures of the proximal tibia simulating malignancy. *Br J Radiol* 1988;61:903–908.
8. Davies SG, Baudouin CJ, King JB, Perry JD. Ultrasound, computed tomography and magnetic resonance imaging in patellar tendonitis. *Clin Radiol* 1991;43:52–56.
9. De Smet AA, Fisher DR, Graf BK, Lange RH. Osteochondritis dissecans of the knee: Value of MR imaging in determining lesion stability and the presence of articular cartilage defects. *AJR* 1990;155:549–553.
10. De Smet AA, Norris MA, Yandow DR, Quintana FA, Graf BK, Keene JS. MR diagnosis of meniscal tears of the knee: importance of high signal in the meniscus that extends to the surface. *AJR* 1993;161:101–107.
11. Dunham WK, Marcus NW, Enneking WF, Haun C. Developmental defects of the distal femoral metaphysis. *J Bone Joint Surg* 1980;62A:801–806.
12. Fitch RD. Tibial tubercle avulsions. *J Pediatr Orthop* 1986;6:186–192.
13. Freiberg RH, Kotzen LM. Fracture of the medial margin of the patella, a finding diagnostic of lateral dislocation. *Radiology* 1967;88:902.
14. Green NE. Tibia valga caused by asymmetrical overgrowth following a nondisplaced fracture of the proximal tibial metaphysis. *J Pediatr Orthop* 1983;3:235–237.
15. Grogan DP, Carey TP, Leffers D, Ogden JA. Avulsion fractures of the patella. *J Pediatr Orthop* 1990;10:721–730.
16. Gronkvist H, Hirsch G, Johansson L. Fracture of the anterior tibial spine in children. *J Pediatr Orthop* 1984;4:465–468.
17. Hall F. Radiographic diagnosis and accuracy in knee joint effusions. *Radiology* 1975;115:49–54.
18. Hayden CK Jr, Swischuk LE. Para-articular soft tissue changes in infants and trauma of the lower extremity in children. *AJR* 1980;134:307–311.
19. Helms CA, Laorr A, Cannon WD Jr. The absent bow tie sign in bucket-handle tears of the menisci in the knee. *AJR* 1998;170:57–61.
20. Iwaya T, Takatori Y. Lateral longitudinal stress fracture of the patella: Report of three cases. *J Pediatr Orthop* 1985;5:73–75.
21. Jordan SE, Alonson JE, Cook FF. The etiology of valgus angulation after metaphyseal fractures of the tibia in children. *J Pediatr Orthop* 1987;7:450–457.
22. Kirchner SG, Pavlov H, Heller RM, Kay JJ. Periosteal chondromas of the anterior tibial tubercle: Two cases. *AJR* 1978;131:1088–1089.
23. Lancourt JE, Cristini JA. Patella alta and patella infera: Their etiologic role in patellar dislocation, chondromalacia and apophysitis of the tibial tubercle. *J Bone Joint Surg* 1975;57:1112–1115.
24. Lanning P, Heikkinen E. Ultrasonic features of the Osgood-Schlatter lesions. *J Pediatr Orthop* 1991;11:538–540.

25. Lynch MC, Walsh HPJ. Tibia recurvatum as a complication of Osgood-Schlatter's disease: A report of two cases. *J Pediatr Orthop* 1991;11:543–544.

26. Malghem J, Maldague B. Depth insufficiency of the proximal trochlear groove on lateral radiographs of the knee: Relation to patellar dislocation. *Radiology* 1989;170:507–510.

27. McCauley TR, Kier R, Lynch KJ, Jokl P. Chondromalacia patallae: Diagnosis with MR imaging. *AJR* 1992;158:101–105.

28. Neitosvaara Y, Aalto K, Kallio PE. Acute patellar dislocation in children: Incidence and associated osteochondral fractures. *J Pediatr Orthop* 1994;4:513–517.

29. Nelson DW, DiPaola J, Colville M, Schmidgall J. Osteochondritis dissecans of the talus and knee: Prospective comparison of MR and arthroscopic classifications. *J Comp Assist Tomogr* 1990;14:804–808.

30. Ogden JA, McCarthy SM, Jokl P. The painful bipartite patella. *J Pediatr Orthop* 1982;2:263–269.

31. Resnick D, Greenway G. Distal femoral cortical defects, irregularities and excavations: A critical review of the literature with the addition of histologic and paleopathologic data. *Radiology* 1982;143:345–354.

32. Robert M, Khouri N, Carlioz H, Alain JL. Fractures of the proximal tibial metaphysis in children: Review of a series of 25 cases. *J Pediatr Orthop* 1987;7:444–449.

33. Rogers LF, Jones S, Davis AR, Dietz G. "Clipping injury" fracture of the epiphysis in the adolescent football player: An occult lesion of the knee. *AJR* 1974;121:69–78.

34. Rosenberg ZS, Kawelblum M, Cheung YY, Beltran J, Lehman WB, Grant AD. Osgood-Schlatter lesion: fracture or tendonitis: Scintigraphic, CT, and MR imaging features. *Radiology* 1992;185:853–858.

35. Safran MR, Mcdonough P, Seeger L, Gold R, Oppenheim WL. Dorsal defect of the patella. *J Pediatr Orthop* 1994;14:603–607.

36. Rosewarne MD. Synovial rupture of the knee joint: Confusion with deep vein thrombosis. *Clin Radiol* 1978;29:417–420.

37. Sinding-Larson MF. A hitherto unknown affliction of the patella in children. *Acta Radiol [Diagn.] (Stockh.)* 1921;1:171–173.

38. Swischuk LE, John SD, Tschoepe EJ. Upper tibial hyperextension fractures in infants: Another occult toddler's fracture. *Pediatr Radiol* 1999;29:6–9.

39. Tschoepe EJ, John SD, Swischuk LE. Tibial fractures in infants and children: Emphasis on subtle injuries. *Emerg Radiol* 1998;5:245–252.

40. Vahey TN, Hunt JE, Shelbourne KD. Anterior translocation of the tibia at MR imaging: A secondary sign of anterior cruciate ligament tear. *Radiology* 1993;187:817–819.

41. Zionts LE, Harcke T, Brooks KM, MacEwen GD. Posttraumatic tibia valga: A case demonstrating asymmetric activity at the proximal growth plate on technetium bone scan. *J Pediatr Orthop* 1987;7:458–462.

Lower Leg (Midshafts of the Tibia and Fibula)

Injuries of the Lower Leg

Overt fractures of the midshafts of the tibia and fibula are not difficult to recognize. It should be noted, however, that such fractures show a distinct tendency to occur in the tibia but not in the fibula. In some of these cases, even though this might be one's initial impression, with closer perusal of the films often it is noted that the fibula actually is bent (Fig. 4.214). In other words, the overt fracture of the tibia is accompanied by an associated acute, bending, plastic fracture of the fibula, which occurs at the same level as the transverse fracture of the tibia. These plastic bending fractures of the fibula probably are more common than generally appreciated (6), and in some cases the fibula may be bent outward rather than inward (Fig. 4.214C).

In young infants, a very common fracture of the tibia is the so-called toddler's fracture (1). This fracture characteristically is a spiral, hairline fracture and often is invisible, or

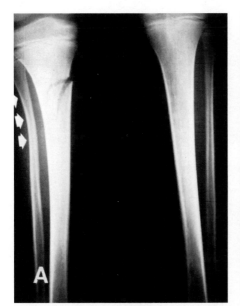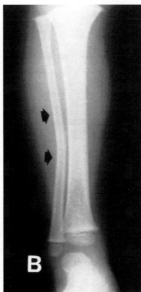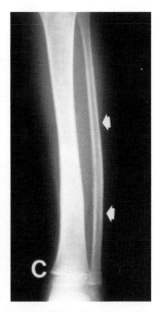

FIGURE 4.214. *Bending fractures of the fibula.* **(A)** Note the clear-cut fracture of the tibia, but also note localized bending of the upper fibula (*arrows*). (Courtesy of J. Bjelland, M.D.) **(B)** Marked inward bending of the right fibula (*arrows*). This is the common direction of bending. **(C)** Unusual outward bending of the fibula (*arrows*).

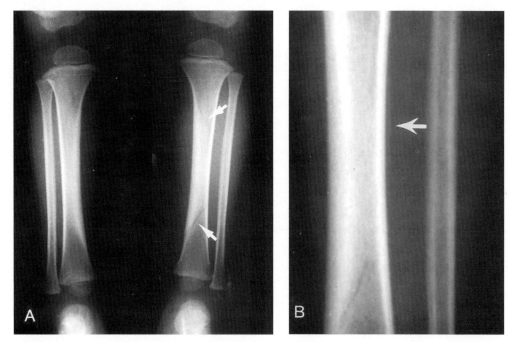

FIGURE 4.215. *Spiral fracture of the tibia (toddler's fracture).* **(A)** Note that the calf on the left is a little bigger and slightly more opaque than that on the right. This is because of edema. Then note the two limbs of the typical spiral fracture of the tibia (*arrows*). **(B)** Follow-up film 2 weeks later again demonstrates the fracture line, but this time early periosteal new bone is visible (*arrow*).

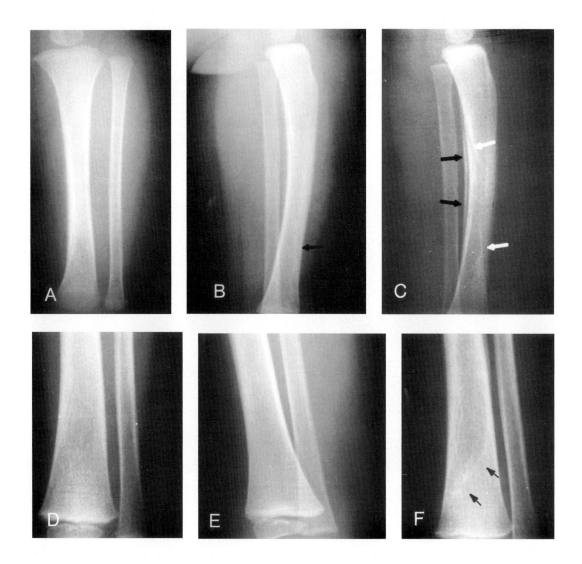

nearly invisible, on initial roentgenograms. It behaves almost like a stress fracture, and even in those cases in which it is visible, it often appears clearer on one view than the other (Fig. 4.215). In other cases, soft-tissue swelling of the muscles around the tibia can bring attention to the fracture, but it cannot be overstressed that many of these children present with normal or very subtle findings (Fig. 4.216). Because of this, the situation can become quite puzzling. Couple this with the fact that no fracture is visible roentgenographically, and one has a definite diagnostic puzzle (i.e., these children do not walk, or if they walk they do so with a limp, and yet on physical examination the findings are relatively negative). ***If torque stress is placed on the tibia (one hand on the knee and one on the ankle, twisting in opposite directions), however, pain is evoked and the diagnosis clarified.***

A somewhat similar fracture has been recorded in ballet dancers. These individuals, in general, are prone to stress injuries of the lower extremities (5). Of course, as with any stress fracture, if these fractures are identified in their advanced healing phase, profound periosteal new-bone deposition may erroneously suggest the presence of a bone tumor. Stress fractures of the fibula also occur (3), and all of these fractures are readily discovered with bone scintigraphy.

Another unusual fracture of the tibia is a longitudinal fracture (4). The findings in these cases can mimic those of early

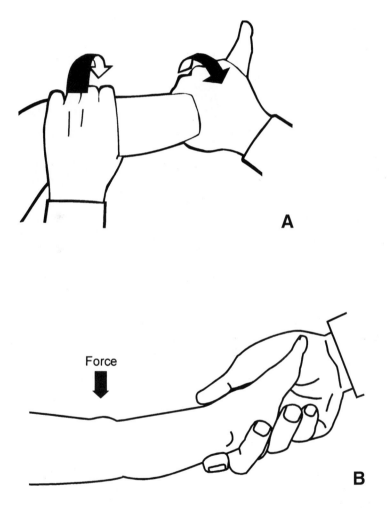

Force

A

B

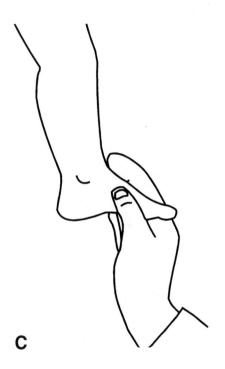

C

FIGURE 4.217. *Toddler's fracture expanded: physical examination.* **(A)** To detect the typical spiral toddler's fracture, twist the tibia in opposite directions. **(B)** To detect the hyperextension-type upper tibial toddler's fracture, put hyperextension forces on the knee. **(C)** To detect cuboid and first metatarsal fractures, apply focal pressure to these bones. (Adapted from John SD, Moorthy CS, Swischuk LE. Expanding the concept of the toddler's fracture. *RadioGraphics* 1997;17:367–376, with permission.)

FIGURE 4.216. *Occult toddler's fractures.* **(A)** In this infant, a little soft tissue swelling is seen, but no fracture can be noted. **(B)** On lateral view there is subtle suggestion of a fracture line (*arrow*). **(C)** Two weeks later, periosteal new bone is seen along the posterior aspect (*black arrows*). The fracture line still is difficult to visualize (*white arrows*). **(D)** Another patient in whom no fracture is seen on the frontal view. **(E)** On the lateral view no fracture is seen. **(F)** Two weeks later, there is evidence of a healing fracture with a fine, white sclerotic fracture line (*black arrows*) now visible.

malignancy such as Ewing's sarcoma. This fracture is similar to the classic toddler's fracture of infancy, but it occurs in older children. As with the toddler's fracture in infancy, however, if healing occurs, malignancy can be mimicked.

Toddler's Fracture Expanded

The original toddler's fracture, as described by Dunbar et al. in 1964 (1), still is the most common toddler's fracture seen in infants. Other fractures presenting in the same age group leading to unexplained limping, however, also can be encountered. These include subtle buckle and epiphyseal fractures in the distal tibia and fibula, buckle

fractures of the base of the first metatarsal, compression fractures of the cuboid bone, and hyperextension-induced fractures of the upper tibia (7,8). The fractures of the first metatarsal and cuboid bone often are referred to as "bunkbed fractures." Any of these injuries can lead to limping in an infant, in whom the fracture may go undetected because one is not familiar with its site and appearance (2). If one knows where to look for these fractures radiographically, however, and how to demonstrate them clinically (Fig. 4.217), one can detect most of them. This is especially true if comparative films are obtained. These fractures are illustrated throughout various places in this chapter, but their findings are summarized in Figs. 4.218 and 4.219.

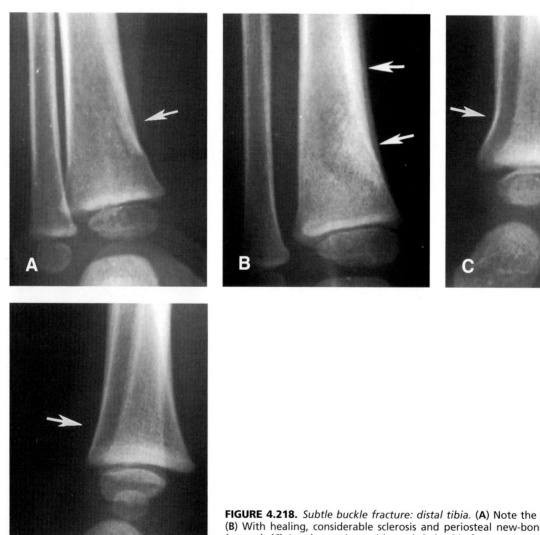

FIGURE 4.218. *Subtle buckle fracture: distal tibia.* (**A**) Note the subtle buckle (*arrow*). (**B**) With healing, considerable sclerosis and periosteal new-bone deposition are seen (*arrows*). (**C**) Another patient with a subtle buckle fracture (*arrow*). (**D**) Normal side for comparison. Note the smooth cortex (*arrow*). (Adapted from Tschoepe EJ, John SD, Swischuk LE. Tibial fractures in infants and children: Emphasis on subtle injuries. *Emerg Radiol* 1998;5:245–252, with permission.)

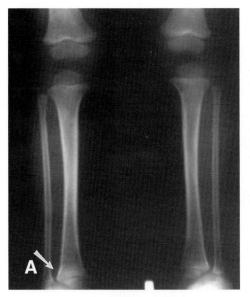
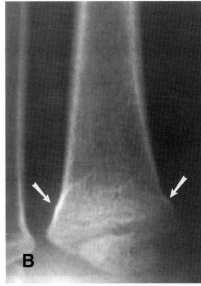
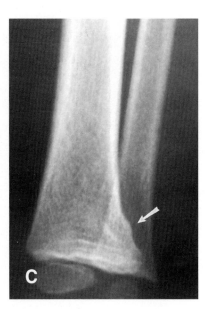

FIGURE 4.219. *Subtle distal tibial buckle fracture.* **(A)** The fracture is difficult to see and barely included on the film (*arrow*). The lower extremities were examined *in toto* because a fracture of the ankle was not suspected clinically. **(B)** Focused view demonstrates the fracture (*arrows*) to better advantage. **(C)** Lateral view confirms the buckle through the distal tibia (*arrow*).

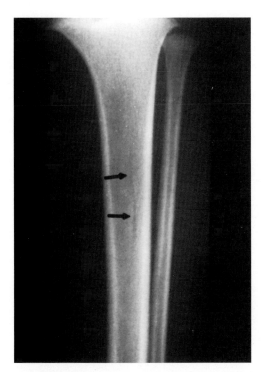

FIGURE 4.220. *Tibial vascular groove: pseudofracture.* Note the vascular groove (*arrows*) in the upper tibia. This vascular groove is quite common and should not be misinterpreted as a spiral fracture of the tibia.

Normal Findings Causing Problems

About the only normal finding in the midshaft of the tibia or fibula that can be confused with an underlying lesion is a normal vascular groove (Fig. 4.220). These vascular grooves appear no different from those in other long bones, but in the tibia they can be misinterpreted as a spiral toddler's type fracture.

REFERENCES

1. Dunbar JS, Owen HF, Nogrady MB, McLeese R. Obscure tibial fracture of infants: The toddler's fracture. *Can J Assoc Radiol* 1964; 15:136–144.
2. John SD, Moorthy CS, Swischuk LE. Expanding the concept of the toddler's fracture. *RadioGraphics* 1997;17:367–376.
3. Kozlowski K, Azouz M, Hoff D. Stress fracture of the fibula in the first decade of life: Report of eight cases. *Pediatr Radiol* 1991; 21:381–383.
4. Miniaci A, McLaren AC, Haddad RG. Longitudinal stress fracture of the tibia: Case report. *Can J Assoc Radiol* 1988;39: 221–223.
5. Nussbaum AR, Treves ST, Micheli L. Bone stress lesions in ballet dancers: Scintigraphic assessment. *AJR* 1988;150:851–855.
6. Stenstrom R, Gripenberg L, Bergius AR. Traumatic bowing of forearm and lower leg in children. *Acta Radiol* 1978;19:243–249.
7. Swischuk LE, John SD, Tschoepe EJ. Upper tibial hyperextension fractures in infants: Another occult toddler's fracture. *Pediatr Radiol* 1999;29:6–9.
8. Tschoepe EJ, John SD, Swischuk LE. Tibial fractures in infants and children: Emphasis on subtle injuries. *Emerg Radiol* 1998; 245–252.

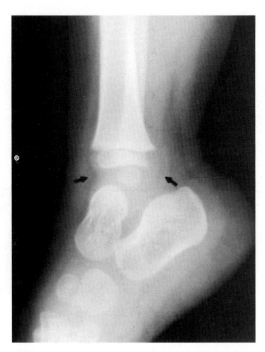

FIGURE 4.221. *Normal soft tissues and fat pads of the ankle.* The pre-Achilles fat pad is clearly visible but not utilized for joint-fluid detection. The anterior (*anterior arrow*) and posterior (*posterior arrow*) fat pads are readily visualized and, as seen, normally are tucked tightly against the joint capsule. With joint fluid, they are displaced outwardly (see Fig. 4.222).

Ankle

Normal Soft Tissues and Fat Pads of the Ankle

In the infant and child, three fat pads around the ankle usually are visualized on lateral view. The largest is the pre-

Achilles fat pad, located just anterior to the Achilles tendon, but this fat pad is not utilized for the detection of joint fluid. Rather, the anterior and posterior fat pads lying against the joint capsule are the ones that are assessed for joint-fluid detection (Fig. 4.221). In the older child, the anterior fat pad may be comprised of two pads; it is the inner one that should be assessed. With soft-tissue edema, both the anterior and posterior fat pads are obliterated; with joint-fluid accumulations they are displaced outwardly (5).

Detecting Fluid in the Ankle Joint

In determining whether fluid is present in the ankle joint, it is best to study the lateral view (5,18). On frontal view, only soft-tissue swelling around the ankle is seen, but on lateral view outward displacement of the anterior or posterior fat pads is seen (Fig. 4.222). In older children, bulging of the capsule, in a more discrete fashion, leads to the "teardrop" sign (18) (Fig. 4.223). No joint space widening is seen, for the ligaments around the ankle joint are very sturdy and usually do not allow for much in the way of joint distraction.

Injuries of the Distal Tibia and Fibula

A variety of injuries can be sustained in the distal tibia and fibula, and most often these result from a combination of inversion, eversion, and rotational forces. In the young infant, cortical buckle (torus) fractures through the distal tibia and fibula are very common (Fig. 4.224). In the older child, however, the more common injury is some type of Salter–Harris epiphyseal–metaphyseal fracture. In the ankle, injuries of all Salter–Harris types, with the exception of the type V injury,

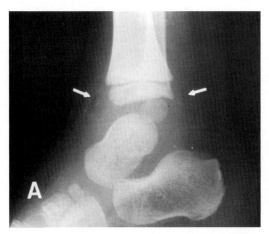
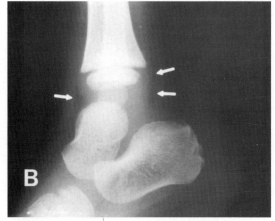

FIGURE 4.222. *Detecting fluid in the ankle joint.* **(A)** Note outward displacement of both the anterior and posterior fat pads (*arrows*). **(B)** Normal side for comparison. Note normal position of the fat pads (*arrows*).

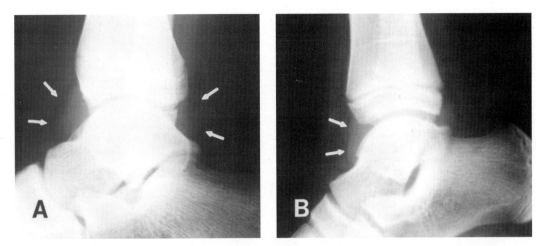

FIGURE 4.223. *Teardrop configuration of ankle fluid.* **(A)** Note typical teardrop sign anteriorly (*anterior arrows*). A similar configuration exists posteriorly (*posterior arrows*). **(B)** Another patient with a less pronounced teardrop sign anteriorly (*arrows*). Similar subtle findings are present posteriorly.

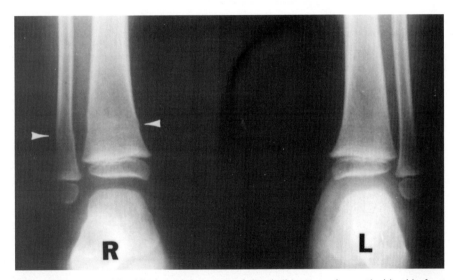

FIGURE 4.224. *Cortical buckle (torus) fractures of distal tibia.* Note the cortical buckle fracture along the inner aspect of the distal right tibia (*arrow*). A more subtle cortical buckle fracture is present on the opposite side of the tibia. Also note the fracture of the distal fibula at the same level (*arrow*).

are common. Salter–Harris type III and IV injuries often are associated with some degree of epiphyseal displacement and generally are not difficult to identify (Fig. 4.225), but if displacement of the epiphysis is not present, they may be just as difficult to identify as type I and II injuries. The key to detecting these more subtle fractures lies in comparing the width of the epiphyseal lines in the injured ankle to those on the normal side and in assessing the soft tissues for evidence of swelling (Fig. 4.226). The Salter–Harris type III injury is quite common in the distal tibia and often is missed on initial inspection. Oblique views may be required for its delineation. The reason for this is that the distal tibial epiphysis fuses earlier medially than it does laterally. Consequently, with an inversion injury of the ankle there is separation of the epiphysis laterally but not medially (Fig. 4.227A). These fractures, the equivalent of the Tillaux fracture (4), are best assessed with CT scans (Fig. 4.227). These are required to define the degree of fracture fragment displacement and to determine whether internal fixation is required. The usual maximum allowable limit of the diastatic fracture is 3 mm.

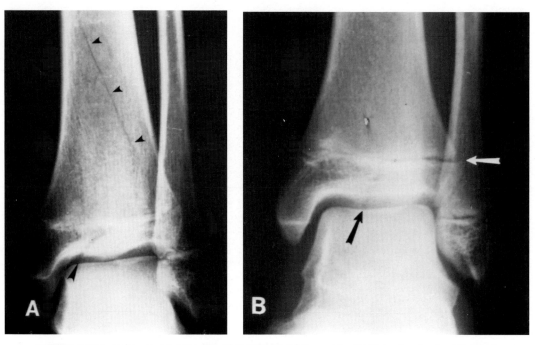

FIGURE 4.225. *Salter–Harris type III and IV injuries of the ankle.* (**A**) Note the fracture through the distal tibial epiphysis (*lower arrow*) and the fracture through the metaphysis (*upper arrows*). This is a Salter–Harris type IV injury. (**B**) Note the fracture through the distal tibial epiphysis (*lower arrow*). Also note slight separation of the lateral epiphyseal fragment from the metaphysis (*lateral arrow*). This is a Salter–Harris type III injury.

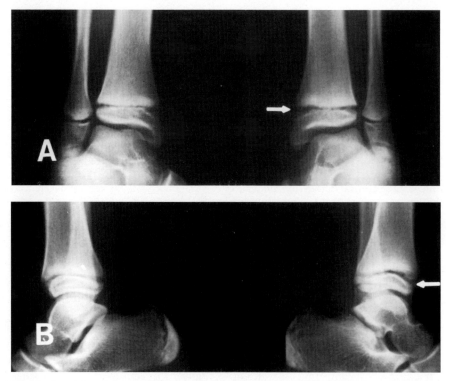

FIGURE 4.226. *Salter–Harris type I injury of the ankle.* (**A**) Note that the epiphyseal line through the distal tibia is wider on the left (*arrow*) than on the right. (**B**) Lateral view confirms widening of the epiphyseal line on the left (*arrow*). These findings are those of a Salter–Harris type I injury.

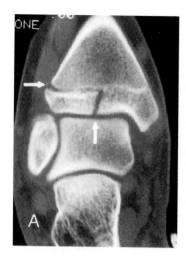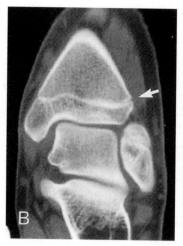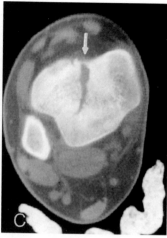

FIGURE 4.227. *Salter–Harris type III fracture of tibia: value of computed tomographic scanning.* **(A)** Coronal view demonstrates the fracture (*lower arrow*). Note that the epiphyseal line is widened laterally (*upper arrow*). Also note that the epiphyseal line through the medial aspect has closed. **(B)** On the normal side, note that, although medially the epiphyseal line is completely closed, it is still a little open on the lateral side (*arrow*). This leads to the common occurrence of a type III Salter–Harris fracture with an inversion injury. **(C)** Axial computed tomographic scan demonstrates the fracture through the epiphysis (*arrow*).

Inversion–rotation injuries of the ankle are very common, and although in most cases they result only in a sprained ankle, in other instances Salter–Harris injuries result. In adults, the Ottawa ankle rules can, if applied, significantly reduce the number of ankle injuries requiring radiographic examination (20). ***This also probably is true in children, but there is no uniform adherence to these rules.***

Specifically, one may see an epiphyseal–metaphyseal separation of the distal fibular epiphysis and an associated fracture through the medial malleolus of the tibial epiphysis (Fig. 4.228A). Less commonly, one may encounter only a small

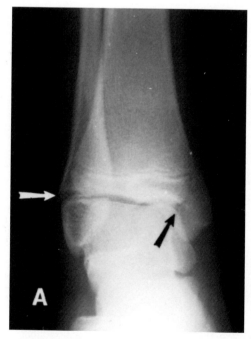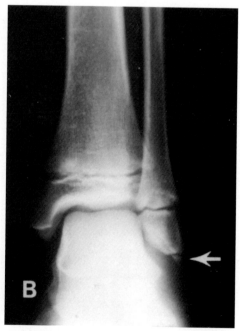

FIGURE 4.228. *Inversion injuries of the ankle.* **(A)** Bimalleolar fracture. First note the fracture through the medial malleolus (*black arrow*), and then note that the distal fibular epiphysis has been separated from the metaphysis (i.e., there is widening of the epiphyseal line and a small metaphyseal avulsion fracture [*white arrow*]). The fibular fracture is a Salter–Harris type II injury; the medial malleolar fracture is a type III injury. **(B)** Small avulsion fracture of the distal fibula. Note the small avulsed distal fibular bony fragment (*arrow*). *(continued on next page)*

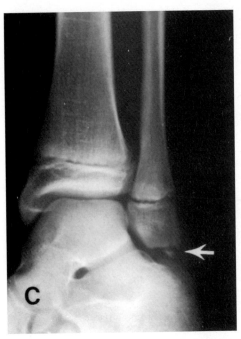

FIGURE 4.228. *(continued)* **(C)** Oblique view demonstrates the fragment *(arrow)* to better advantage. There is no epiphyseal–metaphyseal injury of either the tibia or fibula in this patient. The small avulsion fracture should be differentiated from the normal ossicle (os subfibulare) commonly occurring in this area (see Fig. 4.243B).

sliverlike cortical avulsion of the distal fibular metaphysis or epiphysis (Fig. 4.228B). These latter fractures must be differentiated from normal accessory ossicles occurring in this area (see Fig. 4.242). In all of these injuries, there is a certain degree of soft tissue swelling over the lateral malleolus. Obviously, if an underlying fracture is visualized, the soft tissue thickening is of lesser consequence, but many times there is nothing more to see than soft tissue thickening. In such cases, I have found it useful to assume that an occult Salter–Harris epiphyseal–metaphyseal injury has been sustained if soft tissue thickening is greater than 1 cm.

With eversion injuries, the ankle mortise often is seriously disturbed, and a wide range of relatively severe injuries can be encountered (Fig. 4.229). So-called posterior malleolar fractures actually are Salter–Harris type II epiphyseal–metaphyseal fractures (Fig. 4.230), and many times the fracture is visible only on lateral view. If these fractures occur with fractures through the medial and lateral malleoli, the term **trimalleolar fracture** is applied. These posterior malleolar fractures often are associated with a type III epiphyseal–metaphyseal fracture as part of a Tillaux fracture (4).

Injuries of the Tarsal Bones

Fractures and dislocations of the tarsal bones are generally less common in childhood than in adulthood. This is especially true in the infant and young child. In the older child, one can encounter fractures of bones such as the tarsal navicular and talus (Figs. 4.231 and 4.232). With

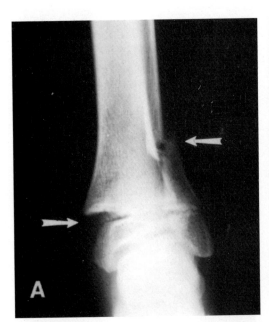
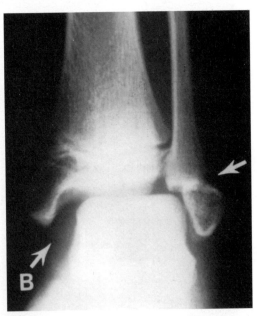

FIGURE 4.229. *Eversion injuries of the ankle.* **(A)** Note the displaced fracture of the distal fibula *(upper arrow)* and the displaced Salter–Harris type II epiphyseal–metaphyseal fracture of the distal tibia *(lower arrow).* The ankle mortise is not disturbed. **(B)** Note the displaced Salter–Harris type I injury of the distal fibula *(lateral arrow)* and the widely opened joint space medially *(medial arrow).* The ankle is dislocated and the ankle mortise grossly disturbed. Note, however, that there is no epiphyseal–metaphyseal fracture of the distal tibia.

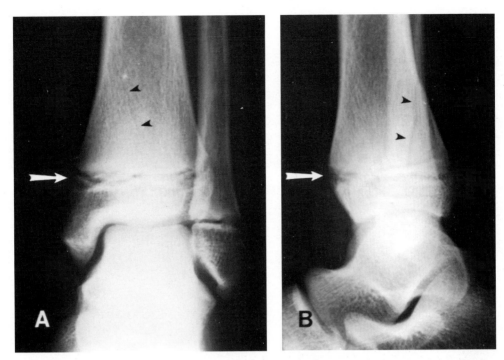

FIGURE 4.230. *Posterior malleolar fracture.* **(A)** On frontal view, the fracture line is just barely visible (*upper arrows*). Note, however, that the epiphyseal line is a little wider medially (*lower arrow*) than laterally. **(B)** Lateral view demonstrating the posterior malleolar metaphyseal fracture with greater clarity (*upper arrows*). The epiphyseal line is slightly wider than normal anteriorly (*lower arrow*), and overall the findings constitute a Salter–Harris type II epiphyseal–metaphyseal injury.

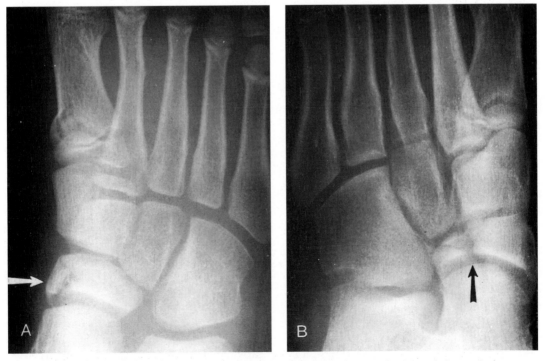

FIGURE 4.231. *Tarsal navicular fractures.* **(A)** Note the compression fracture of the navicular (*arrow*). An impaction–compression fracture of the base of the first metatarsal also is present, and there is an angulated cortical fracture through the midshaft of the second metatarsal. **(B)** Another patient with a compression fracture of the navicular (*arrow*).

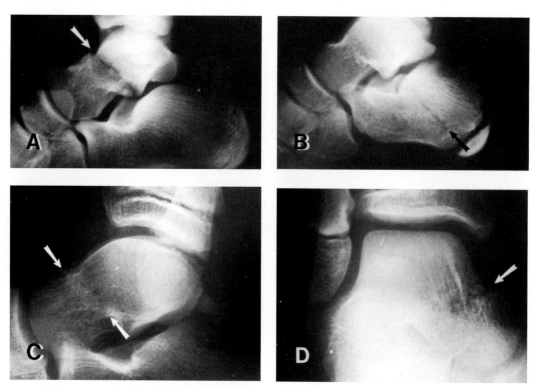

FIGURE 4.232. *Talar and calcaneal fractures.* **(A)** Note the clear-cut talar fracture (*arrow*). **(B)** Linear fracture through the calcaneus (*arrow*). **(C)** Subtle fracture through the neck of the talus (*arrows*). **(D)** Oblique view demonstrates offsetting of the fracture (*arrow*).

fractures through the talus, dislocation of one of the fragments can occur and, in addition, subsequent aseptic necrosis is a known complication. Rotation of the anterior fragment is common and results in a distorted talocalcaneal joint. These fractures of the talus more frequently occur in adolescents and adults and may be difficult to detect. In such cases MR imaging (19) has proven useful.

Cuboid fractures are more common than generally realized and tend to occur in younger children and infants. They can be considered as part of the expanded toddler's fracture concept (1,2,9), for these patients frequently present with limping, the cause of which remains unclear until the fracture is detected. As with all toddler's fractures, diagnosis is a matter of knowing ***what to look for and where to look for it.***

With cuboid fractures, the most significant finding is a transverse area of sclerosis in the involved cuboid bone secondary to impaction and healing. These fractures usually are detected a few days after they occur, but if one is careful in examining the cuboid bone for increased sclerosis, one is likely to detect the injury (Fig. 4.233). Of course, nuclear scintigraphy also can detect these injuries (Fig. 4.233C).

Fractures of the calcaneus usually result from patients jumping or falling on their heels, and because one often is not thinking of the possibility of such fractures, they may remain occult (8,11,15,17). Nuclear scintigraphy is helpful in detecting some of these fractures, but in other cases a clear-cut fracture line may be visible (Fig. 4.232B). Otherwise, one must look for indirect findings such as soft tissue swelling, loss of Boehler's angle, decreased height of the calcaneus, or increased density (impaction) of the calcaneus (Fig. 4.234). In addition, if a calcaneal fracture is suspected, it is mandatory that tangential views of the calcaneus be obtained. On this view, the most productive in calcaneal injuries, compression fractures almost always are visualized with clarity, and previously unsuspected fractures also may become visible (Fig. 4.234C). Finally, with calcaneal fractures, it is most important that the normally sclerotic and irregular calcaneal apophysis not be misinterpreted as such a fracture (see Fig. 4.243A).

Small avulsion fractures of the various tarsal bones and other bones around the ankle also can be encountered. These are more common than generally appreciated, and although they may be visible on standard views, very often oblique views first bring these fractures to light (Fig. 4.235). Indeed, in some cases visualization of these fractures is

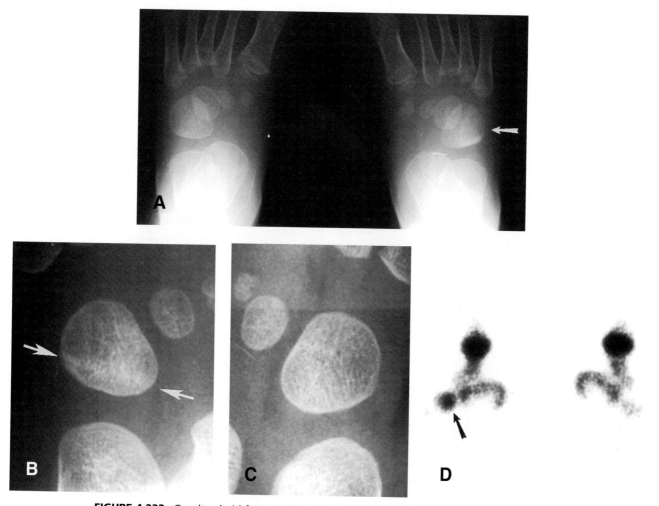

FIGURE 4.233. *Occult cuboid fracture.* **(A)** Note slight sclerosis of the left cuboid bone (*arrow*). **(B)** In this patient a line of sclerosis (*arrows*) is seen in the cuboid bone. **(C)** Normal side for comparison. **(D)** Bone scan demonstrates increased activity in the involved cuboid bone (*arrow*). (Courtesy of Joanna Seibert, M.D.).

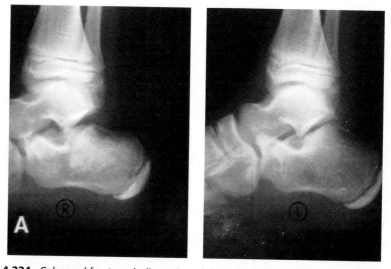

FIGURE 4.234. *Calcaneal fracture: indirect signs.* **(A)** On the right, (R) note that the calcaneus has lost considerable height, and that there is an area of central sclerosis due to impaction. The left (L) calcaneus appears normal.

(continued on next page)

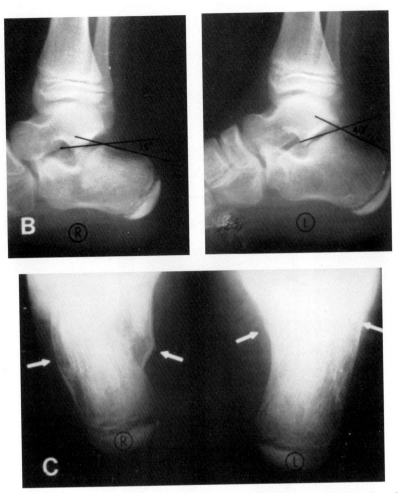

FIGURE 4.234. *(continued)* **(B)** Boehler's angle on the right has been markedly reduced; on the left it is within normal range. Normally, it measures between 30 and 40 degrees. Anything smaller than 28 degrees is considered abnormal. **(C)** Tangential view of the calcanei demonstrates the previously documented compression fracture of the calcaneus on the right (*arrows*) but in addition detects the presence of a previously unsuspected, noncompressed, subtle calcaneal fracture on the left (*arrows*).

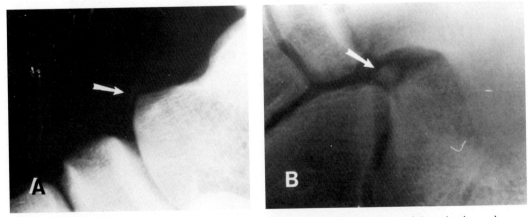

FIGURE 4.235. *Avulsion fractures around the ankle.* **(A)** Note small avulsion of the talus (*arrow*). This is a common fracture. **(B)** Small corner avulsion of the calcaneus (*arrow*), seen only on oblique view.

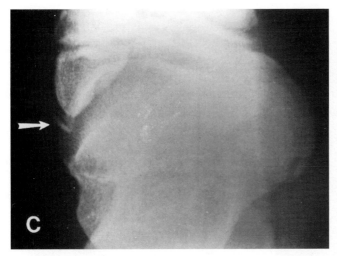
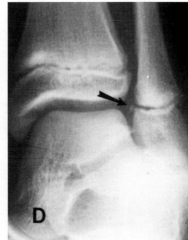

FIGURE 4.235. *(continued)* **(C)** Avulsion fracture of the distal fibular epiphysis (*arrow*). **(D)** Another avulsion fracture of the fibula (*arrow*), seen only on oblique view.

strictly fortuitous, and all of them must be differentiated from normal accessory ossification centers of the various bones around the ankle (see Fig. 4.243).

Sprained Ankle

Unlike the sprained wrist, a sprained ankle most often turns out to be nothing more than a sprained ankle. Of course, this is not to say that fractures never occur, but only to point out that the high incidence of underlying fracture that accompanies wrist sprains is not present with ankle sprains. Another important aspect of a sprained ankle resulting from an inversion injury is that very often there is an associated fracture of the base of the fifth metatarsal. The peroneus brevis muscle inserts into this bone, and with inversion injuries, an avulsion fracture frequently occurs. This fracture usually is overlooked clinically but almost always is detectable roentgenographically (see Fig. 4.255).

Achilles Tendonitis

Children very commonly develop acute or chronic pain over the insertion of the Achilles tendon into the calcaneus. Actually the condition represents bursitis or tenosynovitis and usually is considered to be the result of subclinical tendon injury in the active child (6,10,12). It frequently is associated with plantar fasciitis (3), because the plantar fascia and Achilles tendon are a continuous tendonomembranous structure wrapping around the heel.

Some children are more prone to develop this problem than others, and frequently it is recurrent. It is similar to Osgood–Schlatter disease of the knee, and conservative measures are in order. There are no roentgenographic findings except for localized swelling over the area. This usually manifests in thickening of the Achilles tendon and plantar fascia along with obliteration of the pre-Achilles fat pad (Fig. 4.236). Unless one appreciates this injury when a patient presents with heel pain there is a great tendency to attribute the problem to the nearby, normally sclerotic and irregular-appearing calcaneal apophysis. Such a diagnosis should be avoided, because this is the expected appearance of the normal calcaneus (see Fig. 4.244) and never is involved in Achilles tendonitis. Frequently, the findings are described as those of Sever's disease, indicating aseptic necrosis of the calcaneal apophysis. The problem is not aseptic necrosis, however, and it is doubtful that aseptic necrosis of the calcaneal apophysis exists.

Ultrasonography and MR imaging can be used to detect plantar fasciitis and Achilles tendonitis (3,6) but usually are superfluous. Plain films should suffice.

Osteochondritis Dissecans of the Tarsal Bones

Osteochondritis dissecans of the tarsal bones is not particularly common in childhood but does occur and most often involves the talus (7). The findings are similar to those of osteochondritis dissecans elsewhere in that there is a bony defect with slight peripheral sclerosis (Fig. 4.237). An intraarticular piece of bone may or may not be visualized. It might be noted, however, that as with osteochondritis dis-

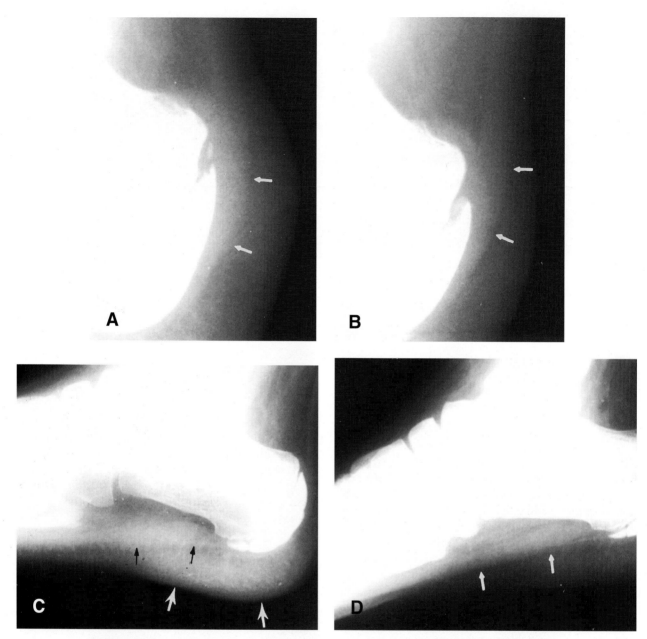

FIGURE 4.236. *Tendonitis and fasciitis.* (**A**) *Achilles tendonitis.* Note swelling over the posterior aspect of the heel and thickening of the insertion of the Achilles tendon into the calcaneus (*arrows*). The edge of the tendon is indistinct. (**B**) Normal side demonstrates no swelling and a distinct edge to the tendon (*arrows*) as it inserts into the calcaneus. (**C**) *Plantar fasciitis.* Note extensive swelling of the heel (*white arrows*) and thickening and indistinctness of the plantar fascia (*black arrows*). (**D**) *Normal side for comparison.* Note the normal appearance of the plantar fascia (*arrows*). Also note that no swelling is present.

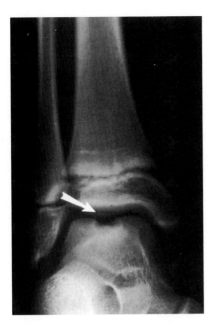

FIGURE 4.237. *Osteochondritis dissecans of talus.* Note the characteristic defect (*arrow*) in the articular surface of the talus.

secans elsewhere, the lesion may or may not be symptomatic at the time of detection. MR imaging can be utilized to detect the degree of fragment displacement.

Aseptic Necrosis of the Tarsal Bones

Aseptic necrosis of the various tarsal bones can be a cause of foot pain, and in this regard the tarsal navicular is the most commonly involved bone. ***Köhler's disease*** is the term applied to aseptic necrosis of the navicular. The roentgenographic features consist of irregularity and sclerosis of the bone (Fig. 4.238A and B). In addition, one can utilize the soft tissues (21) for detection of less-than-classic Köhler's disease. The soft tissues over the aseptically necrotic bone are edematous (Fig. 4.238C), whereas if normal irregular ossification mimics Köhler's disease, the soft tissues are normal (Fig. 4.238D).

In Köhler's disease, it should be appreciated that the tarsal navicular, along with other tarsal bones, can demonstrate normal irregular ossification. These findings should not be misinterpreted as those of Köhler's disease (see Fig.

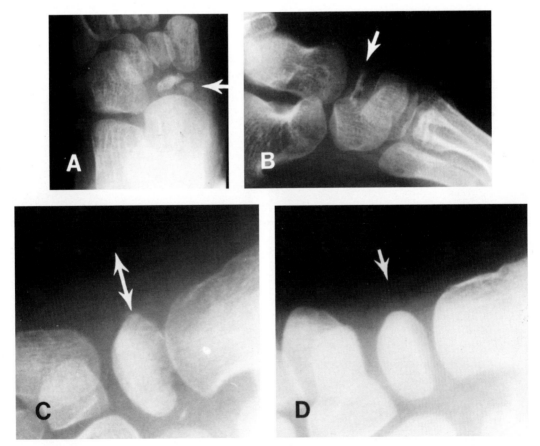

FIGURE 4.238. *Köhler's disease: tarsal navicular.* **(A)** Note the small, irregular, fragmented navicular bone (*arrow*). **(B)** Lateral view showing similar fragmentation. **(C)** In this case the navicular bone is a little sclerotic, but note mostly that the soft tissues over the bone are thickened because of edema (*arrows*). **(D)** *Normal side for comparison.* Note the normal appearance of the navicular bone and lack of swelling of the soft tissues.

4.246), and once again absence of overlying soft tissue swelling should aid in proper diagnosis.

Septic Arthritis, Osteomyelitis, and Cellulitis

Septic arthritis of the ankle manifests primarily in joint-space distension, causing outward displacement of the fat pads (Fig. 4.239). Cellulitis around the ankle manifests primarily in edema of the soft tissues and obliteration of the various fat pads. The fat pads are not displaced outwardly unless there is pus in the joint (i.e., septic arthritis). With osteomyelitis of the distal tibia and fibula, similar deep soft tissue swelling and obliteration of fat–muscle interfaces occur, but no joint-space distension is seen. Of course, if septic arthritis accompanies the problem, fluid is present in the joint.

Unfortunately, the deep soft tissue changes of osteomyelitis around the ankle are not particularly different from those seen with cellulitis. To be sure, in the ankle, differentiation of superficial from deep edema is more difficult than around the other large joints of the body. Whatever the cause of edema, however, the anterior and posterior fat pads remain in normal position unless joint fluid (pus) is present (Fig. 4.240).

Eventually, with osteomyelitis, bone destruction is seen (Fig. 4.241A and B), but the disease may be present for some time before this becomes evident. This is especially true of the tarsal bones, and consequently, bone scans are indispensable in looking for early osteomyelitis in and around the ankle (Fig. 4.241C and D). In this regard calcaneal osteomyelitis can be very subtle in terms of radiographic findings (14). Often it is the result of puncture wounds, and in such cases, peripheral cortical erosion and demineralization of the calcaneus is seen. This can occur in the calcaneus proper or in the calcaneal apophysis, but in either case the findings are subtle and require close scrutiny of the films (Fig. 4.241E and F). Of courst, once again nuclear scintigraphy can be very helpful.

Normal Variations Causing Problems

Numerous accessory ossicles occur in the ankle, and to illustrate all of them would be excessive. The most common are those occurring at the distal ends of the lateral and medial malleoli and the posterior aspect of the talus (Fig. 4.242). However, many more commonly occur in the ankle and a diagrammatic representation of these accessory ossicles is

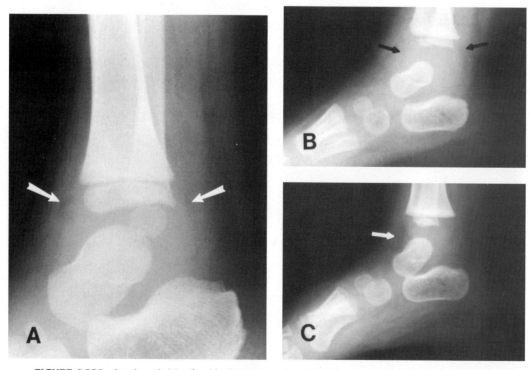

FIGURE 4.239. *Septic arthritis of ankle.* **(A)** Note outward displacement of the anterior and posterior fat pads (*arrows*). **(B)** Another patient with just barely visible outwardly displaced fat pads (*arrows*). The reason for poor visualization of the fat pads is that there is marked associated edema of the soft tissues. Note also that the pre-Achilles fat pad, behind the posterior fat pad, is outwardly displaced and curved. **(C)** *Normal side for comparison.* Note especially the normal anterior fat pad (*arrow*).

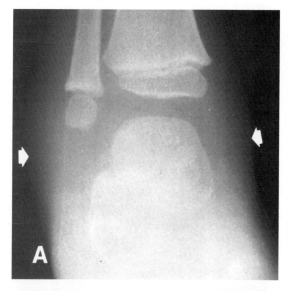
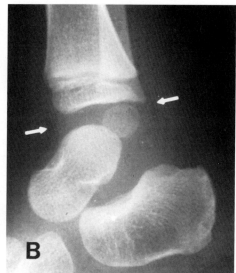
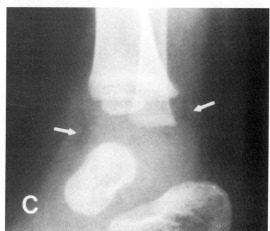

FIGURE 4.240. *Deep edema of the soft tissues of the ankle.* (**A**) Note marked swelling of the ankle (*arrows*). (**B**) Lateral view, however, demonstrates normal position of the anterior and posterior fat pads (*arrows*). This excludes fluid in the joint and suggests that the findings are caused by soft-tissue edema alone. (**C**) Another patient with edema around the ankle and persistent visualization of the anterior and posterior fat pads in their normal location (*arrows*). It is important in these cases to note that the fat pads are in normal position. If they were outwardly displaced, fluid (pus) in the joints should be suspected.

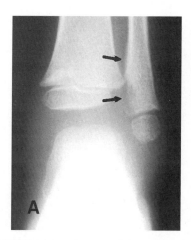
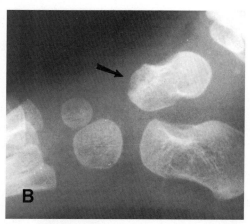

FIGURE 4.241. *Osteomyelitis around the ankle.* (**A**) Note bony destruction and periosteal new-bone reaction in the distal fibula (*arrows*). (**B**) Another patient with a destructive lesion (*arrow*) with some reactive sclerosis in the talus. *(continued on next page)*

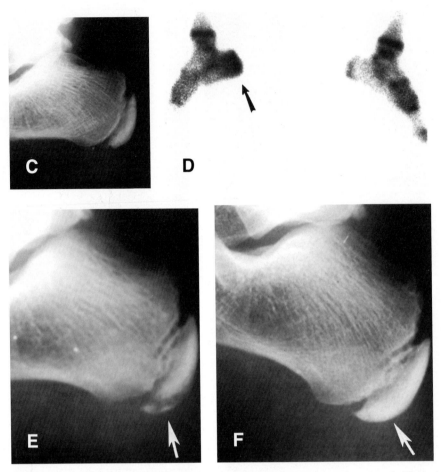

FIGURE 4.241. *(continued)* **(C)** *Patient with heel pain.* The calcaneus appears normal. **(D)** Nuclear scintigraphy demonstrates markedly increased activity in the involved calcaneus (*arrow*). This patient had osteomyelitis. **(E)** *Another patient with heel pain after a puncture wound.* Note irregularity and destruction of the inferior aspect of the calcaneal apophysis (*arrow*). **(F)** *Normal side for comparison.* The calcaneal apophysis is smooth and sclerotic (*arrow*).

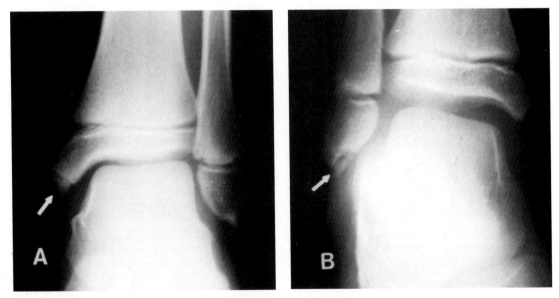

FIGURE 4.242. *Common accessory ossicles about the ankle.* **(A)** Accessory ossicle (os subtibiale) of medial malleolus (*arrow*). **(B)** Accessory ossicle (os subfibulare) of the distal fibular epiphysis (*arrow*).

presented in Fig. 4.243. It is most important not to misinterpret these secondary ossification centers and accessory ossicles as avulsion fractures, even though avulsion of the secondary centers themselves can occur (13).

The normal, sclerotic, irregular calcaneal apophysis (16) is notoriously misinterpreted as resulting from aseptic necrosis of the calcaneus. ***Indeed, its normal appearance is often so frightening that is it almost impossible not to assign some type of pathologic condition to the bone*** (Fig. 4.244A). ***This is especially true in cases of Achilles tendonitis.*** Another problem with the calcaneal apophysis is that with certain degrees of obliquity its fragmented appearance can suggest a calcaneal fracture (Fig. 4.244B).

Another normal finding frequently misinterpreted for abnormality is the apparently offset distal fibular epiphysis on oblique views of the ankle (Fig. 4.245). This is a normal finding on this view. In addition, the distal tibial epiphyseal–metaphyseal junction tends to be very irregular in normal children and can suggest a fracture (Fig. 4.245). Finally,

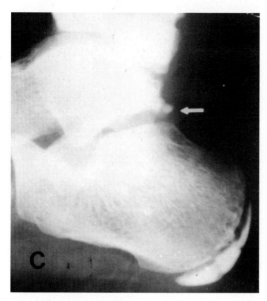

FIGURE 4.242. *(continued)* **(C)** Os trigonum *(arrow)* of talus.

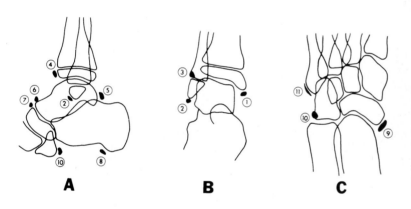

A   **B**   **C**

FIGURE 4.243. *Accessory ossicles about the ankle: diagrammatic representation.* **(A–C)** Accessory center of medial malleolus or os subtibiale *(1)*; accessory center of distal fibular epiphysis or os subfibulare *(2)*; accessory metaphyseal fibular ossicle *(3)*; os talotibiale *(4)*; os trigonum *(5)*; os supratalare *(6)*; os supranaviculare *(7)*; os subcalcis *(8)*; os subtibiale externum *(9)*; os peroneum *(10)*; and os vesalianum *(11)*.

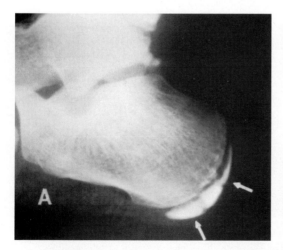
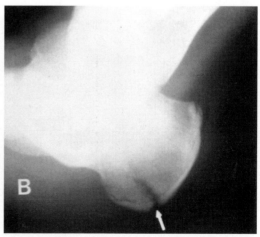

FIGURE 4.244. *Normal calcaneal apophysis.* **(A)** Note the typical sclerotic, irregular appearance of the fragmented calcaneal apophysis *(arrows)*. **(B)** With obliquity, the normal defects through the calcaneal apophysis can suggest a calcaneal fracture *(arrow)*.

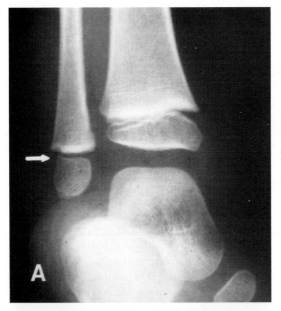

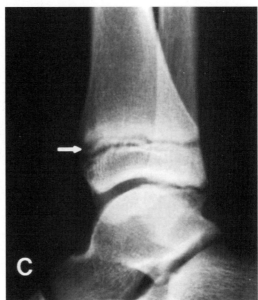

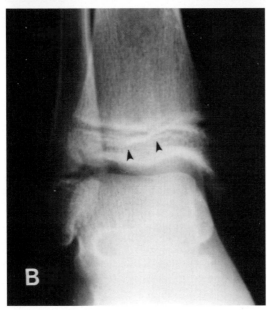

FIGURE 4.245. *Normal distal fibular and tibular epiphyseal–metaphyseal configurations.* **(A)** Note normal offsetting of the distal fibular epiphysis (*arrow*). This is a common finding on oblique views of the normal ankle. It should not be misinterpreted as a displaced epiphyseal fracture. Also note slight irregularity along the inner aspect of the fibula. This also is normal. **(B)** Note the typically irregular appearance of the epiphyseal–metaphyseal junction of the normal distal tibia (*arrows*). This should not be misinterpreted as a Salter–Harris epiphyseal–metaphyseal fracture. **(C)** Lateral view of another ankle demonstrating what appears to be a metaphyseal avulsion (*arrow*). The finding, however, is normal. Of all the epiphyseal–metaphyseal junctions in the body, the one through the distal tibia is most prone to such normal variations.

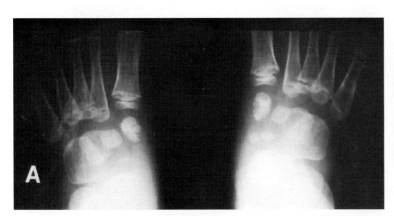

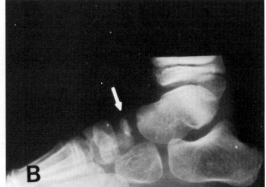

FIGURE 4.246. *Normal irregular ossification of various tarsal bones and pseudoepiphyses of the metatarsals.* **(A)** Note the various irregular configurations of the tarsal bones and pseudoepiphyses of the third through fifth metatarsals. **(B)** Lateral view demonstrating underossification and irregular sclerosis of the normal navicular bone (*arrow*). The findings should not be misinterpreted as those of aseptic necrosis.

it should be noted that tarsal bones are especially prone to irregular ossification, which should not be misinterpreted as fracturing or aseptic necrosis (Fig. 4.246).

REFERENCES

1. Bauer G, Kinzl L. Fracture of the cuboid in children: Case report and review of the literature. *J Pediatr Orthop* 1998;18:466–468.
2. Blumberg K, Patterson RJ. The toddler's cuboid fracture. *Radiology* 1991;179:93–94.
3. Cardinal E, Chhem RK, Beauregard CG, Aubin B, Pelletier M. Plantar fasciitis: Sonographic evaluation. *Radiology* 1996;201: 257–259.
4. Felman AH. Tillaux fractures of the tibia in adolescents. *Pediatr Radiol* 1989;20:87–89.
5. Hayden CK Jr, Swischuk LE. Para-articular soft tissue changes in infections and trauma of the lower extremity in children. *AJR* 1980;134:307–311.
6. Heneghan MA, Wallace T. Heel pain due to retrocalcaneal bursitis-radiographic diagnosis. *Pediatr Radiol* 1985;15:119–122.
7. Higuera J, Laguna R, Peral M, Aranda E, Soleto J. Osteochondritis dissecans of the talus during childhood and adolescence. *J Pediatr Orthop* 1998;18:328–332.
8. Inokuchi S, Usami N, Hiraishi E, Hasmimoto T. Calcaneal fractures in children. *J Pediatr Orthop* 1998;18:469–474.
9. John SD, Moorthy CS, Swischuk LE. Expanding the concept of the toddler's fracture. *RadioGraphics* 1997;17:367–376.
10. Kainberger FM, Engel A, Barton P, Huebsch P, Neuhold A, Salomonowitz E. Injury of the Achilles tendon: Diagnosis with sonography. *AJR* 1990;155: 1031–1036.
11. Laliotis N, Pennie BH, Carty H, Klenerman L. Toddler's fracture of the calcaneum. *Injury* 1993;24:169–170.
12. Micheli LJ, Ireland ML. Prevention and management of calcaneal apophysitis in children: An overuse syndrome. *J Pediatr Orthop* 1987;7:34–38.
13. Ogden JA, Lee J. Accessory ossification patterns and injuries of the malleoli. *J Pediatr Orthop* 1990;10:306–316.
14. Puffinbaarger WR, Gruel CR, Herndon WA, Sullivan JA. Osteomyelitis of the calcaneus in children. *J Pediatr Orthop* 1996;16:224–230.
15. Schindler A, Mason DE, Allington NJ. Occult fracture of the calcaneus in toddlers. *J Pediatr Orthop* 1996;16:201–206.
16. Shopfner CE, Coin CG. Effect of weight-bearing on the appearance and development of the secondary calcaneal epiphysis. *Radiology* 1966;86:201–206.
17. Starshak RJ, Simons GW, Sty JR. Occult fracture of the calcaneus: Another toddler's fracture. *Pediatr Radiol* 1984;14:37–40.
18. Towbin R, Dunbar JS, Towbin J, Clark R. Teardrop sign: Plain film recognition of ankle effusion. *AJR* 1980;134:985–990.
19. Umans H, Pavlov H. Insufficiency fracture of the talus: Diagnosis with MR imaging. *Radiology* 1995;197:439–442.
20. Verma S, Hamilton K, Hawkins HH, Kothari R, Singal B, Buncher R, Nguyen P, O'Neill M. Clinical application of the Ottawa ankle rules for the use of radiography in acute ankle injuries: An independent site assessment. *AJR* 1997;169:825–827.
21. Weston WJ. Köhler's disease of the tarsal scaphoid. *Australas Radiol* 1978;12: 332–337.

Foot

Normal Soft Tissues and Fat Pads

As in the hand, there are no particularly valuable fat pads to evaluate in the foot. Consequently, except for localized edema, there is little else to analyze.

Detecting Fluid in the Small Joints of the Foot

The detection of fluid in the small joints of the foot rests with noting soft tissue swelling around the involved joint. Occasionally, the joint space can be widened because of distension, but this is not a common finding (see Fig. 4.259).

Injuries of the Metatarsals and Phalanges

Dislocation of the various joints of the foot is uncommon except perhaps for dislocation of the great toe. Cortical, buckle, or torus fractures, on the other hand, are quite common and, as in the hand, often require oblique views for adequate visualization (Fig. 4.247). Some of these fractures still can be quite subtle, however, and only telltale soft tissue edema (Fig. 4.248) or meticulous inspection of the films aids one in detecting them (Fig. 4.249). The

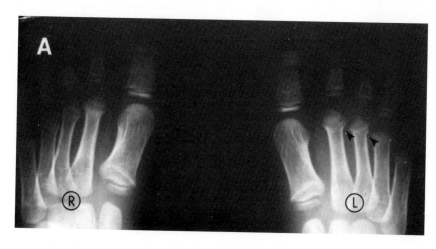

FIGURE 4.247. *Subtle cortical fractures of metatarsals.* **(A)** On the left, note subtle cortical buckling of the second and third metatarsals (*arrows*). Also note that the soft tissues in the area are a little more opaque because of underlying edema.

(continued on next page)

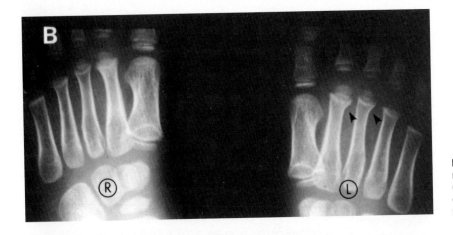

FIGURE 4.247. *(continued)* (B) Oblique view more clearly demonstrates the cortical buckles (*arrows*). Compare these findings with the corresponding cortices on the normal right side.

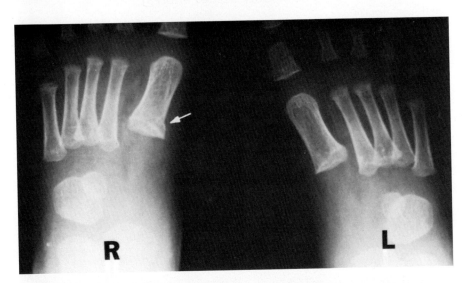

FIGURE 4.248. *Cortical fracture of first metatarsal.* First, note extensive edema of the soft tissues of the right forefoot. Then note the cortical buckle fracture at the base of the first metatarsal (*arrow*).

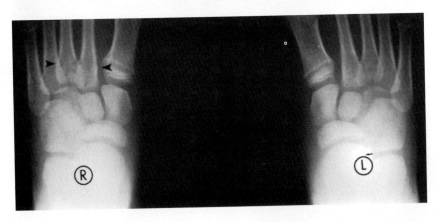

FIGURE 4.249. *Metatarsal fractures, subtle findings.* On the right, note subtle fractures through the base of the second and third metatarsals (*arrows*). These fractures easily could be missed unless the findings are compared with those of the normal bones on the left side.

buckle fracture through the first metatarsal demonstrated in Figure 4.248 also is considered a form of toddler's fracture (3).

This latter fracture also occurs with the bunkbed fracture where the forefoot is jammed into the floor or ground (3,4). This fracture is believed to be the childhood equivalent of the Lisfranc fracture (2), and although there probably is no true dislocation of the first metatarsal from the cuniform bone, (as in adults), a buckle fracture through the base of the first metatarsal is common and the abnormality is to be sought. Comparative views are important here, unless the avulsed fracture fragment is clearly visible (Fig. 4.250A). If these fractures heal they may leave an exostoticlike bone bulge (Fig. 4.250B). This fracture also can be considered

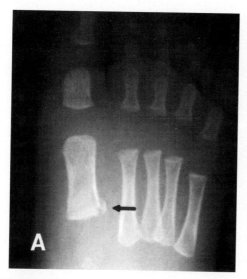
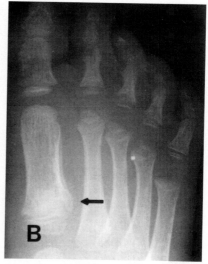

FIGURE 4.250. *"Bunkbed" fracture of first metatarsal.* **(A)** Note typical location of this dislocation–avulsion fracture (*arrow*). **(B)** Healing phase demonstrates an exostotic-like hump (*arrow*).

another form of the toddler's fracture, in the expanded concept of toddler's fractures (3).

Epiphyseal–metaphyseal injuries are much less common in the foot than in the hand and, similarly, fractures of the various epiphyses themselves are less common. A problem, however, can arise in the great toe, where the occasional type III Salter–Harris fracture (Fig. 4.251) can be confused with the more common normal bipartite epiphysis (Fig. 4.252).

Salter–Harris type I, and even type II, epiphyseal–metaphyseal injuries can occur in the small bones of the feet, especially in the great toe. Indeed, these fractures have a propensity to become infected, because there often is a break through the nail bed (5). These fractures usually can be suspected if there is excessive widening of the epiphyseal line; once again, comparative views are indispensable here (Fig. 4.253).

Other fractures of the small bones of the foot include a variety of spiral and transverse fractures, many of which are hairline (Fig. 4.254), and the ***avulsion fracture of the base of the fifth metatarsal.*** Actually, this latter injury is common and usually is sustained with inversion sprains of the ankle. Also called the ***Jones fracture,*** it results from pulling on the base of the fifth metatarsal by the peroneus brevis muscle. Many times, however, swelling around the ankle diverts attention from this fracture, and it is not until the fracture is detected roentgenographically that the injury comes to light. In this regard, it is most fortunate that on almost any roentgenogram of the ankle the base of the fifth metatarsal is included, and ***thus, if one always looks at this area in patients with a sprained***

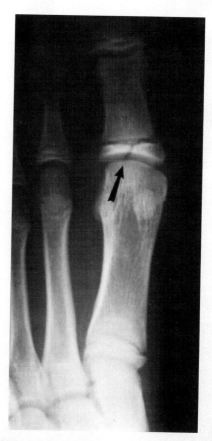

FIGURE 4.251. *Epiphyseal fracture (Salter–Harris type III injury).* Note the fracture through the epiphysis (*arrow*) of the proximal phalanx of the great toe. Also note that the epiphyseal line is a little wider medially, giving further support to the presence of this Salter–Harris type III injury.

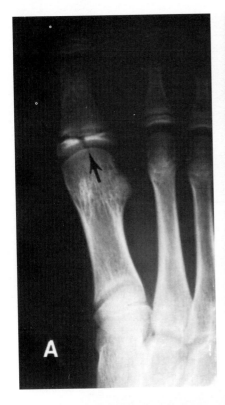

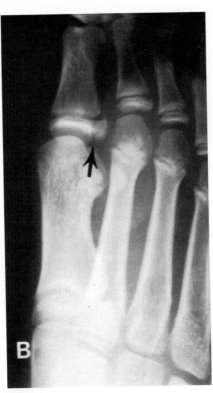

FIGURE 4.252. *Bipartite epiphysis: pseudofracture of the great toe.* **(A)** Note the bipartite epiphysis (*arrow*) of the great toe. The findings are virtually indistinguishable from the fracture demonstrated in Fig. 4.251. **(B)** Another example of an eccentric bipartite epiphysis mimicking a fracture (*arrow*).

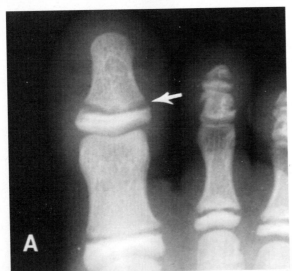

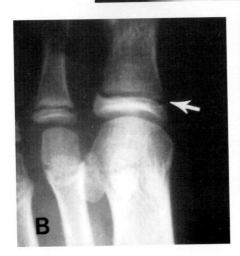

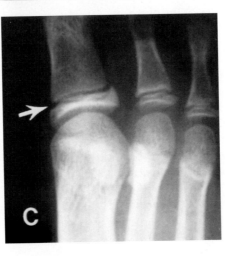

FIGURE 4.253. *Epiphyseal–metaphyseal fractures of the great toe.* **(A)** Note widening of the epiphyseal line of the distal phalanx (*arrow*). Compare it with the width of the other lines. **(B)** Another patient with somewhat subtle widening of the epiphyseal line (*arrow*). **(C)** Compare with the same epiphyseal line on the normal side.

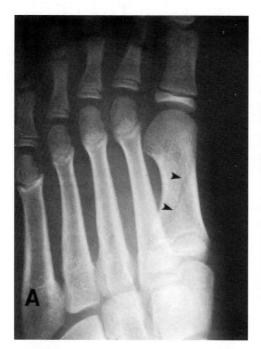
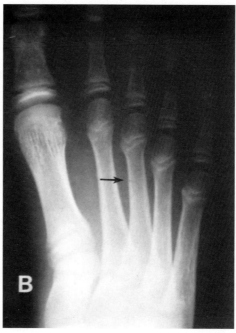

FIGURE 4.254. *Hairline fractures of the metatarsals.* **(A)** Note the oblique hairline fracture of the first metatarsal (*arrows*). **(B)** Very subtle transverse hairline fracture of the third metatarsal (*arrow*).

ankle, one can be the first to detect a good many of these fractures.

In ***differentiating fractures of the base of the fifth metatarsal from the normal os vesalianum,*** it should be noted that the fractures almost always are transverse or near transverse (Fig. 4.255), and the os vesalianum usually is a longitudinal structure (Fig. 4.256). If avulsion of the os vesalianum occurs, a variable degree of separation from the base of the fifth metatarsal is seen, and clinically the findings are accompanied by local tenderness (Fig. 4.257). Occasionally, the os vasalianum can be fractured as part of the Jones fracture.

Miscellaneous Injuries of the Foot

Stress fractures in the foot are reasonably common in the older child but not in the infant. Of these, the best known is the stress fracture of the second metatarsal, the so-called march fracture. As with any stress fracture, the fracture line may be difficult to detect in its early stages, but later on the fracture becomes evident because it causes abundant periosteal new-bone deposition (Fig. 4.258). Stress fractures of the proximal phalanx of the great toe also have been described (6).

Another lesion in the foot that causes pain is aseptic necrosis of the second metatarsal head, or Freiberg's disease.

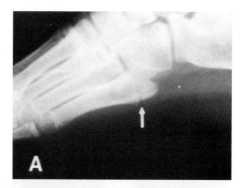
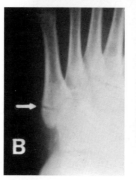
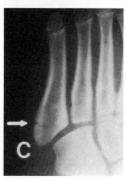

FIGURE 4.255. *Fracture of the base of the fifth metatarsal.* **(A)** Typical transverse fracture (*arrow*) through the base of the fifth metatarsal. **(B)** Same fracture (*arrow*) on anteroposterior view. **(C)** Oblique view of the fracture (*arrow*). Typically, this fracture occurs in the transverse plane.

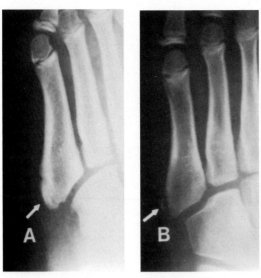

FIGURE 4.256. *Os vesalianum: base of fifth metatarsal accessory center.* **(A)** Large os vesalianum (*arrow*). **(B)** Thin sliver-like os vesalianum (*arrow*). As opposed to a fracture through the base of the fifth metatarsal, the os vesalianum always lies in the longitudinal plane.

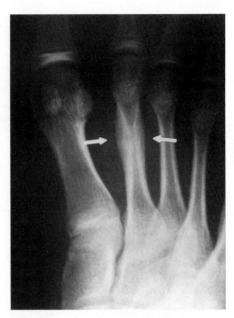

FIGURE 4.258. *Stress fracture of second metatarsal.* Note extensive periosteal new-bone deposition along the second metatarsal (*arrows*). This is a healing stress fracture.

Roentgenographically, the findings range from increased sclerosis to sclerosis interspersed with focal bony resorption of the second metatarsal head. Osteochondritis dissecans in the foot is rare but has been documented in the epiphysis of the first metatarsal (1).

Septic Arthritis, Osteomyelitis, and Cellulitis of the Foot

Septic arthritis is manifest by swelling around the joint space and, occasionally, distension of the joint space (Fig. 4.259). Osteomyelitis and cellulitis, on the other hand, usually present with soft tissue swelling only. Indeed, they are difficult to differentiate from one another, but eventually

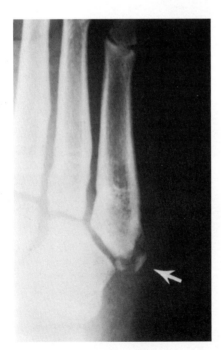

FIGURE 4.257. *Avulsion of the os vesalianum.* Note the fragmented, partially avulsed os vesalianum (*arrow*). Not visible on this reproduction is localized soft tissue swelling over the avulsed bony fragment. Clinically, point tenderness over the area was present.

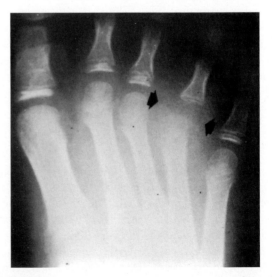

FIGURE 4.259. *Septic arthritis of the small joints of the foot.* Note the widened joint space between the fourth metatarsal and the adjacent proximal phalanx (*arrows*). Also note that the joint is dislocated and that the epiphysis of the phalanx has been partially destroyed.

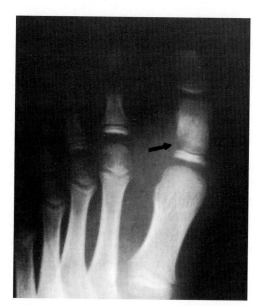

FIGURE 4.260. *Osteomyelitis: small bones of the foot.* Note swelling around the great toe and early bone destruction (*arrow*).

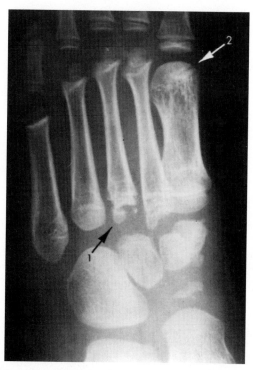

FIGURE 4.261. *Normal irregular ossification of the metatarsal apophyses.* Note the irregular ossification pattern of the apophysis (pseudoepiphysis) of the third metatarsal (*1*). Also note irregular ossification of some of the tarsal bones. The radiolucent defect through the head of the first metatarsal (*2*) should not be misinterpreted as a fracture. It is a residual defect caused by the apophysis (pseudoepiphysis) of the first metatarsal.

osteomyelitis results in bony destruction (Fig. 4.260). Finally, it should be noted that patients with sickle cell disease can present with extensive soft tissue swelling, bony destruction, and periosteal new-bone deposition as part of the hand–foot syndrome. The findings are no different from those seen in the hand (Fig. 4.123) and are difficult to differentiate from osteomyelitis.

Normal Findings Causing Problems

The os vesalianum, or accessory ossification center at the base of the fifth metatarsal, has been dealt with earlier in this chapter and is a common normal finding misinterpreted as a fracture of the base of the fifth metatarsal (Fig. 4.256). Irregular ossifications of the epiphyses or pseudoepiphyses of the metatarsals and phalanges are less commonly misinterpreted as fractures but can be misinterpreted as areas of aseptic necrosis (Fig. 4.261).

The bipartite epiphysis of the great toe, a common normal variation, also has been dealt with earlier (Fig. 4.252) and is a normal finding commonly misinterpreted as a fracture. In addition, bipartite or even tripartite sesamoid bones over the head of the first metatarsal are common and frequently are misinterpreted as fractures of these bones (Fig. 4.262A). Finally, it should be noted that the normal proximal epiphysis of the first metatarsal, seen in oblique projection, can have a very bizarre appearance. In many of these cases, a fracture is suggested (Fig. 4.262B), but knowlege of this phenomenon should enable one to avoid such a misinterpretation.

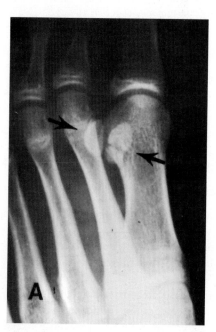

FIGURE 4.262. *Other normal findings causing problems.* (**A**) Note the sesamoid bones of the great toes (*arrows*). One of the bones is bipartite and should not be misinterpreted as a fracture of the sesamoid bone. *(continued on next page)*

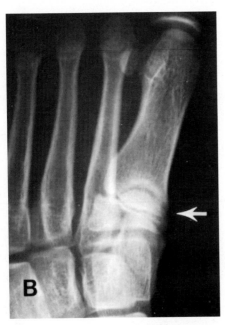

FIGURE 4.262. *(continued)* **(B)** Irregular appearance of the epiphysis of the first metatarsal *(arrow)*. The finding should not be misinterpreted as a fracture.

REFERENCES

1. Falkenberg MP, Dickens DRV, Menelaus MB. Osteochondritis of the first metatarsal epiphysis. *J Pediatr Orthop* 1990;10:797–799.
2. Foster SC, Foster RR. Lisfranc's tarsometatarsal fracture-dislocation. *Radiology* 1976;120:79–83.
3. John SD, Moorthy CS, Swischuk LE. Expanding the concept of the toddler's fracture. *RadioGraphics* 1997;17:367–376.
4. Johnson GF. Pediatric Lisfranc injury: "Bunkbed" fracture. *AJR* 1981;137: 1041–1044.
5. Pinckney LE, Currarino G, Kennedy LA. The stubbed great toe: A cause of occult compound fracture and infection. *Radiology* 1981;138:375–377.
6. Yokoe K, Mannoji T. Stress fracture of the proximal phalanx of the great toe: A report of three cases. *Am J Sports Med* 1986;14: 240–242.

MISCELLANEOUS EXTREMITY PROBLEMS

Battered Child Syndrome

A complete discussion of the battered child syndrome is beyond the scope of this book, but one or two pertinent observations are in order. First, it is not uncommon for a battered infant to first present as an emergency patient, and one should be suspicious if roentgenographic evidence of trauma is greater than the clinical history would suggest, roentgenographic evidence of trauma is poorly correlated with clinical history, and unsuspected fractures are detected. The main job of the physician is to analyze the problem and know when to proceed with further investigation. ***The importance of taking an accurate history in these patients cannot be overstated.*** One needs to know the distance of a fall, the surface involved in the fall, the leading part of the body in the fall, and so forth. The more detailed the history one takes, the more likely one is to uncover discrepancies. Often the individuals bringing the infant to the emergency room say that the infant fell out of bed, but it has been demonstrated (28,32) that it is unlikely that an infant could sustain an extremity fracture from such a fall. Injuries from such a fall are minimal and usually involve the scalp and face (32). Retinal hemorrhages, caused by shaking, are an important finding in the battered child syndrome. Because many of these patients arrive at the trauma center or emergency room unconscious and have received cardiopulmonary resuscitation, the question arises as to whether resuscitation could have caused the retinal hemorrhages. Once again, recent studies (16) have demonstrated that retinal hemorrhages after cardiopulmonary resuscitation alone are uncommon.

Besides the usual patient who presents with bruising and other cutaneous manifestations, extremity deformities, and so forth, there are two other groups of patients that might be considered. The first includes those with burns, often immersion burns in which the lower half of the body is scalded, and the other is those infants presenting to the emergency room dead on arrival, with no visible external injuries. Although associated skeletal injuries in infants sustaining burns can be seen, they are relatively uncommon. We service a large burn population, and this certainly has been our experience.

Infants presenting to the emergency room dead on arrival often are considered to have succumbed to the sudden infant death syndrome. These patients show no overt signs of injury, and usually a CT study of the brain is obtained. This may show nothing, or only the presence of diffuse edema. Often one's first thought is that the problem is diffuse encephalitis. Hypoxia as a cause, in the absence of a history of respiratory distress, often is not considered at first, but it should be remembered that many infants who are asphyxiated on purpose show no signs of injury elsewhere in the body. All that is seen is brain edema. It is in such patients that one should look more closely for occult fractures, especially rib fractures (Fig. 4.263), and in our institution if none are found on ordinary radiographs, nuclear scintigraphy is employed to detect occult bony injuries. On the other hand, if a shaking-type injury has occurred, one may see small cerebral bleeds or contusions, or so-called shearing tears at the junction of the white and gray matter (Fig. 4.264). In addition, one may see evidence of subarachnoid or subdural bleeding. All of these abnormalities can be identified with initial CT studies, but some may remain occult. For this reason follow-up MR studies of the brain are helpful, because they detect previously occult lesions and show progression of already documented lesions.

In terms of skeletal injury, it first should be noted that many battered children present with calvarial injuries and

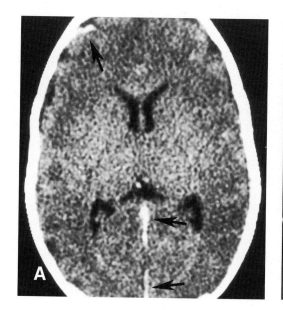

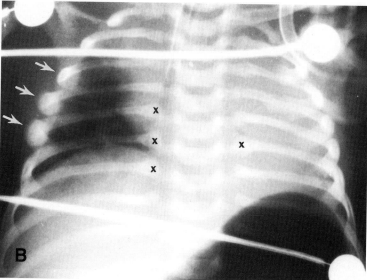

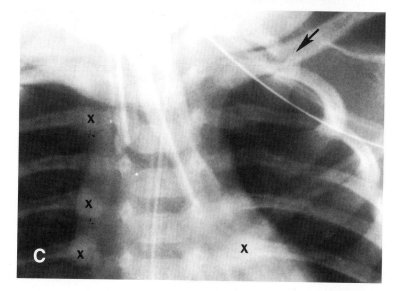

FIGURE 4.263. *Battered child syndrome presenting as sudden infant death syndrom.* **(A)** This patient presented as a sudden infant death problem. Computed tomographic scanning, however, demonstrated blood along the Falx (*posterior arrows*) and some over the right convexity (*upper arrow*). **(B)** Chest film demonstrates three healing fractures on the right (*arrows*) and other healing fractures on both sides (*X*). **(C)** A fresh fracture of the left first rib is seen (*arrow*). Also note healing rib fractures (x).

underlying subdural hematomas. Consequently, any unexplained skull fracture or subdural hematoma should be treated with a great deal of suspicion. Plain skull films are still helpful in the battered child syndrome and should be obtained as part of the bone survey. They are more effective at demonstrating skull fractures than are CT studies. For the most part these fractures are horizontal, linear fractures. Of course, in these cases it is important to obtain subsequent CT studies and eventually MR studies. If no calvarial fractures are present, however, even though other fractures are noted, as long as there are no neurologic findings CT studies have been shown to be of little additional benefit (29).

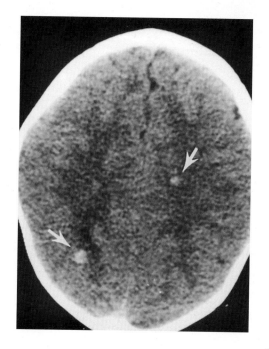

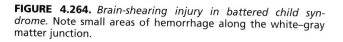

FIGURE 4.264. *Brain-shearing injury in battered child syndrome.* Note small areas of hemorrhage along the white–gray matter junction.

Intracranial injuries can result from direct blows to the calvarium or from violent back-and-forth shaking with acceleration and deceleration of the head. The latter results in dural vein tears and subdural hematomas; the former results in subarachnoid bleeding, contusions, intracranial hemorrhage, and infarction. All of these findings are demonstrable with CT studies (Fig. 4.265), but it is important to appreciate that if these are negative or demonstrate only minimal findings, and the clinical picture suggests more extensive injury, more informative follow-up MR studies are in order (Fig. 4.266).

The most characteristic skeletal lesion in the battered child syndrome is the epiphyseal–metaphyseal fracture (5,17,21). These usually are Salter–Harris type I and II fractures, and their multiplicity along with their different stages of healing are characteristic of this syndrome (Fig. 4.267). Some of these fractures are more subtle than others, and after healing occurs they become more obvious (Fig.

4.268). They result from violent shaking of the infant, as do many of the intracranial injuries and retinal hemorrhages. Although this fracture is the most pathognomonic of the battered child syndrome, however, it is not the most commonly seen. Indeed, it has become increasingly apparent that many infants, perhaps as many as 50%, present with injuries other than those involving the epiphyseal–metaphyseal junction (18,26,27,43). There may be soft tissue injuries, unremarkable-appearing spiral or transverse fractures of the extremity, or no bony injury at all. *Consequently, in the emergency room, any injury that does not seem to fit with the clinical history should be treated with suspicion, and if necessary a bone survey should be obtained* (Fig. 4.269).

Among isolated long bone injuries, the femoral fracture has received a great deal of attention in recent years (3,9,27,34,39,45). More recently the isolated humeral fracture also has received such attention. It is accepted that such

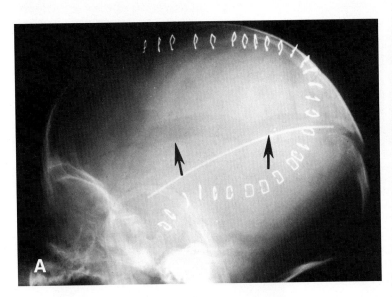

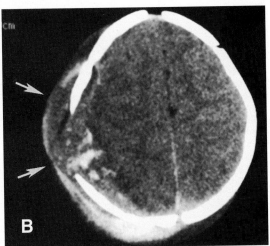

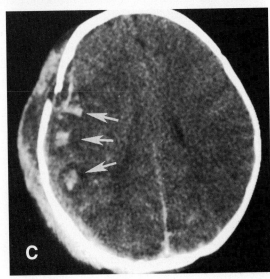

FIGURE 4.265. *Battered child syndrome: extensive cranial injury.* **(A)** Note the diastatic fracture (*arrows*). **(B)** Axial computed tomographic scanning demonstrates extensive subgaleal edema and scattered areas of bleeding in the brain parenchyma, which is herniating through the fracture defect. **(C)** Another slice demonstrating the fracture and a number of parenchymal hemorrhagic foci (*arrows*).

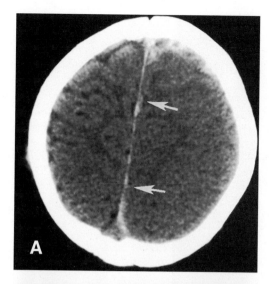

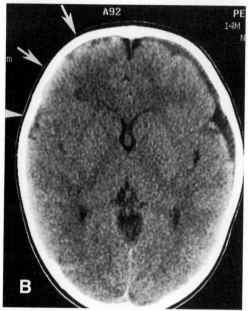

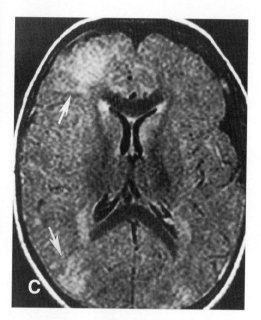

FIGURE 4.266. *Battered child syndrome: intracranial injury, value of magnetic resonance imaging.* **(A)** Note subarachnoid hemorrhage (*arrows*) along the falx. **(B)** A lower slice demonstrates edema of the right frontal lobe (*arrows*). Fluid over the left convexity is normal. White–gray matter distinction is still present. **(C)** A magnetic resonance study (FLAIR sequence), a few days later, demonstrates increased signal in the right frontal and right occipital lobes (*arrows*). These findings confirm the presence of parenchymal contusion at these two sites.

fractures in patients younger than 1 year of age should make the clinician highly suspicious of the battered child syndrome. Indeed, humeral and other long bone fractures, except for femoral fractures should be similarly suspect in patients younger than the age of 2 years. Femoral fractures are excepted, because they are common on a legitimate basis in infants older than 1 year of age. If seen in a child younger than 1 year of age, *however, an isolated, unexplained femoral fracture, or any other long bone fracture should be considered highly suggestive of the battered child syndrome, and a search for other injuries should be initiated* (Figs. 4.270).

If one encounters such an isolated long bone injury, it is most important that a detailed history of how it occurred be obtained (27,39,45). The reason for this is that some of these injuries are legitimate, and one should avoid falsely accusing an individual of inflicting the trauma. For the most part, if trauma is legitimate, the history is detailed and unchanging. *In addition, the individual inflicting the injury admits to the fact that it was inflicted by accident or poor judgment. Of course, there may be some hesitancy on the part of the party in coming forth truthfully to begin with, but eventually the consistent detailed story of how the fracture was inflicted comes to bear.*

Finally, a comment about the outwardly angulated transverse or spiral fracture of the humerus or femur (Fig. 4.271) is in order. I have found that this fracture in children younger than 2 years is highly suggestive of abuse. It is not always part of generalized abuse of the infant, and in fact *it often is an isolated injury inflicted in a fit of anger or*

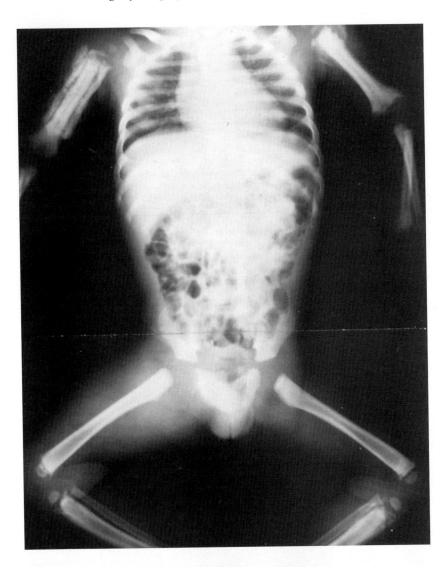

FIGURE 4.267. *Battered child syndrome: classic findings.* Note numerous epiphyseal–metaphyseal fractures in numerous stages of healing in the shoulders, elbows, and knees. Periosteal new-bone deposition at certain sites is profound. Also note that the right hip joint is distended and that the femur is displaced laterally. This represents an acute hemarthrosis resulting from an occult hip fracture. On later films, a healing Salter–Harris epiphyseal–metaphyseal injury became evident.

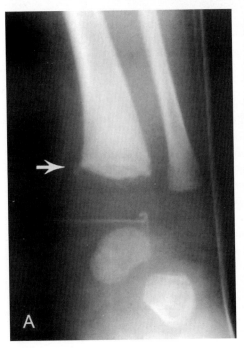
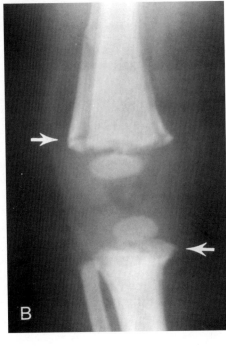

FIGURE 4.268. *Battered child syndrome: epiphyseal–metaphyseal fractures.* **(A)** Subtle, corner epiphyseal–metaphyseal fracture of distal tibia (*arrow*). Note the almost ring-like configuration of the fracture fragment. **(B)** Typical healing epiphyseal–metaphyseal fractures of all bones.

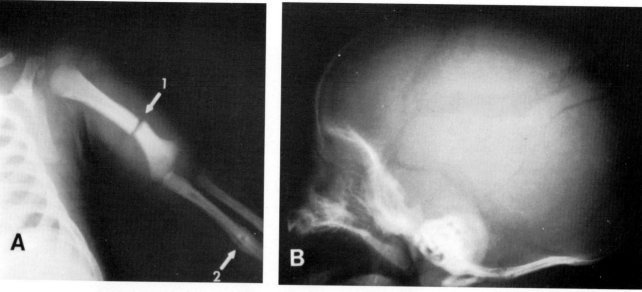

FIGURE 4.269. *Battered child syndrome: incidental identification.* **(A)** This 6-week-old infant was brought to the emergency room by the mother because she thought the infant's arm was broken. A clear-cut fracture through the humerus is visible (*1*), but also note periosteal new-bone deposition around an old distal ulnar fracture (*2*). This latter fracture was unexpected and unexplained. Consequently, a bone survey was obtained. **(B)** Skull film obtained as part of the bone survey demonstrates a number of totally unsuspected calvarial fractures. In addition, this patient demonstrated fractures of the lower extremities and ribs.

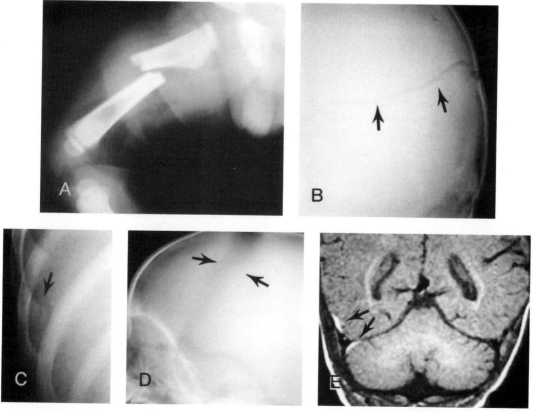

FIGURE 4.270. *Battered child syndrome: various presentations.* **(A)** Note the transverse fracture through the femur of this 4-month-old infant. This was the only fracture present at the time of this admission. **(B)** Two weeks later, the patient returned with an unexplained skull fracture (*arrows*). The skull fracture was not present on the previous bone survey. **(C)** Note the anterior rib fracture (*arrow*). This was the only other bony injury in this child. **(D)** Skull film demonstrates spread coronal sutures (*arrows*). This indicates increased intracranial pressure. **(E)** Magnetic resonance scan, coronal view, demonstrates subdural bleeding at two sites (*arrows*).

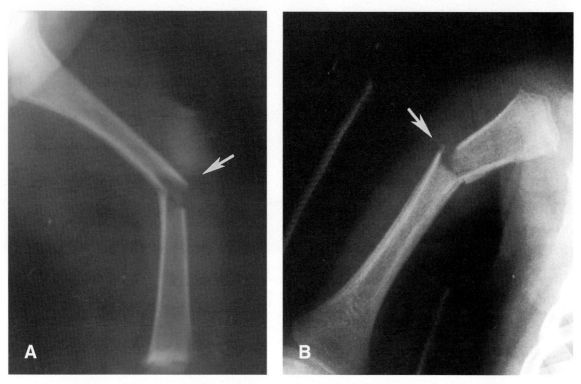

FIGURE 4.271. *Humeral and femoral fractures without outward angulation.* **(A)** Note transverse, outwardly angled fracture (*arrow*) of the femur. **(B)** A similar fracture of the humerus (*arrow*) in another patient. These outwardly angulated fractures are highly suspicious for abuse.

accidentally. This fracture requires that leverage be applied to the femur or humerus from an inward to outward direction, and it is almost impossible for an infant to sustain this type of fracture under any other circumstance. What happens is that the knee or elbow is grabbed by someone and leverage is applied to the long bone, whereupon it fractures with outward angulation through its mid portion. In some cases, the individual inflicting the trauma is very specific and tells exactly how it occurred. If such a history is not forthcoming, then it is almost certain that the injury was inflicted intentionally. *A word of caution, however: This does not necessarily mean that the patient was totally battered, but only that this injury was inflicted on an isolated basis in a fit of anger or misjudgment. Counseling, rather than full accusation, may be in order.*

Bones other than the long bones and skull also are commonly fractured in the battered child syndrome, some more commonly than others. These include the ribs (22,23,26, 39,45) and clavicles (26), and less commonly the spine (7, 10,12,24,25,35,45), pelvis (1), and scapula (26). Rib fractures are very significant, for it is difficult for an infant to sustain rib fractures under almost any other circumstance, including a motor vehicle accident. Therefore, if one sees rib fractures in an infant, no matter what the stage of healing, one should be very suspicious. Often these fractures are

hairline in configuration in their early stages and difficult to detect. Later, as callus formation develops, they are readily visible (Fig. 4.272). Generally, the callus formation produces a round, knotlike appearance at the site of fracture; this eventually smooths out, so that by 8 weeks there is barely any visible evidence of a fracture.

Rib fractures occur posteriorly, laterally, and anteriorly (20,22,23,26). They result from squeezing and shaking. Lateral rib fractures also can result from direct blows. With squeezing and shaking, posteriorly the transverse vertebral process acts as a fulcrom against the posterior rib, and thus fractures occur. Squeezing accounts for most of the lateral fractures; squeezing and shaking account for the anterior fractures. These latter fractures actually are costochondral separations and are manifested in their healing stages by increased cupping of the anterior aspect of the ribs (Fig. 4.273).

Clavicular fractures also are common in the battered child syndrome. Many occur through the midportion of the clavicle and probably result from direct blows. Shaking injuries result in fragmentation fractures of the distal clavicle, which can be considered the equivalent of the classic epiphyseal–metaphyseal fractures of the long bones (Fig. 4.272A). Similar fractures can be seen involving the acromial process (Fig. 4.272B). Both of these fractures can be

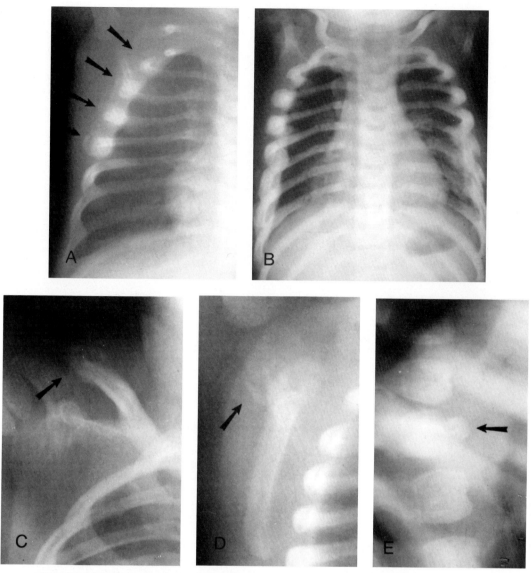

FIGURE 4.272. *Battered child syndrome: other fractures.* **(A)** Note healing fractures (*arrows*), with abundant callus formation, of numerous ribs, laterally. **(B)** Another patient with numerous similar fractures on both sides. In addition, note a number of fractures of the posterior ribs on both sides. **(C)** Epiphyseal–metaphyseal equivalent fracture of the distal clavicle (*arrow*). **(D)** Fragmented acromial fracture (*arrow*). **(E)** Compression fracture with notched vertebra (*arrow*) in another infant. (Parts A and C–E from Kogutt M, Swischuk LE, Fagan CJ. Patterns of injury and significance of uncommon fractures in the battered child syndrome. *AJR* 1974;121:143–149, with permission.)

considered virtually pathognomonic of the battered child syndrome in infants.

Spine fractures and fracture dislocations also can occur but are not particularly common. Of note, however, is that often these fractures are silent (24,35). This is why it is especially important to obtain lateral views of the complete spine as part of the bone survey in these patients. A fracture of the spine is demonstrated in Figure 4.272C.

A number of reviews on imaging of infant abuse are available (19,36), and in addition it has been suggested by

some that initial screening for injury be done with nuclear scintigraphy (14). There is no question that the nuclear scintigraphic study can detect areas of injury, but the findings are nonspecific. There are, however, two opinions regarding this matter, but most institutions still perform the roentgenographic bone survey. It has been suggested that the bone survey be quite detailed (36), but actually most institutions settle for an adequate, more abbreviated screening study. In our institution, we obtain anteroposterior views of the upper extremities and chest and of the pelvis

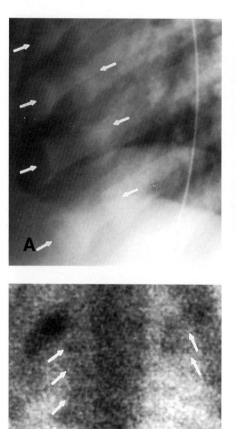

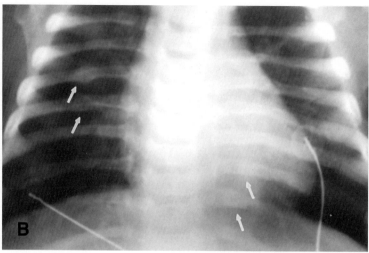

FIGURE 4.273. *Battered child syndrome: rib fractures.* **(A)** Note exaggerated anterior cupping of the ribs (*arrows*) indicating the presence of healing costochondral separations. **(B)** In this patient numerous healing fractures, albeit subtle, are seen on both sides (*arrows*). **(C)** Bone scan demonstrates multiple areas of increased activity (*arrows*).

and lower extremities. We also obtain a lateral view of the complete spine and anteroposterior and lateral views of the skull. If there are any areas of suspicion on these studies whatsoever, whether soft tissue or bony, focused studies of those areas are obtained. The detailed bone survey suggested (36) is very time-consuming, and one must remain somewhat practical about the whole problem. With a good screening sequence, it is doubtful that one would miss any injuries. The key to all of this is to be very astute in one's observations and follow any suspicious finding with focused films.

Nuclear scintigraphic bone surveys can be used in patients older than 5 years of age, to avoid extensive radiographic bone surveys, which usually are unrewarding. *The real role of the nuclear scintigraphic study, however, is in those patients with no visible fractures and in whom battering is suspected.* One characteristic scenario is the infant who is unconscious on arrival and is suspected to have succumbed to an aborted sudden infant death syndrome, but who also could have been asphyxiated. Very often the nuclear scintigraphic study demonstrates fractures in their

healing phases that are not readily visible on radiographs. This is especially true of rib fractures.

Visceral injury (6,31,40) is becoming more common in the battered child syndrome, as is sexual abuse (40). Visceral injury most commonly involves the pancreas and duodenum, but involvement of other intraabdominal organs also is seen. These are best studied with CT scanning. Very often these visceral injuries carry a graver prognosis and mortality rate than do visceral injuries from other causes (6). In most cases no fractures are visible on the bone survey, but one should still inspect the study and especially look for rib fractures (1). Another form of visceral injury is that which occurs with placing objects in the mouth or down the esophagus. In such cases, pharyngeal or esophageal perforations can occur (13,30), and the presenting problem may be drooling (13).

Finally, in assessing the radiographs of battered children one always should keep in mind the possibility that someone will ask the question, "Does the infant suffer from osteogenesis imperfecta or brittle bone disease?" Brittle bone disease is an unproven entity, which probably does not exist, and one should be careful in invoking this entity as a cause for fractures (42). Osteogenesis imperfecta, although leading to multiple fractures in children, does not present with the array of injuries seen in battered children. Specifically, epiphyseal–metaphyseal fractures are not characteristic of osteogenesis imperfecta, and furthermore in osteogenesis imperfecta the bones themselves appear abnormal. In the battered child syndrome, the bones appear normal except for the fractures.

Before concluding discussion of the battered child syndrome, it might be noted that it has been determined that infants suffering from the battered child syndrome also tend to have high blood lead levels (4).

REFERENCES

1. Ablin DS, Greenspan A, Reinhart MA. Pelvic injuries in child abuse. *Pediatr Radiol* 1992;22:454–457.
2. Ablin DS, Sane SM. Non-accidental injury: Confusion with temporary brittle bone disease and mild osteogenesis imperfecta. *Pediatr Radiol* 1997;27:111–113.
3. Beals RK, Tufts E. Fractured femur in infancy: The role of child abuse. *J Pediatr Orthop* 1983;3:583–586.
4. Bithoney WG, Vandeven AM, Ryan A. Elevated lead levels in reportedly abused children. *J Pediatr* 1993;122:719–720.
5. Caffey J. Multiple fractures in long bones of children suffering from chronic subdural hematoma. *AJR* 1946;56:163–173.
6. Cameron CM, Lazoritz S, Calhoun AD. Blunt abdominal injury: Simultaneously occurring liver and pancreatic injury in child abuse. *Pediatr Emerg Care* 1997;13:334–336.
7. Carrion WV, Dormans JP, Drummond DS, Christofersen MR. Circumferential growth plate fracture of the thoracolumbar spine from child abuse. *J Pediatr Orthop* 1996;16:210–214.
8. Chapman S, Hall CM. Non-accidental injury or brittle bones. *Pediatr Radiol* 1997;27:106–110.
9. Dalton HJ, Slovis T, Helfer RE, Comstock J, Schuerer S, Riolo S. Undiagnosed abuse in children younger than 3 years with femoral fracture. *Am J Dis Child* 1990;144:875–878.
10. Diamond P, Hansen CM, Christofersen MR. Child abuse presenting as a thoracolumbar spinal fracture dislocation: A case report. *Pediatr Emerg Care* 1994;10:83–86.
11. Feldman KW, Brewer DK. Child abuse, cardiopulmonary resuscitation and rib fractures. *Pediatrics* 1984;73:339.
12. Gabos PG, Tuten HR, Leet A, Stanton RP. Fracture-dislocation of the lumbar spine in an abused child. *Pediatrics* 1998;101:473–477.
13. Golova N. An infant with fever and drooling: Infection or trauma? *Pediatr Emerg Care* 1997;13:331–333.
14. Haase GM, Ortiz VN, Sfakianakis GN, Morse TS. Value of radionuclide bone scanning in the early recognition of deliberate child abuse. *J Trauma* 1980;20:873–875.
15. Harles JR. Disorders of coagulation misdiagnosed as nonaccidental bruising. *Pediatr Emerg Care* 1997;13:347–349.
16. Kanter RK. Retinal hemorrhage after cardiopulmonary resuscitation or child abuse. *J Pediatr* 1986;108:430–432.
17. Kempe CH, Silverman FN, Steel BF, Droegenmueller W, Silver HK. Battered child syndrome. *JAMA* 1962;181:17–24.
18. King J, Diefendorf D, Apthorp J, Negrete VF, Carlson M. Analysis of 429 fractures in 189 battered children. *J Pediatr Orthop* 1988;8:585–589.
19. Kleinman PK. Diagnostic imaging in infant abuse. *AJR* 1990;155:703–712.
20. Kleinman PK, Marks SC, Adams V. Factors affecting the visualization of anterior rib fractures in abused infants. *AJR* 1987;150:635.
21. Kleinman PK, Marks SC, Blackbourne B. The metaphyseal lesion in abused infants: A radiologic-histopathologic study. *AJR* 1986;146:895–905.
22. Kleinman PK, Marks SC Jr, Nimkin K, Rayder SM, Kessler SC. Rib fractures in 31 abused infants: Post-mortem radiologic-histopathologic study. *Radiology* 1996;200:807–810.
23. Kleinman PK, Schlesinger AE. Mechanical factors associated with posterior rib fractures: Laboratory and case studies. *Pediatr Radiol* 1997;27:87–91.
24. Kleinman PK, Shelton YA. Hangman's fracture in an abused infant: Imaging features. *Pediatr Radiol* 1997;27:776–777.
25. Kleinman PK, Zito JL. Avulsion of the spinous processes caused by infant abuse. *Radiology* 1984;151:389–392.
26. Kogutt MS, Swischuk LE, Fagan CJ. Patterns of injury and significance of uncommon fractures in the battered child syndrome. *AJR* 1974;121:143–149.
27. Leventhal JM, Thomas SA, Rosenfield NS, Markowitz RI. Fractures in young children: Distinguishing child abuse from unintentional injuries. *Am J Dis Child* 1993;147:87–92.
28. Lyons TJ, Oates RK. Falling out of bed: A relatively benign occurrence. *Pediatrics* 1993;92:125–127.
29. Mogbo KI, Slovis TL, Canady AI, Allasio DJ, Arfken CL. Appropriate imaging in children with skull fractures and suspicion of abuse. *Radiology* 1998;208:521–524.
30. Morzaria S, Walton J, MacMillan A. Inflicted esophageal perforation. *J Pediatr Surg* 1998;33:871–873.
31. Ng CS, Hall CM. Costochondral junction fractures and intra-abdominal trauma in non-accidental injury. *Pediatr Radiol* 1998;28:671–676.
32. Nimityongskul P, Anderson LD. The likelihood of injuries when children fall out of bed. *J Pediatr Orthop* 1987;7:184–186.
33. Reece RM. Fatal child abuse and sudden infant death syndrome: A critical diagnostic decision. *Pediatrics* 1993;91:423–429.
34. Rivera FP, Kamitsuka MD, Quan L. Injuries to children younger than one year of age. *Pediatrics* 1988;81:93–97.
35. Rooks VJ, Sisler C, Burton B. Cervical spine injury in child abuse: Report of two cases. *Pediatr Radiol* 1998;28:193–195.
36. Rosenberg NM, Marino D. Frequency of suspected abuse/neglect in burn patients. *Pediatr Emerg Care* 1989;5:219–221.
37. Schweich P, Fleisher G. Rib fractures in children. *Pediatr Emerg Care* 1985;1:187–189.
38. Section on Radiology: Diagnostic imaging of child abuse. *Pediatrics* 1991;87:262–264.
39. Shaw BA, Murphy KM, Shaw A, Oppenheim WL, Myracle MR. Humerus shaft fractures in young children: Accident or abuse? *J Pediatr Orthop* 1997;17:293–297.
40. Sivit CJ, Taylor GA, Eichelberger MR. Visceral injury in battered children: A changing perspective. *Radiology* 1989;173:659–661.
41. Spevak MR, Kleinman PK, Belanger PL, Primack C, Richmond JM. Cardiopulmonary resuscitation and rib fractures in infants: A post-mortem radiologic-pathologic study. *JAMA* 1994;272:617–618.
42. Stewart GM, Rosenberg NM. Conditions mistaken for child abuse: Part I. *Pediatr Emerg Care* 1996;12:116–121.
43. Strait RT, Siegel RM, Shapiro RA. Humeral fractures without obvious etiologies in children less than 3 years of age: When is it abuse? *Pediatrics* 1995;96:667–671.
44. Strouse PJ, Owings CL. Fractures of the first rib in child abuse. *Radiology* 197:763–765.
45. Swischuk LE. Spine and spinal cord trauma in the battered child syndrome. *Radiology* 1969;92:733–738.

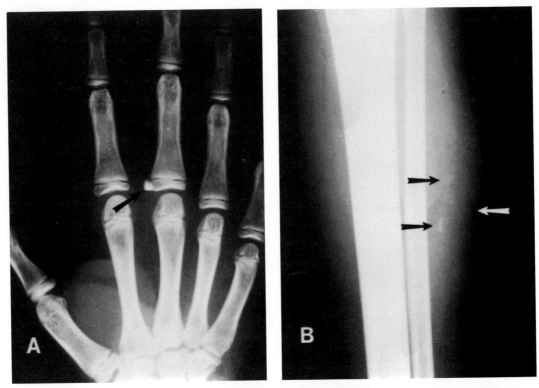

FIGURE 4.274. *Glass in the soft tissues.* **(A)** Clearly visible glass fragment (*arrow*) in the soft tissues of the third digit. **(B)** Less clearly visualized fragments of glass (*black arrows*) in the soft tissues of the leg. Also note edema in the leg and air in the soft tissues (*white arrow*).

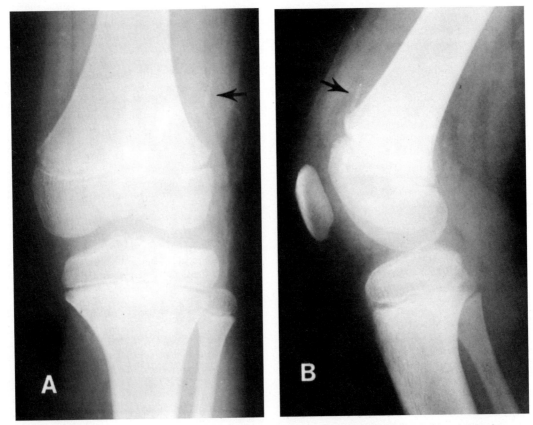

FIGURE 4.275. *Pencil lead in soft tissues.* **(A)** Note the barely visible lead-pencil fragment in the soft tissues of the knee (*arrow*). **(B)** Lateral view demonstrating the same lead-pencil fragment (*arrow*).

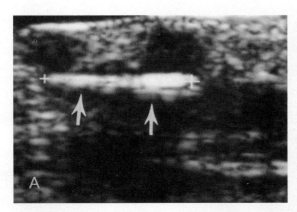

FIGURE 4.276. *Foreign body: ultrasound detection.* **(A)** Note the echogenic palm thorn (*arrows*). **(B)** Transverse image also demonstrates the thorn (*arrow*). There is a surrounding collar of hypoechoic fluid.

Foreign Bodies in the Soft Tissues

Soft tissue foreign bodies are a common problem in childhood. Metallic foreign bodies and pebbles or dirt, of course, are readily demonstrable, but less-opaque or totally nonopaque foreign bodies present more of a problem. Pieces of glass may or may not be visible, although most are visible (1,5,11); visibility depends entirely upon the amount of lead in the glass. In some cases, the glass fragment is readily demonstrable; in others it is more difficult to see (Fig. 4.274). Lead from a lead pencil is another foreign body commonly embedded in the soft tissues, and in some cases it may be demonstrable roentgenographically (Fig. 4.275). Plastic generally is invisible (5), but all foreign bodies now can be readily identified if needed, with ultrasound (3,6,8,9) and CT scanning (3). Examples of such foreign bodies are presented in Figs. 4.276 and 4.277. Most foreign bodies, however, can be detected with ultrasound, and CT examination seldom is needed.

Of special interest is the thorn, wooden or other organic foreign body that becomes embedded in the soft tissues on a chronic basis (2–4,7,10,12,13). In such instances, most often one is dealing with a toothpick, although thorns, tree twigs, and so forth also have been encountered. Most of these foreign bodies, of course, are not visible roentgenographically, but they now usually are detected readily with ultrasound. Until such studies can be obtained, one must rely on secondary findings consisting of widening of the soft tissues between the adjacent bones and, eventually, periosteal new-bone deposition; that is, reactive periostitis (Fig. 4.278). In some cases, the resulting periosteal new bone and adjacent demineralization of the bones can lead to a pseudoosteomyelitis or tumorlike appearance.

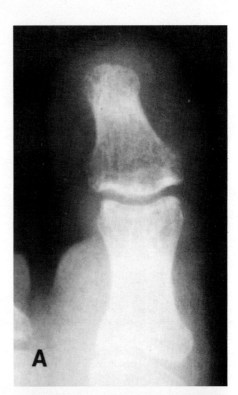

FIGURE 4.277. *Soft tissue foreign body: Computed tomographic scan.* **(A)** This big toe was swollen for a prolonged period of time. No clear-cut foreign body is seen, but one was suspected medially. **(B)** Computed tomographic scan clearly demonstrates the foreign body (*arrow*) and the swollen soft tissues around the big toe.

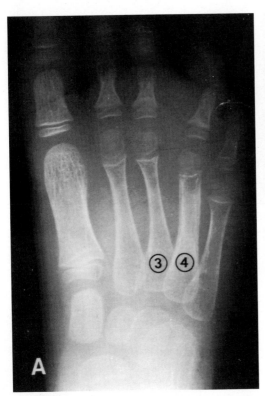
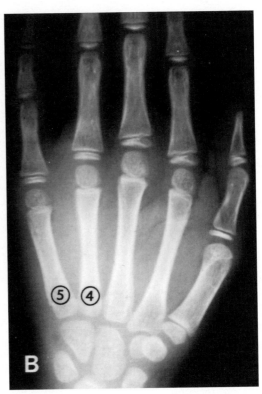

FIGURE 4.278. *Chronically embedded toothpick.* **(A)** Note widening of the soft tissues between the third (*3*) and fourth (*4*) digits, and periosteal new bone deposition along the fourth metatarsal. This patient presented with a chronically draining lesion between the third and fourth toes. A toothpick was extracted. **(B)** Note increased density of the soft tissues around the fourth (*4*) and fifth (*5*) metacarpals, and that the soft tissue space between the fourth and fifth metacarpals is widened. Also note periosteal new-bone deposition along the shaft of the fourth metacarpal. This patient had a toothpick embedded between these bones.

REFERENCES

1. Avner JR, Baker D. Lacerations involving glass: The role of routine roentgenograms. *Am J Dis Child* 1992;146:600–602.
2. Barton LL, Saied KR. Thorn-induced arthritis. *J Pediatrics* 1978; 93:322–323.
3. Bray H, Stringer DA, Poskitt K, Newman DE, MacKenzie WG. Maple tree knee: A unique foreign body—value of ultrasound and CT examination. *Pediatr Radiol* 1991;21:457–458.
4. Cahill N, King JD. Palm thorn synovitis. *J Pediatr Orthop* 1984; 4:175–179.
5. DeLacey G, Evans R, Sandin B. How easy is it to see glass (and plastic) on radiographs? *Br J Radiol* 1985;58:27–30.
6. Fornage BD, Schernberg FL. Sonographic diagnosis of foreign bodies of the distal extremities. *AJR* 1986;147:567–569.
7. Gerle RD. Thorn-induced pseudo-tumors of bone. *Br J Radiol* 1971;44:642–645.
8. Gooding GAW, Hardiman T, Sumers M, Stess R, Graf P, Grunfeld C. Sonography of the hand and foot in foreign body detection. *J Ultrasound Med* 1987;6:441–447.
9. Shiels WE II, Babcock DS, Wilson JL, Burch RA. Localization and guided removal of soft-tissue foreign bodies with sonography. *AJR* 1990;155:1277–1281.
10. Swischuk LE, Jorgenson F, Jorgenson A, Capen D. Wooden splinter induced "pseudotumors" and "osteomyelitis-like lesions" of bone and soft tissue. *AJR* 1974;122:176–179.
11. Tandberg D. Glass in hand and foot: Will X-ray film show it? *JAMA* 1982;248:1872–1874.
12. Weston WJ. Thorn and twig-induced pseudotumors of bone and soft tissues. *Br J Radiol* 1963;36:323–326.
13. Yousefzadeh DK, Jackson JR Jr. Organic foreign body reaction: Report of two cases of thorn-induced "granuloma" and review of literature. *Skeletal Radiol* 1978;3:167–176.

Soft Tissue Infections, Edema, and Air in the Soft Tissues

Many times, children come to the emergency room with extensive soft tissue swelling secondary to trauma or infection. Roentgenographically, the findings in both cases consist of thickening of the soft tissues, obliteration of the fat–muscle interfaces, and a characteristic reticulation of the fatty tissues. Reticulation is caused by the accumulation of fluid within the fibrous septae of the fatty tissues and is seen primarily with cellulitis and superficial contusions (Fig. 4.279). In other instances, deep soft tissue infections are associated with gas-producing organisms, and gas is seen in the soft tissues (Fig. 4.280). Air also can be seen in the soft tissues in association with extensive lacerations and blast injuries.

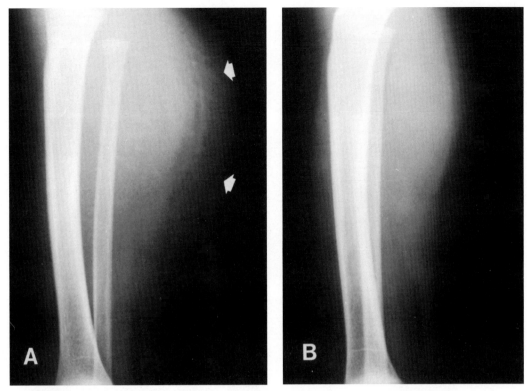

FIGURE 4.279. *Superficial cellulitis.* **(A)** Note typical reticulated appearance of the edematous soft tissues of the posterior aspect of the calf (*arrows*). **(B)** Compare with normal side.

As noted in the preceding paragraph, superficial edema produces reticulation of the subcutaneous fatty tissue; this finding also can be seen on ultrasound, on which the soft tissue structures are separated and become more echogenic while all along looking more reticular. If edema is deeper, however,

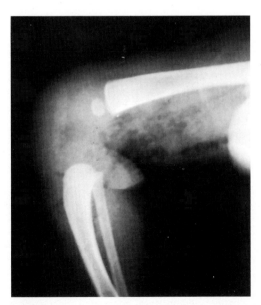

FIGURE 4.280. *Air on the soft tissues: gas-forming organism.* Young infant with cellulitis of the thigh. Note numerous air bubbles and linear collections of air in the soft tissues of the thigh.

a problem arises as to whether it is caused by osteomyelitis or soft tissue infection (e.g., pyomyositis, abscess). In the past, often it was difficult to make this determination, but with ultrasound, CT, and MR imaging (1,3,8,9) it has become increasingly easier. Ultrasound can clearly identify soft tissue abscesses and should be used whenever soft tissue infection is suspected. The findings are not difficult to define or interpret (Figs. 4.281 and 4.282). Such soft tissue abscesses, often involving the muscles, are more common than generally appreciated. The term ***pyomyositis*** (1,2,4,5,9) is applied to this condition. Isotope studies frequently are helpful in identifying these sites of infection (Fig. 4.283), but, as already noted, ultrasonography is the most valuable study.

Inflammatory adenopathy often is a presenting problem in the emergency room. In the past, it was difficult to document, but currently ultrasonography can readily document the presence of enlarged, inflamed lymph nodes (Fig. 4.284). These lymph nodes can suppurate or become necrotic (6); this also can be readily identified with ultrasonography. Color flow Doppler frequently demonstrates increased blood flow to inflamed lymph nodes (Fig. 4.284B). Such increased blood flow to lymph nodes is a nonspecific phenomenon and occurs with both inflammatory and tumoral adenopathy (7). Ultrasonographically, lymph nodes appear as oval or round, relatively hypoechoic structures. With suppuration, their centers become more hypoechoic (Fig. 4.284D).

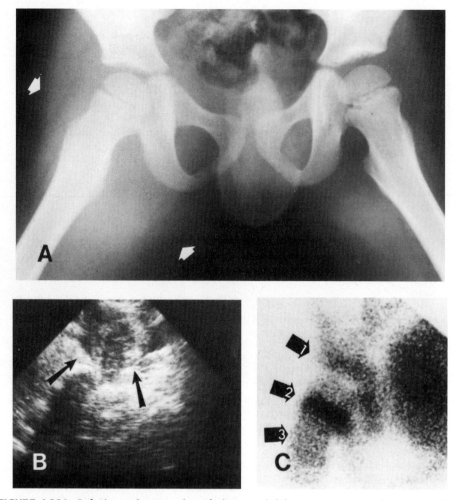

FIGURE 4.281. *Soft tissue abscess: value of ultrasound.* (**A**) Note extensive soft tissue swelling around the upper femur (*arrows*). (**B**) Ultrasound study clearly identifies an abscess in the medial soft tissues of the thigh (*arrows*). (**C**) Isotope study performed previously is normal. Normal uptake in acetabular roof (*1*), epiphyseal–metaphyseal junction (*2*), and upper femur (*3*). There is no increased uptake at any of these sites.

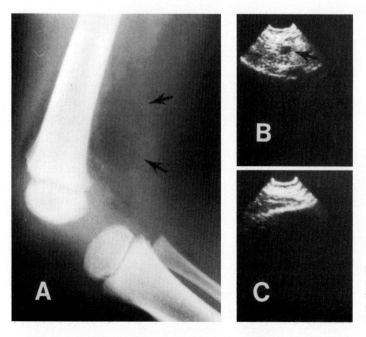

FIGURE 4.282. *Soft tissue abscess: ultrasound study.* (**A**) This patient demonstrates edematous reticulation of the soft tissues posterior to the knee (*arrows*). (**B**) Ultrasound study demonstrates a sonolucent abscess in the area (*arrow*). (**C**) Normal side for comparison.

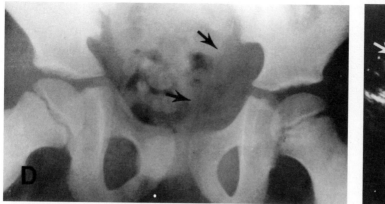
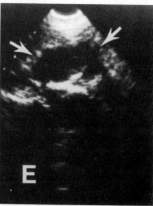

FIGURE 4.282. *(continued)* **(D)** Another patient with deep soft tissue swelling in the pelvis (*arrows*). **(E)** Ultrasonography over the buttocks demonstrates a large abscess (*arrows*).

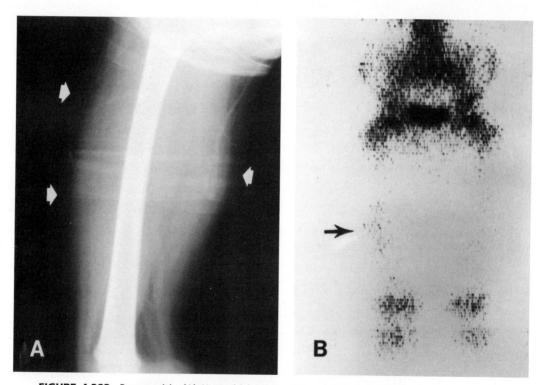

FIGURE 4.283. *Pyomyositis.* **(A)** Note thickening of the soft tissues of the thigh (*arrows*). **(B)** Nuclear scintigraphy demonstrates increased, albeit vague, tracer accumulation in the area of muscle inflammation (*arrow*).

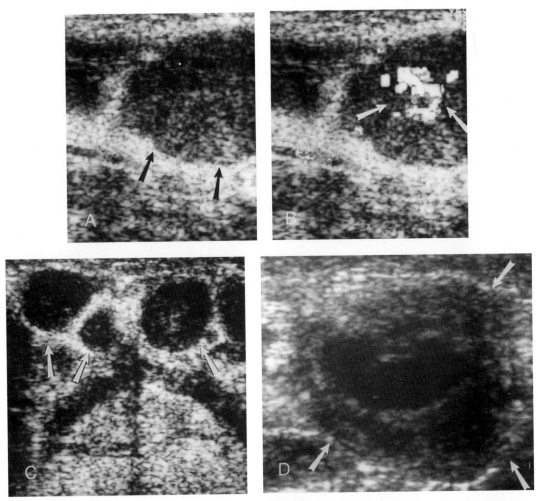

FIGURE 4.284. *Adenopathy.* **(A)** Note the enlarged lymph node (*arrows*). **(B)** Color flow Doppler demonstrates exuberant blood flow (*arrows*) within the lymph node. **(C)** Another patient with multiple enlarged, relatively hypoechoic lymph nodes (*arrows*). **(D)** Enlarged lymph node (*arrows*) with central hypoechoic suppuration. (From Swischuk LE, Desai PB, John SD. Exuberant blood flow in enlarged lymph nodes: Findings on color flow Doppler. *Pediatr Radiol* 1992;22:419–421, with permission.)

A special situation in which the identification of adenopathy is helpful is if it is seen in the epitrochlear region (Fig. 4.83). In such cases, the enlarged nodes and edema can be seen on plain films but are vividly demonstrable with ultrasound. Many times the problem in such a case is cat-scratch disease, and the lymph nodes demonstrate exuberant increased blood flow on color flow Doppler ultrasound.

Soft tissue hematomas also can be demonstrated with ultrasound. Initially, they produce an area of vague echogenicity, but later, as liquefaction of the hematoma occurs, central fluid collections can be seen (Fig. 4.285). Hematomas also can be demonstrated with CT and MR imaging, but MR imaging is more exquisite and informative.

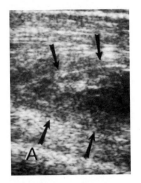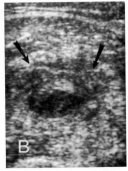

FIGURE 4.285. *Soft tissue hematoma.* **(A)** Note the heterogeneous texture of the hematoma (*arrows*) dissecting in between muscle planes. **(B)** Cross-sectional view demonstrates the hematoma (*arrows*) with a liquifying relatively hypoechoic center.

REFERENCES

1. Gibson RK, Rosenthal SJ, Lukert BP. Pyomyositis: Increasing recognition in temperate climates. *Am J Med* 1984;77:768–772.
2. Grose C. Staphylococcal pyomyositis in south Texas. *J Pediatr* 1978;93:457–458.
3. Hernandez RJ, Leim DR, Chenevert TL, Sullivan DB, Aisen AM. Fat-suppressed MR imaging of myositis. *Radiology* 1992;182: 217–219.
4. Hirano T, Srinivasan G, Jamakiraman N, Pleviak D, Mukhopadhyay D. Gallium-67 citrate scintigraphy in pyomyositis. *J Pediatr* 1980;97:596–598.
5. Sirinavin S, McCraken GH Jr. Primary supporative myositis in children. *Am J Dis Child* 1979;133:263–265.
6. Smith HL II. Necrotizing lymphadenitis (Kikuchi's disease). *Pediatrics* 1993;91:152.
7. Swischuk LE, Desai PB, John SD. Exuberant blood flow in enlarged lymph nodes: Findings on color flow Doppler. *Pediatr Radiol* 1992;22:419–421.
8. Tang JSH, Gold RH, Bassett LW, Seeger LL. Musculoskeletal infection of the extremities: Evaluation with MR imaging. *Radiology* 1988;166:205–209.
9. Yousefzadeh DK, Schumann EM, Mulligan GM, Bosworth EE, Young CS, Pringle KC. The role of imaging modalities in diagnosis and management of pyomyositis. *Skeletal Radiol* 1982;8:285–289.

5

THE HEAD

HEAD TRAUMA

Trauma to the calvarium and intracranial structures is common in childhood, but roentgenographic examination of the skull in most cases is relatively unrewarding. Indeed, it has been demonstrated that at most only about 25% of patients demonstrate skull fractures (2) and that most injuries are minor (1). For these reasons, the use of skull roent-genograms has virtually vanished in the evaluation of head trauma. The only exception is the use of the skull film in the battered child syndrome, in which it is more rewarding than the computed tomographic (CT) study for demonstrating fractures (Fig. 5.1). Overall, however, rather than assessing fractures, it is more important to assess intracranial injuries, and CT scans are best for demonstrating these injuries. Magnetic resonance (MR) images also can be used

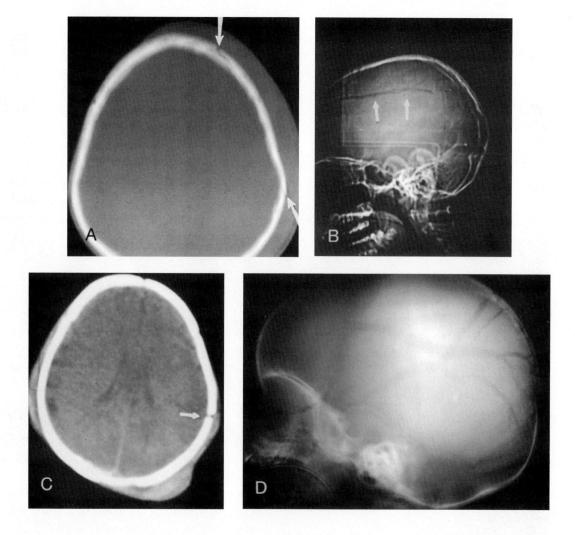

TABLE 5.1. CLINICAL FINDINGS PREDISPOSING TO CT EXAMINATION

History
- Age less than 1 year[a]
- Unconsciousness or amnesia of greater than 5-min duration
- Gunshot wound or skull penetration
- Focal neurologic symptoms

Physical Examination
- Focal neurologic or ocular signs
- Skull depression
- CSF discharge from ear or nose
- Blood in middle ear
- Battle's sign
- Blackeye (hematoma)
- Lethargy, coma, or stupor

[a]With more severe trauma only.

to image intracranial problems (4,6), but they are not obtained as easily and are not dependable in detecting fresh bleeding. MR imaging is most rewarding with chronic or subacute bleeds that are more than 3 days old (4,6).

Indications for obtaining CT scans in patients with head injury, interestingly enough, are really no different from those utilized for obtaining skull films in the past (Table 5.1). These criteria parallel the Glasgow coma scale, on which a score of 12 or greater signifies the presence of a minor injury (3,5,7). Some studies, however, have demonstrated that even in patients in whom the Glasgow score is 12 or more, significant intracranial injury can still be present (5,7). Therefore, final decisions are individual, generally guided by the criteria outlined in Table 5.1.

REFERENCES

1. Duhaime AC, Alario AI, Lewander WJ, Schut L, Sutton LN, Seidel TS, Nudelman S, Budenz D, Hertle R, Tsiaras W, Loporcio S. Head injury in very young children: Mechanisms, injury types, and ophthalmologic findings in 100 hospitalized patients younger than 2 years of age. *Pediatrics* 1992;90:179–185.
2. Harwood-Nash DC, Hendrick EB, Hudson AR. The significance of skull fractures in children: A study of 1,187 patients. *Radiology* 1971;101:151–155.
3. Hennes H, Lee M, Smith D, Sty JR, Losek J. Clinical predictors of severe head trauma in children. *Am J Dis Child* 1988;142: 1045–1047.
4. Hesselink JR, Dowd CF, Healy ME, Hajek P, Baker LL, Luerssen TG. MR imaging of brain contusions: A comparative study with CT. *AJR* 1988;150:1133–1142.
5. Rivara F, Tanaguchi D, Parish RA, Stimac GK, Mueller B. Poor prediction of positive computed tomographic scans by clinical criteria in symptomatic pediatric head trauma. *Pediatrics* 1987;80: 579–584.
6. Snow RB, Zimmerman RD, Gandy SE, Deck MDF. Comparison of magnetic resonance imaging and computed tomography in the evaluation of head injury. *Neurosurgery* 1986;18:45–52.
7. Stein SC, Ross SE. The value of computed tomographic scans in patients with low-risk head injuries. *Neurosurgery* 1990;26: 638–640.

Which Skull Views Should Be Obtained?

Skull films certainly are not obtained as often as they were in the past, but still it is important to know which ones to obtain if they are necessary. Generally speaking, lateral, posteroanterior, and Towne's views suffice. In addition, if facial injuries are being assessed, the Water's view should be included. In most instances, there is little reason to obtain a view of the base of the skull, but in some cases special tangential or oblique views may be necessary to fully visualize a suspected fracture. In the patient who is not alert or in whom a neck injury also is suspected, one should confine the initial calvarial study to cross-table lateral, anteroposterior, and Towne's views; all should be obtained without moving the patient.

Importance of Site and Fracture Type

Much more important than the mere detection of a fracture is the determination of the type and site of the fracture. For example, compound skull fractures and fractures through air-filled structures such as the paranasal sinuses and mastoid air cells are important because they can lead to complications such as meningitis, pneumocephalus (1,2), and cerebrospinal fluid leaks. Depressed fractures are clearly important and place the patient into a markedly higher risk category. Most of these fractures require elevation and repair of underlying dural tears, and associated brain damage and long-lasting complications such as focal seizures are definite additional problems. Multiple calvarial fractures (eggshell fractures) such as might be sustained in automobile accidents or from falls on the head from great heights are of obvious significance, and linear fractures traversing vascular structures such as the middle meningeal artery and deep venous sinuses are more significant than the same linear fractures not traversing these sites. Fractures of the base of the skull also generally are considered significant frac-

FIGURE 5.1. *Skull films and computed tomographic scans.* **(A)** On this computed tomographic scan, note subtle suggestion of a left parietal fracture (*arrow*). **(B)** Tomogram more clearly delineates the fracture (*arrows*). **(C)** Another patient with brain edema and a left parietal fracture (*arrows*). Note extensive subcutaneous thickening caused by subgaleal hematomas. This is a battered child. **(D)** Lateral view of the skull reveals the extensive degree of fracturing present. This is an eggshell fracture. In the battered child syndrome especially, it is important to obtain a combination of the two studies, that is, plain films and computed tomographic scan.

tures, for they tend to extend into the mastoid air cells, sphenoid sinus, cribriform plate, ethmoid sinuses, nasal cavity, or foramen magnum.

Can One Predict the Site and Fracture Type from the Site and Type of Injury?

There is usually good correlation of the site of fracture with the site of injury, for the contrecoup phenomenon associated with brain injury is not applicable to calvarial fractures. To restate this: If trauma occurs over the forehead, then the fracture is most likely to be in this location. Furthermore, if the blow is delivered with a small, high-velocity object such as a baseball bat, hammer, or dashboard knob, the fracture usually lies immediately under the point of impact (Fig. 5.2A). On the other hand, if the blow is delivered by a broad-surface, high-velocity object such as the flat surface of a door, floor, or windshield, the fracture may be somewhat removed from the center of impact (Fig. 5.2D). The same general information is useful in predicting the actual type of fracture present. For example, in the first instance, in which a small, high-velocity object delivers the blow, the fracture often is focally depressed; in the other instance, linear or broad

curvilinear fractures result (Fig. 5.2C and D). All of these considerations are important in the assessment of calvarial fractures, and the specific types of fractures produced are dealt with in later sections.

How Important Is the Mode of Injury?

Knowledge of the mode of injury is very important, especially in the battered child syndrome, for often it leads to information regarding severity of injury. For example, an infant falling backward and striking his or her occiput on a well-cushioned floor represents a problem very different from that of an infant falling backward on a concrete floor, sidewalk, or the edge of a sink or bathtub. Clearly, one would not expect a fracture in the first instance, but in the latter case the possibility of calvarial fracturing is much greater. Consequently, it is very important to determine just how the patient was injured, for this knowledge may foretell the type and site of fracture.

Fracture Types

As stated previously, the type of fracture depends on the mode of injury, but generally speaking, one encounters lin-

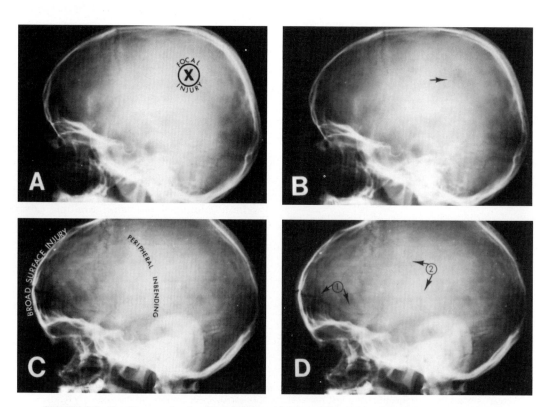

FIGURE 5.2. *Fracture mechanics.* **(A** and **B)** Focal injury. High-velocity focal injury results in dissipation of forces over a small area (*X*). The resulting fracture is a small, stellate, depressed fracture (*arrow*). **(C** and **D)** Broad-surface injury. High-velocity broad-surface injury results in a central, diastatic, V-shaped fracture (*1*), and a more peripheral curvilinear arclike fracture at the zone of peripheral inbending (*2*).

ear, curvilinear, stellate, eggshell, depressed, and diastatic sutural fractures. Linear fractures are perhaps the most common type encountered. Many of these are hairline fractures (Fig. 5.3A), and some may be more difficult to see on one view than another. If linear fractures result from greater forces, they often spread at the end closest to the point of impact, and the fracture assumes a V-shaped configuration (Fig. 5.3B). Another interesting feature of these fractures is that they usually do not cross sutures (Fig. 5.3B).

Linear fractures that are not widely diastatic are not a cause for alarm unless they cross a critical area such as the middle meningeal artery groove or the deep venous sinuses or extend into the paranasal sinuses or mastoid air cells. If they cross a vascular structure, intracranial bleeding can be a problem, and if they extend into the paranasal sinuses or mastoid air cells, meningitis can be a complication. If linear fractures are widely diastatic (Fig. 5.4), they often are associated with underlying dural or meningeal tears, subdural hematomas, or cerebral injury. In those

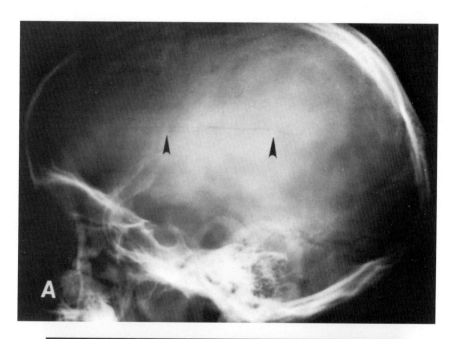

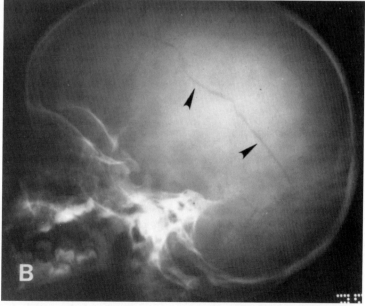

FIGURE 5.3. *Linear fractures.* **(A)** Hairline linear fracture (*arrows*) crossing middle meningeal artery area anteriorly. **(B)** Slightly diastatic linear fracture (*arrows*). Note that the fracture is wider in the center than at either end, and that the fracture stops at the coronal and lambdoid sutures.

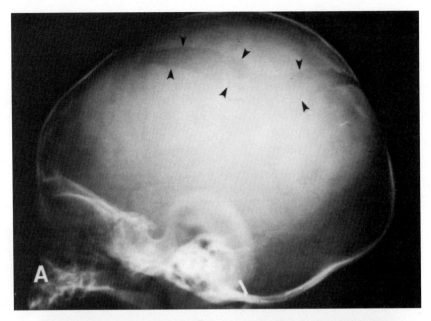

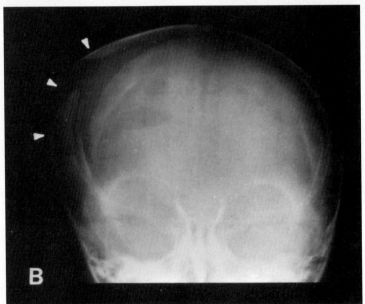

FIGURE 5.4. *Widely diastatic linear fracture.* **(A)** Note the widely diastatic fracture (*arrows*) on this lateral view. **(B)** Frontal view demonstrating how the bone edges have been displaced outwardly and how the cranial contents bulge outward (*arrows*).

cases in which a dural tear only occurs, the leptomeninges may herniate through the tear and cause the fracture to become progressively wider. This often is termed a ***growing fracture,*** and eventually the bulging, pulsating leptomeningeal sac causes calvarial erosion and a round or oval, scalloped calvarial defect around a leptomeningeal cyst (Figs. 5.5 and 5.6).

Broad, curvilinear fractures, that is, fractures with broad, peripheral arcs, usually result from high-velocity,

broad-surface injuries, and the curvilinear arclike portion of the fracture outlines the peripheral-most points of bony inbending. In many cases, these peripheral curvilinear fractures are associated with linear fractures originating from the point of impact (Fig. 5.2B). Stellate fractures are classic examples of such fractures, because the fracture lines radiate from the center of impact, and circumferentially a peripheral arc demarcates the zones of maximal inbending. Stellate fractures usually are depressed (Fig. 5.7).

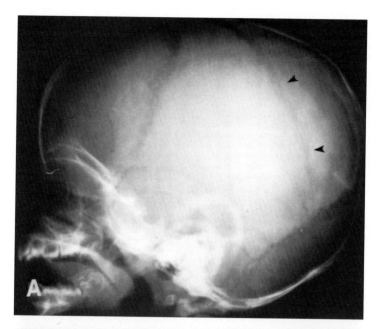

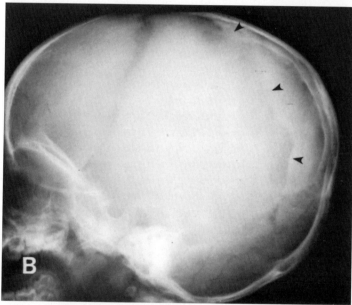

FIGURE 5.5. *Diastatic fracture with subsequent leptomeningeal cyst.* (**A**) Note the moderately diastatic linear fracture of the parietal bone (*arrows*). (**B**) Months later note how the fracture has grown, and how its edges have become scalloped (*arrows*). These findings are characteristic of a leptomeningeal cyst.

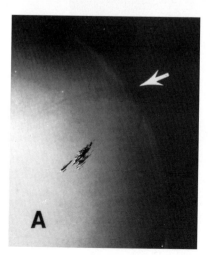
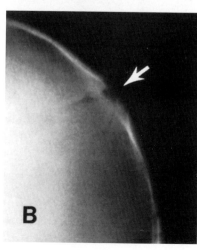

FIGURE 5.6. *Leptomeningeal cysts, varying configurations.* (**A**) Note initial fracture (*arrow*). (**B**) Months later, note a small leptomeningeal cyst (*arrow*).　*(continued on next page)*

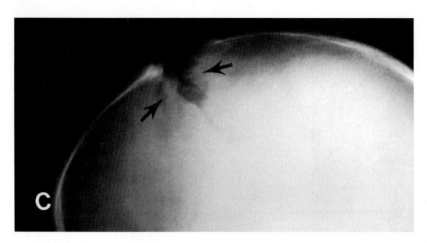

FIGURE 5.6. *(continued)* (C) Large leptomeningeal cyst *(arrows)*. (Part C courtesy of Virgil Graves, M.D.)

With ***depressed fractures,*** the injury usually results from a high-velocity impact dissipating its forces over a relatively small area of the skull (e.g., injuries sustained from baseball bats, hammers, dashboard knobs) or a high-velocity broad-surface blow. In those cases in which the impact site is over a small area, a relatively small stellate–peripheral arc type of fracture results (Fig. 5.7A). Very often these fractures are visualized better on one view than another, and tangential views are required for adequate evaluation of the degree of depression (Fig. 5.7B). Seen *en face,* sclerosis along the edge of one of the fracture fragments, undue widening of the space between two fracture fragments, or disproportionate widening of the peripheral arc portion of the fracture can serve to alert one

to the presence of the depressed element of these fractures (Fig. 5.8). Nonetheless, it cannot be overstated that depressed fractures can be most elusive on the *en face* view, and in such cases, one must learn to suspect the slightest degree of sclerosis, disproportionate radiolucency, or so forth and to pursue these findings with tangential views (Fig. 5.9). Of course, currently CT scans usually are obtained for the delineation of these fractures (Fig. 5.10); tangential views then become superfluous.

With depressed fractures resulting from broad-area injuries, the stellate–peripheral arc appearance is replaced by irregular rectangular- or triangular-shaped bony fragments seen at various angles (Fig. 5.11). Because these fragments are rotated and tilted, one or more may appear

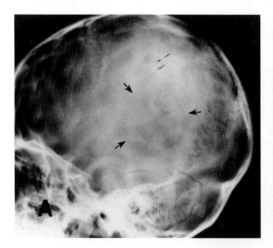

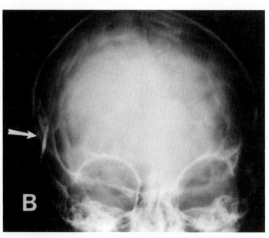

FIGURE 5.7. *Stellate, depressed skull fracture.* **(A)** Note the round peripheral zone of inbending producing a complete circle *(arrows)*. Also note stellate fractures radiating outward from the center of the circle. **(B)** Frontal view. Note degree of depression of the central fragments *(arrow)*.

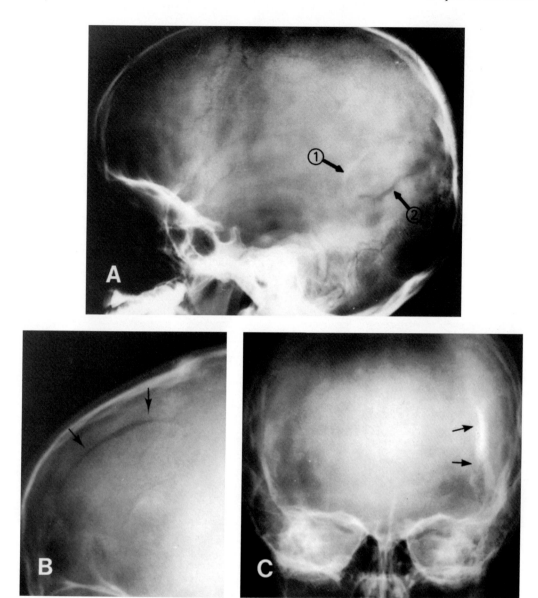

FIGURE 5.8. *Depressed fractures: other findings.* **(A)** Stellate, depressed fracture similar to the one demonstrated in Fig. 5.7. Note the area of increased sclerosis resulting from overlapping of the bony fragments (*1*), and the radiolucent, diastatic portion (*2*) of this circular, depressed fracture. Also note the typical diastatic, central, stellate limbs of the fracture. **(B)** Note the curvilinear frontal-bone fracture (*arrows*), and that it is wider in the center than at either end. This denotes depression. **(C)** Frontal view demonstrating the profound degree of depression of the central fragment (*arrows*). The degree of depression is not suspected from the lateral view in **B**.

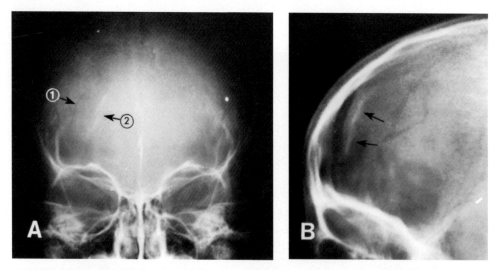

FIGURE 5.9. *Depressed fracture: subtle findings.* (**A**) Once again, note the combination of a central vertical radiolucent line (*1*) and a vertical area of increased sclerosis just medial to it (*2*). These findings represent a depressed fracture. (**B**) Lateral, tangential view more clearly demonstrates the depressed fracture fragment (*arrows*).

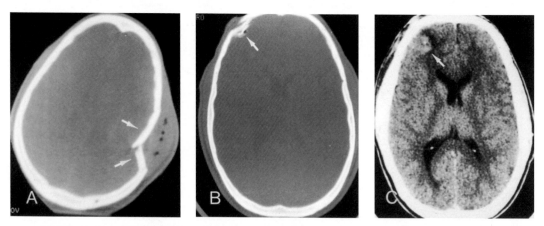

FIGURE 5.10. *Depressed skull fracture: computed tomographic findings.* (**A**) Note the markedly depressed left parietal skull fracture (*arrows*). There is a subcutaneous hematoma present, with a few bubbles of air within it. (**B**) Another patient with a focally depressed right frontal fracture (*arrow*). There is a small bubble of air along the inner table representing a mild degree of pneumocephalus. (**C**) Same patient demonstrating an underlying contusion (*arrow*).

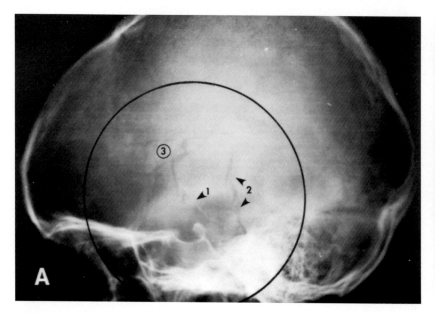
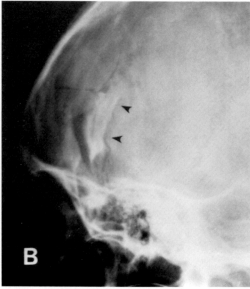

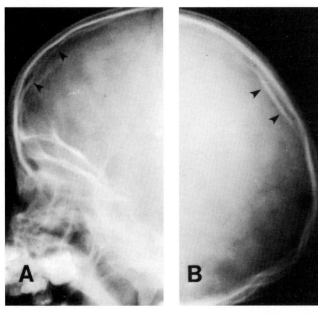

FIGURE 5.12. *Inner-table convolutions: "pseudodepressed" fractures.* Note frontal and posterior parietal inner-table sclerosis mimicking fracture fragment depression (*arrows*).

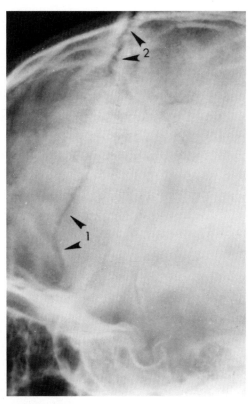

FIGURE 5.13. *Fracture causing diastasis of suture.* Note the fracture (*1*) in the lower frontal parietal region. Then note the associated spread (diastasis) of the ipsilateral coronal suture (*2*). The radiolucent line above the sella is the normal groove of the middle meningeal artery.

unduly sclerotic, or, once again, one side of a fragment may be sclerotic (overlap) and the other wide and radiolucent (diastasis). The normal finding most commonly misinterpreted as a depressed fracture is a normal inner-table convolutional marking. This can occur anywhere over the calvarium (Fig. 5.12).

Diastatic Sutural Fractures

Diastatic sutural fractures can occur in isolated form or in association with a linear fracture. In these latter cases, the fracture often runs directly into the suture (Fig. 5.13). Diastatic sutural fractures can involve any suture but are especially likely to occur in the posterior fossa, where unilateral sutural spread can serve to alert one to the presence of underlying intracranial injury (Fig. 5.14). *Generalized sutural diastasis* in the young infant or child with a closed head injury is a common problem and can occur with or without associated fracturing of the calvarium (Fig. 5.15). The explanation for this phenomenon is most likely that the sutures spread because of an

associated acute increase in cerebral mass resulting from posttraumatic hyperemia. This has been shown to be the most common intracranial manifestation of head trauma in childhood. Of course, generalized sutural diastasis also can be seen with other intracranial space-occupying problems such as subdural or epidural hematomas, but spread because of posttraumatic hyperemia alone is more common.

Finally, a few comments on the so-called *eggshell fracture of the calvarium* are in order. This fracture presents a startling roentgenographic picture (Fig. 5.16A and B), and obviously in most of these cases the fracture is not a surprise. *There is one practical aspect to these fractures, however, and that is that their findings should not be confused with similar roentgenographic findings in nor-*

FIGURE 5.11. *Depressed skull fracture: multiple fragments.* (**A**) A broad-surface, high-velocity injury has resulted in a mosaic pattern of depressed fracture fragments (*large circle*). Note linear sclerosis resulting from overlapping (*1*), diastasis caused by depression (*2*), and a generalized increase in density of one of the fragments because of depression and tangential positioning (*3*). (**B**) Tangential view demonstrating the degree of depression of one of the fragments (*arrows*). Depression of this fragment causes the fracture to appear wide and radiolucent.

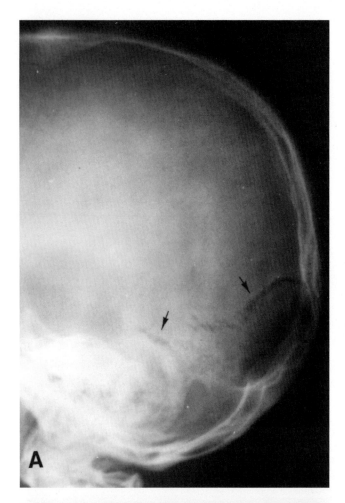

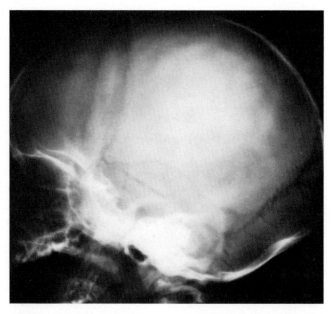

FIGURE 5.15. *Generalized suture diastasis.* This infant suffered a blow to the head. No fractures were detected, but all of the sutures showed moderate spreading. The linear lines extending posteriorly from the lambdoid and occipitomastoid sutures are normal mendosal and other accessory sutures. They are not fractures.

mal infants with numerous intraparietal accessory sutures (Fig. 5.16C and D). In the latter patients, there often is discrepancy between the clinical history and the apparent extent of calvarial fracturing. Roentgenographic differentiation often still is a problem, but it is of some assistance to note that multiple intraparietal accessory sutures usually are very symmetric (Fig. 5.16D).

When Should Follow-up Films be Obtained?

Generally speaking, the mere presence of a linear fracture does not mandate a follow-up roentgenogram. Widely or even mildly diastatic fractures, however, should be followed up with repeat roentgenograms a few weeks or months later. The reason for this is to check for the development of a posttraumatic leptomeningeal cyst (Fig. 5.6). Of course, these cysts often first are suspected clinically (i.e., a soft, pulsatile bulge is palpable), but before such a cyst becomes palpable, the radiologist often is able to detect that the fracture is spreading.

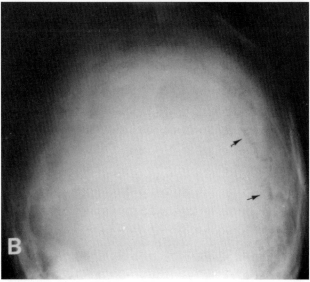

FIGURE 5.14. *Unilateral posterior fossa suture diastasis.* **(A)** Note unilateral diastasis of the lambdoid and parietomastoid sutures (*arrows*). **(B)** Towne's projection confirms unilateral spreading of these sutures (*arrows*). No fracture, however, is present.

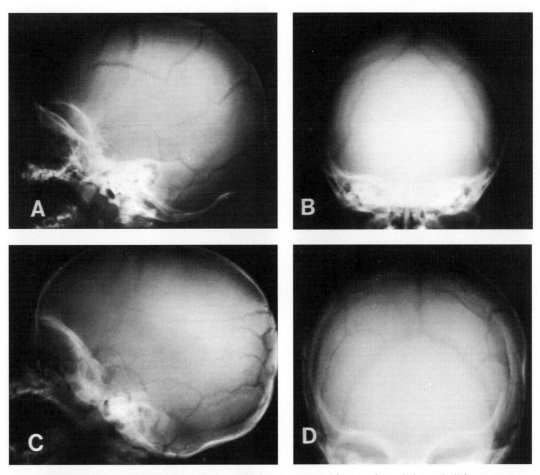

FIGURE 5.16. *Eggshell fracture versus multiple intraparietal fissures.* (**A** and **B**) Eggshell fracture. On the lateral view, note the numerous, moderately diastatic fractures and generalized spreading of the sutures. On frontal view, note asymmetry of the fractures. (**C** and **D**) Multiple intraparietal fissures. Note fracturelike appearance of the numerous intraparietal fissures on lateral view. On frontal view, note how symmetric these accessory fissures are.

REFERENCES

1. Bhimani S, Virapongse C, Sabshin JK, Sarwar M, Paterson RH Jr. Intracerebral pneumatocele: CT findings. *Radiology* 1985;154: 111–114.
2. Genieser N, Becker M. Head trauma in children. *Radiol Clin North Am* 1974;12:333–342.

Intracranial Manifestations of Head Injuries

Intracranial manifestations of head injuries are numerous and consist of acute epidural hematomas, acute subdural hematomas, vascular lacerations and aneurysms, cerebral contusions, intracerebral bleeds, focal or generalized cerebral edema, and traumatic pneumocephalus (1). Traumatic pneumocephalus can be seen on plain films (Fig. 5.17) but is more clearly visualized on CT scans (Fig. 5.18). Indeed, CT scanning is the main imaging modality for the evaluation of any intracranial injury. MR imaging also can be used but is not as useful in the early stages, because it does not detect fresh blood (6). Overall, CT scanning is the preferred modality, and it also is excellent for detecting occult intracranial damage in the battered child syndrome. In addition, it is very useful in demonstrating the phenomenon of the contrecoup injury. In these cases, although the blow to the head is sustained on one side, cerebral contusion and hemorrhage occur on the side directly opposite (Fig. 5.19). CT scanning, of course, also is excellent in delineating subdural, epidural, intra-

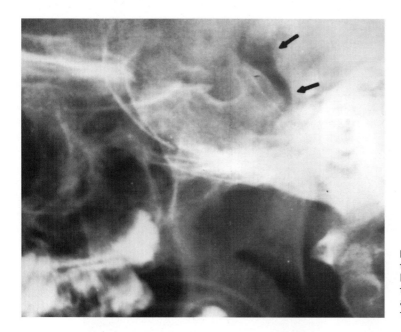

FIGURE 5.17. *Traumatic pneumocephalus.* Note air in the basal cistern (*arrows*), and that the sphenoid sinus has been obliterated by blood. Also note disruption of the base of the skull just anterior to the anterior clinoids and unilateral depression of one of the anterior fossa floors.

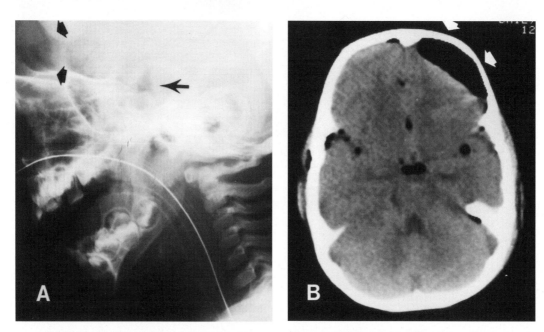

FIGURE 5.18. *Intracranial air: computed tomographic scan.* **(A)** Cross-table lateral view demonstrates large collection of air in the frontal region (*anterior arrows*). Air also is seen in the middle fossa (*single arrow*). **(B)** Computed tomographic scan more vividly demonstrates the large collection of air over the frontal region (*arrows*) and scattered throughout the calvarium.

cerebral, and subarachnoid bleeding (Fig. 5.20). Subarachnoid bleeding is characterized by an increase in density along the falx and tentorium (9). A similar appearance can be seen with the normal falx if there is pronounced cerebral edema. In these cases the brain becomes hypodense and the falx is seen in relief. With subarachnoid bleeding the cerebral tissue usually has normal density, and it is important to appreciate a subtle scalloped appear-

ance of the dense falx (Fig. 5.21). Scalloping results from blood creeping into the neighboring sulci (4). Similar collections of blood can be seen in the sylvian fissures and around the brainstem.

Brain edema, with resultant intracranial pressure, manifests in loss of the sulci and decrease in ventricular size (Fig. 5.22). It is decrease in third-ventricular size and obliteration of the basal cisterns (Fig. 5.22), however, that are most

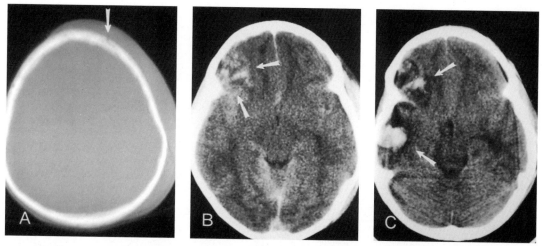

FIGURE 5.19. *Contrecoup injury.* **(A)** Note extensive edema of the scalp on the left and an underlying fracture (*arrow*). **(B)** Focal area of contusion and bleeding in the right frontal region (*arrows*). There is slight contralateral midline shift, representing a contrecoup injury. **(C)** The next day, evidence that bleeding and edema are more extensive is apparent throughout the frontal and temporal lobes (*arrows*).

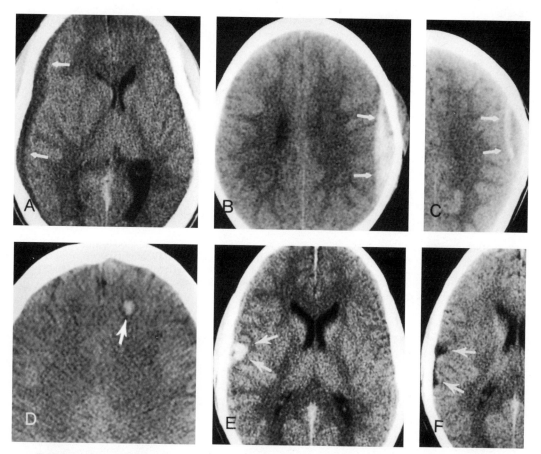

FIGURE 5.20. *Intracranial manifestations of head injury.* **(A)** Note the hypodense subdural hematoma (*arrows*). There is ipsilateral compression of the ventricles and contralateral midline shift. **(B)** Epidural bleeding (*arrows*), with some soft-tissue swelling of the scalp. **(C)** A slightly higher cut demonstrates the more characteristic elliptical appearance of the epidural bleeding. **(D)** Focal small parenchymal bleed (*arrow*). **(E)** Another patient with a focal parenchymal bleed (*arrows*). **(F)** Later, gliosis is seen in the region (*arrows*).

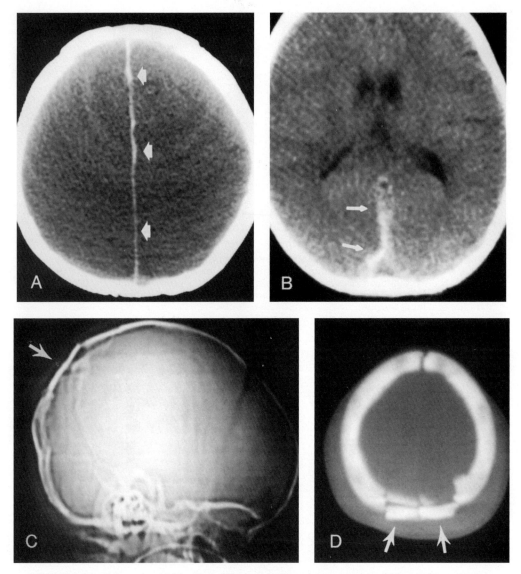

FIGURE 5.21. *Subarachnoid bleeding.* (**A**) Note scalloped appearance of blood along the falx (*arrows*). (**B**) Another patient with bleeding along the posterior falx. Brain edema also is present. (**C**) Same patient demonstrating a fracture fragment over the posterior parietal occipital region (*arrow*). (**D**) Computed tomographic scan through the upper calvarium demonstrates the comminuted posterior parietal fracture (*arrows*).

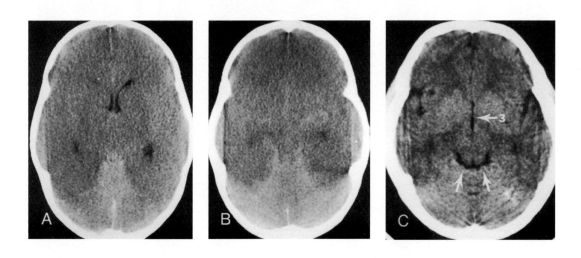

important in detecting early brain edema. It is important to appreciate these early findings of brain edema, because they may be the first findings heralding impending brainstem herniation.

It should be remembered that midway through the course of a subdural hematoma it may appear isodense on CT studies and under such circumstances may be missed unless one notices other findings such as ipsilateral ventricular compression and shift of the midline structures. Of course, if the subdurals are bilateral, such shift may not be present. Rapid, high-dose contrast CT scanning has been suggested as a method useful in circumventing this problem (5). Isodense subdural hematomas also are a problem in anemic patients, in whom the decreased iron content of the blood is the cause of the problem (9).

Finally, CT scanning, and even moreso MR imaging, have brought to light the so-called white–gray matter interface tears, or shearing injuries (2,3,7,8) resulting in small foci of increased density in the parenchyma. They are seen with accidental trauma and in the battered child syndrome (see Fig. 4.228). In the battered child syndrome it is believed that such tears are sustained from violent shaking of the child, much as are subdural hematomas and retinal hemorrhages.

REFERENCES

1. Arkins TJ, McLennan JE, Winston KR, Strand RD, Suzuki Y. Acute posterior fossa epidural hematomas in children. *Am J Dis Child* 1977;131:690–692.
2. Besenski N, Jadro-Santel D, Grevic N. Patterns of lesions of corpus callosum in inner cerebral trauma visualized by computed tomography. *Neuroradiology* 1992;34:126–130.
3. Dharker SR, Mittal RS, Bhargava N. Ischemic lesions in basal ganglia in children after minor head injury. *Neurosurgery* 1993;33: 863–865.
4. Dolinskas CA, Zimmerman RA, Bilaniuk LT. A sign of subarachnoid bleeding on cranial computed tomograms of pediatric head trauma patients. *Radiology* 1978;126:409–411.
5. Hayman LA, Evans RA, Hinck VC. Rapid-high-dose contrast computed tomography of isodense subdural hematoma and cerebral swelling. *Radiology* 1979;131:381–383.
6. Hayman LA, Pagani JJ, Kirkpatrick JB, Hinck VC. Pathophysiology of acute intracerebral and subarachnoid hemorrhage: Applications to MR imaging. *AJR* 1989;153:135–139.
7. Mendelsohn DB, Levin HS, Harward H, Bruce D. Corpus callosum lesions after closed head injury in children: MRI, clinical features and outcome. *Neuroradiology* 1992;34:384–388.
8. Mittl RL Jr, Grossman RI, Hiehle JF Jr, et al. Prevalence of MR evidence of diffuse axonal injury in patients with mild head injury and normal head CT findings. *AJR* 1994;15:1583–1589.
9. Smith WP Jr, Batnitzky S, Rengachary SS. Acute isodense subdural hematomas: A problem in anemic patients. *AJR* 1981;136: 543–546.

BASAL SKULL FRACTURES

Fractures through the base of the skull often are most difficult to detect roentgenographically. Clinically, they can be suspected if nasal discharge of cerebral spinal fluid is present, if there is bleeding from the ear, or if there is blood behind the eardrum. Roentgenographically, in looking for these fractures it is best to divide the skull into three zones: the anterior fossa, the middle fossa, and the posterior fossa. Fractures through the floor of the anterior fossa frequently involve the orbital roof and are best visualized on frontal views. In such cases, discontinuity of the cortex of the roof of the orbit, a clearly visible fracture line, or a depressed orbital fracture fragment usually alerts one to the problem (Fig. 5.23). CT scans, in some cases, can considerably augment the data obtained regarding these fractures (Fig. 5.24). In other instances, air may be present in the orbit (i.e., from the adjacent paranasal sinuses), or opacification of, or an air–fluid level in the adjacent paranasal sinuses may be noted. On lateral view, these fractures can be seen to extend through the cribriform plate into the ethmoid sinuses (Fig. 5.25A and B), but they are not always easy to detect. Furthermore, they must be differentiated from the normal, unfused planum sphenoidal (4), a commonly occurring "pseudofracture" in this area (Fig. 5.25C).

Fractures through the floor of the middle fossa also frequently are best visualized on frontal projection, but of course they also are visible on lateral view. Many of these

FIGURE 5.22. *Brain edema.* **(A)** Pronounced cerebral edema in this patient results in the absence of visualization of the various gyri and sulci. Furthermore, the lateral ventricles are markedly compressed, and there is no visualization of the third ventricle. The posterior fossa contents remain opaque; the supratentorial portion of the brain is hypodense (edema). This is characteristic of cerebral edema. **(B)** A slightly lower slice demonstrates the same findings. There is no visualization of the third ventricle or of the quadrigeminal plate cistern. **(C)** Normal patient for comparison. This slice of a computed tomographic scan is about the same level as that shown in **B** demonstrates the normal appearance of the third ventricle (*3*) and the quadrigeminal plate cistern (*lower arrows*).

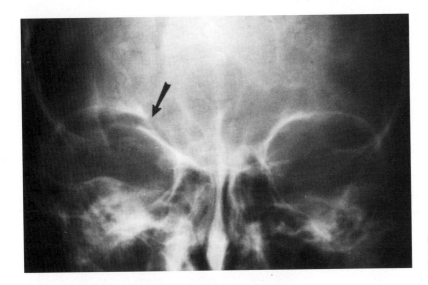

FIGURE 5.23. *Anterior fossa floor fracture: frontal view.* Note depressed supraorbital (anterior fossa floor) fracture (*arrow*).

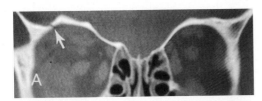

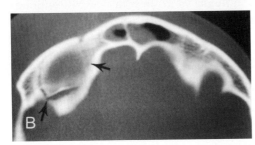

FIGURE 5.24. *Anterior fossa floor fracture: computed tomographic visualization.* **(A)** Note the supraorbital rim fracture (*arrow*). **(B)** Axial view demonstrates the fracture fragment (*arrows*) as it involves the upper wall of the orbit. Blood is seen in the frontal sinuses.

fractures also extend into the region of the sella turcica (1,2), and one may see complete disruption of the sella, fracturing through the various sellar structures, or an air–fluid level in the sphenoid sinus (Fig. 5.26). The air–fluid levels, of course, usually are visualized on crosstable lateral views of the skull or axial CT scans, and the fluid represents blood in the sphenoid sinuses. If air from the sphenoid sinuses escapes into the calvarium, one may see air in the basal cisterns (Fig. 5.17).

Fractures through the posterior fossa floor involve the temporal bone and may be associated with hearing and equilibrium problems (3). In some cases one can clearly see the linear fracture extending through the temporal bone (Fig. 5.27), but in other cases one first is alerted to the problem by the presence of unilateral opacification of the mastoid air cells only. Obliteration of the mastoid air cells results from bleeding, and even if a fracture is not

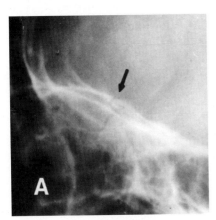

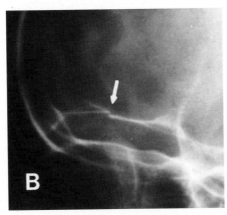

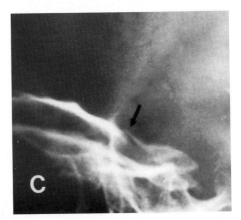

FIGURE 5.25. *Anterior fossa floor fracture versus ununited planum sphenoidale.* **(A)** Basal fracture through anterior fossa floor. Note the irregular radiolucent fracture (*arrow*) extending into the ethmoid sinus. **(B)** Another basal fracture (*arrow*). **(C)** Normal defect (*arrow*) resulting from unfused planum sphenoidale.

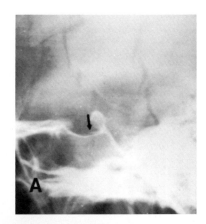

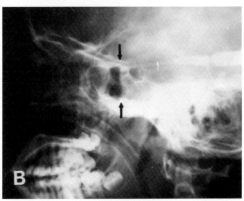

FIGURE 5.26. *Middle fossa basal fractures.* **(A)** Injured patient demonstrating a barely discernable fracture extending to the base of the skull (*arrow*). **(B)** Indirect evidence of a basal fracture extending into the sphenoid sinus is present in this patient in the form of an air–fluid level in the sphenoid sinus (*arrows*). This was a cross-table lateral view of the cervical spine with the face pointing upward.

visible, the presence of such obliteration should cause one to assume that an occult fracture is present. Thereafter, clinical correlation determines whether opacification is in fact caused by acute bleeding or by the inflammatory changes of coincidental mastoid and middle ear infection. This, of course, is very important, for middle ear infections, with mastoid involvement, are common in children. Consequently, if one does not take the time to determine whether opacification of the air cells truly is caused by bleeding, one could overdiagnose these injuries. Fractures through the tympanic portion of the temporal bone or, for that matter, any fractures through the temporal bone usually are best detected with CT scanning (Fig. 5.27C and D).

The other common fracture of the base of the skull in the posterior fossa is the vertical occipital bone fracture.

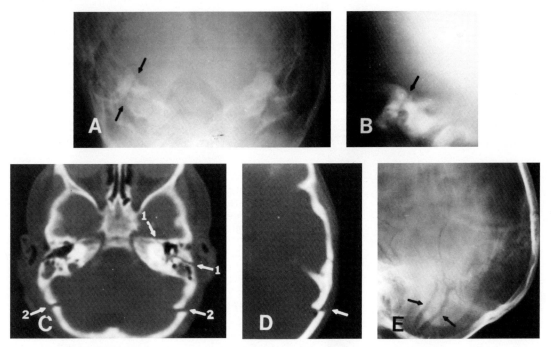

FIGURE 5.27. *Posterior fossa basal fractures.* **(A)** Note the fracture through the petrous bone on the right. Note also that the mastoid air cells are hazy because of bleeding. **(B)** Tomogram demonstrates the fracture to better advantage (*arrow*). **(C)** Computed tomographic study in another patient demonstrates a basal fracture (*1*) and bilateral occipitomastoid sutural diastatic fractures (*2*). The one on the left is offset. Also note that both mastoid air cells are hazy, because of bleeding. Another fracture was present on the other side, on another cut. **(D)** Slightly higher cut demonstrates a small bubble of air under the left occipitomastoid fracture (*arrow*). **(E)** Radiograph demonstrates numerous occipital fractures and the bilateral occipitomastoid suture diastatic fractures (*arrows*).

Most often these fractures are midline, but they may be set off to one side or the other(Fig. 5.28). The midline fracture must be differentiated from the fortuitous superimposition of the normally open metopic suture. In the latter instance, of course, the apparent fracture line crosses the foramen magnum; with a true occipital bone fracture the fracture line stops at the posterior lip of the foramen magnum (Fig. 5.29). These fractures also must be differentiated from the infrequently occurring, unusually prominent median occipital bone fissure. Normally, these fissures are short and extend upward from the lip of the foramen magnum or downward from the region of the posterior fontanel. In some cases, however, these fissures are unusually long and are misinterpreted as occipital bone fractures (see Fig. 5.49).

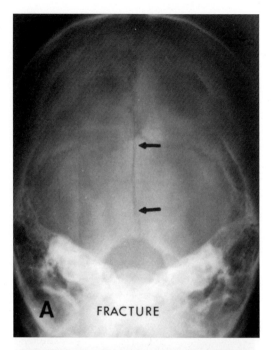

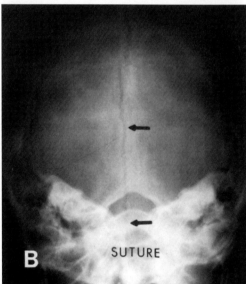

FIGURE 5.29. *Midline occipital fracture versus metopic suture.* **(A)** Note the typical appearance of a midline occipital fracture (*arrows*). Note that it stops at the posterior lip of the foramen magnum. **(B)** Metopic suture mimicking occipital fracture (*arrows*). Note that the metopic suture crosses the foramen magnum.

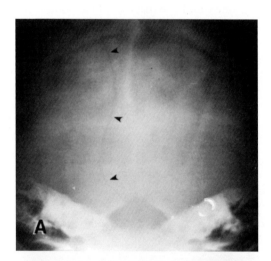

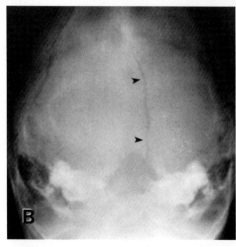

FIGURE 5.28. *Posterior occipital basal skull fractures.* **(A)** Note the typical appearance of a slightly diastatic occipital fracture (*arrows*). **(B)** Another patient demonstrating a thin linear posterior occipital fracture (*arrows*).

REFERENCES

1. Archer CR, Sundaram M. Uncommon sphenoidal fractures and their sequelae. *Radiology* 1977;122:157–161.
2. Dublin AB, Poirier VC. Fracture of the sella turcica. *AJR* 1976; 127:969–972.
3. Harwood-Nash DC. Fractures of the petrous and tympanic parts of the temporal bone in children. *AJR* 1970;110:598–607.

4. Smith TR, Kier EL. The unfused planum sphenoidal: Differentiation from fracture. *Radiology* 1971;98:305–309.

FRACTURES VERSUS NORMAL SUTURES, FISSURES, AND VASCULAR GROOVES

So common is the problem of a normal suture, fissure, or vascular groove mimicking a fracture that it is just as important to be familiar with these structures as with the fractures themselves. In this regard, it is best to become familiar with the direction in which these normal sutures, fissures, and vascular grooves travel (1,8–10). The sutures and fissures more than the vascular grooves are remarkably consistent from patient to patient and almost always appear in the same place. Consequently, if one sees a radiolucent line that does not conform to the site and location of one of these structures, then one should consider it to represent a fracture. These normal variations are considered in three general areas: the frontal region, the temporoparietal region, and the occipital region.

Frontal Region Fractures and Pseudofractures

One of the most common structures misinterpreted as a fracture in the frontal bone is the vascular groove produced by the supraorbital branch of the ophthalmic artery. The problem is not so great on frontal view (Fig. 5.30), but on lateral view, often it is almost impossible to differentiate the two (Figs. 5.31 and 5.32). A few general rules can be applied, however: (a) Most vascular grooves are located in the anterior third of the frontal bone; (b) most vascular grooves run in a vertical fashion with a gentle, posterior curve; (c) vascular grooves tend to have sclerotic edges, but fractures have sharp, nonsclerotic edges; and (d) vascular grooves seldom run in a horizontal or anteriorly sloping direction.

Another problem arising in the anterior fossa, but this time on frontal view, is the misinterpretation of a persistently open metopic suture (11) as a fracture. This suture commonly is open in children and to the unwary can suggest a midline frontal bone fracture (Fig. 5.33A). This is an even greater problem if the suture is partially closed (Fig. 5.33B). The metopic suture also is notorious for mimicking an occipital bone fracture on Towne's projection (Fig. 5.29B). On lateral view, a less common problem in the frontal region is the misinterpretation of the fissure representing the unfused planum sphenoidal (7) as a basal, anterior fossa floor skull fracture (Fig. 5.25C).

Temporoparietal Region Fractures and Pseudofractures

In terms of vascular grooves in this portion of the skull, it is the outer-table groove of one of the branches of the superficial temporal artery that causes most problems (Fig. 5.34B). In some cases, these vascular grooves virtually defy distinction from fractures, except perhaps through the fact that often the grooves show sclerosis along their edges. These grooves can be seen projected over the entire sellar region and, in addition, one also can encounter similar problems with the posterior branch of

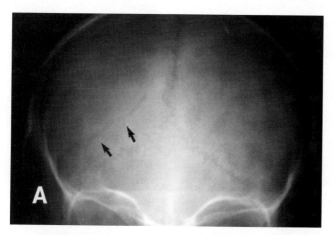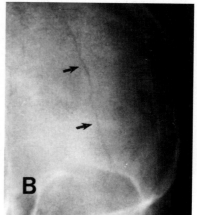

FIGURE 5.30. *Frontal vascular groove versus fracture.* **(A)** Note the radiolucent line resulting from a normal frontal vascular groove (*arrows*). **(B)** Thin, long radiolucent line representing a frontal fracture extending into the left orbital roof (*arrows*). Distinction between a vascular groove and fracture on frontal view usually is not difficult.

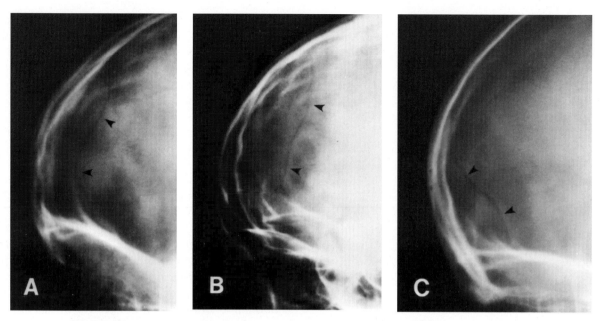

FIGURE 5.31. *Frontal vascular grooves: lateral view.* **(A)** Note typical appearance of a vascular groove in the frontal region (*arrows*). Characteristically it assumes a gentle posteriorly curving course. **(B)** Another vascular groove, somewhat less typical (*arrows*), and one that might easily be misinterpreted as a frontal-bone fracture. **(C)** Unusual direction of another normal vascular groove (*arrows*). In this case, however, the slight sclerosis along the edge of the groove identifies it as a vascular groove.

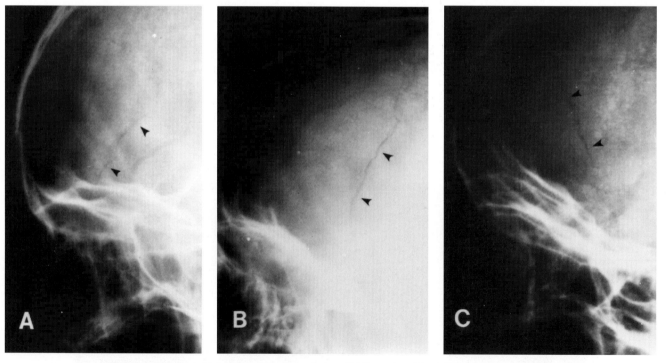

FIGURE 5.32. *Frontal bone fractures: lateral view.* **(A)** Note the thin radiolucent line representing a frontal-bone fracture (*arrows*). Its gentle posteriorly curving course could cause one to misinterpret it as a vascular groove. A true vascular groove of the middle meningeal artery lies just posterior to the fracture. **(B)** Frontal bone fracture located in the posterior third of the frontal bone (*arrows*). Frontal vascular grooves are quite uncommon in this area. **(C)** Anteriorly sloping frontal fracture (*arrows*). Vascular grooves usually do not head in this direction.

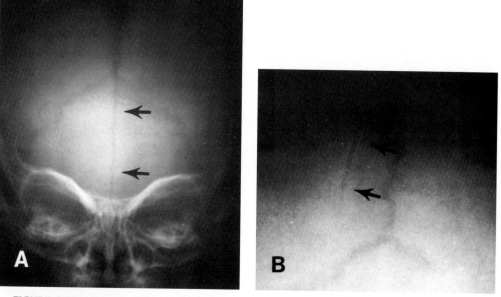

FIGURE 5.33. *Metopic suture: pseudofracture.* **(A)** Note the typical location of the metopic suture (*arrows*). **(B)** Partially obliterated metopic suture (*arrows*) extending from the anterior aspect of the anterior fontanel. The fontanel is not visualized on this reproduction. Note slight sclerosis along the suture edge, identifying it as a normal suture and not a fracture.

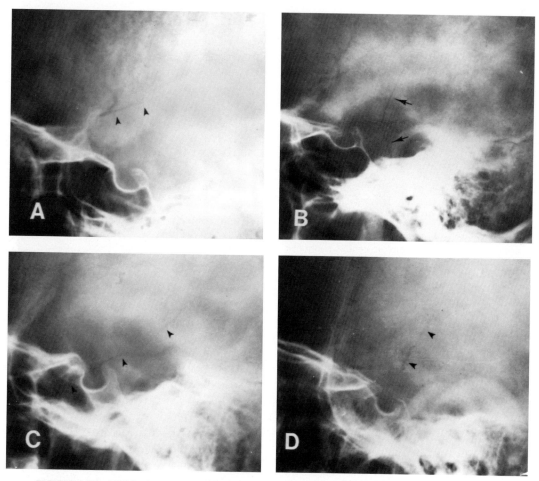

FIGURE 5.34. *Middle fossa vascular grooves versus fracture.* **(A)** Typical appearance of a vascular groove produced by the posterior branch of the middle meningeal artery (*arrows*). **(B)** Fracture-like appearance of a vascular groove produced by one of the branches of the superficial temporal artery (*arrows*). It would be difficult to differentiate this groove from a fracture. **(C)** True fracture (*arrows*) of the middle fossa. The fracture line is somewhat sharper than the vascular groove in **B**, but still the two might be confused. **(D)** Small linear fracture in the lower parietal bone (*arrows*). Irregularity of the bone edges suggests a fracture.

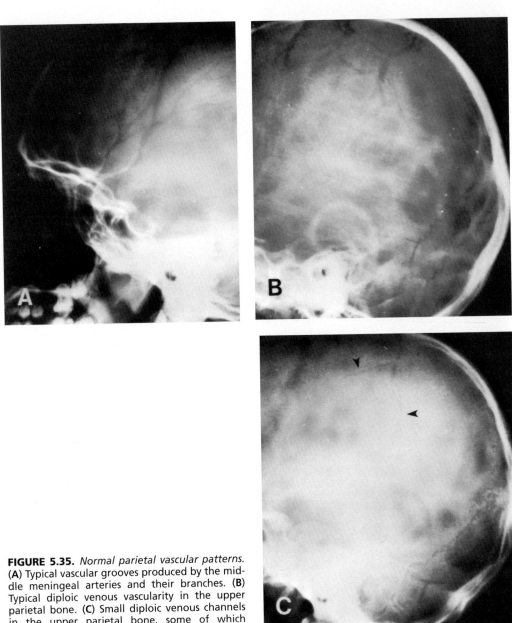

FIGURE 5.35. *Normal parietal vascular patterns.* (A) Typical vascular grooves produced by the middle meningeal arteries and their branches. (B) Typical diploic venous vascularity in the upper parietal bone. (C) Small diploic venous channels in the upper parietal bone, some of which (*arrows*) could be misinterpreted as a fracture.

the middle meningeal artery (Fig. 5.34A). Parietal diploic vascular grooves are not easily confused with calvarial fractures, nor are the inner-table vascular grooves produced by the main branches of the middle meningeal artery (Fig. 5.35). It is only if either of these vascular grooves is very thin that confusion with calvarial fractures can occur (Fig. 5.35).

As far as sutures in this area are concerned, although a number exist (Fig. 5.36), it is the squamosal suture that causes most difficulty. Indeed, with slight degrees of rotation of the calvarium, either from front to back or top to bottom, this suture can appear so like a fracture that it is impossible to convince oneself that it simply represents a normal suture (Fig. 5.37). This is less of a problem with

the other sutures in the area (Fig. 5.37C). On frontal view, the squamosal suture also is a problem and commonly mimics a fracture (Fig. 5.38). Fortunately, however, almost always the sclerotic line along either side of the suture identifies it as such. Either the posterior or anterior limbs of the squamosal suture can present in this fashion.

In the young infant, accessory fissures along the posterior parietal bone can mimic small wedgelike linear fractures. Generally speaking, these fissures occur in the lower two thirds of the parietal bone and often are multiple. In some cases, they are associated with a posterior parietal bony defect, the so-called third fontanel (2). If these fissures occur over the lower two thirds of the parietal bone and if no soft tissue swelling overlies them, then they most likely are normal fissures. If they lie in the upper third of the posterior parietal bone, however, and soft tissue swelling overlies them, then a fracture is most likely (Fig. 5.39). This rule, of course, is not 100% foolproof, for obviously one can encounter fractures in the lower two thirds of the parietal bone and normal fissures in the upper third, but still it is useful in most cases.

Another problem with accessory sutures in the parietal bone is so-called intraparietal sutures or fissures (5). The fissures have a great propensity to mimic parietal bone fractures, especially if they are unilateral (Fig. 5.40). It is of some value, however, to note that these fissures usually are relatively horizontal in position, and because of this if a vertical, radiolucent line is encountered, it should represent a fracture. In addition, if the radiolucent line truly

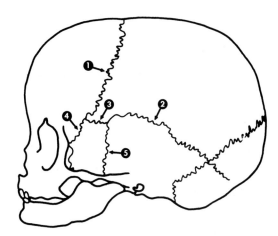

FIGURE 5.36. *Normal anterior and middle fossa sutures: diagrammatic representation.* Coronal suture (*1*), squamosal suture (*2*), sphenoparietal suture (*3*), sphenofrontal suture (*4*), and sphenosquamosal suture (*5*).

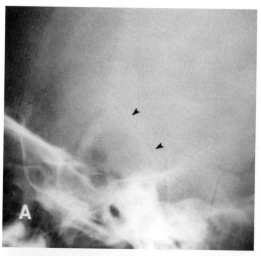

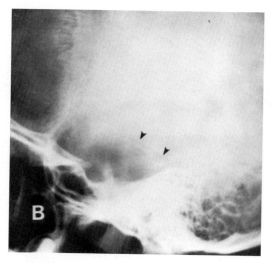

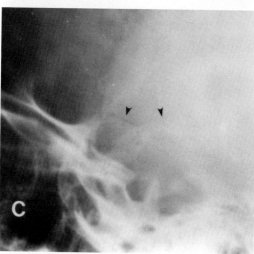

FIGURE 5.37. *Squamosal suture pseudofractures: lateral view.* (**A**) Note fracturelike appearance of the normal squamosal suture (*arrows*). The near-vertical radiolucent line about an inch posteroinferior to it is the occipitomastoid suture, which also appears fracturelike because of rotation of the skull. (**B**) Another normal squamosal suture (*arrows*) that is virtually indistinguishable from a fracture. (**C**) Normal sphenoparietal suture (*arrows*) mimicking a fracture. Compare these findings with true fractures in this area demonstrated in Figs. 5.34C and D.

represents a fracture, overlying soft tissue edema usually is present (Fig. 5.41). Of course, if the fissures are bilateral, as they commonly are, their remarkable symmetry usually serves to identify them correctly (Fig. 5.42). Nonetheless, if multiple, these sutures can mimic multiple, eggshell calvarial fractures.

Along the base of the skull in the middle fossa, the only normal structures to be misinterpreted as fractures are the sphenooccipital and intersphenoid synchondroses (Fig. 5.43). The intersphenoid synchondrosis usually disappears by the age of 2 years (6), but the sphenooccipital synchondrosis remains open until the late teens and early adulthood (4).

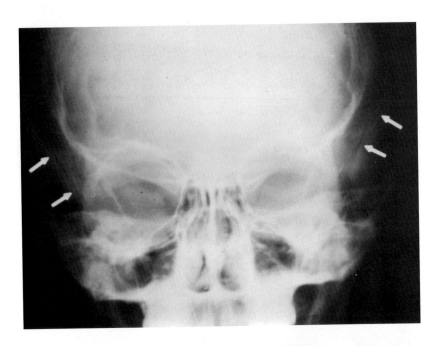

FIGURE 5.38. *Squamosal suture pseudofractures: frontal view.* In certain patients, the anterior or posterior limbs of the squamosal suture can appear slitlike on frontal projection (*arrows*) and suggest a fracture. In this case, note typical sclerosis on either side of the radiolucent lines identifying them as normal squamosal sutures. On the left, both anterior and posterior limbs of the squamosal suture are demonstrated.

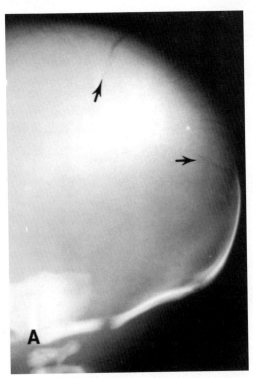
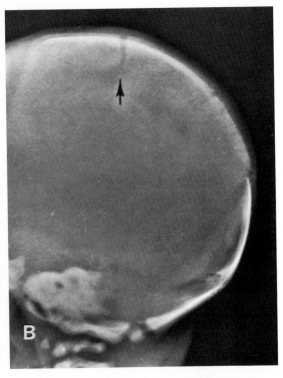

FIGURE 5.39. *Posterior parietal fissures versus fracture.* **(A)** Typical posterior parietal fissuring. This is a normal. Two of the fissures stand out more prominently (*arrows*), and either one could be misinterpreted as a fracture. **(B)** True parietal bone fracture (*arrow*). Note slight degree of soft tissue swelling over the fracture site. (Reproduction enhanced to bring out soft tissues.)

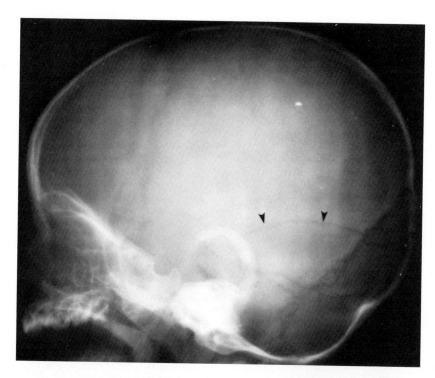

FIGURE 5.40. *Unilateral intraparietal fissure mimicking fracture.* Note the fracturelike appearance of this normal intraparietal fissure (*arrows*). All of the sutures in the occipital bone also are normal.

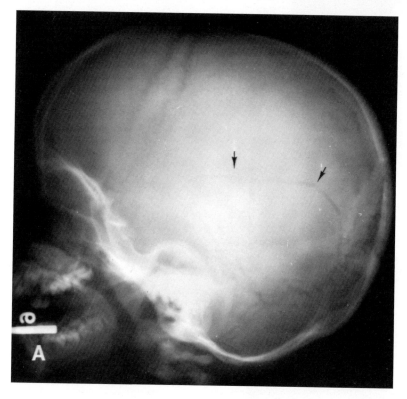

FIGURE 5.41. *Transverse parietal fracture.* **(A)** Note the transverse parietal bone fracture (*arrows*). Also note that all of the sutures show minimal diastasis.

(continued on next page)

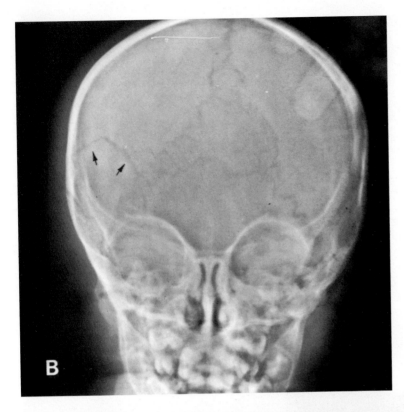

FIGURE 5.41. *(continued)* **(B)** Frontal view demonstrating the fracture *(arrows)*. Also note extensive soft tissue edema over the right side of the calvarium. Such edema is not present with normal intraparietal accessory fissures. (Frontal view altered to bring out soft tissues.)

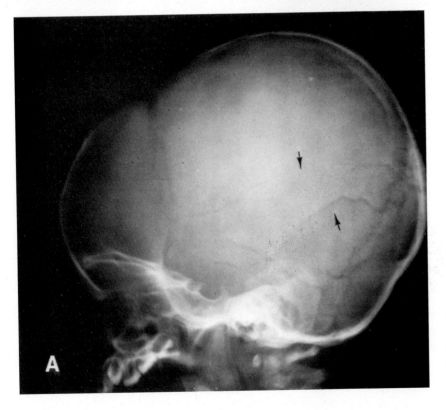

FIGURE 5.42. *Bilateral intraparietal accessory fissures.* **(A)** Either one of these normal fissures can be misinterpreted as a fracture *(arrows)*.

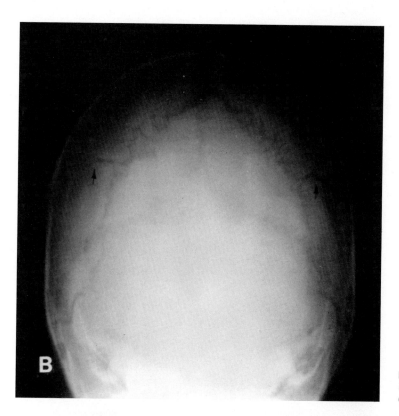

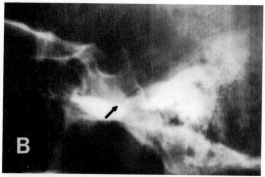

FIGURE 5.42. *(continued)* **(B)** Frontal view demonstrating characteristic symmetry of these normal fissures (*arrows*).

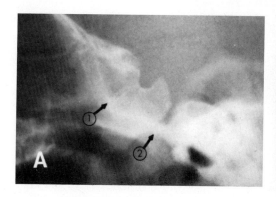

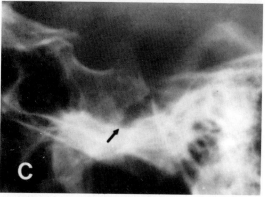

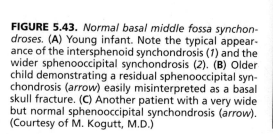

FIGURE 5.43. *Normal basal middle fossa synchondroses.* **(A)** Young infant. Note the typical appearance of the intersphenoid synchondrosis (*1*) and the wider sphenooccipital synchondrosis (*2*). **(B)** Older child demonstrating a residual sphenooccipital synchondrosis (*arrow*) easily misinterpreted as a basal skull fracture. **(C)** Another patient with a very wide but normal sphenooccipital synchondrosis (*arrow*). (Courtesy of M. Kogutt, M.D.)

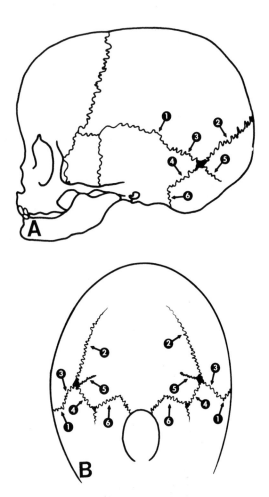

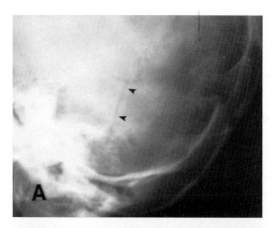

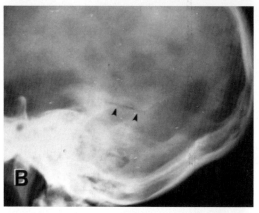

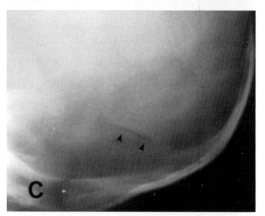

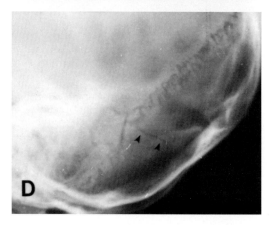

FIGURE 5.44. *Posterior fossa sutures: diagrammatic representation.* Lateral (**A**) and Towne's (**B**) projections. Squamosal suture (*1*), lambdoid suture (*2*), parietomastoid suture (*3*), occipitomastoid suture (*4*), mendosal suture (*5*), and innominate synchondrosis complex (*6*).

Occipital Region Fractures and Pseudofractures

The only vascular groove that can cause confusion in the occipital region of the skull is the groove for the mastoid emissary vein, but usually it is so tortuous that it presents no real problem. Sutures, on the other hand, are a significant problem in this area, for the occipital region of the skull is cluttered with normal and accessory sutures and synchondroses (Fig. 5.44). Familiarity with all of them is mandatory, for otherwise one is sure to misinterpret one of them as a fracture.

FIGURE 5.45. *Posterior fossa pseudofractures: lateral view.* (**A**) Note fracturelike appearance of the normal occipitomastoid suture (*arrows*). (**B**) Fracturelike appearance of the normal parietomastoid suture (*arrows*). (**C**) Isolated visualization of one mendosal suture (*arrows*) in a young infant. To the uninitiated, this is virtually indistinguishable from a fracture. (**D**) Mendosal suture pseudofracture (*arrows*) in an older child.

On lateral view, the sutures most commonly visible are the lambdoid, parietomastoid, occipitomastoid, and mendosal; the visible synchondrosis is the innominate synchondrosis. The four sutures radiate outward from the region of the posterolateral fontanel, but the mendosal suture usually is visible more in infancy. The problem with these sutures is not that they are difficult to identify in the average patient, but rather that with slight degrees of rotation any one of them can appear absolutely fracturelike (Fig. 5.45). This is not to say that true fractures in this area do not occur, for indeed they do (Fig. 5.46), and because of this one must be able to differentiate a fracture from a suture. If one believes that a radiolucent line represents a normal suture, one should look for its mate on the other side. Whether this contralateral suture appears fracturelike or not, if only two radiolucent lines heading in the same direction are identified, then one can be confident that the fracturelike line is simply a normal suture. However, if an extra line exists (i.e., a third radiolucent line), or if one finds these radiolucent lines to be traveling in unusual directions, then one should consider them to be fractures (Figs. 5.46 and 5.47). These sutures also are problems on frontal and Towne's projections, on which slight degrees of rotation also can cause them to appear absolutely fracturelike (Fig. 5.48).

In the posterior fossa, if one remembers that most of the sutures are paired, a third radiolucent line, even though

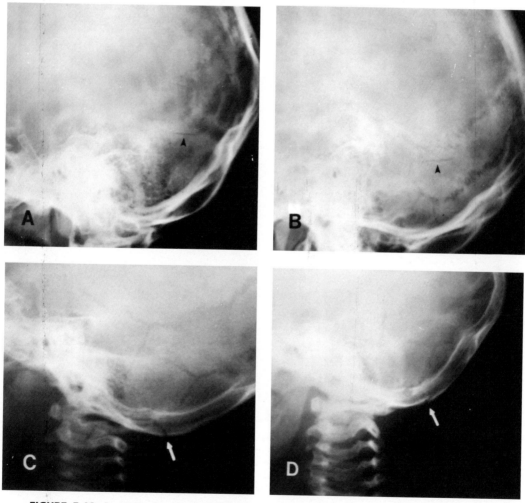

FIGURE 5.46. *Posterior fossa pseudofractures versus true fracture.* **(A)** Note the fracturelike appearance of the normal parietomastoid suture (*arrow*). **(B)** Fracture of the posterior fossa (*arrow*) mimicking a parietomastoid suture. If one lines this radiolucent line up with the two true parietomastoid sutures, however, one finds that it represents an extra radiolucent line and hence is probably a fracture. **(C)** Normal innominate synchondrosis (*arrow*). **(D)** Diastatic, slightly offset fracture of innominate synchondrosis (*arrow*). Normal fissures and synchondroses are not offset, and thus this probably is a fracture.

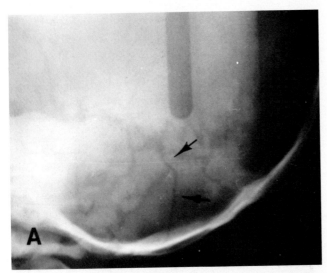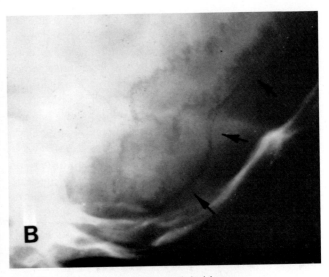

FIGURE 5.47. *True occipital fractures: lateral view.* **(A)** Note the fracture in the occipital bone (*arrows*). There are no normal sutures in this area. **(B)** Another patient demonstrating a long linear fracture of the occipital bone (*arrows*). All of the normal sutures are identified, and this represents an extra radiolucent line, or in other words a fracture.

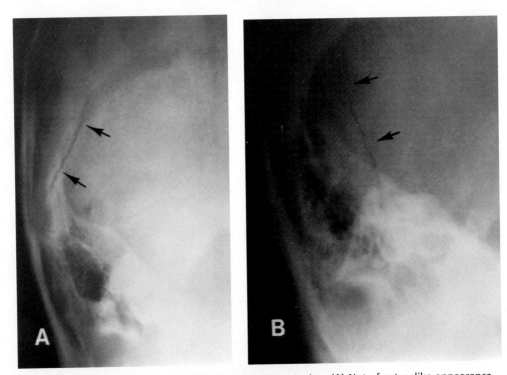

FIGURE 5.48. *Occipital suture pseudofractures: Towne's view.* **(A)** Note fracturelike appearance and characteristic slope of the normal parietomastoid suture (*arrows*). **(B)** Pseudofracture appearance and characteristic slope of the occipitomastoid suture (*arrows*).

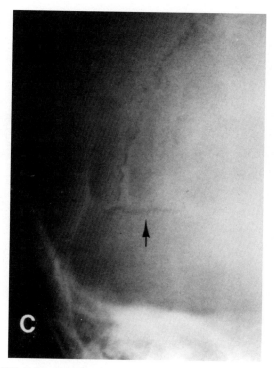

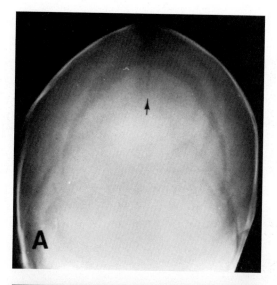

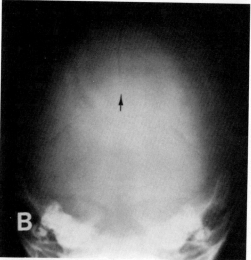

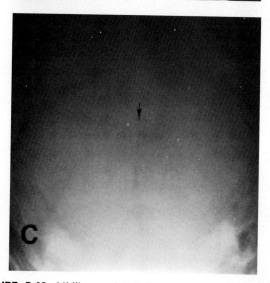

FIGURE 5.48. *(continued)* **(C)** Small residual mendosal suture *(arrow)* mimicking a fracture.

heading in a direction suggestive of a normal suture, should be considered a fracture. In addition, of course, if a radiolucent line is located in a totally unexpected place, a fracture should be considered.

In addition to these problems, the occipital bone also is prone to irregular ossification over the posterior lip of the foramen magnum. Furthermore, the median occipital fissure (3) visualized just below the posterior fontanel commonly is misinterpreted as a fracture. This fissure usually is seen in young infants only and is not more than 1 to 2 cm in length (Fig. 5.49A). Very rarely it is longer, and then it is more likely to suggest a midline occipital fracture (Fig. 5.49B). A similar problem can occur with an abnormally long but normal, fissure extending upward from the posterior lip of the foramen magnum (Fig. 5.49C).

Finally, one should note that a number of interparietal accessory bones can be seen in the occipital bone, just at the junction of the lambdoid and sagittal sutures. On frontal view, this bone (inca bone) or bones are of characteristic appearance and location and usually are not misinterpreted as fractures (Fig. 5.50). On lateral view, however, they often appear very sclerotic and frequently are misinterpreted as a depressed fracture (Fig. 5.50).

FIGURE 5.49. *Midline occipital fissures: pseudofractures.* **(A)** Note typical appearance and length of the median occipital fissure *(arrow)* visualized on Towne's projection in young infants. **(B)** Unusually long but normal median occipital fissure *(arrow)* in another infant. Also, note residual mendosal sutures on both sides. **(C)** Unusually long occipital fissure *(arrow)* arising from the posterior lip of the foramen magnum.

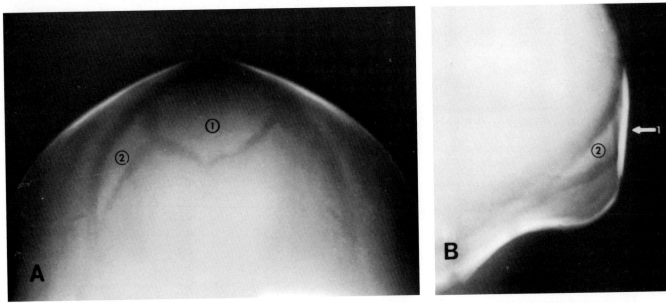

FIGURE 5.50. *Interparietal bone.* **(A)** Note the large interparietal (inca) bone (*1*) and the other accessory bone (*2*). These usually are not misinterpreted as fractures on this view. **(B)** On lateral view, however, their extremely sclerotic appearance (*arrow*) can strongly suggest a depressed fracture, especially if the skull is slightly obliqued.

Base of Skull Pseudofractures

On basal skull views, almost any of the normal sutures mentioned, with certain degrees of obliquity, can be projected so as to mimic a fracture. Most often, this occurs with the coronal suture or one of the posterior fossa sutures (Fig. 5.51). The various sutures and synchondroses posing problems on plain films are not nearly as troublesome on CT scans. They still can be problematic, however, and most of them are demonstrated in Fig. 5.52.

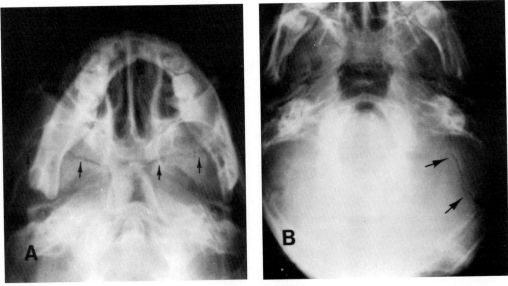

FIGURE 5.51. *Sutural pseudofractures on basal views.* **(A)** Note the coronal suture crossing the base of the skull (*arrows*). **(B)** Occipitomastoid suture (*arrows*) appearing as though it were a fracture on basal view.

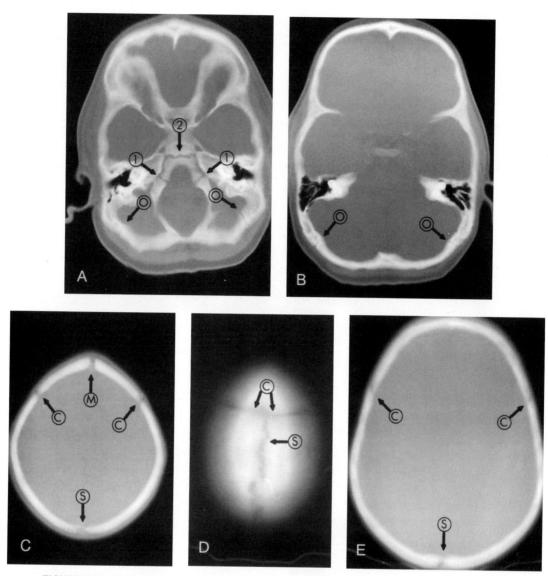

FIGURE 5.52. *Normal sutures, and synchondroses: computed tomographic study.* **(A)** Base of the skull view. **(B)** Lower calvarial posterior fossa view. **(C)** Upper calvarial view. **(D)** Another upper calvarial view. **(E)** Midcalvarial view. Coronal suture, *C*; sagittal suture, *S*; metopic suture, *M*; occipito-mastoid suture, *O*; innominate synchondrosis, *1*; sphenooccipital synchondrosis, *2*.

REFERENCES

1. Allen W, Kier E, Rothman S. Pitfalls in the evaluation of skull trauma: A review. *Radiol Clin North Am* 1973;11:479–503.
2. Chemke J, Robinson A. Third fontanelle. *J Pediatr* 1969;75: 617–622.
3. Franken EA Jr. The midline occipital fissure: Diagnosis of a fracture versus anatomic variants. *Radiology* 1969;93:1043–1046.
4. Irwin AL. Roentgen demonstration of the time of closure of the spheno-occipital synchondrosis. *Radiology* 1960;75:451–452.
5. Shapiro R. Anomalous parietal sutures and the bipartite parietal bone. *AJR* 1972;115:569–577.
6. Shopfner CE, Wolfe TW, O'Kell RT. The intersphenoid synchondrosis. *AJR* 1968;104:184–193.
7. Smith TR, Kier EL. The unfused planum sphenoidal: Differentiation from fracture. *Radiology* 1971;98:305–309.
8. Swischuk LE. The growing skull. *Semin Roentgenol* 1974;9: 115–124.
9. Swischuk LE. The normal newborn skull. *Semin Roentgenol* 1974;9:101–113.
10. Swischuk LE. The normal pediatric skull: Variations and artifacts. *Radiol Clin North Am* 1972;10:277–290.
11. Torgerson J. A roentgenologic study of the metopic suture. *Acta Radiol* 1950;33:1–11.

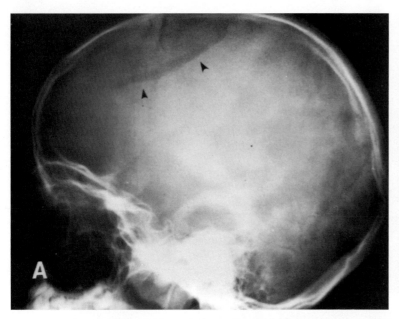

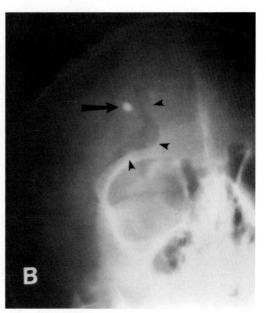

FIGURE 5.53. *Scalp laceration and pebble artifacts.* **(A)** Note the radiolucency secondary to a deep laceration over the calvarium (*arrows*). **(B)** Another patient with a laceration over the forehead (*small arrows*) and a pebble embedded in the laceration (*large arrow*). Such a laceration should not be misinterpreted as a depressed skull fracture.

ARTIFACTS MIMICKING CALVARIAL FRACTURES

A number of artifacts can be mistaken for calvarial abnormalities (1). One of the most common is the laceration that projects as a radiolucent defect or pseudofracture of the cal-

varium (Fig. 5.53A). Clinical correlation is the rule here, and it is most important that such correlation be accomplished, for if the laceration suggests a fracture, it often suggests a depressed one. Other artifacts that can cause problems in the interpretation of skull roentgenograms include dirt and pebbles over the scalp and in the hair (Fig. 5.53B),

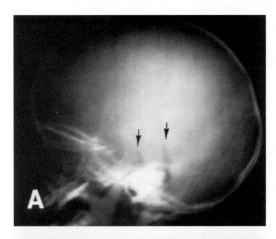

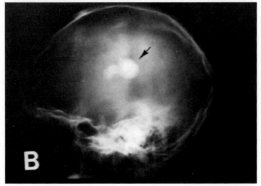

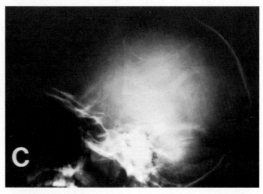

FIGURE 5.54. *Other artifacts.* **(A)** Note accumulations of air in the pinnae of both ears (*arrows*). These air collections should not be misinterpreted as pneumocephalus. **(B)** Tightly braided hair mimicking an intracranial calcification (*arrow*). **(C)** Whorl-like configurations of strands of wet hair.

hair soaked with water or blood (Fig. 5.54C), hair braids, air trapped in the pinna of the ear so as to suggest pneumocephalus, and abnormal shadows produced by the pinna and the earlobe itself (Fig. 5.54).

REFERENCE

1. Swischuk LE. The normal pediatric skull: Variations and artifacts. *Radiol Clin North Am* 1972;10:277–290.

FACIAL, ORBITAL, AND MANDIBULAR FRACTURES

Fractures of the face, orbit, and mandible are certainly not as common in the infant and young child as they are in the adult. Nasal fractures might be considered an exception, but generally speaking, facial fractures do not become a major problem until the child is older, and at this age, the considerations are not different from those in the adult. The presence or absence of symmetry is the key to the assessment of facial bone fractures. Most faces are very symmetrical, and thus if one encounters any asymmetry of cortical continuity or contour, one should suspect a fracture. In terms of which views to obtain, one usually obtains frontal, posteroanterior, lateral, and Water's views.

The Water's view, however, is the most productive and the single most important view in the assessment of facial injuries. Thereafter, one might require special orbital, zygomatic arch, or mandibular views for complete assessment. These views now often are supplanted by CT scans (6,21), but still, in most cases of facial trauma, standard plain films are the starting point and thus require expertise in assessment.

Fracture Types

Facial fractures generally can be divided into nasal fractures, orbital fractures, zygomatic–maxillary fractures, and mandibular fractures (1,2).

Nasal Bone Fractures

Nasal bone fractures usually are best demonstrated with moderately penetrated lateral views of the nasal bone and a Water's view for assessment of nasal septal deviation. Fractures of the nasal bone can be simple linear fractures, depressed fractures, or comminuted fractures, and all can be associated with other facial fractures or fractures of the spine or the maxillary bone (Fig. 5.55). Linear fractures must be differentiated from three normal radiolucent lines commonly seen around the nose: the nasomaxillary suture,

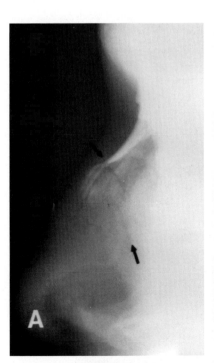
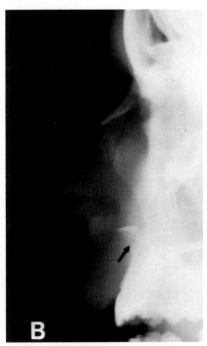
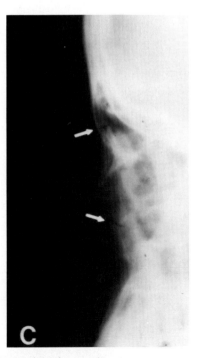

FIGURE 5.55. *Nasal fractures.* **(A)** Note the comminuted nasal fracture. Two of the fracture lines are identified with arrows. **(B)** Note the comminuted fracture of the nasal bone. The vertical radiolucent line is a fracture. It is too far anterior to be the nasomaxillary suture and too sharp and radiolucent to be the nasociliary groove. Both of these normal structures are shown in Fig. 5.56. Also note the fracture through the spinous process of the maxillary bone (*arrow*). **(C)** This patient was hit in the nose and face. Note fractures through the anterior wall of the frontal sinus (*upper arrow*) and the maxillary bone below the nose (*lower arrow*).

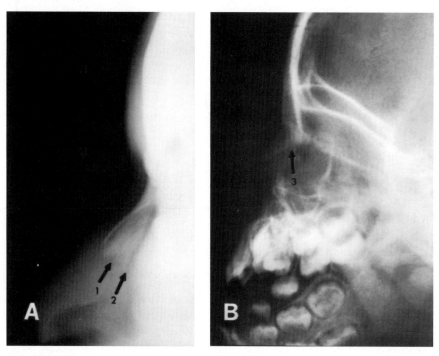

FIGURE 5.56. *Pseudofractures of nasal bone.* Note the barely visible groove for the nasociliary nerve (*1*) and the more prominent vertical radiolucent line representing the nasomaxillary suture (*2*). Both of these structures can be misinterpreted as fractures. (**B**) Normal nasofrontal suture (*3*).

the groove for the nasociliary nerve, and the nasofrontal suture (Fig. 5.56). The lines produced by the nasomaxillary suture and groove for the nasociliary nerve are straight and more or less parallel the anterior aspect of the nasal bone. This is not to say that fractures do not occur in this plane, but only to indicate that if one sees a radiolucent line traveling in the opposite direction or, even better, in the horizontal plane, then one should assume the line to represent a fracture.

Orbital Fractures

Fractures of the orbits can be linear or depressed and often occur in conjunction with frontal bone or other facial fractures. They also occur alone, however, and Caldwell, Water's, lateral, or oblique (optic foramen) views may be required for their complete demonstration (Fig. 5.57). CT scans, however, eventually are obtained and more precisely demonstrate these fractures (Fig. 5.58).

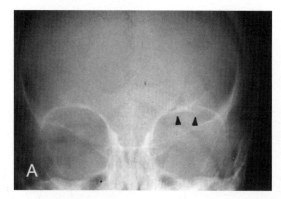
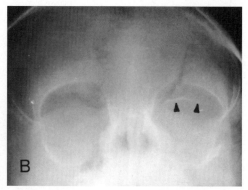

FIGURE 5.57. *Superior orbital rim fracture.* (**A**) Note generalized increase in soft tissue density over the left orbit and also note discontinuity of the left orbital roof (*arrows*). A depressed fracture fragment and a fracture extending into the frontal bone above the orbit are suggested. (**B**) Water's view more clearly demonstrates the depressed fragment (*arrows*) and clearly demonstrates the fracture extending into the frontal bone.

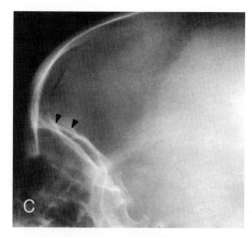 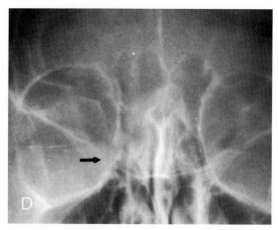

FIGURE 5.57. *(continued)* **(C)** Lateral view demonstrating the fracture of the frontal bone and the malaligned left anterior orbital roof (*arrows*). Compare the configuration of the left orbital roof with the normal right orbital roof beneath it. **(D)** Medial orbital wall fracture. Note suble discontinuity of the cortex of the medial orbital wall on the right (*arrow*). Also note that the ethmoid air sinuses are obliterated because of associated bleeding.

A special type of fracture of the orbit is the ***blowout fracture.*** This fracture occurs through the floor of the orbit and results from blunt trauma to the eye (2,5). Usually it occurs in isolated form, but it can be associated with other facial fractures, especially the tripod fracture of the maxillary bone. In the blowout fracture, the hydrostatic pressure produced within the globe blows out, or displaces, the orbital wall at its weakest point. This point is along the inferior aspect, or floor, of the orbit and the orbital contents decompress through it. Because of this, the globe becomes partially fixed and cannot move in all directions. Typically,

diplopia secondary to lack of upward gaze is present in these patients.

Roentgenographically, the best view for detecting blowout fractures is the Water's view. On this view, one should look for asymmetry of the floors of the orbits, and in some cases one may see actual downward displacement of the bony fragments. In other cases, one can note only that a soft tissue mass (usually just intraorbital fat) has prolapsed into the maxillary antrum (Fig. 5.59). The prolapsed soft tissue mass has been referred to as the "teardrop" sign and the depressed bony fragments have been

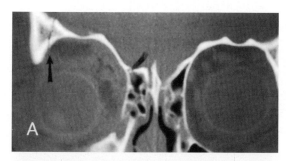 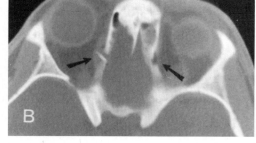

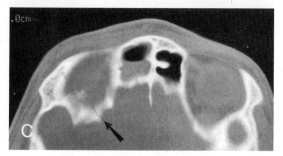

FIGURE 5.58. *Orbital fractures: computed tomographic findings.* **(A)** Note the fracture through the lateral aspect of the superior orbital rim (*arrow*). **(B)** Another patient with extensive facial fractures demonstrating bilateral fractures of the medial walls of the orbits (*arrows*). The fracture fragment on the right is displaced. **(C)** Another patient demonstrating an irregular fracture (*arrow*) through the right orbital roof.

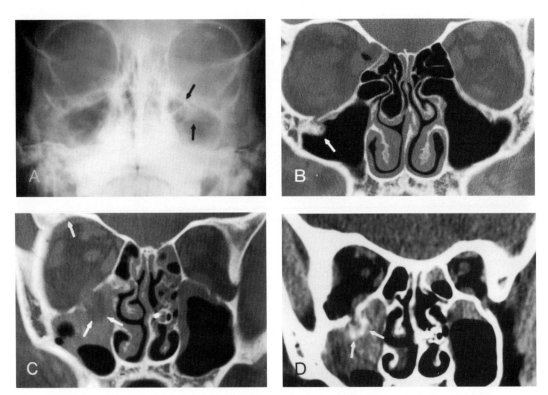

FIGURE 5.59. *Blowout fracture.* **(A)** Suspicious plain-film findings. Note an indistinct mass (*lower arrow*) in the roof of the left maxillary sinus. In addition, there is a depressed fracture fragment involving the floor (*upper arrow*). **(B)** Coronal computed tomographic study in another patient demonstrates a small blowout fracture (*arrow*) on the right. **(C)** Another patient with a blowout fracture on the right demonstrating fat (*arrows*) herniating into the blood-filled maxillary sinus. The floor of the orbit is disrupted. The upper arrow points to an associated superorbital fracture (*arrow*). **(D)** Soft tissue windows in the same patient demonstrate the blowout fracture (*arrows*), with fragments of bone displaced into the blood-filled sinus. Some fluid is also present in the other maxillary sinus cavity and the ethmoid sinuses on the left.

referred to as the "open bomb bay door" sign. The maxillary sinus may be totally clear or obliterated by blood, and, once again, this fracture is best demonstrated on CT scanning (Fig. 5.59). Plain films (Water's and Caldwell views), however, still are quite reliable in initially detecting this fracture.

Most often blowout fractures occur through the floor of the orbit, but occasionally they can occur medially and extend into the ethmoid sinus cavities. They also can extend into the frontal sinuses, and fractures in all of these latter sites are more difficult to detect. This is precisely the time to use CT scanning.

Fractures of the Zygomatic and Maxillary Bones

These include solitary zygomatic arch fractures, tripod fractures of the zygomaticomaxillary bone complex, isolated maxillary fractures, and Le Fort's fractures of the face. Of course, many times these fractures occur in conjunction with one another, but they also occur in isolated form. Of all the fractures of the maxillary bone, the most common is the ***tripod fracture.*** This fracture results from a direct blow to the cheek (7), and characteristically fracturing occurs at three sites: the zygomatic–frontal suture,

FIGURE 5.61. *Tripod fracture in infant: subtle findings.* **(A)** First note a generalized increase in soft tissue density over the right orbit and maxillary sinus region. Then note asymmetry of the inferior aspects of the orbits. On the right, there is downward and outward orbital floor displacement (*arrows*). **(B)** Same patient demonstrating bony detail. Note the fracture through the zygomaticofrontal suture (*1*); a distorted, fractured zygomatic arch (*2*); and a poorly defined, although obligatorily present, fracture through the orbital floor and maxillary sinus (*3*). Very often, in young infants, these fractures are difficult to define on plain films.

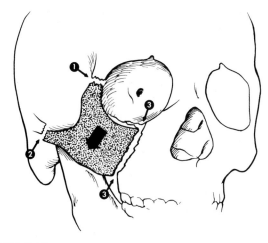

FIGURE 5.60. *Tripod fracture: diagrammatic representation.* Characteristically, fractures occur through the zygomaticofrontal suture (*1*), the zygomatic arch (*2*), and the junction of the zygoma and maxillary bone (*3*). In addition, the fracture fragment is displaced downward and outward (*large arrow*).

the inferior orbital rim and maxillary bone (i.e., junction of the zygoma and maxillary bone), and the zygomatic arch (Fig. 5.60). Depending on the severity of the injury and the extent of the fracture through the inferior orbital rim and maxillary sinus, more or less lateral and downward displacement of the fracture fragment occurs. In actual fact, this fracture fragment is the entire zygoma, and roentgenographically its depression results in a variable degree of asymmetry of the lower orbital rims (Fig. 5.61). In children, it is important not to misinterpret the normal zygomatic–frontal suture as the most superior fracture of the tripod fracture complex.

Other fractures of the maxillary bone are less common but also result from direct blows to the cheek. Many of these fractures extend into the alveolar process of the maxilla, and in so doing produce a loose fragment with separation of the teeth.

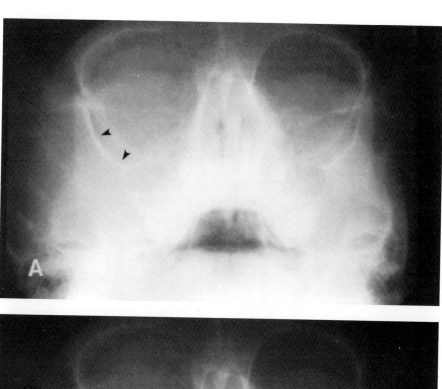

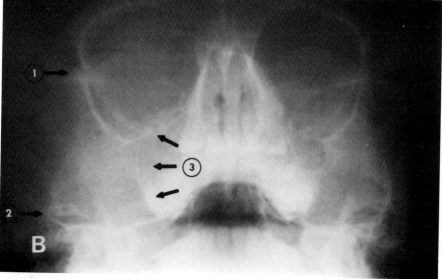

Fractures isolated to the **zygomatic arch** usually result from direct blows to the side of the face. These fractures can be depressed or nondepressed; in those cases in which depression occurs, the zygomatic arch fractures at three sites. Depression occurs at the middle site (Fig. 5.62). Zygomatic arches can be visualized on Towne's projections (see Fig. 5.65), Water's projection, and posteroanterior projections with the chin tucked tightly against the neck. If these views do not suffice, special tangential views or better still, CT studies should be obtained.

One of the more serious facial injuries is the Le Fort's fracture. This fracture is a transverse maxillary fracture extending across the face (2,5–7) and often is associated with a fracture of the pterygoid process. Le Fort's fractures usually are classified into three types, depending on the level of fracture (Fig. 5.63). The lowermost of these fractures is the Le Fort I or transverse maxillary fracture. The fracture line is located above the level of the teeth but below the nose; there is separation of the teeth and the hard palate from the upper portions of the maxilla. In the Le Fort II fracture, the fracture line is located at a higher level and generally runs along the upper aspect of the maxillary bones and nose. Laterally, it may extend along the infraorbital ridge. This fracture often is referred to as the **pyramidal fracture** because of the shape of the main fracture fragment. In Le Fort III injuries, there is craniofacial separation. The fracture is high in position and is located somewhere upward of the bridge of the nose. It usually extends into the orbits, and to a varying degree separates the face from the base of the skull. The main fracture fragment is the entire face. Le Fort's fractures usually are complex and serious

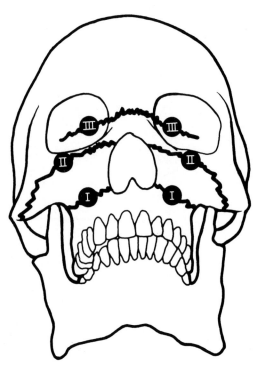

FIGURE 5.63. *Le Fort's fractures: diagrammatic representation.* Note the characteristic position of the Le Fort I, II, and III fractures.

injuries and are sustained from head-on blows to the face such as those sustained in automobile accidents. All of these and other facial fractures, once suspected, require further delineation with CT scanning (Fig. 5.64).

Mandibular Fractures

These fractures usually result from direct blows to the lower jaw, and often, because of the ringlike configuration of the mandible, fractures occur at two sites. Single fractures also commonly occur, however, and usually are not very difficult to detect (Fig. 5.65A). In other cases, fractures can occur through the condylar processes of the mandible. These fractures can be unilateral or bilateral and in young infants often are of the greenstick or bending variety (1,3,4) (Fig. 5.65B). Usually, these fractures are best demonstrated on Towne's or Caldwell views of the head. On the latter view, if one has the patient tuck the chin tightly against his or her chest, the mandibular condyles become readily visible. With more extensive fractures of the mandible, that is, those in which fracturing might occur at three sites, the mandible often is noted to be wider than it should be: In other words, the mandible appears magnified and too large for the remainder of the face (Fig. 5.65). Mandibular fractures, of course, now are readily demonstrable with CT scanning, and the study is obtained in virtually all cases. It

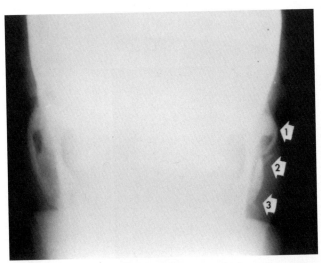

FIGURE 5.62. *Zygomatic arch fracture.* Note the typical configuration of the fractured zygomatic arch (*arrows*). The fracture occurs at three sites (*1, 2, 3*) and is depressed in the middle site (*2*). Other zygomatic arch fractures are demonstrated in Figures 5.61B and 5.65B.

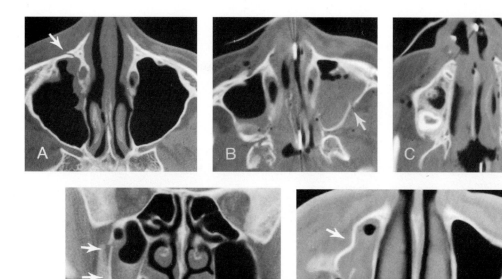

FIGURE 5.64. *Maxillary fractures: appearance on computed tomographic scan.* **(A)** Note the nondisplaced fracture (*arrow*) through the maxillary bone on the right. There is some underlying mucosal edema in the sinus cavity. **(B)** Another patient with extensive facial injuries demonstrates a slightly displaced fracture (*arrow*) through the posterior wall of the left maxillary sinus. Air and fluid are seen in the sinus cavity. A fluid level is seen in the contralateral maxillary sinus, and a few air bubbles are seen in the soft tissues overlying the right maxillary sinus. **(C)** An adjacent cut demonstrates a markedly displaced anterior maxillary fracture (*arrow*). Again, air and fluid are seen in the maxillary sinus, and air bubbles are scattered in the soft tissues on the right side of the face. **(D)** Another patient whose coronal CT scan demonstrates an inwardly displaced lateral maxillary wall fracture (*arrows*). Blood is present in the sinus cavity. **(E)** Axial view demonstrates the depressed lateral wall (*upper arrow*). In addition, there are one or two displaced bony fragments lying in the sinus cavity (*lower arrow*). Blood virtually fills the sinus cavity. Note the normal sinus on the other side.

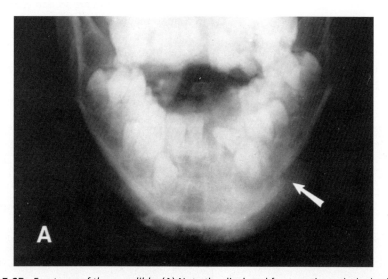

FIGURE 5.65. *Fractures of the mandible.* **(A)** Note the displaced fracture through the body of the mandible (*arrow*). Alignment of the teeth is disrupted.   *(continued on next page)*

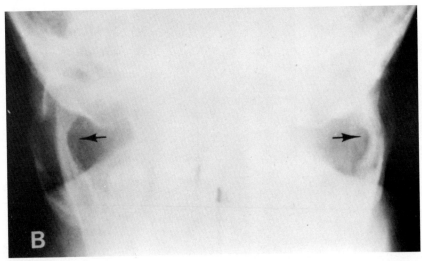

FIGURE 5.65. *(continued)* **(B)** Bilateral greenstick (bending) fractures of the mandibular condyles (*arrows*) in a young infant. The zygomatic arch, on the right, also is fractured but not depressed. It merely is separated at the zygomatic frontal suture.

is much easier to assess bone alignment on CT scans (Fig. 5.66).

Dislocation of the mandible is not particularly common but can occur. Of course, clinically it should be readily apparent, because the patient is unable to open and close the mouth. On Law's projection and subsequent regular or computed tomography, the condyles are visualized with considerable clarity, and it can be determined that in the dislocated joint the condyle lies anterior to the articular fossa.

Soft Tissue Changes with Facial Injury

Very often the soft tissues are swollen and distorted with facial injury. This can occur with or without underlying

bony abnormality, and it is important to appreciate these changes. In some instances, considerable edema and swelling are present and can distract one from a more serious underlying problem (Fig. 5.67). One of the more distracting soft tissue changes is that produced if air is trapped between the palpebral fissures. In such cases, air within the orbit might be erroneously suggested (Fig. 5.67B).

Normal Findings Causing Problems

The facial bones are so complexly constructed and united by so many sutures that it is no surprise that many normal structures are misinterpreted as fractures. This can occur both on plain films and CT scans. The most common of these are dealt with at appropriate places elsewhere in this

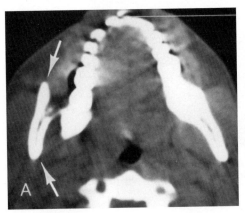
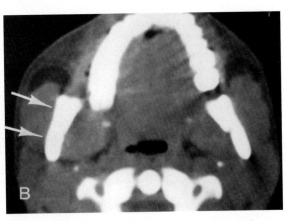

FIGURE 5.66. *Mandibular fracture: computed tomographic findings.* **(A)** Note the comminuted fracture through the right mandibular angle (*arrow*). The mandibular ramus is displaced outwardly. **(B)** Another cut demonstrates the same displaced fracture (*arrows*).

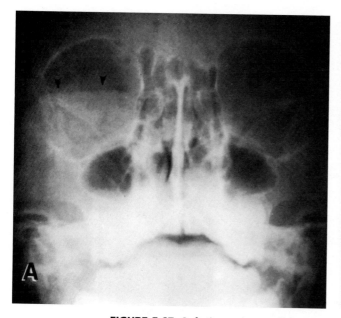
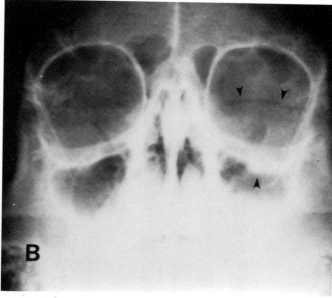

FIGURE 5.67. *Soft tissue abnormalities in facial trauma.* **(A)** Note extensive swelling of the soft tissues above the right maxillary sinus (*arrows*). All of the bony structures, however, are normal. **(B)** Another patient who sustained a blow to the left orbit. Note some generalized increase in soft-tissue density over the lower left orbit and the slitlike transverse radiolucency caused by air being trapped in the palpebral fissure (*upper arrows*). Swelling of the lower eyelid causes the trapped air to appear slitlike. Note its normal appearance on the right side. In addition, note a minimal blowout fracture on the left (*lower arrow*).

chapter, and perhaps at this point *it is best merely to underscore the value of assessing symmetry in the face.* If one notes a finding that suggests that a fracture might be present, then one immediately should compare this area with the same one on the other side. If the finding is normal, chances are that it can be seen and appears the same on the other side. Of course, this is with the understanding that the examination is performed with proper positioning, that is, without rotation, obliquity, or so forth.

In the mandible, the most commonly misinterpreted normal structure is the synchondrosis of the symphysis menti. This is a radiolucent, vertical line in the middle of the mandible and usually is seen in infants and young children. Knowledge of its midline position should avoid its misinterpretation as a fracture. The groove for the mandibular branch of the trigeminal nerve also can be misinterpreted as a fracture of the body of the mandible.

REFERENCES

1. Ahrendt D, Swischuk LE, Hayden CK Jr. Incomplete (bending?) fractures of the mandibular condyle in children. *Pediatr Radiol* 1984;14:140–141.
2. Dolan KD, Jacoby C, Smoker W. The radiology of facial fractures. *RadioGraphics* 1984;4:577–663.
3. Hubbard KA, Klein BL, Hernandez M, Forrester D, Chamberlain JM. Mandibular fractures in children with chin lacerations. *Pediatr Emerg Care* 1995;11:85–86.
4. Lee CYS, McCullom C III, Blaustein DI. Pediatric chin injury: Occult condylar fractures of the mandible. *Pediatr Emerg Care* 1991;7:160–162.
5. Le Fort R. Etude experimentale sur les fractures de la machoire superieure. *Rev Chir Orthop Reparatrice Appar Mot* 1901;23: 208–209.
6. Le Fort R. Fracture de la machoire superieure. *Congr Internat Med Paris Sect Chir Gen* 1900;275–278.
7. Unger JD, Unger FG. Fracture of the pterygoid processes accompanying severe facial bone injury. *Radiology* 1971;98:311–316.

DETECTING INCREASED INTRACRANIAL PRESSURE (SPREAD SUTURES)

In infancy and early childhood, increased intracranial pressure is manifest primarily in widening or spreading of the calvarial sutures. The coronal suture usually is the first to spread, and in the infant younger than 3 months of age no valid measurements are available. Consequently, one must rely on one's objective observation that the coronal suture is wider and more V-shaped than normal (4). In addition to this finding, one may note that the anterior fontanel is bulging (Fig. 5.68). In the older infant and child, it has been suggested that if the coronal suture measures more than 3 mm at its uppermost aspect, then spread probably is present (2). This measurement is the most useful one avail-

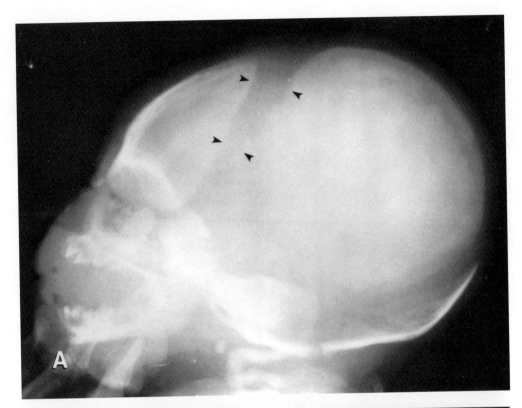

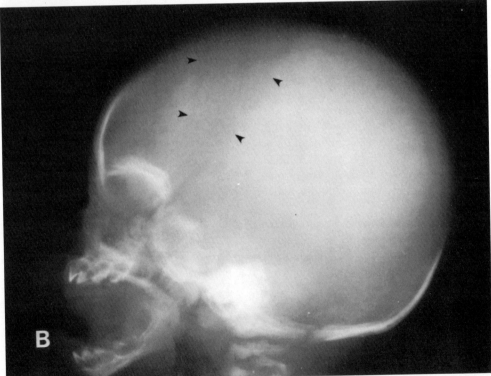

FIGURE 5.68. *Spread sutures in infancy.* **(A)** Normal infant demonstrating upper limits of normal of the coronal suture (*arrows*). Note that the coronal suture is slightly V-shaped. **(B)** Exaggerated V-shaped configuration of the coronal suture (*arrows*) caused by markedly increased intracranial pressure. Also note that the anterior fontanel is bulging. In **A** the anterior fontanel is not bulging.

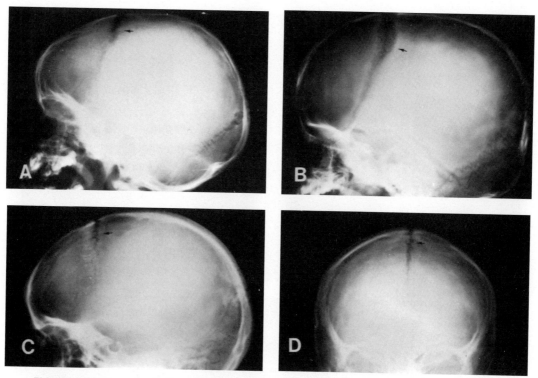

FIGURE 5.69. *Spread sutures in older infants and children.* **(A)** Note clearly spread coronal suture (*arrow*). **(B)** Gross spreading with an exaggerated V-shaped configuration of the coronal suture (*arrow*) in an infant with meningitis. All of the other sutures also are spread. **(C)** Questionably spread coronal suture (*arrow*). Such a configuration often is difficult to differentiate from normal. **(D)** Frontal view demonstrating definite spread of the sagittal suture (*arrow*). This should suggest that the coronal suture in Fig. **C** truly is spread. This patient had an intracranial bleed.

able, but in some cases borderline measurements still cause uncertainty. It is in such cases that I have found it worthwhile to examine the sagittal suture as well (3). The reason for this is that although the normal coronal suture often appears spread but in truth is not, seldom does this occur with the sagittal suture. Consequently, if the sagittal suture is judged to be spread, then increased intracranial pressure is likely (Fig. 5.69).

Spread of the cranial sutures is a nonspecific finding and can be seen with increased intracranial pressure secondary to cerebral edema, subdural hematomas, cerebral hematomas, meningitis (1), and brain tumors. In the emergency setting, however, one usually is confronted with sutural spread secondary to calvarial injury with intracranial bleeding, cerebral edema, or meningitis.

REFERENCES

1. Holmes RD, Kuhns LR, Oliver WJ. Widened sutures in childhood meningitis: Unrecognized sign of an acute illness. *AJR* 1977;128:977–979.

2. Segal HD, Mikity VG, Rumbaugh CL, et al. Cranial sutures in the first year of life: Limits of normal and the "sprung suture." Paper presented at the 57th Annual Meeting of the Radiological Society of North America, Chicago, 1971.

3. Swischuk LE. The growing skull. *Semin Roentgenol* 1974;9: 115–124.

4. Swischuk LE. The normal newborn skull. *Semin Roentgenol* 1974; 9:101–113.

MISCELLANEOUS SKULL AND FACE PROBLEMS

Ocular Foreign Body Localization

Ocular foreign bodies are a common problem in the emergency room. Nonopaque ones pose obvious problems, but most opaque foreign bodies are relatively easily localized on plain films and CT scans (2) (Fig. 5.70). Orbital ultrasonography also is useful in detecting ocular foreign bodies (1).

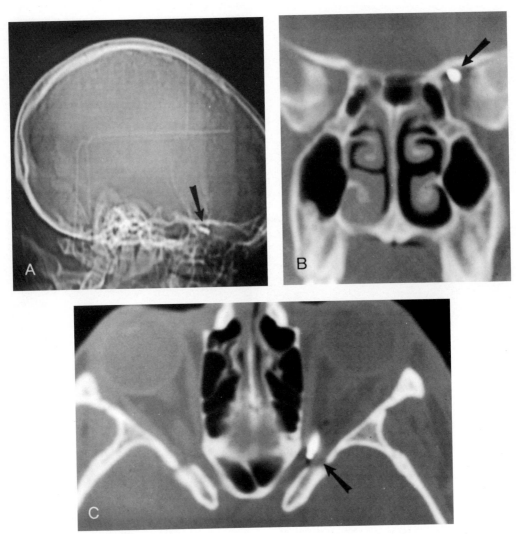

FIGURE 5.70. *Ocular foreign body: computed tomographic (CT) scan.* **(A)** Tomogram demonstrates the opaque foreign body (*arrow*). **(B)** Axial CT cut demonstrates the metallic pellet (*arrow*) embedded deep in the orbit just next to the optic nerve. **(C)** Coronal CT cut demonstrates the foreign body (*arrow*) again.

REFERENCES

1. Coleman DJ, Trokel SL. A protocol for B-scan and radiographic foreign body localization. *Am J Ophthalmol* 1971;71:84–89.
2. Tate E, Cupples H. Detection of orbital foreign bodies with computed tomography: Current limits. *AJR* 1981;137:493–495.

Proptosis and Orbital Cellulitis

Proptosis can result from a number of causes, but in the child, acute unilateral proptosis usually is secondary to trauma or orbital inflammatory disease. Trauma, of course, is self-evident, and with orbital inflammatory disease, most often the problem is preorbital cellulitis (1). If that is not the case, one should consider orbital inflammation sec-ondary to sinusitis (3,7,8,10). In most of these cases, there is no true osteomyelitis of the bones of the orbit, but rather adjacent, sympathetic, intraorbital soft tissue inflammation. Less common causes of proptosis associated with orbital swelling include orbital bone infarction in sickle cell disease (2,12,14), pseudotumor of the orbit (11), and nonspecific orbital cellulitis.

In the past, periorbital and intraorbital inflammatory diseases often were difficult to differentiate clinically (5), but now they are differentiated readily with CT scanning (4,6,9). On CT scanning, preorbital cellulitis presents with normal intraorbital contents and swelling over the front of the eye. Intraorbital inflammatory disease associated with sinusitis usually presents with displacement of the medial rectus muscle and adjacent collections of intraorbital fluid

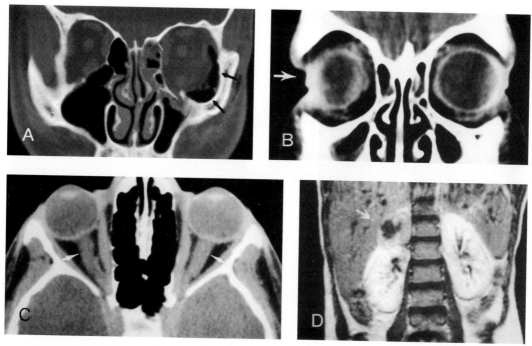

FIGURE 5.71. *Computed tomographic scanning of orbital disease.* **(A)** Intraorbital air (*arrows*) resulting from facial trauma. Note the associated blowout fracture through the floor of the orbit. **(B)** Penetrating injury to the right globe has resulted in its decompression (*arrow*). **(C)** Bilateral thickened optic nerves (*arrows*) in a patient with acute systemic hypertension. This patient had papilledema, and such optic-nerve thickening commonly is seen with papilledema. **(D)** Same patient demonstrating a suprarenal mass (*arrow*) that turned out to be a pheochromocytoma presenting with acute systemic hypertension. (Parts C and D courtesy of C. Keith Hayden, Jr., M.D.)

or an actual abscess. In addition, bone destruction may be seen, but the most common findings are displacement of the medial rectus muscle and adjacent edema. All of these findings are demonstrated in Fig. 2.28.

Other Intraorbital Problems

Bleeding into the globe can occur with trauma (13) and is readily demonstrable with CT scanning. Similarly, retinal hemorrhages, characteristic of the battered child syndrome, also can be identified with CT scans. Thick optic nerves are seen with optic neuritis and also with papilledema (Fig. 5.71C and D). Penetrating injuries to the globe may result in decompression of the globe (Fig. 5.71B), and in addition, air in the orbit also is readily demonstrable on CT scanning (Fig. 5.71A).

REFERENCES

1. Barkin RM, Todd JK, Amer J. Periorbital cellulitis in children. *Pediatrics* 1978;62:390–392.
2. Blank JP, Gill FM. Orbital infarction in sickle cell disease. *Pediatrics* 1981;67:879–881.
3. Chandler JR, Langenbrunner DJ, Stevens ER. The pathogenesis of orbital complications in acute sinusitis. *Laryngoscope* 1970;80:1414.
4. DeSilva M, Lam V, Broadfoot J. CT findings of orbital inflammation in children. *Australas Radiol* 1987;31:241–245.
5. Gellady AM, Shulman ST, Ayoub EM. Periorbital and orbital cellulitis in children. *Pediatrics* 1978;61:272–277.
6. Goldberg F, Berne AS, Oski FA. Differentiation of orbital cellulitis from preseptal cellulitis by computed tomography. *Pediatrics* 1978;62:1000–1005.
7. Hawkins DB, Clark RW. Orbital involvement in acute sinusitis: Lessons from 24 childhood patients. *Clin Pediatr* 1977;16:464–471.
8. Haynes RE, Crambleth HG. Acute ethmoiditis, its relationship to orbital cellulitis. *Am J Dis Child* 1967;114:261.
9. Hirsch M, Lifshitz T. Computerized tomography in the diagnosis and treatment of orbital cellulitis. *Pediatr Radiol* 1988;18:302–305.
10. Jarret WH II, Gutman FA. Ocular complication of infection in the paranasal sinuses. *Arch Ophthalmol* 1969;81:83.
11. Nugent RA, Rootman J, Robertson WD, Lapointe JS, Harrison PB. Acute orbital pseudotumors: Classification and CT features. *AJR* 1981;137:957–962.
12. Seeler RA. Exophthalmos in hemoglobin SC disease. *J Pediatr* 1983;102:90–91.
13. Tomasi LG, Rosman NP. Purtscher's retinopathy in the battered child syndrome. *Am J Dis Child* 1975;129:1335–1337.
14. Wolff MH, Sty JR. Orbital infarction in sickle cell disease. *Pediatr Radiol* 1985;15:50–52.

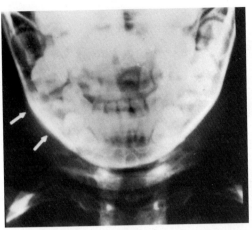

FIGURE 5.72. *Mandibular periostitis.* Note early deposition of periosteal new bone on the right (*arrows*). This patient presented with soft-tissue swelling of the mandible in this area. No osteomyelitis is present. (Courtesy of V. Mikity, M.D.)

febrile seizures. In either case, skull roentgenograms are most unproductive (1,3). In addition, although transient postictal edema can be seen on CT scanning (4), CT scans for childhood seizures also are relatively unproductive (2). MR scans, however, are becoming more helpful but generally are not obtained on an emergent basis.

REFERENCES

1. Committee on Radiology: Skull roentgenography of infants and children with convulsive disorders. *Pediatrics* 1978;62:835–837.
2. Harwood-Nash DC. Computed tomography and seizures in children. *J Neuroradiol* 1983;10:130–136.
3. Ogunmekan AO. Routine skull roentgenography in the clinical evaluation of children with febrile convulsions. *Br J Radiol* 1980; 53:815.
4. Rumack CM, Guggenheim MA, Fasules JW, Burdick D. Transient positive postictal computed tomographic scan. *J Pediatr* 1980;97: 263–264.

Swollen Jaw

Very often, children presenting with a "swollen jaw" have as their underlying problem submandibular adenopathy, and in some of these patients periosteal new-bone deposition along the body of the mandible can be seen (Fig. 5.72). These findings, however, do not represent osteomyelitis but rather a reactive periostitis secondary to the soft tissue inflammation (1). Other causes of swelling of the mandible include Caffey's disease, submandibular salivary gland inflammations, and primary bone tumors and infections. The most common cause, however, is submandibular adenopathy. Currently, such adenopathy is most expediently confirmed with ultrasonography.

REFERENCE

1. Suydam MJ, Mikity VC. Cellulitis with underlying inflammatory periostitis of the mandible. *AJR* 1969;56:133–135.

Seizures

Seizures are a common problem in the pediatric population, and although the occasional seizure can herald the presence of an intracranial tumor, most are idiopathic or

ACUTE INTRACRANIAL VASCULAR AND INFLAMMATORY DISEASES

In the past, the diagnosis of meningitis, for the most part, was nonradiologic. With CT scanning, however, one now can see early brain edema and later, with contrast enhancement, increased definition (enhancement) of the meninges or areas of associated cerebritis (Fig. 5.73). It might be noted, however, that posterior fossa encephalitis, usually of viral origin (6), can have an appearance similar to a posterior fossa tumor.

Enhancement of the meninges is especially profound with tuberculous and fungal meningitis. Brain abscess characteristically produces an area of hypodensity on plain CT scans and a ring of enhancement on contrast studies (Fig. 5.74). Epidural abscesses also can be identified with CT and, as with parenchymal abscesses, demonstrate a hyperemic rim (Fig. 5.74). A similar hyperemic rim with surrounding edema can be seen with cysticercosis in its active stages (Fig. 5.75). Later, as the lesion heals, a punctate calcification remains.

As far as acute vascular problems are concerned, spontaneous intracranial bleeding in children is quite uncommon. Nonetheless, it does occur, either with angiomas, aneurysms, or blood dyscrasias (Fig. 5.76). Deep venous thrombosis is readily identified with CT scanning. On

FIGURE 5.74. *Intracranial inflammatory disease: computed tomographic finding.* **(A)** Brain abscess. Nonenhanced scan demonstrates an area of hypodensity in the right posterior parietal–occipital region (*arrows*). There is some contralateral midline shift, and the occipital horn of the right lateral ventricle has been compressed and is not visible. **(B)** After administration of contrast, a brain abscess with an enhancing rim (*arrows*) is seen.

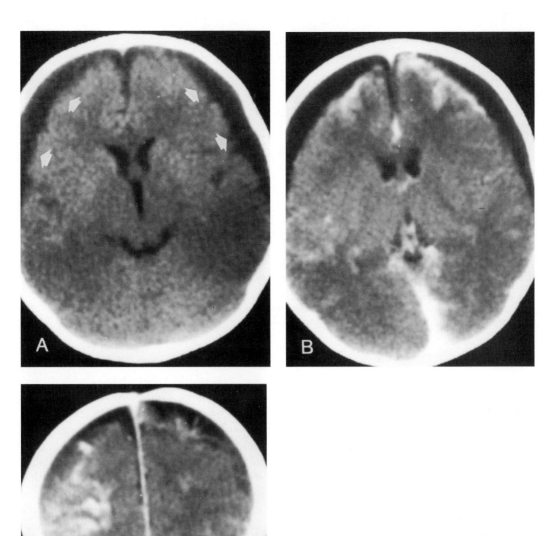

FIGURE 5.73. *Meningitis: cerebritis.* (A) Nonenhanced scan demonstrates subdural effusions on both sides (*arrows*). (B) Contrast study demonstrates diffuse enhancement of the meninges over the frontal regions and along the falx. (C) A higher cut demonstrates diffuse enhancement of the meninges over the various sulci of the brain.

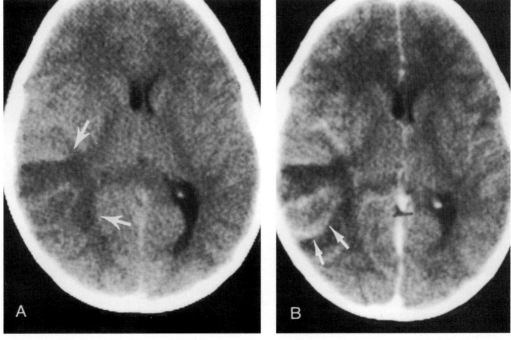

(continued in next page)

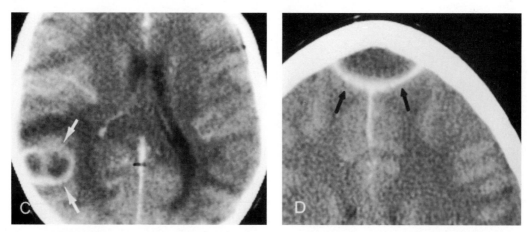

FIGURE 5.74. *(continued)* **(C)** A slightly higher slice demonstrates the characteristic ringlike appearance of the enhancing rim of the brain abscess *(arrows)*. **(D)** Enhancing rim *(arrows)* of a frontal epidural abscess secondary to sinus disease.

contrast-enhanced studies, a radiolucent, triangular defect is seen at the confluence of the straight and transverse sinuses (1,5). Stroke resulting from vascular occlusive disease also is uncommon in children but on CT scanning produces an area of hypodensity (infarction–edema), which later is followed by luxury perfusion around the infarcted area on contrast-enhanced scans (Fig. 5.77). Such infarcts can occur spontaneously (infantile hemiplegia) or as a complication of trauma or intracranial infection such as meningitis. Brain death resulting from acute hypoxia to

the brain usually is best defined with nuclear scintigraphy or angiography (Fig. 5.78). Nuclear scintigraphy is preferred, however, because it is easier to obtain.

With the battered child syndrome, CT of the brain is invaluable (3). The findings are quite variable and may be very extensive. On the other hand, they may consist of nothing more than brain edema or subtle evidence of a shearing injury between the white and gray matter (see Fig. 4.228). If more profound injury occurs, the findings are not difficult to identify (Fig. 5.79). In addition to intra-

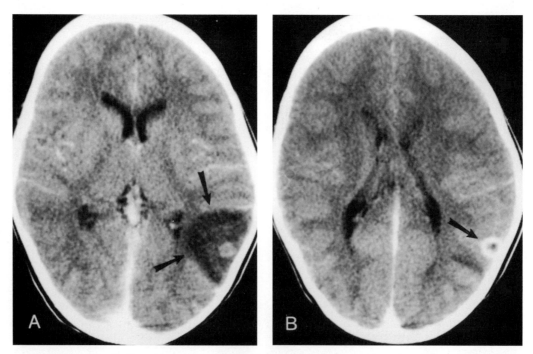

FIGURE 5.75. *Cysticercosis.* **(A)** Note the focal area of edema *(arrows)* in the posterior parietal region on the left. A central enhancing ringlike lesion is visible. **(B)** Slightly higher cut demonstrates the enhancing ring to better advantage. Later, as these lesions heal, a small focus of calcification will remain.

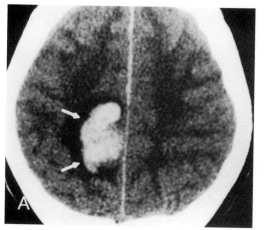
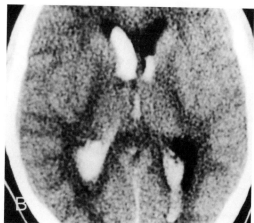

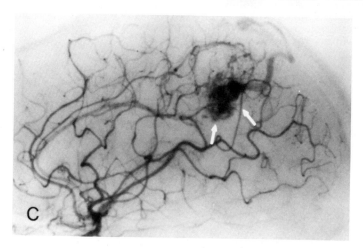

FIGURE 5.76. *Acute intracranial bleeding.* **(A)** Note the parasagittal hematoma (*arrows*) in this patient with acute apoplexy. **(B)** Another computed tomographic scan demonstrates widespread blood in both ventricles. **(C)** Angiogram demonstrates an arteriovenous malformation (*arrows*), with early filling of the veins.

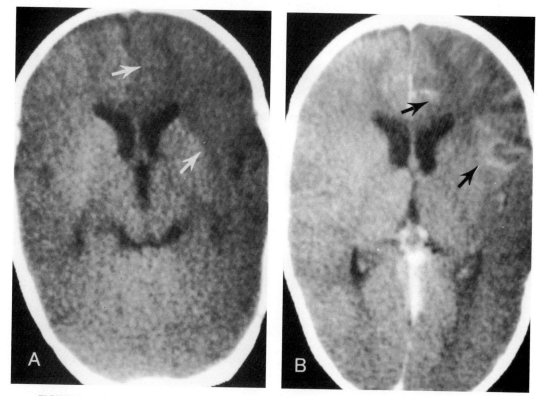

FIGURE 5.77. *Cerebral infarction.* **(A)** Note area of hypodensity in the left frontal lobe (*arrows*). **(B)** Contrast enhancement shows luxury perfusion in the area of the infarction (*arrows*).

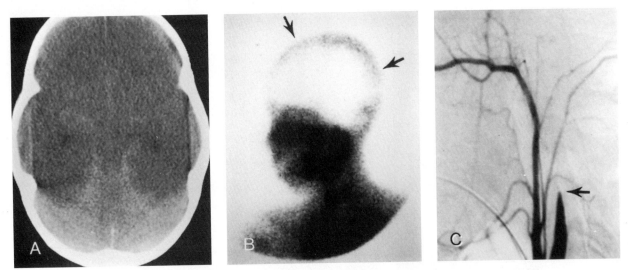

FIGURE 5.78. *Brain death.* (**A**) Computed tomographic scan demonstrates diffuse edema of the cerebral hemispheres. There are no sulci, gyri, or ventricles visible. (**B**) Nuclear scintigraphy demonstrates normal distribution of isotope over the face and scalp (*arrows*) but no evidence of distribution to the brain. (**C**) Another patient with an arteriogram demonstrating no flow in the internal carotid artery (*arrow*).

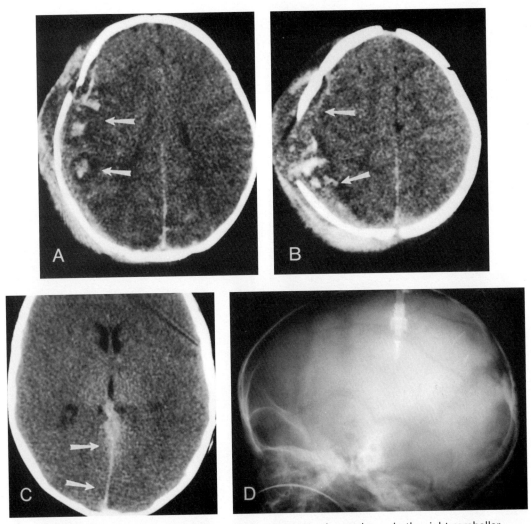

FIGURE 5.79. *Battered child syndrome.* (**A**) Note extensive hemorrhages in the right cerebellar hemisphere (*arrows*). There is midline shift of the falx and evidence of subarachnoid bleeding along it. There is also extensive scalp edema and bleeding and an underlying fracture. (**B**) A slightly higher cut demonstrates the extensive nature of the intracranial bleed (*arrows*), the diastatic fracture, and the associated subgaleal hematoma. (**C**) Another patient demonstrating diffuse edema of the brain and bleeding along the falx (*arrows*). (**D**) Skull film demonstrates the numerous fractures and spread sutures.

cranial hemorrhage and other abnormalities, retinal hemorrhages also can be demonstrated with CT scanning.

Finally a note regarding hypernatremic dehydration is in order. In such cases, damage to the brain can be devastating in the form of edema and hemorrhage (2,4). It is important to appreciate this, because often damage to the brain is overlooked in these patients until later in their clinical courses.

REFERENCES

1. Eick JJ, Miller KD, Bell KA, Tutton RH. Computed tomography of deep cerebral venous thrombosis in children. *Radiology* 1981; 140:399–402.

2. Han BK, Lewe M, Yoon HD. Cranial ultrasound and CT findings in infants with hypernatremic dehydration. *Pediatr Radiol* 1997; 27: 739–742.

3. Merten DF, Osborne DRS, Radkowski MA, Leonidas JC. Craniocerebral trauma in the child abuse syndrome: Radiological observations. *Pediatr Radiol* 1984;14:272–277.

4. Mocharla R, Schexnayder SM, Glasier CM. Fatal cerebral edema and intracranial hemorrhage associated with hypernatremic dehydration. *Pediatr Radiol* 1997;27:785–787.

5. Rao KCVG, Knipp HC, Wagner EJ. Computed tomographic findings in cerebral sinus and venous thrombosis. *Radiology* 1981;140: 391–398.

6. Unsal E, Olgun N, Sarialioglu F, Cevik N. Posterior fossa pseudotumour due to vital encephalitis in a child. *Pediatr Radiol* 1997; 27:788–789.

6

THE SPINE AND SPINAL CORD

CERVICAL SPINE INJURIES

Injuries of the cervical spine are less common in the infant and young child than in the older child and adult, but if they occur, injuries involving C1, C2, and C3 are more common (1,5,6,8,16). In older children and adolescents the distribution is the same as in adults, that is, over the middle and lower cervical spine (6,7). In the end, however, one's approach to the analysis of the roentgenograms should be the same whatever the age of the patient. One's most important job is to determine whether the cervical spine is stable or unstable. To do this, one must understand all of the mechanisms of cervical spine injury and the abnormal findings they produce. It is to this end that this chapter is primarily devoted.

There is no question that the evaluation of the cervical spine in trauma, be it overt or subtle, is a problem. It has been demonstrated that delay in adequate diagnosis often stems from not obtaining a flexion view, *not having an experienced radiologist review the roentgenogram* and, of course, the inherent difficulty in obtaining adequate films in many of these patients (4,12). In addition, it has been demonstrated that protocol-driven imaging regimens for suspected cervical spine injuries are generally unrewarding (9). *In other words, there should be some attempt to evaluate the patient clinically before he or she is sent to the radiography suite to be examined. Certainly this has become a great problem in terms of the so-called EMS collar. Most emergency-ambulance operators are instructed to place a collar on a patient at the slightest indication of a neck injury and, indeed, even if there is no such indication. These patients should be evaluated clinically before they are sent to the radiography suite, for many will not require roentgenographic examination. A carefully executed physical examination is easy to accomplish in the patient who is coherent, and if it is negative, it can save enormous amounts of time and dollars in the evaluation of these patients (9,14,17,18). This seems such a practical approach, and yet it is ignored over and over again.*

What Views Are Necessary?

Of all of the views of the cervical spine, the lateral view is the most important. It is on this view that one makes most

of one's observations and decisions regarding stability or instability of the spine. Patients with cervical spine injuries fall into two groups: those who are fully coherent and can move their necks, and those who are compromised, incoherent, or unconscious. In the latter group, one should confine the examination to cross-table lateral, frontal, and open-mouth odontoid views; all should be obtained without moving the patient. If an open-mouth odontoid view is not obtainable (e.g., in an intubated patient), one should proceed to computed tomographic (CT) scanning.

In the coherent patient, lateral, frontal, and open-mouth odontoid views also should be obtained. Oblique views generally are not needed and are time-consuming. Although some still favor obtaining these views, it is probably better to proceed to CT scanning for further evaluation of the cervical spine.

Flexion views also are very helpful (12,22) and are quite safe in the responsive patient (21). The reason flexion views are so helpful is that if the flexion view is normal, it is highly unlikely that any significant underlying problem exists. *They are not always required but are useful in demonstrating occult posterior ligamentous injuries and confirming normality.* We use it if required but not in every case.

Once one adopts the attitude that a flexion view should be obtained, then one must develop some type of protocol for obtaining this view. *Obviously this view is not advised in patients who are incoherent or comatosed.* Flexion views usually require that patients be communicative and alert, and under these circumstances it is best for the patients to perform the flexion maneuver themselves. In this way, it is highly unlikely that they will sustain significant neurologic injuries. If they have a fracture or, indeed, if they have a neck sprain, they will not flex their neck to the point at which neurologic injury results. *Forced flexion of the spine in a patient who is incoherent or unconscious can lead to such a problem, and certainly initially one would not think of obtaining a flexion view in such a patient. This contraindication, however, has been transferred overexuberantly to the patient who is coherent but simply has been placed in a collar because emergency medicine ambulance services require it.* Of course, this is understandable, but one must decide where to abort this sequence of events: in the initial examination room or the radiology suite. Ideally this should be accomplished with physical examination, during the initial encounter with the patient. On a practical basis, however, one might approach the problem as follows.

First, it must be underscored that the patient must be coherent. If the patient is coherent, one should ask if he or she has any pain. If the answer is no, one can remove the collar, and if motion is normal no roentgenograms are necessary. If pain is present, the regular spine series should be obtained. If it is normal one can remove the collar and see what spontaneous movements occur. Thereafter, the patient should be asked to move the neck through a full range of motion, knowing that being able to fully flex the neck is the most important maneuver. With underlying injury a patient cannot move the neck freely, if at all, and certainly does not want to flex the neck. At this point one should make a judgment as to whether the patient really has pain or is merely frightened. If one suspects that the patient is frightened, then he or she should be asked to flex his or her neck further. Usually this requires some gentle but positive and judicious encouragement. This can be done by placement of the examiner's hand on the occiput and gently urging flexion of the neck. It is important to remember that flexion should be encouraged, not forced. If one adheres to this, there is little chance that a patient will get into trouble. Indeed, if a patient can fully flex his or her neck spontaneously or with encouragement, it is unlikely that a significant injury is present. Certainly an unstable fracture is unlikely. Patients with such lesions usually have so much pain that they do not flex their neck even with encouragement. These latter patients obviously constitute a different group than the former. With the former group, once flexion of the neck has been accomplished clinically, the patient should be examined roentgenographically just to make sure that a subtle, nondisplaced fracture is not present.

With patients who are compromised or unconscious one should proceed directly to the regular c-spine series i.e., lateral, anteroposterior, and open-mouth odontoid views. A flexion view can be obtained after these initial views are reviewed and the spine is judged to be stable. Flexion views should be accomplished in small increments with multiple exposures until one is convinced that no abnormality is present. Forced flexion should not be utilized, and should be performed by a physician.

Visualize All of the Cervical Spine

Visualization of all of the cervical spine is necessary; if this is not achieved, that is, if the shoulder covers the lower cervical spine, one can miss significant lesions in this area. Consequently, it is very important to count the vertebral bodies to ensure that all of them are included on any given film. Always count seven cervical vertebrae and one thoracic vertebra. In terms of the latter, often it is only the upper half that is visible, and one must make a judgment as to whether this is acceptable. In most cases it is. If seven vertebrae cannot be visualized, the swimmer's view can be obtained, but

this is difficult to accomplish and evaluate, and in fact we have discontinued it. The reason for this is that CT scans are much more productive in this area and should be obtained whenever any doubt exists (10). This also applies to the upper cervical spine (3,10,13); CT scanning solves many problems and also reveals occult fractures of the vertebrae and the occipital condyles (3,10). For the upper cervical spine, once again one makes one's initial and most important observations on the lateral view. Thereafter, the open-mouth odontoid view should be obtained, but if on the basis of these two views one cannot come to the conclusion that the upper cervical spine is normal, one should proceed to CT scanning.

In infants and young children up to the age of 5 years, a question often arises as to whether the open-mouth odontoid view should be pursued until it is obtained (19). This is an important consideration, because often numerous attempts at obtaining the view produce no useful information. Indeed, there is some preliminary evidence suggesting that omitting the open-mouth odontoid view, as long as the lateral view is normal, in patients 5 years of age or younger, could come to pass (21). Most fractures of the odontoid in this age group occur through the dens body synchondrosis and are easily detected on lateral view. Furthermore, most result in anterior tilting or displacement of the dens (1,11), and the lateral view usually detects these fractures. Therefore, if the lateral view is normal and the open-mouth odontoid view is not obtainable, it may not be necessary to pursue obtaining it in plain films or shifting to CT scanning (20).

Finally, one or two other aspects of cervical spine injury should be considered. First, in a patient with severe head trauma it probably is worthwhile to extend the CT examination to the upper cervical spine, because associated fractures in this area have been demonstrated to be significantly common (2). *This also is probably a wise maneuver in those infants and young children in whom the mechanism of injury could produce a Jefferson fracture, and the open-mouth odontoid view is unsatisfactory (20).*

It is also important to remember that spinal injuries may occur at multiple levels. They can occur in the cervical spine alone, or throughout the entire vertebral column (3). In addition, it might also be recalled that facial injuries often are associated with hyperextension spinal injuries, and that force to the back of the head can induce concomitant flexion injuries of the cervical spine.

Magnetic resonance (MR) imaging, for the most part, is reserved for evaluation of complicating soft tissue injuries, spinal canal injuries, and spinal cord injury (21). It is especially useful if neurologic findings are present but no bony abnormality is seen on the preliminary roentgenograms (i.e., spinal cord injury without radiographic abnormalities [SCIWORA]). On the other hand, if no abnormalities are seen on the initial radiographic study and no neurologic findings are seen, it has been demonstrated that MR scanning is of minimal or no use (15). Protocols, of course, for obtaining cervical spine studies in the emergency room vary

TABLE 6.1B

PATIENT NAME _____ UH # _____

	N	A
1. Anterior arch C1		
2. Posterior arch C1		
3. Predental distance		
4. Anterior cortex C2		
5. Posterior cortex C2		
6. Ring of Harris		
7. Posterior arch of C2		
8. Body of C3		
9. Alignment C2-C3		

	N	A
1. Dens		
2. Lat. mass C1		

	N	A
1. Superior plate C6		
2. Superior and inferior plate C6,7		
3. Superior and inferior plate C7-T1		
4. Alignment C6,7		
5. Alignment C7,T1		
6. Posterior element C6		
7. Posterior element C7		

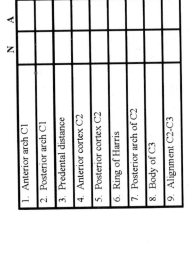

RESIDENT _____

TABLE 6.1A DEPARTMENT OF RADIOLOGY: C-SPINE PROTOCOL

1. ADULT AND CHILDREN OVER 5 YEARS*

THREE view cervical spine: if normal, stop

If open-mouth odontoid or C7-T1 view not visualized, repeat study once; if unsatisfactory, stop. Go to CT.

If open-mouth view not obtainable (i.e., patient intubated); go to CT.

2. INFANT AND CHILDREN 5 YEARS AND UNDER*

THREE view cervical spine; if normal, stop.

If opne-mouth odontoid view unsatisfactory or unobtainable, repeat once, and stop if lateral view normal. No CT needed.

If C7-T1 unsatisfactory, repeat once and stop. Go to CT.

If open-mouth odontoid view unsatisfactory and Jefferson fracture suspected by mechanism of injury or history, extend regular head CT down to C4. If head CT is not obtained, perform CT of upper cervical spine.

3. In any case, if abnormality is detected on the three-view cervical spine study in any age group, CT is mandatory. CT should also be performed **if there is any clinical or imaging question** as to whether the patient is abnormal, especially if symptoms are present or there is altered sensorium on consciousness.

4. If neurologic signs or symptoms are or were present (radiculopathy or spinal cord symptoms) perform cervical MRI.

*Flexion views as required. See page 533 for flexion protocols.

slightly from institution to institution. Our protocol is outlined in Table 6.1A, and a diagrammatic checklist for the upper and lower cervical spine areas appears in Table 6.1B. The latter was designed to force the observer to check all the significant areas outlined.

REFERENCES

1. Apple JS, Kirks DR, Merten DF, Martinez S. Cervical spine fractures and dislocations in children. *Pediatr Radiol* 1987;17: 45–49.
2. Blacksin MF, Lee HJ. Frequency and significance of fractures of the upper cervical spine detected by CT in patients with severe head trauma. *AJR* 1995;165:1201–1204.
3. Bloom AI, Neeman Z, Floman Y, Gomori J, Bar-Ziv J. Occipital condyle fracture and ligament injury: Imaging by CT. *Pediatr Radiol* 1996;26:786–790.
4. Davis JW, Phreaner DL, Hoyt DB, Mackersie RC. The etiology of missed cervical spine injuries. *J Trauma* 1993;34:342–346.
5. Dietrich AM, Ginn-Pease ME, Barkowski HM, King DR. Pediatric cervical spine fractures: Predominantly subtle presentation. *J Pediatr Surg* 1991;26:995–1000.
6. Ehara S, El-Khoury GY, Sato Y. Cervical spine injury in children: Radiologic manifestations. *AJR* 1988;151:1175–1178.
7. Givens TG, Polley KA, Smith GF, Hardin WD Jr. Pediatric cervical spine injury: A three year experience. *J Trauma* 1996;4: 310–314.
8. Hadley MN, Zabramski JM, Browner CM, Rekate H, Sonntag VKH. Pediatric spinal trauma: Review of 122 cases of spinal cord and vertebral column injuries. *J Neurosurg* 1988;68:18–24.
9. John SD, Moorthy C, Swischuk LE. The value of routine cervical spine, chest, and pelvis radiographs in children after trauma. *Emerg Radiol* 1996;3:176–180.
10. Nunez DB Jr, Quencer RM. The role of helical CT in the assessment of cervical spine injuries. *AJR* 1988;171:951–957.
11. Odent T, Langlais J, Glorion C, Kassis B, Bataille J, Pouliquen JC. Fractures of the odontoid process: A report of 15 cases in children younger than 6 years. *J Pediatr Orthop* 1999;19: 51–54.
12. Orenstein JB, Klein BL, Ochsenschlager DW. Delayed diagnosis of pediatric cervical spine injury. *Pediatrics* 1992;89: 1185–1188.
13. Poirier VC, Greenlaw AR, Beatty CS, Seibert JA, Ablin DS. Computed tomographic evaluation of C1-C2 in pediatric cervical spine trauma. *Emerg Radiol* 1:195–199.
14. Roberg RJ, Weaars RC, Kelly M, Evans TC, Kenny MA, Daffner R, Kremen R, Murray K, Cottington EC. Selective application of cervical spine radiography in alert victims of blunt trauma: A prospective study. *J Trauma* 1988;28:784–788.
15. Ronnen HR, de Korte PJ, Brink PRG, van der Bijl HJ, Tonino AJ, Franke CL. Acute whiplash injury: Is there a role for MR imaging? A prospective study of 100 patients. *Radiology* 1996; 201:93–96.
16. Ruge JR, Sinson GP, McLone DG, Cerullo LJ. Pediatric spinal injury: The very young. *J Neurosurg* 1988;68:25–30.
17. Schwartz GR, Wright SE, Fein JA, Sugarman J, Salhanick S. Pediatric cervical spine injury sustained in falls from low heights. *Ann Emerg Med* 1997;30:249–252.
18. Stiell IG, Wells GA, Vandemheen K, Laupacia A, Brison R, Eisenhauer MA, Greenberg GH, MacPhail I, McKnight RD, Reardon M, Verbeek R, Worthington J, Lesiuk H. Variation in emergency department use of cervical spine radiography for alert, stable trauma patients. *CMAJ* 1997;156:1352.
19. Swischuk LE. Pursuing the odontoid fracture in infants. *Emerg Radiol* 1996;3:54–55.
20. Swischuk LE, John SD, Hendrick EP. Is the open mouth odontoid view necessary in children under five years? *Pediatr Radiol* 2000;30:186–189
21. Terk MR, Hume-Neal M, Fraipent M, Ahmade J, Colleti PM. Injury of the posterior ligament complex in patients with acute spinal trauma: Evaluation by MR imaging. *AJR* 1997;168: 1481–1486.
22. Woods WA, Brady WJ, Pollock G, Kini N, Young JS. Flexion-extension cervical spine radiography in pediatric blunt trauma. *Emerg Radiol* 1998;5:381–384.

What to Look for in Cervical Spine Injuries

One should have some system for analyzing the cervical spine, and I have found it best to start with the lateral view. This view is the most informative one, and a number of assessments should be made before turning to the frontal and oblique views. First, one should note the general curvature of the spine, and then one should assess the individual structures from front to back. These structures include the prevertebral soft tissues, predental space (C1-to-dens distance), odontoid process, individual vertebral bodies, disc spaces, apophyseal joints, neural arches, and spinous tips.

Loss of Normal Cervical Spine Curvature

On lateral view, the cervical spine in the normal, neutral position assumes a gentle lordotic curve (Fig. 6.1), and on

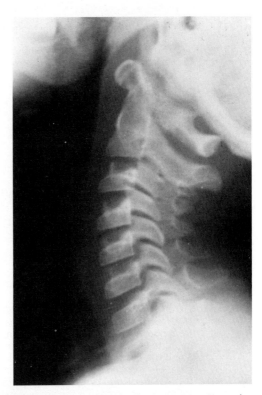

FIGURE 6.1. *Normal cervical spine curvature.* Note the gentle lordosis of the cervical spine. Also note the normal predental distance, the normal synchondrosis (*horizontal radiolucent line*) between the dens and body of C2, and the normal prevertebral soft tissues. In addition, note the high position of the anterior arch of C1. This occurs during extension and is normal.

frontal view it is straight. Deviation from these normal alignments usually reflects the presence of underlying muscle spasm or bony or ligament injury. Spasm usually produces a straight spine on lateral view, but in many children it may lead to a mild to striking anterior, kyphotic angulation of C2 on C3 (Fig. 6.2). In such cases, there is no associated anterior displacement of the body of C2 on the body of C3, and although the overall configuration may appear worrisome, it is quite reversible and not representative of a fracture or dislocation. Localized kyphosis at lower levels, on the other hand, is significant and usually indicates the presence of ligamentous laxity secondary to a hyperflexion injury.

Prevertebral Soft Tissue Thickening

Prevertebral soft tissue swelling or thickening resulting from edema or hematoma formation is an important ancillary finding in cervical spine injuries. It should be noted, however, that it is not present in all cases (2). There is good reason for this: In those cases in which no significant anterior spinal ligament or vertebral-body injury occurs, there is no reason for the prevertebral soft tissues to become widened. Consequently, in a good many significant cervical spine injuries, the prevertebral soft tissues are normal. This lack of prevertebral soft tissue thickening also frequently occurs with minimal fractures of the dens (2).

Another problem with the assessment of the prevertebral soft tissues in the infant and young child is that, if the airway is not fully distended or the spine is not fully extended, pseudothickening can be suggested (Fig. 6.2). True soft tissue swelling should be reproducible from film to film and also should cause "smooth" anterior displacement of the airway (Fig. 6.3). In the upper cervical spine, however, even these considerations may not solve the problem, for normal adenoidal lymphoid tissue extending into the retropharyngeal space can interfere significantly with interpretation (Fig. 6.4). Over the lower cervical spine, in those cases in which soft tissue thickening is borderline, it may be helpful to note whether the prevertebral fat stripe is displaced anteriorly (3). Displacement of this fat stripe can be taken to indicate the presence of an underlying vertebral injury, but

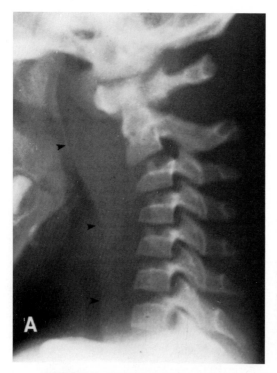
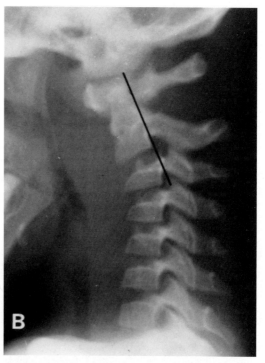

FIGURE 6.2. *C2-3 angulation pseudoabnormality and pseudoprevertebral soft-tissue thickening.* **(A)** Note that the prevertebral soft tissues appear thickened (*arrows*). Such thickening results from poor roentgenographic technique (i.e., inadequate distension of the airway and hyperflexion of the spine). Also note that C2 is angled forward on C3. In **B**, however, note that a line drawn along the posterior aspect of the dens and body of C2 demonstrates that there is no associated anterior displacement of C2 on C3. In the absence of such displacement, angulation of C2 on C3 is of no particular consequence and can be seen with both voluntary and involuntary muscle spasm. Finally, note that the predental distance is wide (4–5 mm in this patient), and that the distance between the spinous tips of C1 and C2 also is unusually wide. Both of these findings also are normal.

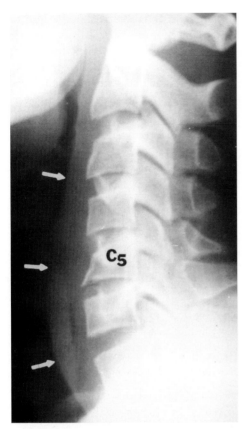

FIGURE 6.3. *Prevertebral soft-tissue swelling.* Note prevertebral soft-tissue swelling (*arrows*) anterior to a compression fracture of C5. Not only are the tissues thickened, but they also produce continuous, arcing anterior displacement of the airway. Compare these prevertebral soft tissues with the normal ones shown in Figure 6.4.

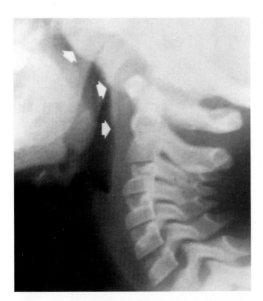

FIGURE 6.4. *Normal prevertebral soft tissues.* Note prominent prevertebral soft tissues extending into the retropharyngeal space (*arrows*). This type of soft-tissue thickening should not be misinterpreted as pathologic thickening. Note preservation of the normal stepoff of the posterior walls of the hypopharynx and trachea. Compare to the smooth arcing configuration of these two walls with true soft-tissue thickening seen in Figure 6.3.

it is of limited value in the pediatric age group, for it is not readily visible in the infant and young child.

In children, far too much variability exists for normal measurement guidelines for prevertebral soft tissue thickening to be useful. Nonetheless, it has been suggested that, above the glottis, soft-tissue thickness of 7 mm or more be considered abnormal, and that below the glottis more than 14 mm of soft tissue space be considered abnormal (1). These measurements are reasonably dependable in the older child but must be adjusted upward in younger children and infants, in whom vertebral body ossification is incomplete, and even greater width variations occur. In general, however, the measurements do define a rule that I have followed for years: Below the level of the glottis the normal soft tissues double in thickness (Fig. 6.4). This occurs because below this level the esophagus separates from the airway and becomes part of the airless prevertebral soft-tissue mass.

REFERENCES

1. Clark WM, Gehweiler JA Jr, Laib R. Twelve significant signs of cervical spine trauma. *Skeletal Radiol* 1979;3:201–205.
2. Penning L. Prevertebral hematoma in cervical spine injury: Incidence and etiologic significance. *AJR* 1981;136:553–561.
3. Whalen JP, Woodruff CL. The cervical prevertebral fat stripe. *AJR* 1970;109:445–451.

Increase in the Predental Space (C1-to-Dens Distance)

Before beginning any discussion of the predental distance, one must realize that normal variations are much more pronounced in children than in adults. In the adult, a distance greater than 2.5 mm usually is considered abnormal, but in children distances of 3 to 4 mm are commonplace and normal. Indeed, a few children demonstrate a predental distance of 5 mm and still are normal (Fig. 6.5). This was demonstrated by Locke et al. (6) a number of years ago and duplicated in our own survey of 100 consecutive cervical spine roentgenograms in normal children (Table 6.2). In addition to these differences, it should be noted that the predental distance can widen significantly between flexion and extension (Fig. 6.6), often with variations of up to 2 mm (1). Consequently, one must be cautious not to overinterpret an apparently abnormally wide predental space in children.

Abnormal widening of the predental space occurs if there is disruption of the transverse ligament between C1 and the dens (3–5), but this is not a common injury, even with dens fractures. The reason for this is that the dens and C1 move as a unit, and thus the predental distance is not altered. Actually, widening of the predental space occurs more often with atlantoaxial instability caused by underlying abnormalities such as rheumatoid arthritis (7) or congenital hypoplasia of the dens (2). In either case, these

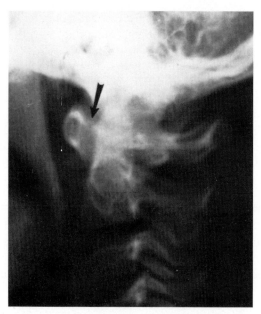

FIGURE 6.5. *Normal wide predental space.* Note the wide (4–5 mm) predental space (*arrow*) in this normal 8-year-old child.

TABLE 6.2. NORMAL PREDENTAL (C₁ TO DENS) DISTANCES

Predental Distance (mm)	No. of Patients
1–1½	7
2–2½	54
3–3½	27
4–4½	9
5	3
Total	100

patients are prone to abnormal atlantoaxial and transverse ligament laxity and hypermobility. As a result, chronic dislocation without fracture is more likely to occur (see page 584). Other injuries that can be associated with an increase in the predental distance include rotatory subluxation of C1 on C2 and some Jefferson bursting fractures of C1.

REFERENCES

1. Cattell HS, Filtzer DL. Pseudosubluxation and other normal variations in the cervical spine in children. *J Bone Joint Surg* 1965;47A:1295–1309.
2. Dawson EG, Smith L. Atlanto-axial subluxation in children due to vertebral anomalies. *J Bone Joint Surg* 1979;61A:582–587.
3. deBeer J. deV, Hoffman EB, Kieck CF. Traumatic atlantoaxial subluxation in children. *J Pediatr Orthop* 1990;10:397–400.
4. Floman Y, Kaplan L, Elidan J. Transverse ligament rupture and atlanto-axial subluxation in children. *J Bone Joint Surg* 1991;73B:640–643.
5. Harouchi A, Padovani JP, Elandaloussi M. Atlanto-axial dislocation in children: A review of 9 cases. *Chir Pediatr* 1984;25:136–144.
6. Locke GR, Gardner JI, Van Epps EF. Atlas-dens interval (ADI) in children: A survey based on 200 normal cervical spines. *AJR* 1966;97:135–140.
7. Reid GD, Hill RH. Atlantoaxial subluxation in juvenile ankylosing spondylitis. *J Pediatr* 1978;93:531–532.

Hypermobility of C1

In infants and young children, both during flexion and extension, C1 tends to stay in close apposition to the base of the skull and thus may appear hypermobile in relation to

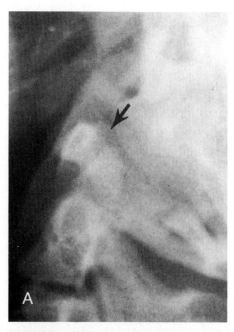
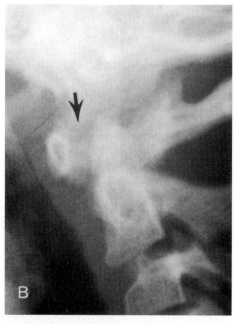

FIGURE 6.6. *Predental distance: variation with extension and flexion.* **(A)** On extension, note the normal appearance of the predental space (*arrow*). **(B)** With flexion, note how much widening has occurred (*arrow*). This patient was normal. A 2-mm increase in the predental space is normal.

C2. In extension, high positioning of the anterior arch of C1 results but is normal (Fig. 6.1). Similarly, an apparently wide intraspinous distance between the spinous tips of C1 and C2 seen on flexion also is normal (Fig. 6.2; see also 6.15B). Both of these configurations, however, to the uninitiated can appear very abnormal. In explaining this phenomenon, it might be recalled that the ligamentous attachments between the base of the skull and C1 are very firm, but in the upper cervical spine, in general, they are quite lax. Therefore, if any excessive motion occurs, it occurs from C1 downwards.

Displacement of the Vertebral Bodies

In most instances, displacement of one vertebral body on another is a significant abnormal finding and reflects underlying instability of the spine. Anterior displacement is much more common than posterior displacement and usually occurs with flexion or rotational injuries. Almost invariably, anterior displacement of a vertebral body indicates a significant underlying injury, but caution must be exercised in the upper cervical spines of infants and young children, in whom normal anterior displacement can occur.

Anterior displacement of the vertebral bodies in the upper cervical spine of infants and young children is a well-known phenomenon and is physiologic (2,4). Such displacement may involve all four upper vertebral bodies or occur at the C2-3 level only. In those cases in which multiple vertebral bodies are involved, the findings are not difficult to interpret (Fig. 6.7), but if isolated anterior displacement of C2 on C3 occurs, interpretation can be a problem. Indeed, in some children, the degree of displacement is so pronounced that it is almost impossible to accept that it is physiologic (Fig. 6.8). Nonetheless, it is, and it results from the fact that the fulcrum for flexion of the upper cervical spine in the infant is at the C2-3 level (see Fig. 6.75). The cervical spine generally is a lax structure in infants and children, and consequently a great deal of excessive normal motion can occur at this site (3). This often is exaggerated in the traumatized patient, because it has been demonstrated that the spine usually is flexed when the patient is immobilized on the emergency medical service's boards (5).

As an aid to this problem, I have devised the **posterior cervical line** (4), and this line has proven to be most helpful in differentiating physiologic from pathologic displacement of C2 on C3 (Fig. 6.8). The line is drawn from the anterior aspect of the cortex of the spinous process of C1 to the same point on C3, and its relationship to the anterior cortex of C2 is noted. If it misses the anterior cortex of C2 by 2 mm or more, a true dislocation, associated with an underlying hangman's fracture, should be present. A measurement of 1.5 mm is borderline, but if it is less than 1.5 mm the findings represent physiologic displacement only (Fig. 6.8). A diagrammatic representation of the normal limits for the posterior cervical line is shown in Figure 6.9, but before one examines these limits, *it must be underscored that the posterior cervical line should be applied only in those cases in which anterior displacement of C2 on C3 is present (4).* If there is mere angulation of C2 on C3, as demonstrated in Figure 6.2, the line will be normal. The posterior cervical line is designed for use if there is actual anterior displacement of C2 on C3 (Fig. 6.10). In the neutral or extended position (see Fig. 6.12), the spinous tip of C2 lies posterior to both C1 and C3; this is normal (4). This posterior positioning is retained if a hangman's fracture of C2 occurs. With this fracture, motion is transferred from the normal apophyseal joints at the C2-3 level to the fracture site. As a result, C1 and the anterior fracture fragment of C2 move forward, and the posterior portion of the arch of C2 remains in the extended position. It is for this reason that the posterior cervical line measures abnormally in these cases. Anterior displacement of the body of C2 results from associated ligament disruption between the bodies of C2 and C3.

Conversely, however, *a normal posterior cervical line measurement does not exclude underlying ligamentous injury at the C2-3 level.* Many times such injury becomes evident at a later date. In such cases, there is enough muscle spasm to keep the vertebral bodies in normal alignment; it is only in subsequent weeks, as muscle spasm subsides, that hypermobility resulting from the underlying ligament injury is appreciated (see Fig. 6.24). On the other hand, in some cases ligamentous injury is acute, and there is clear-cut apophyseal joint separation (Fig. 6.11). Because motion in these cases is not trans-

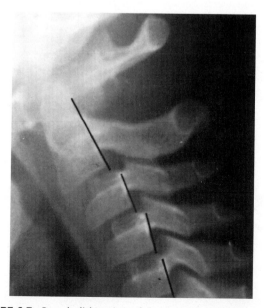

FIGURE 6.7. *Pseudodislocation of the upper cervical spine: multiple levels.* Note that each of the vertebral bodies from C2 through C5 demonstrates anterior displacement. Such displacement is normal and physiologic.

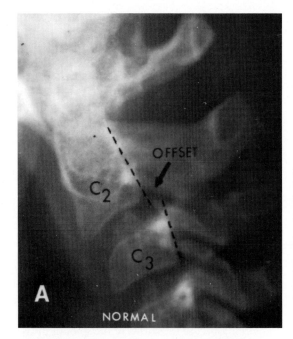

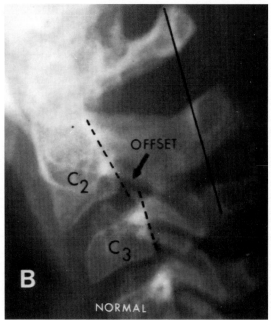

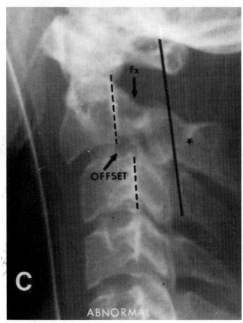

FIGURE 6.8. *Physiologic dislocation of C2 on C3: use of posterior cervical line.* **(A)** Note that C2 is anteriorly displaced on C3 (*dotted lines*). **(B)** The posterior cervical line is drawn from the anterior cortex of the spinous process of C1 to the anterior cortex of the spinous process of C3. In this case, it passes directly through the anterior cortex of C2. This is normal, and thus the findings represent physiologic displacement of C2 on C3 only. **(C)** Pathologic dislocation of C2 on C3 secondary to hangman's fracture: use of posterior cervical line. Note that the body of C2 is displaced forward on the body of C3 and that offsetting is present. Also note that the posterior cervical line is abnormal in that it misses the cortex of C2 (*star*) by more than 2 mm. The actual measurement was 4 mm. The fracture (Fx) is barely visible.

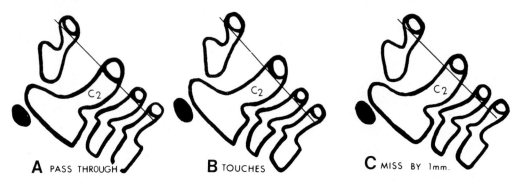

FIGURE 6.9. *Posterior cervical line: normal limits.* The posterior cervical line is normal if it passes through or just behind the cortex of C2 (**A**), touches the anterior cortex of C2 (**B**), or passes within 1 mm of the anterior aspect of the cortex of C2 (**C**). If it passes 1.5 mm in front of the cortex, it is borderline in significance, but if it misses the cortex by 2 mm or more, an underlying pathologic dislocation with an associated hangman's fracture should be present. (From Swischuk, L.E.: Anterior displacement of C2 in children: Physiologic or pathologic? A helpful differentiating line. *Radiology* 1977;122:759–763, with permission.)

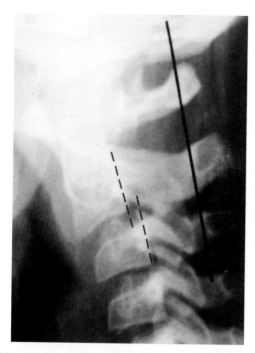

FIGURE 6.10. *Pseudodislocation: C2 on C3.* Note that C2 and C3 are offset (*arrows*). Once this determination has been made, one can apply the posterior cervical line along the spinous tips of C1 and C3. In this case, the posterior cervical line measures normal.

ferred from the C2-3 apophyseal joint to the fracture site of a hangman's fracture, the posterior cervical line remains normal. ***It is important to appreciate this potential pitfall in using the posterior cervical line.*** The phenomenon of physiologic anterior displacement of C2 on C3 is common in childhood but tends to disappear around the age of 16 years. It has been documented in young adults (1), but generally it is a phenomenon of the early and midpediatric age group.

Pathologic posterior displacement of one vertebral body on another is not particularly common but probably occurs during the acute phase of certain extension injuries. Such displacement, however, does not seem to persist for long, and the reason may be that, with subsequent return to a more neutral position or with hyperflexion secondary to whiplashing, normal alignment tends to reestablish itself. Normal physiologic posterior displacement also is not particularly common (1,4), but it does occur (Fig. 6.12). In such cases, I have not seen the displacement to result in more than 1 or 2 mm of offsetting.

Displacement of the vertebral bodies in a lateral direction also can occur but usually is associated with severe fracture dislocations, with significant changes clearly visible on the lateral view.

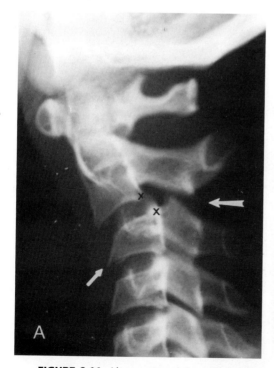

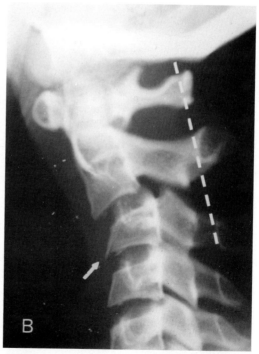

FIGURE 6.11. *Ligamentous injury: C2-3.* **(A)** Note that C2 and C3 are offset (*X*). In addition, the apophyseal joint is V-shaped (*large arrow*) and subluxation is present. There may be a small teardrop fracture of C3 present (*small arrow*). The ring epiphysis seen on edge in this area commonly appears tipped and should not be misinterpreted as a fracture (see Fig. 6.73A). **(B)** The posterior cervical line measures normal. The reason for this is that flexion motion still is occurring through the apophyseal joint. The teardrop fracture of C3 is a little more clearly visualized (*arrow*). The intraspinous distance between the spinous tips of C2 and C3 also is markedly increased, attesting to the hyperflexion injury. (Courtesy of A.M.O. Gorman, M.D.)

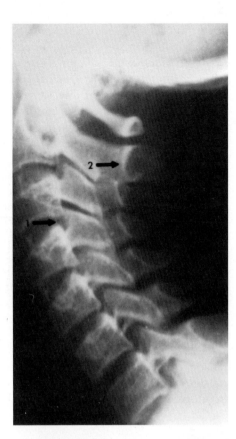

FIGURE 6.12. *Normal posterior vertebral body dislocation and posterior position of the spinous process of C2.* Note the normal posterior displacement of C3 on C4 (*1*) and the normal posterior position of the spinous process of C2 (*2*). In the neutral or extended position, this is the normal location of the spinous process of C2. With flexion, it moves forward and lines up with the spinous processes of C1 and C3. In so doing, it constitutes the basis for the application of the posterior cervical line, as delineated in Figures 6.8 and 6.9.

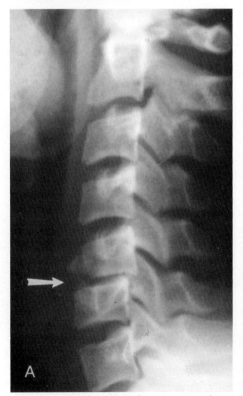
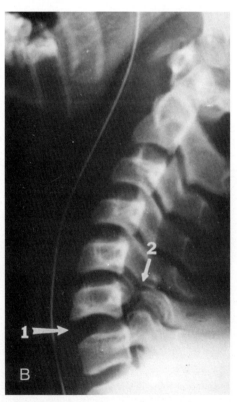

FIGURE 6.13. *Disc-space abnormalities.* (**A**) Note the narrowed disc space (*arrow*) associated with a compression fracture of C5. The vertebral body is retropulsed into the spinal canal, and there is associated widening of the apophyseal joint and widening of the interspinous distance at the C5-6 level. (**B**) Wide disc space (*1*) resulting from hyperextension injury, which also has resulted in bilateral fractures through the neural arch of C6 (*2*).

Alterations in the Width of the Disc Space

In most normal patients, the width of the intervertebral disc spaces is the same from one level to another. This is very important to note, for if there is a level at which gross discrepancy occurs, underlying ligament injury with cervical spine instability should be inferred. Narrowing of the disc space occurs with flexion and rotation injuries (Fig. 6.13A), but widening of the disc space signifies the presence of an underlying extension injury (Fig. 6.13B). Disc space narrowing or widening is best assessed on lateral views of the cervical spine.

REFERENCES

1. Harrison RB, Keats TE, Winn HR, Riddervold HO, Pope TL Jr. Pseudosubluxation in the axis in young adults. *Can J Assoc Radiol* 1980;31:176–177.
2. Kattan KR. Backward "displacement" of the spinolaminal line at C2: A normal variation. *AJR* 1977;129:289–290.
3. Kriss VM, Kriss T. Imaging of the cervical spine in infants. *Pediatr Emerg Care* 1997;13:44–49.
4. Swischuk LE. Anterior displacement of C2 in children: Physiologic or pathologic? A helpful differentiation. *Radiology* 1977;122:759–763.
5. Treloar DJ, Nypaver M. Angulation of the pediatric cervical spine with and without cervical collar. *Pediatr Emerg Care* 1997;13:5–8.

Abnormal Apophyseal Joint Configurations

On a true lateral view of the cervical spine, all of the apophyseal joints are superimposed on one another and clearly visualized (Fig. 6.14A), but with rotation the apophyseal joints are thrown off of each other. If all are rotated to the same general degree, however, rotation should be the cause (Fig. 6.14B). If, however, there is an abrupt discrepancy in the configuration of the joints at one level, that is, if the apophyseal joints are visualized in true lateral position to a certain point, and then above that point they are visualized in oblique position, one should suspect rotatory subluxation with or without a locked facet (Fig. 6.14C).

In other cases, the apophyseal joints can be frankly dislocated or subluxed; almost always this occurs with flexion–rotation injuries. In such cases, the joints, in addition to being anteriorly dislocated, may appear unduly wide or V-shaped (Fig. 6.14D and F). Either configuration is abnormal and should infer ligamentous injury with instability.

Widening of the Joints of Luschka

On normal frontal projection, with lateral bending the contralateral joints of Luschka uniformly increase in width. This phenomenon is quite common and renders evaluation of the joints of Luschka somewhat difficult. If one sees undue widening at one or two levels, however, then one should suspect underlying ligamentous injury.

Widening of the Interspinous Distance

Widening of the interspinous distance is seen with hyperflexion injuries that result in tearing of the posterior spinal ligaments. It is most important to determine whether such an increase in distance is present (Fig. 6.15A), for if it is, the

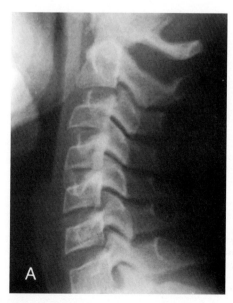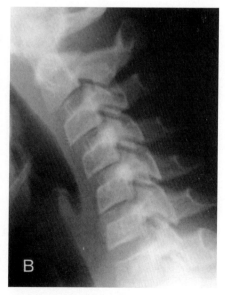

FIGURE 6.14. *Apophyseal joint alignment: normal and abnormal.* **(A)** In this normal patient, all of the apophyseal joints are superimposed one on the other, and all are normal. **(B)** With flexion, and slight rotation because of a stiff neck, universal offsetting of the apophyseal joints is seen. This still is normal.

(continued on next page)

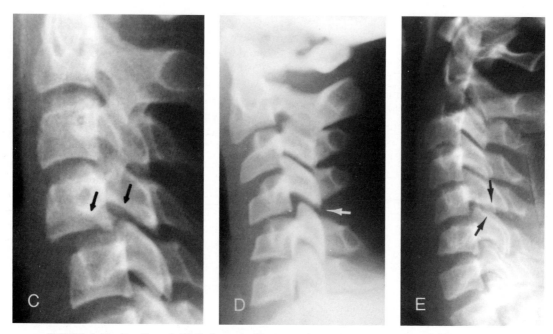

FIGURE 6.14. *(continued)* **(C)** Unilateral offsetting of the apophyseal joints (*arrows*) resulting from rotatory dislocation. Note that C4 is anteriorly displaced on C5. **(D)** Wide apophyseal joint (*arrow*) secondary to hyperflexion injury at the C4-5 level. The interspinous distance also is increased. C5 is fractured and compressed. **(E)** Another patient with a hyperflexion injury leading to a V-shaped or "fanned" apophyseal joint (*arrows*). The interspinous distance at this level also is increased. C6 is compressed.

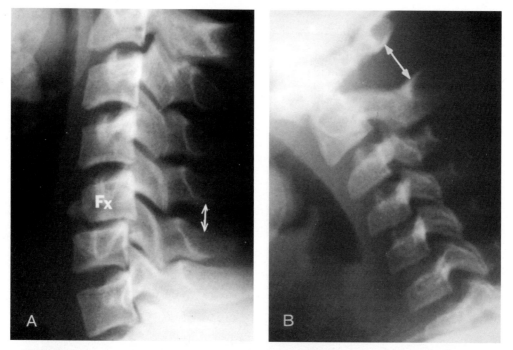

FIGURE 6.15. *Increased interspinous distance.* **(A)** Flexion injury. Note the increased interspinous distance (*arrows*) between the spinous processes of C5 and C6. The apophyseal joint through the same level is also a little widened, and there is a compression fracture of C5 with retropulsion of the vertebral body into the spinal canal. The intravertebral disc space between C5 and C6 is narrowed. **(B)** Normally wide intraspinous distance between C1 and C2 (*arrows*).

injury is unstable. Such widening also can be appreciated on frontal views (2).

With flexion of the upper cervical spine, however, it should be noted that very commonly the distance between the spinous tips of C1 and C2 appears unusually wide but is entirely normal (Fig. 6.15B). In such cases, I believe that tight ligamentous attachments between the base of the skull and C1 cause the pseudoabnormal configuration. It is a very common finding in children (1) and should not be misinterpreted as pathologic separation of the spinous processes of C1 and C2.

REFERENCES

1. Cattell HS, Filtzer DL. Pseudosubluxation and other normal variations in the cervical spine in children. *J Bone Joint Surg* 1965; 47A:1295–1309.
2. Naidich JB, Naidich TP, Garfein C, Liebeskind AL, Hyman RA. The widened interspinous distance: A useful sign of anterior cervical dislocation in the supine frontal projection. *Radiology* 1977; 123:113–116.

Lateral Deviation of the Spinous Processes

On frontal view, in most normal patients the spinous tips are lined up in a straight line. As long as no anomalies such as bifid or unfused spinous tips are present, the tips are easy to visualize. If rotation secondary to positioning occurs, the spinous tips are deviated to the opposite side, but the degree of deviation is progressive and more pronounced in the upper spine. If deviation of the spinous tips is abrupt at one level, one should suspect underlying rotatory subluxation with a locked facet (see Fig. 6.53).

Widening of the Interpedicular Space

Widening of the interpedicular space occurs with bursting fractures of the vertebral bodies. In such cases, on frontal view, the pedicles are displaced laterally and the distance between them is increased. In addition, the apophyseal joints also may widen.

Relationships of Lateral Mass of C1 to Dens

A number of offsetting abnormalities of the lateral masses of C1 have been described (1–3), and to say the least the subject is confusing. One of the reasons for this is that almost any type of offsetting can be produced by varying degrees of rotation and tilting of the upper cervical spine in normal individuals. Because of this, I believe that the only significant abnormal configuration is that of bilateral or unilateral outward offsetting of the lateral masses, as seen with Jefferson bursting fractures of C1 (Fig. 6.16). Indeed, it has been demonstrated that "asymmetric odontoid-lateral mass interspaces on properly centered open mouth [odontoid] x-rays in the absence of otherwise abnormal cervical spine x-rays, in conscious patients without fixed deformity,

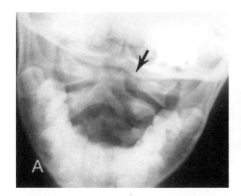 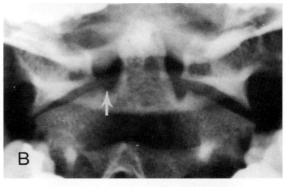

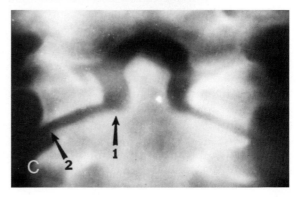

FIGURE 6.16. *Lateral mass of C1 to dens distance.* **(A)** Tilting of the head caused by wryneck results in rotation of the spine and widening of the C1-to-dens distance on the left (*arrow*). **(B)** Another patient with neck spasm demonstrates a wide C1-to-dens distance on the right (*arrow*). Even though one might believe that displacement of the lateral mass should be present, there really is little if any present. There is, however, some narrowing of the atlantoaxial joint and on the contralateral side; note that the lateral mass has shifted medially. This type of arrangement usually is caused by rotation or spasm. **(C)** True widening of the C1-to-dens distance (*1*) resulting from a unilateral Jefferson fracture of C1, which has caused the lateral mass of C1 on the right to be offset on the body of C2 (*2*). The contralateral side shows no offsetting in either direction and is normal.

appear to be incidental" (2). The observation, of course, should be made on a nonrotated film only. With rotation, one lateral mass may appear to be displaced outward and its mate inward, but this is not indicative of a fracture, only rotation. Such rotation may be positional only, secondary to spasm, or associated with rotatory dislocation of C1 on C2.

REFERENCES

1. Fielding JW, Hawkins RJ. Atlanto-axial rotatory fixation (fixed rotatory subluxation of the atlanto-axial joint). *J Bone Joint Surg* 1977;59:37–44.
2. Iannacone WM, DeLong WG Jr, Born CT, Bednar JM, Ross SE. Dynamic computerized tomography of the occiput-atlas-axis complex in trauma patients with odontoid lateral mass asymmetry. *J Trauma* 1990;30:1501–1505.
3. Shapiro R, Youngberg AS, Rothman SLG. The differential diagnosis of traumatic lesions of the occipito atlanto-axial segment. *Radiol Clin North Am* 1973;11:505–526.

TABLE 6.3. SIGNS OF INSTABILITY OF CERVICAL SPINE INJURIES[a]

Anterior, posterior or lateral dislocation of a vertebral body
Widened or narrowed intervertebral disc spaces
Widened, narrowed or dislocated apophyseal joint
Focally widened (dislocated) joints of Luschka
Bilateral or unilateral locked facets
Separation of the spinous processes with or without associated avulsion fractures[b]
Flexion or extension teardrop fractures
Anterior wedge compression fracture with posterior displacement of involved vertebral body
Widened predental (C_1-dens) space
Outward displacement of the lateral masses of C_1 (Jefferson fracture—especially unilateral)
Unilateral anterior displacement of one of the lateral masses of C_1 (rotatory dislocation)
Fracture of the dens, with or without displacement
Bursting fracture of vertebral body

[a]More than one may be present in any case.
[b]May require flexion views for demonstrable instability.

Actual Fracture Visualization

I have left assessment of the cervical spine for the detection of fractures to the end, not because I feel it is unimportant, but because I think it is more important to first assess the spine in other ways. If one looks for fractures first, then one is more likely to miss the other, perhaps more important, findings. However, once one does look for fractures in the cervical spine, it is very important to appreciate those that are associated with instability. Many of these fractures are clearly visible on regular views, but others may remain occult until CT scans are obtained.

Determining Instability of a Cervical Spine Injury

In the final analysis, one's most important mission in evaluating cervical spine injuries is to determine whether the injury is stable or unstable, and in this regard the lateral plain film of the cervical spine is the single most valuable study. Instability results from severe ligamentous injury, with or without a bony fracture, and certain plain-film findings should signify the presence of such injury. These findings are summarized in Table 6.4, and only a few pitfalls exist. These include the flexion injury that appears normal on extension (see Fig. 6.23), the patient with a central cord syndrome and a normal-appearing cervical spine (see Fig. 6.66), and the patient with a nondisplaced or minimally displaced fracture through the base of the dens (see Fig. 6.28). In all of these cases, although a significant, even unstable, injury is present, the cervical spine may appear remarkably normal on initial inspection. Other than under these circumstances, however, one should be able to corre-

late the abnormal findings listed in Table 6.3 with the presence of cervical spine instability.

Types and Mechanisms of Cervical Spine Injuries

Injuries to the cervical spine range from minimal soft-tissue and ligamentous injury to complete fracture dislocation with spinal cord injury. Basically, however, the spine is subject to five forces: flexion, extension, lateral flexion, rotation, and axial compression (35). The types of injuries resulting if these forces become excessive are discussed in detail in the following paragraphs.

Flexion Injuries of the Lower Cervical Spine

These injuries usually produce abnormality in three areas: the vertebral body and its ligaments, the apophyseal joints and their ligaments, and the spinous processes and their ligaments (Fig. 6.17). Overall, compressive forces are in effect anteriorly and distraction forces posteriorly. Anteriorly, this results in vertebral-body compression (Fig. 6.18) and, in many cases, a triangular, corner, avulsion, or "teardrop" fracture (Fig. 6.19A). This fracture results from buckling of the anterior longitudinal ligament during hyperflexion, and most often it is the lower, anterior corner of the vertebral body that is avulsed (16,26). With extension injuries, the teardrop involves the upper anterior corner (see Fig. 6.35). If a teardrop fracture is noted, an unstable hyperflexion injury can be assumed. In children, the equivalent of the teardrop fracture often consists of displacement of a fragment of the normal vertebral epiphyseal ring (9). An example of such an injury is seen in Figure 6.19C. In other cases,

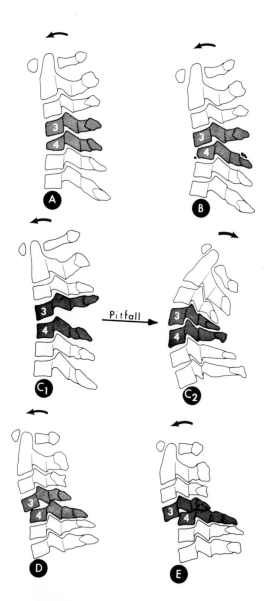

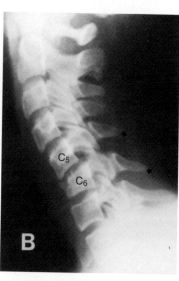

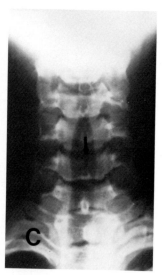

FIGURE 6.17. *Flexion injuries of the lower cervical spine: diagrammatic representation.* **(A)** Minimal flexion causes anterior compression of C4. **(B)** More pronounced flexion causes dislocation of the apophyseal joints between C3 and C4, narrowing of the disc space between the two vertebral bodies, and widening of the interspinous distance between the two vertebrae. Also note an anterior–inferior teardrop fracture of C4 and an avulsion fracture of the spinous process of C4. **(C)** Flexion injury pitfall. On flexion (*C1*) note that there is separation of the apophyseal joints between C3 and C4. Also note that the spinous processes have been separated. On extension (*C2*), however, note that the vertebrae align normally and that no injury is apparent. This is an important pitfall to avoid in the interpretation of flexion injuries and is illustrated in Figure 6.23. **(D)** More pronounced flexion causes marked dislocation of C3 on C4 and locking of the facets. **(E)** Severe anterior dislocation of C3 on C4, with locking of the vertebral bodies.

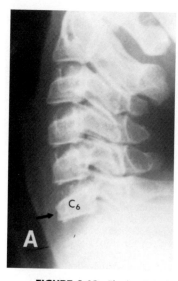

FIGURE 6.18. *Flexion injuries with compressed vertebrae.* **(A)** Note subtle anterior wedging of C6 (*arrow*). There is no corresponding soft-tissue swelling and no other findings of injury. **(B)** More severe injury demonstrates localized kyphosis at the level of C5-6. The corresponding spinous processes are separated (*asterisk*), leading to an increase in the interspinous distance. There is anterior apophyseal joint dislocation, narrowing of the intervening disc space, anterior compression and fragmentation of C6, anterior dislocation of C5 on C6, and clear-cut prevertebral soft-tissue swelling. In addition, note that the posterior portion of C6 has been displaced into the spinal canal. **(C)** Frontal view demonstrating associated vertical fracture (*arrow*) through the body of C6.

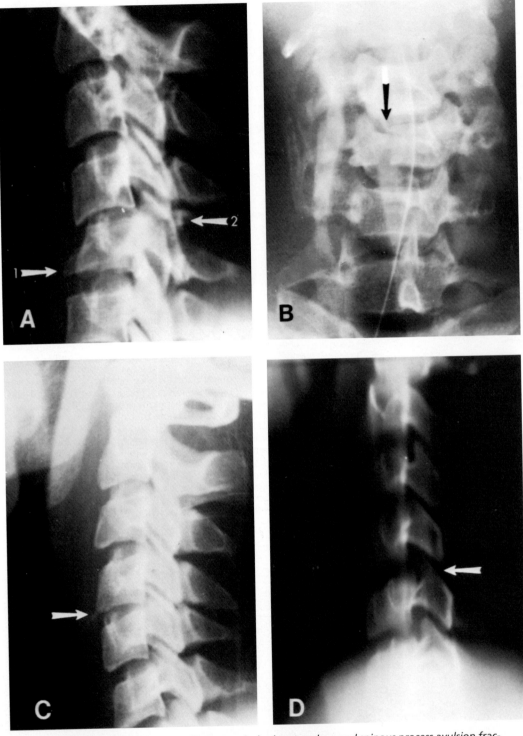

FIGURE 6.19. *Flexion injuries of lower cervical spine: teardrop and spinous process avulsion fractures.* **(A)** Note the large teardrop fracture (*1*) of C5. Also note that C5 is compressed anteriorly and that the disc space between C4 and C5 is narrowed. The interspinous distance between C4 and C5 also is increased, and there is an associated avulsion fracture (*2*) of the posterior elements of C5. **(B)** Frontal view demonstrating associated vertical fracture (*arrow*) of the compressed and expanded body of C5. Note again that the disc space between C4 and C5 is narrowed. **(C)** Small teardrop fracture along the inferoanterior aspect of C4 (*arrow*). Actually, this fragment probably represents an avulsed fragment of the ring epiphysis. Also note marked prevertebral soft-tissue swelling and narrowing of the disc space between C4 and C5. All of these findings should indicate the presence of an unstable flexion injury. **(D)** Subsequent laminagraphy demonstrates associated anterior dislocation of the apophyseal joint (*arrow*) at the involved level, attesting to the presence of a hyperflexion injury.

the corner fracture may be very subtle. In addition to the findings just noted, accompanying ligamentous injury in and around the disc space can lead to disc disruption and narrowing of the disc space (Figs. 6.19 and 6.20).

Prevertebral soft tissue swelling also is a common finding with flexion injuries but does not occur in all cases. Often it is not present with mere anterior compression fractures. With more severe injuries, however, the soft tissues appear thickened.

In those cases in which significant vertebral body compression occurs, a vertical fracture (26) through the involved vertebra frequently is present (Fig. 6.19B). Actually, this fracture attests to the presence of the vertebral compression forces. The presence of such forces causes the involved vertebra to become squashed or burst, and the vertical fracture is one manifestation of this phenomenon. On lateral view, if anterior compression is pronounced there is associated posterior displacement of the compressed vertebral body into the spinal canal (Fig. 6.20). The various fractures of the vertebral body usually are vividly demonstrable with CT scanning; posterior impingement of the spinal canal can be seen with both CT and MR scanning (Fig. 6.21). MR imaging also is very useful in detecting associated spinal cord injury.

The posterior distracting forces associated with hyperflexion injuries lead to ligamentous injury through the apophyseal joints and between the neural arches and spinous processes. At the level of the apophyseal joints, this can lead to widening of the involved joints and variable degrees of subluxation (Fig. 6.22). Vertebral-body displacement can be minimal, and displacement of 3 mm or more definitely is considered abnormal. Correspondingly, anterior angulation of more than 12 to 15 degrees also is considered abnormal. Apophyseal joint dislocation also can be demonstrated with oblique views (Fig. 6.22C). Greater degrees of dislocation can lead to perched or frankly locked facets (Fig. 6.22), or even locked vertebral bodies (Fig. 6.17E).

At the level of the neural arch and spinous processes, ligamentous injury results in separation of the involved spinous processes with widening of the interspinous distance (22) (Fig. 6.22) and, in some cases, avulsion fractures of the posterior elements (Fig. 6.19A). Once all of these features of flexion injuries of the cervical spine are appreciated, it is easy to understand why the spine becomes unstable. Clearly, if there is damage to the anterior and posterior longitudinal ligaments, the ligaments of the apophyseal joints, neural arches, and spinous processes, instability must result.

A significant pitfall in the interpretation of flexion injuries of the lower cervical spine is seen in the patient whose cervical spine shows little or no abnormality in the neutral or extended position (Fig. 6.23A). In these patients, until the spine is flexed (Fig. 6.23B), the lesion can escape

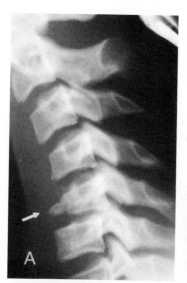 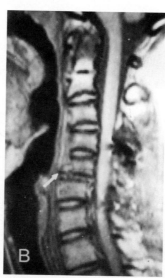 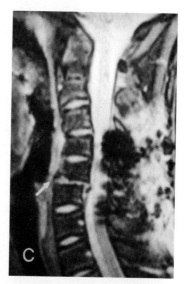

FIGURE 6.20. *Hyperflexion injuries with magnetic resonance imaging.* **(A)** Note the compression and teardrop fracture of C5 (*arrow*). There may be a small teardrop fracture of the inferior anterior corner of C4. The disc space between C5 and C6 is narrowed, and C5 is retropulsed into the spinal canal. The apophyseal joints are widened. **(B)** T1-weighted magnetic resonance image demonstrates the compressed vertebra with the teardrop fracture (*arrow*). **(C)** T2-weighted image more clearly identifies the teardrop fracture (*arrow*), compressed vertebra, narrowed disc space, and retropulsed vertebral body into the spinal canal. There also is a small posterior fragment of bone that has been avulsed off of the posterior aspect of C6. There is minimal impingement of the spinal canal but no impingement of the cord. Extensive soft tissue edema and bleeding are seen in the posterior soft tissues (high signal).

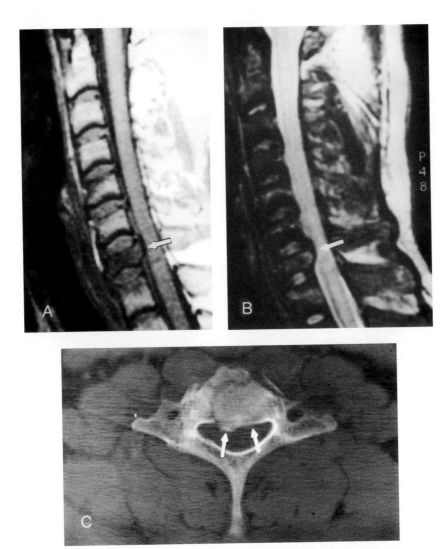

FIGURE 6.21. *Flexion injury with compression fracture: magnetic resonance and computed tomographic findings.* **(A)** T1-weighted image; patient with a compressed vertebra with retropulsion into the spinal canal (*arrow*). **(B)** T2-weighted image more clearly identifies the bulging vertebra (*arrow*). There is minimal impingement on the spinal cord. **(C)** Computed tomographic study in the same patient demonstrates the retropulsed fragment (*arrows*) and the other fractures of the vertebral body.

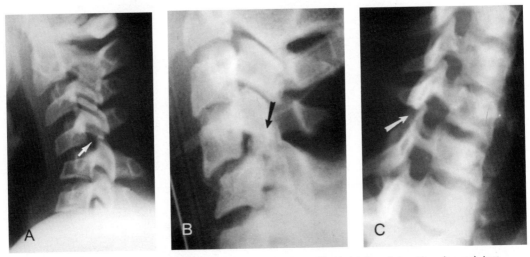

FIGURE 6.22. *Apophyseal-joint dislocation.* Marked apophyseal-joint dislocation (*arrow*) just short of a locked facet. Also note the increased interspinous distance. **(B)** Another patient with actual locked facets (*arrow*). Note that the interspinous distance also has increased and that the disc space between C3 and C4 is narrowed. C3 is displaced anteriorly on C4. **(C)** Oblique view in still another patient demonstrates apophyseal-joint dislocation (*arrow*) with a so-called perched facet. With more flexion it would jump and lock.

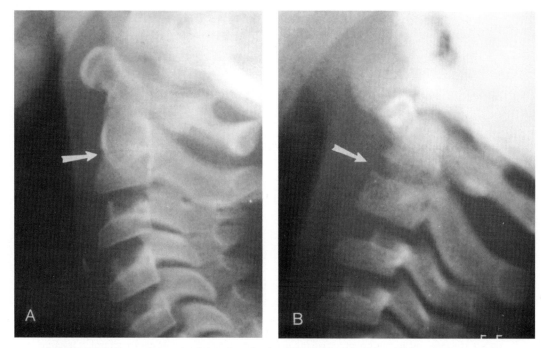

FIGURE 6.27. *Normal dens-body synchrosis of C2.* **(A)** In this older child, note the very thin dens-body synchrosis (*arrow*). Its sclerotic edges should speak towards a normal synchondrosis. **(B)** An infant with a wide but normal dens-body synchrosis (*arrow*). In each of these cases note that the dens is not anteriorly tilted. It is in normal position.

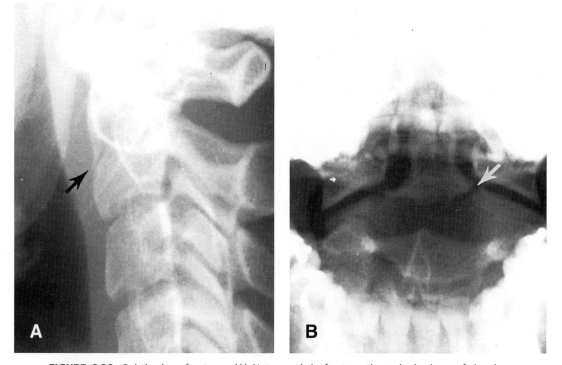

FIGURE 6.28. *Subtle dens fractures.* **(A)** Note a subtle fracture through the base of the dens (*arrow*). There is no displacement of the dens, but the prevertebral soft tissues might be slightly widened. **(B)** Frontal view demonstrating the fracture more clearly (*arrow*); subsequent laminagraphy demonstrated the fracture to extend across the entire base of the dens. (A and B are courtesy of T. Brown, M.D.) *(continued on next page)*

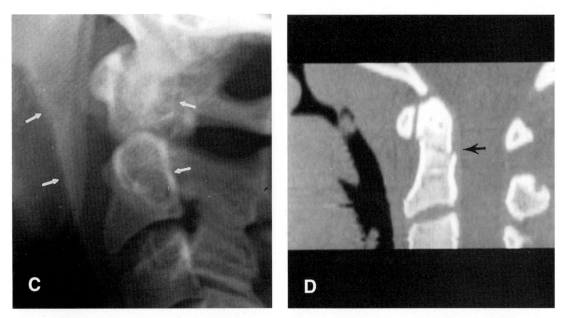

FIGURE 6.28. *(continued)* **(C)** Note suggestion of prevertebral soft-tissue swelling (*anterior arrows*), and that the dens and body of C2 appear slightly angled (*posterior arrows*). Even a defect is suggested in the posterior cortex. **(D)** Sagittal reconstruction demonstrates a fracture through the dens (*arrow*).

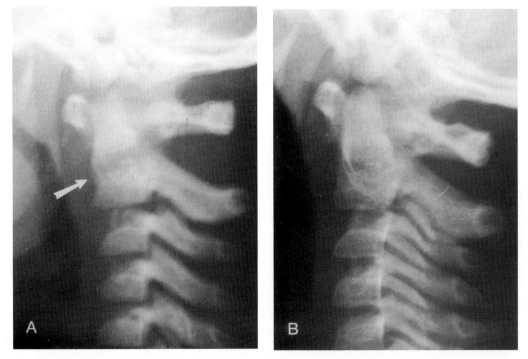

FIGURE 6.29. *Fracture of dens: subtle findings.* **(A)** Note the widened synchondrosis (*arrow*). This becomes important in view of the fact that the dens is also anteriorly tilted. The synchondrosis also is indistinct, and there is some resorption of bone on either side. The reason for this is that the patient sustained this injury 3 weeks previously in an automobile accident. **(B)** One year later the dens and body of C2 have fused, but the dens remains anteriorly tilted.

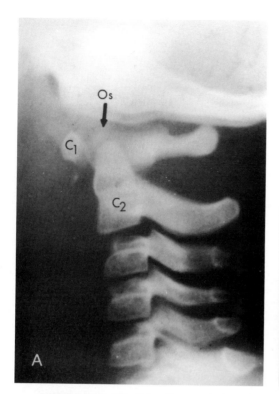 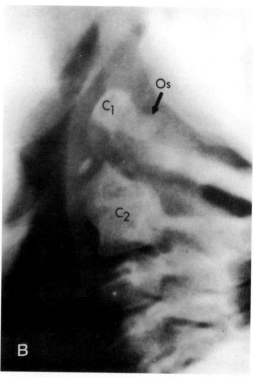

FIGURE 6.30. *C1 dislocation, and dens injury with resorption.* **(A)** Note marked soft-tissue swelling, anterior displacement of C1 with an increased C1-to-dens distance, and an avulsed bony fragment from C1. Not clearly seen but also present is a dislocated os terminale (*Os*). **(B)** Years later, the dens has completely resorbed, and the os terminale has overgrown to produce an acquired os odontoideum (*Os*). (From Ricciardi JE, Kaufer H, and Louis DS: Acquired os odontoideum following acute ligament injury. *J Bone Joint Surg* 1976;58A:410–412.)

patients younger than 13 years of age (13). They may be isolated injuries, or injuries associated with other upper cervical spine injuries (Figs. 6.30 and 6.31). If gross, they usually are inconsistent with survival (Fig. 6.31). It is important to appreciate that in children, atlantoaxial instability and laxity most often result from underlying problems such as rheumatoid arthritis and congenital hypoplasia of the dens (often in the trisomy 21 syndrome). Finally, with some hyperflexion injuries of the upper cervical spine, posterior element avulsion fractures may be seen (Fig. 6.32).

Roentgenographically, if anterior atlantoaxial dislocation is present, no matter what the cause, the predental distance is widened. It should be remembered, however, that the predental distance in children normally is wider than in adults, and that it is not unusual for it to measure as much as 4 or 5 mm and still be normal (Fig. 6.5). In addition to this finding, it should be recalled that the interspinous distance between C1 and C2 also frequently is very prominent in most normal children (Fig. 6.15B) and should not be misinterpreted as being indicative of posterior ligamentous injury at this level.

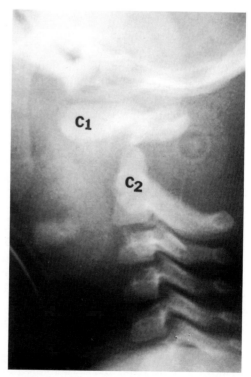

FIGURE 6.31. *Gross atlantoaxial dislocation.* Note that C1 is completely separated and anteriorly displaced from C2. There is extensive prevertebral edema. This patient was dead on arrival.

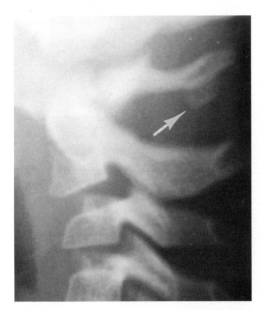

FIGURE 6.32. *Posterior avulsion fracture.* Note the posterior avulsion fracture (*arrow*) of C1.

Extension Injuries of the Lower Cervical Spine

These injuries, as opposed to flexion injuries, result in compressive forces posteriorly and distracting forces anteriorly (Fig. 6.33). Consequently, often there is little in the way of vertebral body fracturing, but considerable evidence of fracturing of the articular facets, pillars, and posterior elements (Fig. 6.34). Disc space widening resulting from anterior ligament disruption also can occur (3) and may be associated with *an extension-type "teardrop" fracture* (Fig. 6.35). This fracture occurs anteriorly, and like the flexion teardrop fracture indicates the presence of a significant ligamentous, unstable injury. As opposed to the flexion teardrop fracture, however, the extension teardrop fracture involves the upper anterior corner of the vertebral body (Fig. 6.35). It results from undue stretching or tearing of the anterior longitudinal ligament during hyperextension (Fig. 6.33C) and, because of this, is associated with a widened disc space (Figs. 6.35 and 6.36).

If an extension teardrop fracture is present, prevertebral soft tissue swelling usually also is present, but if there is no anterior ligamentous injury, the prevertebral soft tissues remain normal. Posteriorly, with hyperextension injuries, a variety of fractures through the neural arches, pedicles, articular facets, pillars, and spinous processes, can occur. If these latter fractures are unilateral and not associated with any other injuries, the spine is not particularly unstable, but if they are bilateral and occur through the neural arch or pedicles, they result in an unstable injury. This injury, of course, is identical to the injury that occurs with the classic hangman's fracture of C2. In these cases, often it is not until CT scanning is performed that the posterior-element frac-

EXTENSION INJURIES
(Lower Cervical Spine)

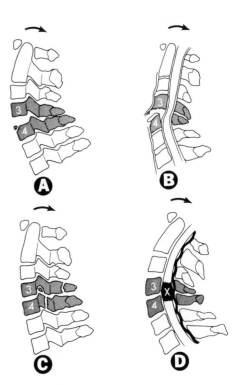

FIGURE 6.33. *Extension injuries of lower cervical spine: diagrammatic representation.* **(A)** Hyperextension causes widening of the disc space between C3 and C4, a characteristic anterior teardrop (corner) fracture of C4, and alteration of the associated apophyseal joint. **(B)** Note how stretching and tearing of the anterior longitudinal ligament leads to the avulsion–teardrop fracture and how cord damage occurs with this type of injury. **(C)** Hyperextension also can produce a variety of posterior element fractures of the involved vertebrae. A combination of disruption of the disc space and posterior-element fractures can lead to slight anterior displacement of the vertebral body (see Fig. 6.36A). **(D)** Central cord (Sciwara) syndrome. In this type of injury no fracture occurs, but buckling of the ligamentum flavum during hyperextension causes compression and injury to the cord (*X*).

tures come to one's attention (Figs. 6.36 and 6.37). Anterior vertebral-body displacement is not as common with extension injuries as with flexion injuries, but if posterior-arch fractures occur in association with ligament and disc disruption, a mild degree of anterior displacement can be seen (Fig. 6.36A). An important pitfall in the evaluation of hyperextension injuries of the lower cervical spine occurs with the so-called central cord or Sciwara syndrome. This syndrome (see Fig. 6.66C) is discussed at a later point, but it should be noted that the cervical spine in these patients usually appears normal. Rather than fracture dislocation, there is buckling of the ligamentum flavum during hyperextension, and focal compression of the spinal cord (Fig. 6.33D). Consequently, although clinically there is definite evidence of cord injury, cervical spine films appear remark-

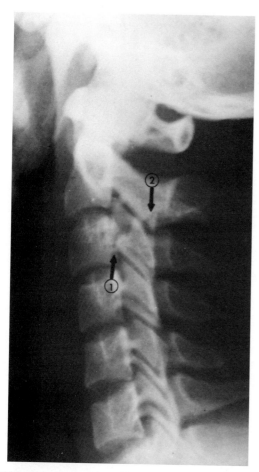

FIGURE 6.34. *Extension injury: multiple posterior element fractures.* Note fractures through the base of the articular facet of C3 (*1*) and the posterior articulating facet of C2 (*2*). The involved facet of C3 is dislocated posteriorly to a slight degree and probably rotated. The injury is most likely the result of a combination of extension and rotation forces.

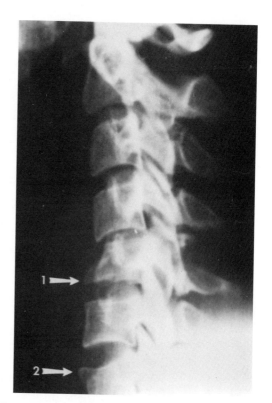

FIGURE 6.35. *Extension and flexion teardrop fractures.* This patient sustained a whiplash injury and on this lateral view shows evidence of both flexion and extension injuries. A typical flexion teardrop fracture of C5 is demonstrated at level 1. Note that the vertebra above is anteriorly displaced and that the intervening disc space is narrowed. An extension teardrop fracture is demonstrated at level 2. Note that it is located at the upper anterior corner of the involved vertebra, and that the disc space above is widened. Such widening is characteristic of extension injuries.

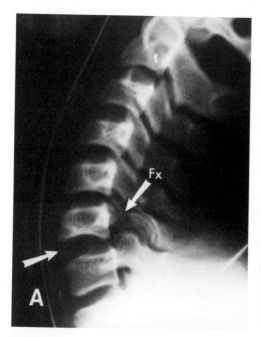
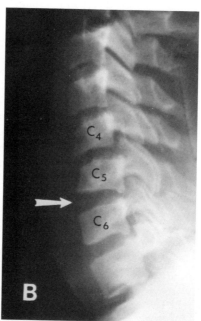

FIGURE 6.36. *Hyperextension injuries: lower cervical spine.* (**A**) Note the fracture through the posterior elements (*Fx*) and the widened disc space (*anterior arrow*). There is slight anterior displacement of the vertebra above the widened disc space. (**B**) Another patient with widening of the disc space between C5 and C6 (*arrow*). Fractures of the posterior elements are not visualized. An associated flexion injury is present at the C4-5 level (i.e., anterior displacement of C4 and apophyseal joint widening or fanning is seen).

(continued on next page)

557

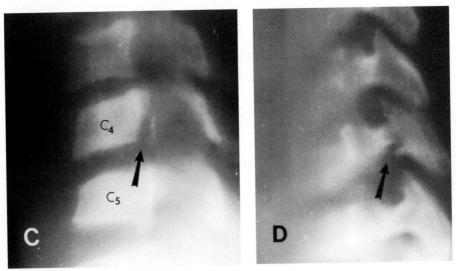

FIGURE 6.36. *(continued)* (**C** and **D**) Tomography, however, demonstrates a number of fractures through the posterior elements *(arrows)*, consistent with a hyperextension injury.

ably negative. In such cases MR imaging (6) is extremely useful in detecting spinal cord and soft-tissue injury (see Fig. 6.66).

Extension Injuries of the Atlas and Axis

These injuries are quite common (Fig. 6.38), and among the most common are fractures through the posterior arch of C1, fractures of the dens, and the classic hangman's fracture of C2 (19,20,34). Fractures through the posterior arch of C1 can be bilateral or unilateral and can be seen alone or in association with other fractures of C1 or C2 (Fig. 6.39). These fractures usually produce narrow defects through the posterior arch of C1, and in this way can be differentiated from commonly occurring congenital defects of the arch. The latter usually are quite wide and associated with triangular, tapered, or otherwise peculiarly shaped residual, ossified fragments of the posterior arch of C1 (Fig. 6.40). At the extreme end of this group of anomalies, posterior-arch

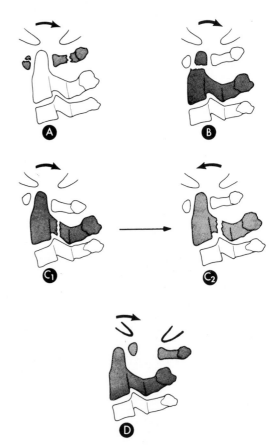

FIGURE 6.38. *Extension injuries of the upper cervical spine.* (**A**) Typical transverse fracture through the anterior arch of C1 and vertical fracture through the posterior arch of C1. (**B**) Fracture of the base of the dens with posterior displacement. (**C1 and C2**) Hangman's fracture of C2. With initial extension bilateral fractures through the arch or pedicles of C2 occur (**C1**). With subsequent return to a more neutral position, abnormal motion through the fracture site occurs, and associated ligament disruption through the C2-3 disc allows the body and dens of C2, and all of C1, to move forward. (**D**) Posterior atlantoaxial dislocation without fracture of the dens. This is a very uncommon injury.

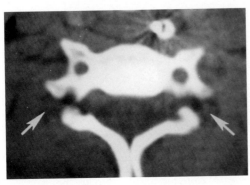

FIGURE 6.37. *Hyperextension injury: computed tomographic findings.* Note the bilateral fractures through the posterior pedicles *(arrows)* of the vertebrae. This is the same patient as shown in Figure 6.36A.

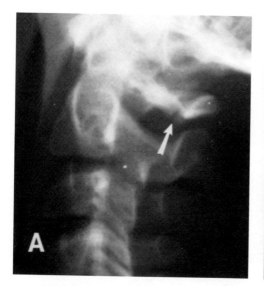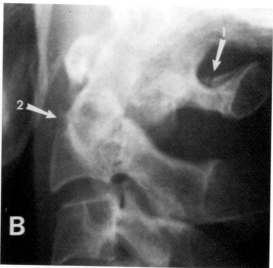

FIGURE 6.39. *Hyperextension, posterior arch of C1 fractures.* (**A**) Note the typical thin radiolucent line of a fracture (*arrow*) through the posterior arch of C1. Such fractures can be unilateral or bilateral. (**B**) Another patient demonstrating a vertical fracture through the posterior arch of C1 (1), but in addition there is a fracture through the base of the dens (2). Note associated posterior tilting and angulation of the dens. Both of these injuries result from hyperextension.

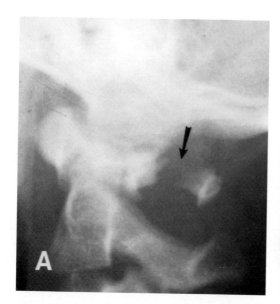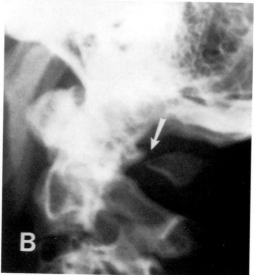

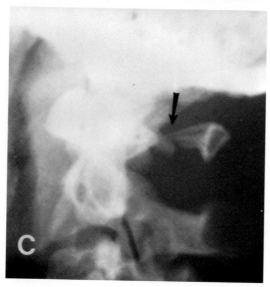

FIGURE 6.40. *Congenital defects of the posterior arch of C1.* (**A**) Wide defect (*arrow*) in a young girl who was in an automobile accident. Note the bizarre appearance of the remaining ossicles of the posterior arch of C1. (**B**) Typical triangular posterior ossicle and tapered ossicle ends seen with congenital defects (*arrow*) of C1. (**C**) Another patient demonstrating a generally thin and hypoplastic posterior arch of C1 and typical tapering of the bone ends on either side of the congenital defect (*arrow*). These defects should not be misinterpreted as posterior arch fractures. (Part C courtesy of P.S. Kline, Jr., M.D.)

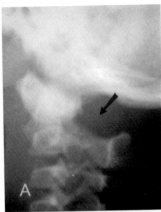
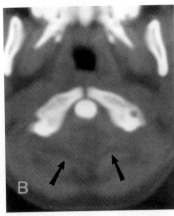
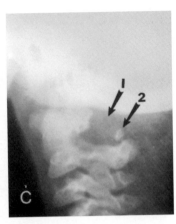

FIGURE 6.41. *Absence of posterior arch of C1.* **(A)** Note complete absence of the bony posterior arch of C1 (*arrow*). **(B)** Computed tomographic study in the same patient demonstrates absence of the posterior arch (*arrows*). **(C)** Another patient with almost complete absence of the posterior arch (1) with only a small ossicle of the spinous tip (2) remaining.

ossification is absent altogether (Fig. 6.41). Less commonly, extension injuries produce transverse fractures of the anterior arch of C1 (Fig. 6.38A). These fractures usually remain occult until CT scanning with reconstruction is performed.

Fractures of the dens secondary to extension injuries often are associated with a variable degree of posterior tilting or displacement of the dens (Fig. 6.42A). Minimal displacements or tilts must be differentiated from the normally tilted or lordotic dens (Fig. 6.42B) occurring with surprising frequency in many normal individuals. As with flexion injuries, some of these fractures are very subtle and come to

light only with subsequent CT scanning with reconstruction (Fig. 6.43).

With the hangman's fracture of C2, initial hyperextension causes bilateral fractures through the neural arch or pedicles and disruption of the ligaments anteriorly. In some such cases, the fracture through the posterior element of C2 is clearly visible; in others it remains obscure. In these latter cases, if any degree of anterior displacement of C2 on C3 is suspected, one should apply the posterior cervical line, for it will be abnormal (i.e., it will miss the posterior arch of C2 by 2 mm or more) (Fig. 6.44). Unilateral neural arch frac-

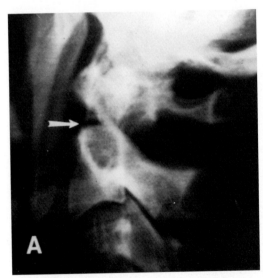
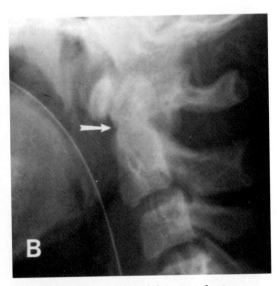

FIGURE 6.42. *Hyperextension fracture of the dens with posterior tilting.* **(A)** Note a fracture through the base of the dens (*arrow*), and readily visible posterior tilting of the dens. A similar fracture is shown in Figure 6.39B. **(B)** Normal posteriorly tilted dens. This patient was in an automobile accident and the normal posteriorly tilted dens was misinterpreted as a fractured dens. This type of misinterpretation often is enhanced by the presence of a slight notchlike defect at the base of the dens (*arrow*).

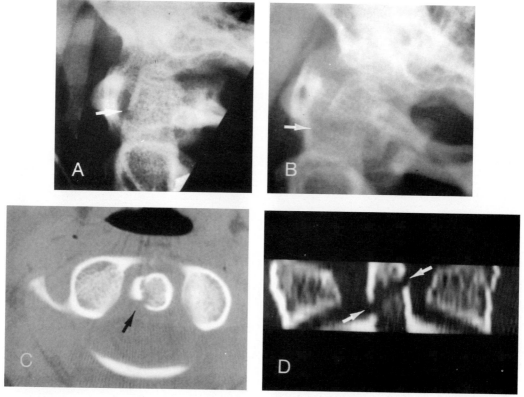

FIGURE 6.43. *Subtle dens fracture.* **(A)** On this view note a subtle fracture (*arrow*) of the dens. It probably would be entirely missed on this view. **(B)** Another view demonstrates a more suspicious-appearing finding (*arrow*) at the base of the dens. Still, nothing is absolutely clear. **(C)** Axial computed tomographic scan demonstrates a clear-cut fracture through the dens (*arrow*). **(D)** Coronal reconstruction demonstrates the fracture (*arrows*) more clearly. The C1-to-dens distance on the right is widened due to rotation. (Courtesy of C. Keith Hayden, M.D., Fort Worth Children's Hospital, Fort Worth, Texas.)

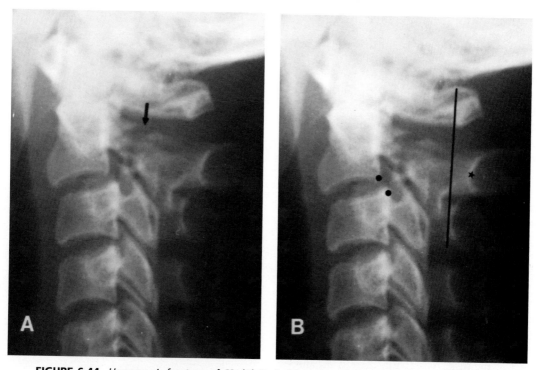

FIGURE 6.44. *Hangman's fracture of C2.* **(A)** Typical location of the bilateral fractures through the neural arch-pedicle junctions of C2 (*arrow*). **(B)** Same patient. Note that C2 is displaced on C3 (*dots*), and that the posterior cervical line lies more than 2 mm anterior to the cortex of the spinous process of C2 (*star*).

(continued on next page)

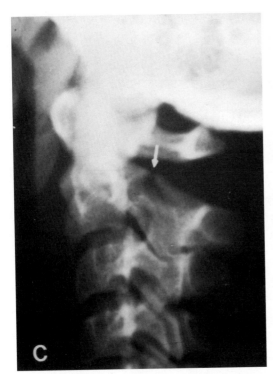

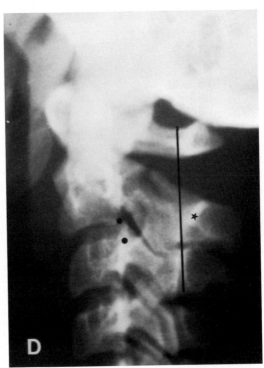

FIGURE 6.44. *(continued)* **(C)** Another patient with more subtle findings. Note, however, the characteristic location of the fracture *(arrow)*. **(D)** Same patient as in **C**. Very little anterior displacement of C2 on C3 is present *(dots)*, but the fact that such displacement is present at all becomes significant. Under these circumstances, the posterior cervical line should be applied, and in this case it misses the anterior cortex of the spinous process of C2 by more than 2 mm. Consequently, the line is abnormal and should reflect the presence of pathologic dislocation of C2 on C3 secondary to a hangman's fracture. For more discussion of the posterior cervical line in normal and abnormal cases, see Figure 6.9.

tures may be more difficult to detect but usually are not associated with cervical spine instability (Fig. 6.45). In young infants, hangman's fractures also may be clinically silent (17). This may occur more often than currently is appreciated (34) (see Fig. 6.48).

The hangman's fracture usually is part of a whiplash injury, in which hyperextension forces lead to the posterior neural arch fracture (unstable) and anterior ligament disruption, and flexion forces lead to posterior ligamentous disruption. As a result of these injuries, normal motion from the apophyseal joints is transferred to the fracture site, and C2 becomes anteriorly displaced on C3 (Fig. 6.44). In those cases in which the hyperextension injury predominates, one may see very little in the way of anterior displacement of C2 on C3 (Fig. 6.44C and D). On the other hand, in children and adolescents, because of normal physiologic laxity of the apophyseal joints of C2 and C3, the flexion component of the injury may result in disruption of the apophyseal joint ligaments and little in the way of disruption of the ligaments along the posterior aspect of the disk. As a result, there is no anterior displacement of C2 on C3 but rather marked motion and instability at the C2-3 apophyseal-joint level (Fig. 6.46).

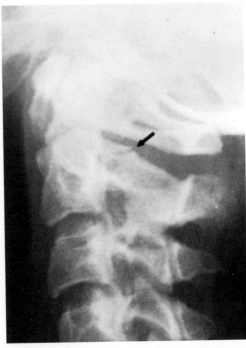

FIGURE 6.45. *Extension injury of C2: unilateral arch fracture.* Note the fracture *(arrow)* through the neural arch–pedicle junction of C2. This was a unilateral fracture, and no instability was present.

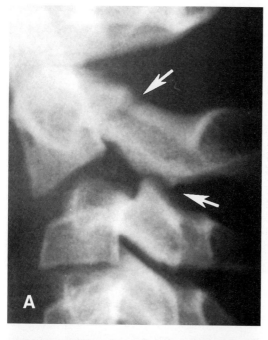

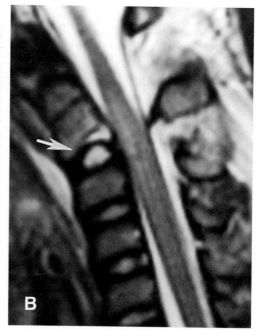

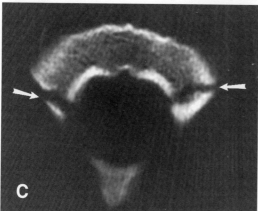

FIGURE 6.46. *Hangman's fracture, whiplash mechanism.* **(A)** Note the fracture (*upper arrow*) through the posterior arch of C2. The C2-3 disk space is widened posteriorly, and the apophyseal joints demonstrate poor coverage and a slight V-shaped configuration (*lower arrow*). **(B)** Sagittal T2-weighted magnetic resonance study demonstrates the disrupted disk at C2-3 with posterior bulging and impingement on the cord. High signal in the cord signifies the presence of a contusion. Note some edema anterior to C2-3, and considerable edema over the posterior ligaments. **(C)** Axial computed tomographic scan demonstrates the bilateral pars fractures (*arrows*).

Congenital defects of the posterior arch of C2 are not as common as those of C1. They do occur, however, and they tend to resemble fractures more than they do if they are seen through the posterior elements of C1. Keys to recognizing these as normal synchondroses are their incidental discovery, sclerosis along their margins, and the fact that they do not change their configuration with flexion (i.e., no abnormal motion) (Figs. 6.47 and 6.72). Hangman fractures are unstable (Fig. 6.48).

Another injury of the cervical spine sustained during hyperextension is the pure posterior atlantoaxial dislocation (Fig. 6.38D). This injury, however, is rare, for the strong transverse ligament usually causes a dens fracture to occur instead. Finally, it should be appreciated that with injuries to the face, in which hyperextension forces are at play, associated hyperextension injuries of the upper cervical spine can coexist (9). This also can occur with airbag injuries (8).

Lateral Flexion Injuries of the Cervical Spine

These injuries can result in simple ipsilateral vertebral body compression, contralateral fractures of the transverse or uncinate processes (27), and contralateral brachial plexus avulsions (Fig. 6.49). With lateral flexion injuries, the contralateral joints of Luschka can be disrupted and appear widened. It should be noted, however, that with normal lateral flexion some widening of the joints of Luschka occurs, and if such widening occurs at numerous adjacent levels, it most likely is normal. If, however, there is marked disparity at one or two levels, significant underlying ligamentous injury with potential instability of the cervical spine should be suspected (Fig. 6.50). Very often, if this finding is present considerable injury to the cervical spine has occurred, and significant findings also are present on the lateral view. In the upper cervical spine, lateral flexion can produce frac-

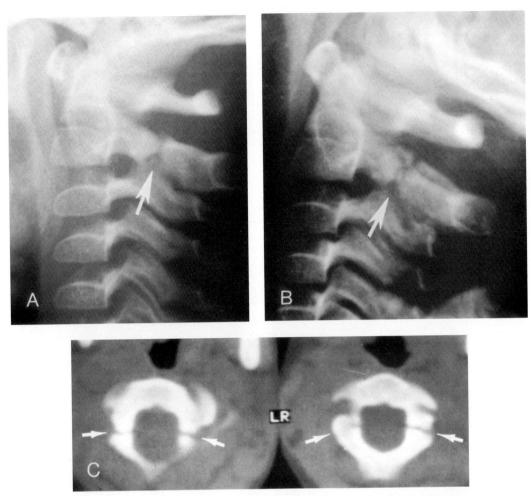

FIGURE 6.47. *Congenital defect through posterior arch of C2.* (**A**) Note the fracture-like appearing defect (*arrow*) through the posterior arch of C2. The edges are somewhat sclerotic. (**B**) Another view with slight rotation makes the defects (*arrow*) appear even more as though they were fractures. (**C**) Axial computed tomographic scan through C2 demonstrates the smooth congenital defects (*arrows*). There was no change with flexion and extension. **B** was obtained during extension; **A** was obtained during partial flexion. Also see Fig. 6.72.

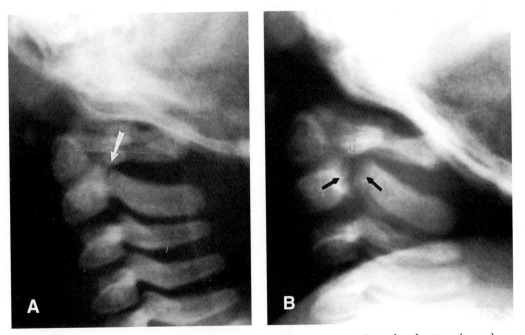

FIGURE 6.48. *Hangman's fracture in an infant.* (**A**) Note suggestion of a fracture (*arrow*) through the pars. (**B**) With flexion the fracture appears widely diastatic (*arrows*). Note that there are no sclerotic smooth edges of the fractured vertebrae. (Courtesy of Jesse Littleton, M.D.).

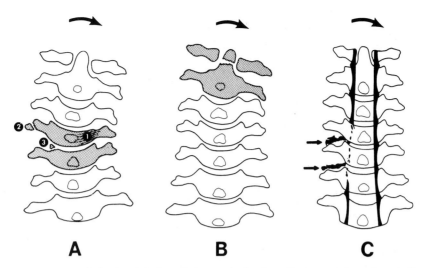

FIGURE 6.49. *Lateral flexion injuries of the cervical spine: diagrammatic representation.* **(A)** With flexion, a fracture (compression) can occur through the ipsilateral side of a vertebral body (*1*). On the contralateral side, avulsion fractures occur through the transverse process (*2*) or through the uncinate process (*3*). **(B)** Fracture of the base of the dens with some lateral displacement to the side of flexion. **(C)** Brachial plexus avulsion. These avulsions occur on the side opposite the side of bending and result in dural tears.

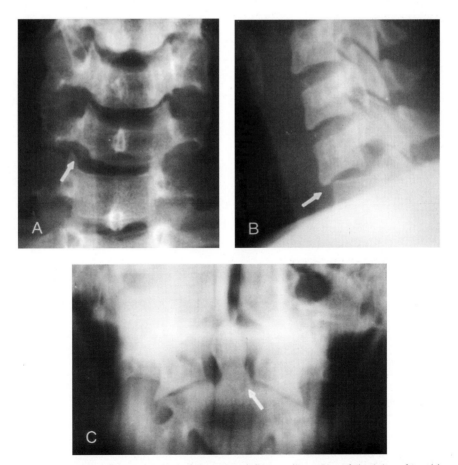

FIGURE 6.50. *Lateral flexion injuries of the spine.* **(A)** Note disruption of the joint of Luschka at the C6-7 level on the right (*arrow*). **(B)** This was caused by a rotatory dislocation at this level. Note the narrowed disc space (*arrow*), anteriorly displaced vertebral body of C6, and malaligned apophyseal joints at that level. **(C)** Laterally tilted dens due to fracture through the base (*arrow*). The C1-to-dens distance on the right is increased by rotation.

tures of the dens, with associated lateral displacement of this structure (Fig. 6.49B). Normal lateral tilting of the dens is rare, and thus any lateral tilting should be treated with suspicion (Fig. 6.50C). Brachial plexus injuries are discussed elsewhere in this chapter (see Fig. 6.66).

Rotation Injuries of the Cervical Spine

These injuries frequently are missed and can occur in both the upper and lower cervical spine (Fig. 6.51). Usually they are associated either with a flexion or extension injury, but most often it is the former. In the lower cervical spine, flexion–rotation injuries result in the so-called unilateral "locked" or "jumped" facet, and associated disruption of the intervening ligaments and disc space. This injury can be suspected on lateral views of the cervical spine if one notes either that the rotated vertebral body is anteriorly displaced on the one below it or that there is an abrupt change in alignment of the apophyseal joints at the level of injury (Fig. 6.52). Anterior displacement of the vertebral body, resulting from disc and ligament disruption, usually is not difficult to detect and most often is associated with narrowing of the disc space and swelling of the soft tissues anterior to the site of injury. Abnormal alignment of the apophyseal joints, on the other hand, may be more difficult to detect and frequently is missed. ***To avoid this, one should recall that for the apophyseal joints to be normal, they either should be all in true lateral projection or all rotated to the same degree.*** Therefore, if one notes an abrupt change in the alignment of the apophyseal joints at one level, one should suspect injury (Fig. 6.52). In addition, with an injury, the space between the posterior cortex of the apophyseal joint and the spinolaminar line (cortex of spinous process) remains normal below the level of rotation. Above the level of rotation, it is reduced (Fig. 6.52).

In many of these cases, associated fractures through the articular facets, pillars, and posterior elements occur, and often there is associated lateral displacement of the upper vertebral body and localized widening and dislocation of the joints of Luschka (Fig. 6.50). Actual demonstration of the associated fractures and the "locked" or "jumped" facet often is best accomplished with oblique views, laminagraphy (in the past), or CT scanning (Fig. 6.52 and 6.53). On frontal view, a unilateral locked facet can be suspected if it is noted that the spinous processes of the rotated vertebra and the vertebrae above it are shifted off midline (Fig. 6.53).

Extension–rotation injuries of the cervical spine usually result in fractures of the articular facets, pillars, and posterior elements (Fig. 6.51C). The resulting injury is not particularly different from that seen with pure hyperextension injuries.

Rotation abnormalities of the atlas and axis consist of rotatory dislocation, rotatory subluxation, and rotatory fixation (13,15,21,25). Rotatory dislocation and subluxation probably represent different degrees of the same problem. Actually, rotatory subluxation of C1 on C2 is the classic problem in the typical wryneck or torticollis abnormality of childhood. Clinically, these patients present with acute onset of a stiff neck, and often with a history of "catching a draft" or previous "minor trauma." Roentgenographically, lateral views of the cervical spine may be relatively normal or may demonstrate a peculiar cocking or dislocated appearance of C1 on C2 (Fig. 6.54). Despite this disturbing appearance of C1, however, there is no evidence of true atlantoaxial dislocation: The predental distance is normal. On frontal view, however, a characteristic alignment of the spinous process of C2 and the tip of the mandible occurs. Normally if the head is turned to one side, the spinous tips of the vertebral bodies rotate to the opposite side (i.e., opposite to the side to which the mandible has rotated or points). With torticollis, on the other hand, the rotated anterior facet of C1 becomes "locked" on the underlying facet of C2, and because of this C2 cannot rotate properly. The end result is that the spinous tip of

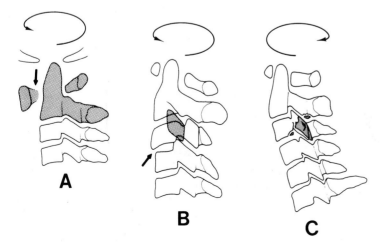

FIGURE 6.51. *Rotation injuries of the cervical spine: diagrammatic representation.* **(A)** Rotatory subluxation of C1 on C2. One of the anterior masses is displaced forward and the predental distance (*arrow*) is increased. **(B)** Unilateral locked facet. In these cases, the involved facet (*shaded area*) comes to lie anterior to its mate. In addition, the involved vertebral body becomes anteriorly displaced on the one below it (*arrow*), and the disc space often is narrowed. **(C)** Associated extension forces usually result in a variety of fractures through the pillars, articular facets, and posterior elements. There also may be disc disruption.

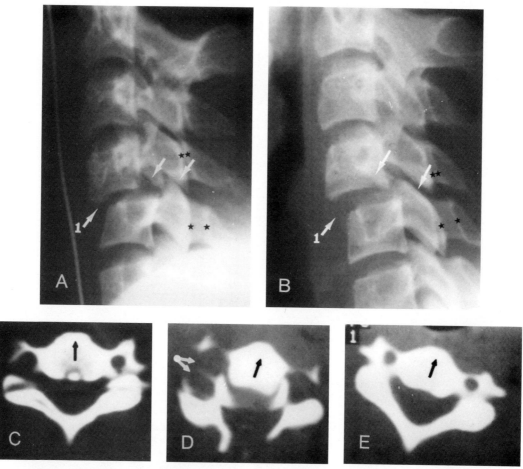

FIGURE 6.52. *Unilateral locked facet: rotation–flexion injury.* **(A)** Note the narrowed disc space between C4 and C5 (*1*). C4 is anteriorly displaced on C5 and the apophyseal joints are offset (*arrows*). Note that the distance between the posterior cortex of the apophyseal joint facet and the anterior cortex of the spinous tip is wider below the level of dislocation than above (*stars*). **(B)** Another patient with similar findings demonstrating a disrupted disc space (*1*) with anterior displacement of the vertebral body above it. The apophyseal joints at the level are offset (*posterior arrows*); the space between the posterior cortex of the articular facet and the anterior cortex of the spinous tip again is wider below the level of rotation than above (*stars*). **(C)** Computed tomographic study in another patient with rotatory dislocation. Note the anteriorly pointing lower vertebral body (*arrow*). **(D)** Just above this level the upper vertebral body is rotated to the left (*black arrow*). The two offset apophyseal joint facets are seen (*white arrows*). **(E)** Slightly higher cut demonstrates the upper vertebral body to be rotated to the left (*arrow*).

C2, rather than rotating to the side opposite to which the mandible has rotated, stays on the same side. This is demonstrable on frontal roentgenograms if a line is dropped from the tip of the dens through the midsagittal plane of the dens (Fig. 6.54). If rotatory subluxation does not correct spontaneously with conservative measures, the patient should be evaluated with dynamic CT scanning (see Fig. 6.56).

With rotatory dislocation of C1 on C2, the same general abnormalities are visualized on frontal view, but on lateral view cocking of C1 on C2 is more pronounced and fixed. In addition, there is visible anterior displacement of the rotated lateral mass of C1 and widening of the predental

space (Fig. 6.55). In this way, the findings are quite different from simple torticollis.

On frontal view, in addition to deviation of the spinous process of C2 off the midline, it has been noted that inward offsetting of the rotated lateral mass of C1 also occurs (13). However, although there is no question that such a malalignment occurs in many cases, similar malalignment can be seen under normal circumstances. Furthermore, it is not uncommon for similar or other offsetting abnormalities of the lateral masses of C1 to occur with simple torticollis (Fig. 6.54B). Consequently, *I have come to the conclusion that it is best to ignore what the lateral masses are doing in these cases, for there are other, more important, find-*

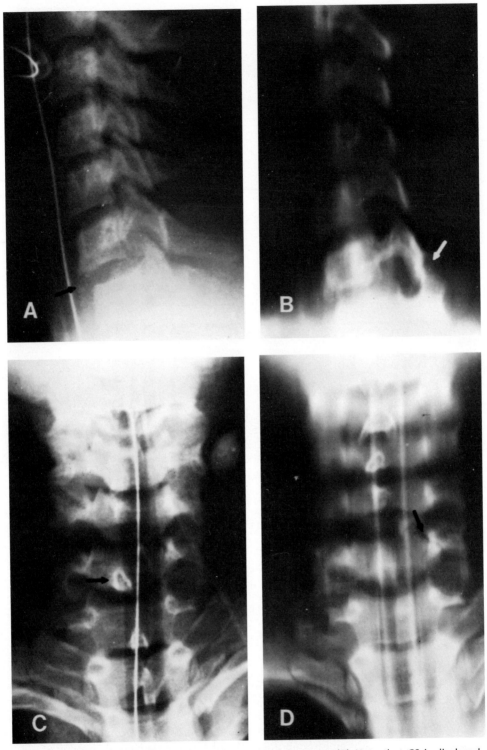

FIGURE 6.53. *Unilateral locked facet with associated fractures.* (**A**) Note that C6 is displaced anteriorly on C7 (*arrow*), and that although above this level the apophyseal joints are seen in pairs, at the level of dislocation only one joint is visualized (the posterior one). Once again, this should signify the presence of a unilateral locked facet. (**B**) Subsequent laminagram demonstrates the locked or jumped facet (*arrow*) at the C6-7 level. (**C**) Frontal view demonstrating the spinous process of C6 to be displaced to the right (*arrow*). The spinous processes above this level all line up with C6; those below the level line up with C7. This is characteristic of a unilateral locked facet. (**D**) Subsequent laminagraphy demonstrates extensive fractures through the lateral aspect of C6 (*arrow*). The bony ossicles just adjacent to the inner aspect of the ribs are normal secondary ossification centers.

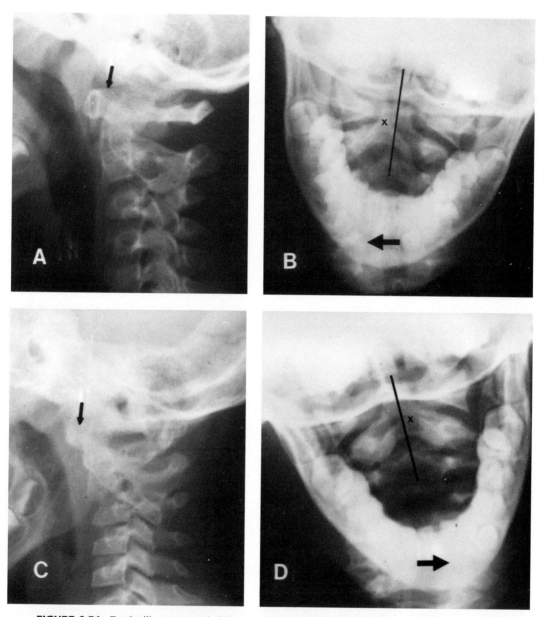

FIGURE 6.54. *Torticollis or wryneck.* (**A**) Note that in this patient the spine is somewhat rotated and C2 is cocked slightly forward on C3. The predental distance, however, is normal (*arrow*). (**B**) Frontal view demonstrating that the spinous process of C2 (*X*) lies to the same side of the midline as the mandible points (*arrow*). The distance from the lateral mass of C1 to the dens is narrow on the right and wide on the left. This is common with rotation. (**C**) Another patient with torticollis showing an apparently completely scrambled upper cervical spine. The predental distance (*arrow*), however, is normal. (**D**) Frontal view demonstrating characteristic findings, in that the spinous process of C2 (*X*) lies to the same side of the midline as the mandible points (*arrow*).

ings to assess. Lateral masses should be assessed only on true anteroposterior films.

Rotatory fixation is a peculiar problem wherein there is persistent subluxation or offsetting of the involved lateral mass of C1 (13,25). The injury is believed to result from fixed invagination of ligaments into the involved joint and, as such, differs from simple subluxation in which the problem is transient. Otherwise, I believe that the two conditions are similar. With rotatory fixation, as with rotatory

subluxation, there is no widening of the predental distance on lateral view. This is different from rotatory dislocation, in which widening is present.

Once rotatory fixation is suspected, dynamic CT scanning with neutral and right and left rotation is best for evaluating the problem (23). The study can be augmented with reconstructed images in the coronal, sagittal, or angled planes, in which the actual apophyseal joints can be seen. The simple dynamic CT study, however, usually serves to alert one to the

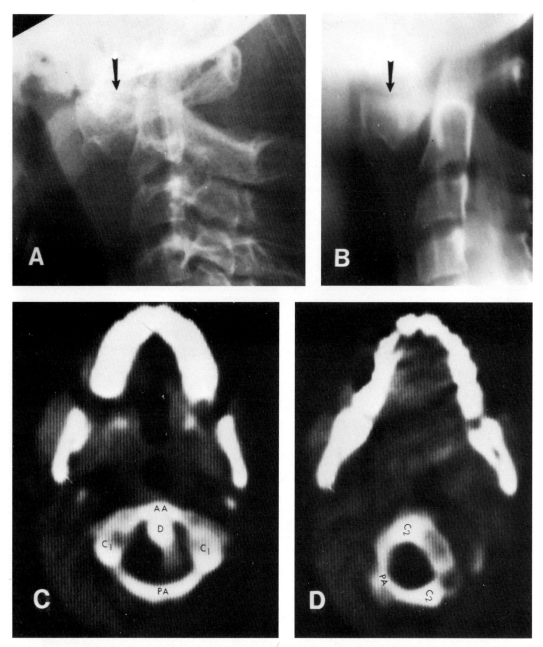

FIGURE 6.55. *Rotatory dislocation of C1 on C2.* (**A**) Note the peculiarly cocked appearance of C1. Also note that the predental distance, although not clearly visualized, appears abnormally wide (*arrow*). A little prevertebral soft-tissue swelling also is present. (**B**) Subsequent laminagrams demonstrate the anterior position of the rotated lateral mass (*arrow*). (**C**) Computed tomographic scan in another patient. Note the position of the lateral masses (*C1*), the anterior arch (*AA*), and the posterior arch (*PA*) of C1. The dens (*D*) is off the midline. (**D**) Lower cut. Note the position of the articular facets of C2 (*C2*) and the position of the posterior arch (*PA*). An almost 90-degree dislocation is present. (Courtesy of F.L.G. Rothman, M.D.)

problem. With this study, the patient, in neutral position, shows C1 angled on C2. C1 points in the direction of the rotation. Thereafter, with rotation to the unaffected side, C1 rotates along with C2. If rotation to the affected side is attempted, C1 does not rotate with C2 and remains fixed in its initially abnormal position (Fig. 6.56). Pseudorotatory dislocation can occur in some infants because of normal ligament laxity in the area (Fig. 6.57). At first the findings in these patients can be quite alarming and confusing.

Axial Compression Injuries of the Cervical Spine

These injuries generally result in bursting of the involved vertebra (Fig. 6.58). In the upper cervical spine, the classic bursting fracture is the Jefferson fracture of C1. In the other vertebral bodies, including the body of C2, axial compression injuries result in bursting and expansion of the vertebral body in all directions, including into the spinal canal (Fig. 6.59).

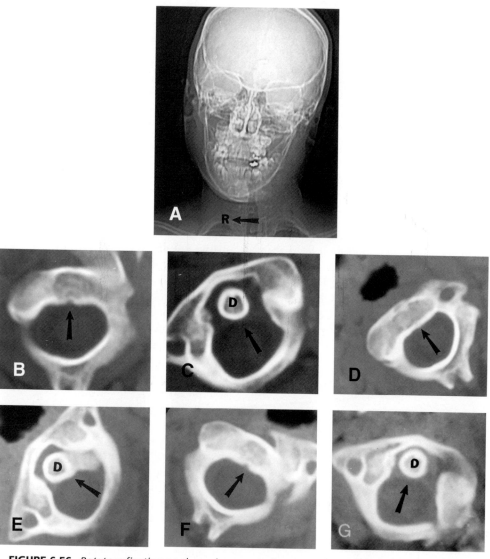

FIGURE 6.56. *Rotatory fixation on dynamic computed tomographic scan.* **(A)** Note that the chin is tilted to the right (*R*). **(B)** In neutral position, C2 points anteriorly (*arrow*). **(C)** C1, however, points to the right (*arrow*). *D*, dens. **(D)** With rotation to the right, C2 points to the right (*arrow*). **(E)** C1 also points to the right (*arrow*). *D*, dens. **(F)** With turning to the left, C2 points to the left(*arrow*). **(G)** C1, however, is fixed and cannot rotate to the left; it points anteriorly (*arrow*). *D*, dens.

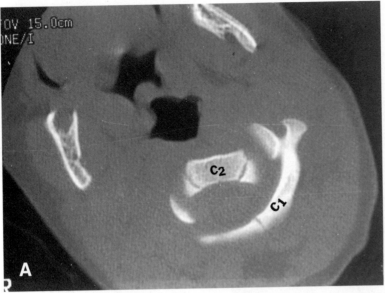
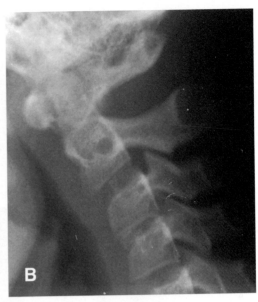

FIGURE 6.57. *Pseudorotatory dislocation.* **(A)** In this patient, C1 (*C1*) is in alignment with the head. C2 (*C2*) appears out of alignment. This patient was heavily sedated during this study. **(B)** Lateral view of the neck obtained later is completely normal. This case attests to the high degree of normal hypermobility of the upper cervical spine in infants and young children.

The Jefferson bursting fracture is unstable and is characterized by bilateral outward displacement of the lateral masses of C1. Instability is more of a problem if fewer than four breaks (two on each side) are present, because transverse ligament tears commonly are associated (18). The fractures through the anterior and posterior arches of C1 usually are not visible unless CT scanning is performed. Consequently, it is most important to detect displacements of the C1 lat-

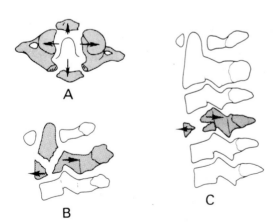

FIGURE 6.58. *Axial compression injuries of the cervical spine.* **(A)** Typical Jefferson bursting fracture of C1. Fractures occur posteriorly and anteriorly, and the fracture fragments are displaced in all directions. **(B)** Bursting fracture of C2. The findings are self-evident. **(C)** Similar findings in a bursting fracture of one of the lower cervical vertebrae.

eral masses on frontal, open-mouth odontoid views. Most often, with four fracture sites (two on each side), both lateral masses are displaced (Fig. 6.59A), but with unilateral displacement of the lateral mass, a unilateral or partial Jefferson fracture (two or three fracture sites) is present. On lateral view, all of these fractures basically are invisible (Fig. 6.60). Less commonly, with compression injuries of C1, one may note an isolated fracture of the medial portion of the lateral mass (Fig. 6.60B). Similarly isolated fractures of the anterior arch have been described (33). These need to be differentiated from normal congenital synchondroses now commonly seen on axial CT studies (2).

A normal variation in infants has been noted to mimic a Jefferson fracture (29). In these patients, on frontal view, the lateral masses appear widely displaced and, as such, suggest a Jefferson fracture (Fig. 6.59E). This is believed to occur because C1 and its lateral masses grow faster than C2 (29). In addition to this normal variation, occasionally one can encounter a normal individual with an increased distance from the dens to the lateral mass (Fig. 6.61). Furthermore, because of normal hypermobility of the upper cervical spine in infants and young children, considerable increase in the distance from the dens to the lateral mass can be seen, and it can change from side to side (Fig. 6.16).

Axial compression injuries of the body and dens of C2 cause vertical or oblique fractures and expansion of the vertebral body in all directions (Fig. 6.62A and B). The same is true of axial fractures of the lower cervical vertebrae (Fig. 6.62C). The configuration of the expanded body of C2 in these cases has been termed the "fat C2" sign (30). It is most

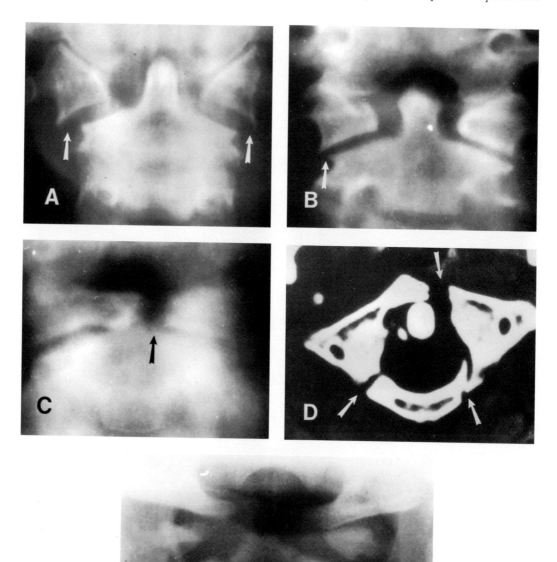

FIGURE 6.59. *Jefferson fracture of C1.* **(A)** Typical outward displacement of both lateral masses of C1 (*arrows*). The one on the right is more displaced than the one on the left. Because of this, the distance between the dens and lateral mass on the right is greater than that on the left. **(B)** Unilateral Jefferson fracture of C1. Note unilateral outward displacement of the right lateral mass of C1 (*arrow*). There is an associated increase in distance between the right lateral mass and the dens. **(C)** Laminagram demonstrates the associated fracture through the anterior arch of C1 (*arrow*). **(D)** Computed tomographic findings: partial fracture. Note how clearly the bursting phenomenon is depicted at the three fracture sites (*arrows*). **(E)** Pseudo-Jefferson fracture in an infant. Note how the lateral masses of C1 (*arrows*) appear laterally displaced in this normal infant.

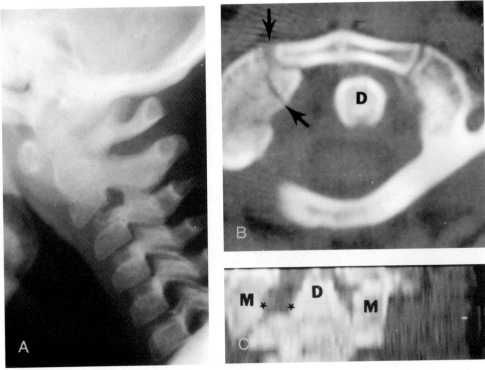

FIGURE 6.60. *Jefferson fracture of C1: computed tomographic detection.* **(A)** On this lateral view, no abnormality is suspected. The anterior C1-to-dens distance is within normal range. **(B)** Computed tomographic scan demonstrates a fracture through the lateral mass of C1 (*arrows*). **(C)** Coronal reconstruction demonstrates the lateral masses of C1 (*M*) and the dens (*D*). The space between the right lateral mass and dens is increased (*stars*).

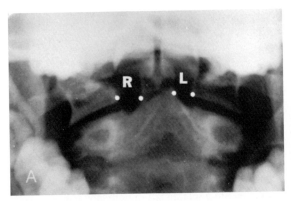

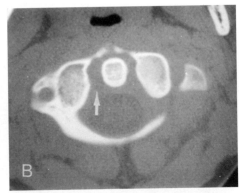

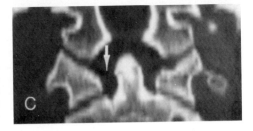

FIGURE 6.61. *Normally wide distance between lateral mass and dens.* **(A)** Note that the distance between the lateral mass and the dens (*dots*) is greater on the right than on the left. This patient had minor cervical spine injury. **(B)** Axial computed tomographic scan demonstrates similar widening (*arrow*). **(C)** Coronal reconstruction again demonstrates unilateral widening (*arrow*). Note, however, that there is no offsetting of the lateral mass on this view or in **A**. This patient had a full range of motion at this time, and the dynamic computed tomographic scan was normal. No fractures or ligamentous injury were identified.

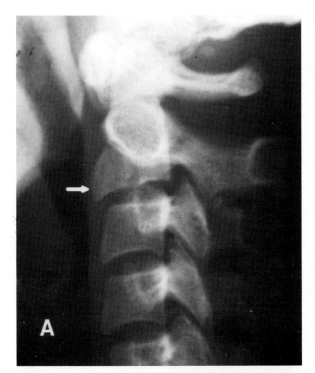

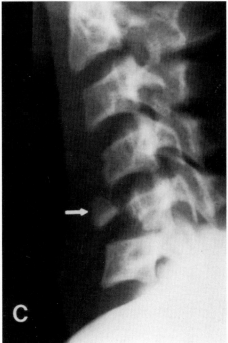

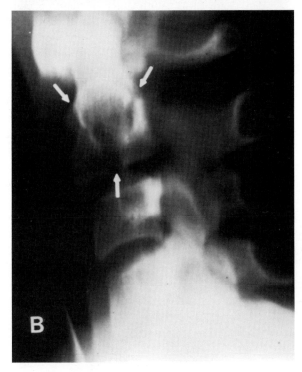

FIGURE 6.62. *Axial compression bursting fractures of the cervical vertebrae: fat vertebra sign.* (**A**) Fat C2 sign. Note anterior displacement of the expanded body of C2 (*arrow*). There is some associated disc-space narrowing, but clear-cut fractures are difficult to define. (**B**) Laminagraphy demonstrates a Y-shaped bursting fracture (*arrows*) involving the body and lower aspect of the dens of C2. (**C**) Bursting fracture of C5 (*arrow*). The findings represent a combination of an axial compression fracture of C5 and a hyperflexion injury at this level. In this regard, note that there is kyphosis at the level of injury, and marked narrowing of the disc space between C5 and C6. Prevertebral soft-tissue swelling is extensive. Very often axial compression injuries of the lower cervical spine are accompanied by a flexion component.

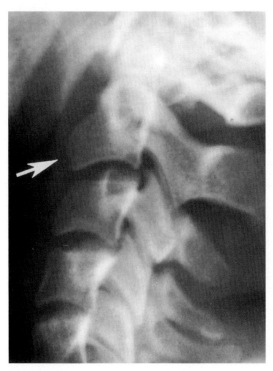

FIGURE 6.63. *Pseudofat C2 sign.* Note the normally wide and plump body of C2 (*arrow*) in this patient with no injuries.

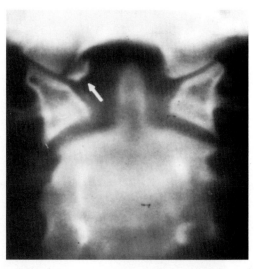

FIGURE 6.65. *Occipital condyle fracture.* Note the fracture (*arrow*) of the occipital condyle on the right. Also note that the right lateral mass of C1 is displaced outwardly, suggesting the associated presence of a unilateral Jefferson fracture.

important not to confuse a similar configuration of C2 occasionally seen in normal individuals (Fig. 6.63).

C1–Occipital Injuries

These injuries, by and large, are not particularly common. Atlanto-occipital dislocations can result from either flexion or extension forces, and both often are associated with sud-

den death (1,4). With anterior atlanto-occipital dislocations, the dens lies anterior to the anterior lip of the foramen magnum; with posterior dislocations, the dens lies posterior to the anterior lip of the foramen magnum. Normally it lies just below the anterior lip of the foramen magnum. Complete atlantooccipital dislocation also can occur (1,4). It has been suggested that, in adults and older children, measurements of both the basion–axial interval and basion–dental interval of 12 mm or less indicate the presence of this injury (10). In children younger than 13 years old, the basion–dental interval is not reliable because of the variable age at which complete ossification and fusion of the

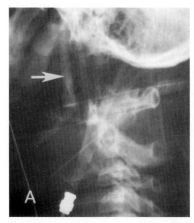
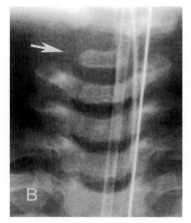
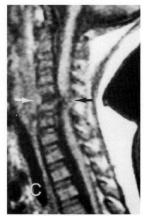

FIGURE 6.64. *Atlantooccipital separation.* **(A)** Note gross separation of the skull and cervical spine (*arrow*). There probably also is some dislocation at the C1-2 level: Note the markedly increased C1-2 interspinous distance. **(B)** Another patient with avulsion of the neural arch from the body of C5 (*arrow*). **(C)** Sagittal, T1-weighted magnetic resonance study in the same patient demonstrates cord compression and virtual transection of the cord (*black arrow*). The completely destroyed disc and altered vertebral bodies in the area also are noted (*white arrow*).

dens occurs (10). C1–occipital separations result from violent distracting rotational forces and also can occur elsewhere in the spine (Fig. 6.64).

Other injuries of the cervical–occipital junction consist of fractures through the occipital condyles (Fig. 6.65), but often these fractures are not detected until subsequent CT scanning is performed . The basic mechanisms through which these fractures occur are poorly understood, but because they can be associated with fractures of C1, they might result from axial compression and hyperextension forces.

REFERENCES

1. Bulas DI, Fitz CR, Johnson DL. Traumatic atlanto-occipital dislocation in children. *Radiology* 1993;188:155–158.
2. Chambers AA, Gaskill MF. Midline anterior atlas clefts: CT findings. *J Comput Assist Tomogr* 1992;16:868–870.
3. Cintron E, Gilula LA, Murphy WA, Gehweiler JA. The widened disk space: A sign of cervical hyperextension injury. *Radiology* 1981;141:639–644.
4. Cohen A, Hirsch M, Katz M, Sofer S. Traumatic atlanto-occipital dislocation in children: Review and report of five cases. *Pediatr Emerg Care* 1991;7:24–27.
5. Connolly B, Emery D, Armstrong D. The odontoid synchondrotic slip: An injury unique to young children. *Pediatr Radiol* 1995;25:S129–S133.
6. Davis SJ, Teresi LM, Bradley WG Jr, Ziemba MA, Bloze AE. Cervical spine hyperextension injuries: MR findings. *Radiology* 1991;180:245–250.
7. Freiberger RH, Wilson PD Jr, Nicholas JA. An acquired absence of the odontoid process: A case report. *J Bone Joint Surg* 1965;47A:1231–1236.
8. Giguere JF, St-Vil D, Turmel A, DiLorenzo M, Pothel C, Manseau S, Mercier C. Airbags and children: A spectrum of C-spine injuries. *J Pediatr Surg* 1998;33:811–816.
9. Gooding CA, Hurwitz ME. Avulsed vertebral rim apophysis in a child. *Pediatr Radiol* 1974;2:265–268.
10. Harris JH, Carson GC, Wagner LK. Radiologic diagnosis of traumatic occipitovertebral dissociation: Normal occipitovertebral relationships on lateral radiographs of supine subjects. *AJR* 1994;162:881–886.
11. Haug RH, Wible RT, Likavec MJ, Conforti PJ. Cervical spine fractures and maxillofacial trauma. *J Oral Maxillofac Surg* 1991;49:725–729.
12. Hawkins RJ, Fielding JW, Thompson WJ. Os odontoideum: Congenital or acquired. A case report. *J Bone Joint Surg* 1976;58A:413–414.
13. Jacobson G, Adler DC. An evaluation of lateral atlanto-axial displacement in injuries of the cervical spine. *Radiology* 1961;61:355–362.
14. Jones ET, Hensinger RN. C2-C3 dislocation in a child. *J Pediatr Orthop* 1981;1:419–422.
15. Kawabe N, Hirotani H, Tanaka O. Pathomechanism of atlantoaxial rotatory fixation in children. *J Pediatr Orthop* 1989;9:569–578.
16. Kim KS, Chen HH, Russell EJ, Rogers LF. Flexion teardrop fracture of the cervical spine: Radiographic characteristics. *AJR* 1989;152:319–326.
17. Kleinman PK, Shelton YA. Hangman's fracture in an abused infant: Imaging features. *Pediatr Radiol* 1997;27:776–777.
18. Lee C, Woodring JH. Unstable Jefferson variant atlas fractures: An unrecognized cervical injury. *AJR* 1992;158:113–118.
19. Lui TN, Lee ST, Wong CW, Yehy YS, Tzaan WC, Chen TY, Hung SY. C1-C2 fracture-dislocations in children and adolescents. *J Trauma* 1996;40:408–411.
20. McGrory BE, Fenichel GM. Hangman's fracture subsequent to shaking an infant. *Ann Neurol* 1977;2:82.
21. Muniz AE, Belfer RA. Atlantoaxial rotary subluxation in children. *Pediatr Emerg Care* 1999;15:25–29.
22. Naidich JB, Naidich TP, Garfein C, Liebeskind AL, Hyman RA. The widened interspinous distance: A useful sign of anterior cervical dislocation in the supine frontal projection. *Radiology* 1977;123:113–116.
23. Odent T, Langlais J, Clorion C, Kassis B, Bataille J, Pouliquen JC. Fractures of the odontoid process: A report of 15 cases in children younger than six years. *J Pediatr Orthop* 1999;19:51–54.
24. Pennecot GF, Leonard P, Des Gachons SP, Hardy JR, Pouliquen JC. Traumatic ligamentous instability of the cervical spine in children. *J Pediatr Orthop* 1984;4:339–344.
25. Phillips WA, Hensinger RN. The management of rotatory atlanto-axial subluxation in children. *J Bone Joint Surg* 1989;71:664–665.
26. Richman S, Friedman RL. Vertical fracture of cervical vertebral bodies. *Radiology* 1954;62:536.
27. Schaaf RE, Gehweiler JA Jr, Miller MD, Powers B. Lateral hyperflexion injuries of the cervical spine. *Skeletal Radiol* 1978;3:73–78.
28. Scher AT. "Tear-drop" fractures of the cervical spine: Radiological features. *S Afr Med J* 1982;61:355–356.
29. Seimon LP. Fracture of the odontoid process in young children. *J Bone Joint Surg* 1977;59A:943–948.
30. Smoker WRK, Dolan KD. The "fat" C2: A sign of fracture. *AJR* 1987;148:609–614.
31. Suss RA, Zimmerman RD, Leeds NE. Pseudospread of the atlas: False sign of Jefferson fracture in young children. *AJR* 1983;140:1079.
32. Swischuk LE, Hayden CK Jr, Sarwar M. The posteriorly tilted dens (a normal variation mimicking a fracture of the dens). *Pediatr Radiol* 1979;8:27–28.
33. Vaughan TE, West OC. Isolated vertical fracture through the anterior atlas arch: A previously unreported fracture. *Emerg Radiol* 1998;5:259–262.
34. Weiss B, Kaufman B. Hangman's fracture in an infant. *Am J Dis Child* 1973;126:268–269.
35. Whitley JE, Forsyth HF. The classification of cervical spine injuries. *AJR* 1960;83:633–644.

Cervical Cord and Nerve Root Injuries

Brachial Plexus Injuries

These injuries are avulsion injuries of the brachial plexus resulting from excessive lateral flexion–rotation of the spine. They also can result from excessive posterior stretching of the arm. In either case, there is paralysis of the affected limb, and with root injuries between C5 and C7, Duchenne-Erb paralysis of the shoulder and upper arm results, while Klumpke's paralysis of the hand results from injuries between C7 and T1. With such injuries, Horner's syndrome also may be present. The diagnosis usually is made clinically and then subsequently confirmed with MR imaging.

Myelography also can be employed but now is used less often than MR or CT myelography. In the past, myelographic findings consisted of extravasation of contrast

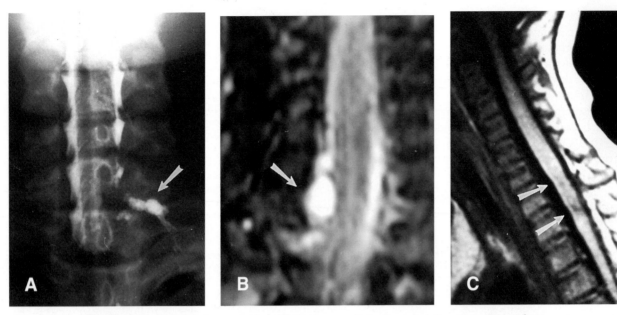

FIGURE 6.66. *Brachial plexus avulsion.* **(A)** Myelogram. Note characteristic extravasation of contrast material along a nerve root. **(B)** In this newborn with a brachial plexus injury, note extravasation of fluid (*arrow*) along the nerve root. **(C)** Central cord syndrome (spinal cord injury without radiographic abnormalities). This patient had no bony abnormality visible, but magnetic resonance scanning demonstrates an area of cord contusion (low signal area) in the midcervical cord (*arrows*).

material along the nerve roots in so-called traumatic meningoceles or cysts (Fig. 6.66A and B).

Central Cord (SCIWORA) Syndrome

The central cord syndrome usually results from hyperextension injuries of the cervical spine. It has also been termed **spinal cord injury without radiographic abnormalities** (SCIWORA) (3,4).

Clinically, there is a definite cord level, with neurologic deficit clearly apparent (1–3). The roentgenograms, however, usually show no fracture or dislocation, but in spite of these rather negative findings, the lesion should be considered unstable and the neck should be immobilized properly. Cord injury results from pinching or squeezing of the cord between the anterior and posterior walls of the spinal canal secondary to buckling of the ligamentum flavum during hyperextension. Currently MR scanning readily detects the subsequent contusion to the spinal cord (Fig. 6.66C).

REFERENCES

1. Daffner RH. Magnetic resonance evaluation of cervical nerve root avulsion injury. *Radiology* 1996;3:172–175.
2. Duprez T, DeMerlier Y, Clapuyt P, de Clety CC, Cosnard G, Adisseux JF. Early cord degeneration in bifocal SCIWORA: A case report. *Pediatr Radiol* 1998;28:186–188.

3. Pang D, Pollack IF. Spinal cord injury without radiographic abnormality in children: The SCIWORA syndrome. *J Trauma* 1989;29:654–664.
4. Yngve DA, Harris WP, Herndon WA, Sullivan JA, Gross RH. Spinal cord injury without osseous spine fracture. *J Pediatr Orthop* 1988;8:153–159.

Cervical Spine Injuries and Apnea

Cardiorespiratory arrest can occur immediately after injury and often is presumed to be due to cerebral injury. However, it is not so uncommon to have these patients present with cardiopulmonary arrest secondary to cervical spine injury to the upper cervical spine and medulla (1).

REFERENCE

1. Bohn D, Armstrong D, Becker L, Humphreys R. Cervical spine injuries in children. *J Trauma* 1990;30:463–469.

Normal Findings and Anomalies of the Cervical Spine Causing Problems

Most of the significant normal findings in the cervical spine are covered at appropriate points in previous sections, but a few others should be discussed for completeness. In this regard, one of the most common normal findings to be misinterpreted as a fracture is the dens–arch synchondrosis of

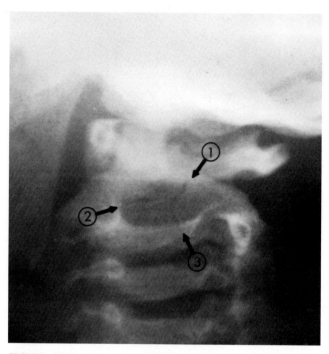

FIGURE 6.67. *Normal synchondroses of C2.* Synchondrosis between the dens and arch (*1*), synchondrosis between the dens and body (*2*), and synchondrosis between the body and arch (*3*). The synchondrosis between the dens and arch is the one most commonly misinterpreted as a fracture of C2.

C2 (7). Actually, this synchondrosis is part of a triad of synchondroses between the dens, body, and arch of C2 (Fig. 6.67). All of these synchondroses lie anterior and are seen only on oblique views of the cervical spine. In the injured child, this most commonly occurs fortuitously on skull roentgenograms. In such cases, although the head is in lateral position, the cervical spine is in the rotated, oblique position (Fig. 6.68).

In assessing these synchondroses, it is important to appreciate that they are anterior structures, and thus visible only if the spine is obliqued. Once this is appreciated, they can be differentiated from fractures through the neural arch of C2 with ease, because these fractures are visible on both oblique and lateral views (Fig. 6.69). Indeed, if one notes a defect in the neural arch of C2 on lateral view, it should be considered a fracture until proven otherwise. Congenital defects in this region are extremely rare (1,2,4,6). The synchondroses between the bodies and arches of the lower cervical vertebrae are less of a problem (Fig. 6.70). The synchondrosis of C2 also can be a problem on lateral parasagittal slices through the spine in sagittal CT reconstruction (Fig. 6.71).

Congenital defects of the posterior arch of C2, as has already been mentioned, are extremely rare. These defects are characterized by smooth margins and lack of separation with flexion (Fig. 6.72). They are fibrous defects and not subject to abnormal motion, and thus if abnormal motion is seen one should suspect a fracture. In the literature, many times these fractures are misinterpreted as congenital defects, even though sclerotic margins are not present. One reason for this is that these fractures may be relatively silent in infants. At any rate *I have always used this rule: If the edges of the fragments are smooth and sclerotic, and there is no change in configuration with flexion, I am satisfied to call it a congenital defect. If the edges are ragged and indistinct and if there is change in configuration (opening of the defect) on flexion, I consider it a fracture.* In the end, whatever one's consideration, the lesion is unstable. In this regard, Currarino (1) has suggested that these defects be considered hangman's fractures with anterior displacement of C2, traumatic spondylosis with no displacement of C2, or congenital defects with no displacement of C2. The first two require treatment.

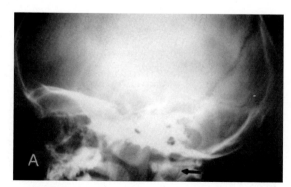

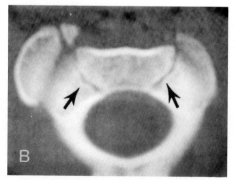

FIGURE 6.68. *Fortuitous visualization of the dens-arch synchondrosis of C2 on a skull film.* Note the fracture-like appearance of the synchondrosis between the dens and arch of C2 (*arrow*). This synchondrosis is visible on oblique views of the cervical spine in infants and young children because it is anterior in location. It is not visible on lateral view. (**B**) Computed tomographic scan demonstrates the anterior position of the synchondroses (*arrows*). Also note the small accessory ossicle on the right.

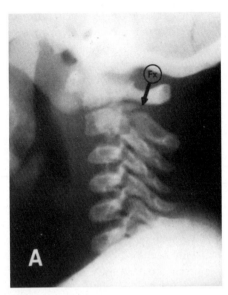
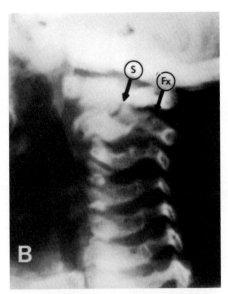

FIGURE 6.69. *Dens–arch synchrosis of C2 versus hangman's fracture.* **(A)** Lateral view demonstrating a defect (*Fx*) through the arch of C2. This is probably a hangman's fracture. **(B)** Oblique view demonstrates the posterior position of the fracture (*Fx*) and the anterior position of the normal dens–arch synchondrosis (*S*) of C2.

Other normal findings causing problems include the transverse processes being projected through the intervertebral disc spaces and the normal ring epiphysis of the growing vertebral body. This ring epiphyises can be misinterpreted as corner (teardrop) fractures of the vertebral bodies, for often they appear "tilted" (Fig. 6.73A). In addition, normal transverse processes can be misinterpreted as intervertebral disc calcifications (Fig. 6.73B).

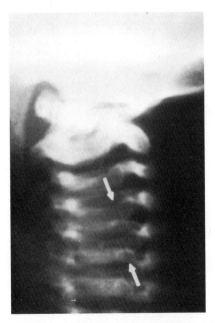

FIGURE 6.70. *Synchondroses of lower cervical vertebrae.* Note the typical appearance of the synchondroses between the bodies and arches of the lower cervical vertebrae (*arrows*).

Wedging of C3 is a normal phenomenon in infants and young children that often is confused with a compression fracture (9). In some of these cases the wedging deformity is quite pronounced (Fig. 6.74). Although it is not precisely known why this occurs, it is believed that it results from the normal hypermobility that occurs at the C2-3 level in young children (9). It has been suggested that the chronic subclinical impaction of the upper anterior corner of C3 leads to impaired bone growth and variable degrees of wedging (9). The phenomenon may occur at the C4 level but basically does not occur at the other levels. Furthermore, it disappears with increasing age. Interestingly enough, with increasing age, as the wedging deformity disappears, there is an associated change in the apex of the flexion curve of the cervical spine. In other words, in infancy the apex occurs in the upper cervical spine, at the C2-3 level (Fig. 6.75), but in the older child the curve is more uniform and curving and the apex is located in the midcervical spine (Fig. 6.75D). It is believed that the apex occurs in the upper cervical spine in infancy and childhood because of normal hypermobility in this area (9). In any case, if there is doubt as to the presence of a fracture one can perform CT scanning of the cervical spine. In cases in which wedging is normal, no fracture is seen (Fig. 6.76).

Although a number of anomalies that can cause problems exist, the most important is the hypoplastic dens associated with an os odontoideum (8,11). In these cases, the os odontoideum can appear as though it were a fractured dens. Actually, the os odontoideum probably is an overgrown os terminale; it overgrows if the dens is hypoplastic (10). The os terminale is a small ossicle occurring in all children, just at the tip of the dens, seated in a V-shaped notch (Fig. 6.77A). By adolescence, the os terminale becomes fused with the

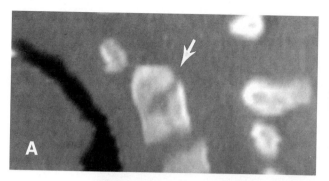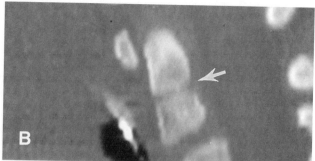

FIGURE 6.71. *Normal dens-body synchondrosis, C2 (computed tomographic findings).* **(A)** On this far parasagittal cut the synchondrosis (*arrow*) mimics a fracture. **(B)** Midsagittal reconstruction demonstrates the normal dens-body synchondrosis (*arrow*).

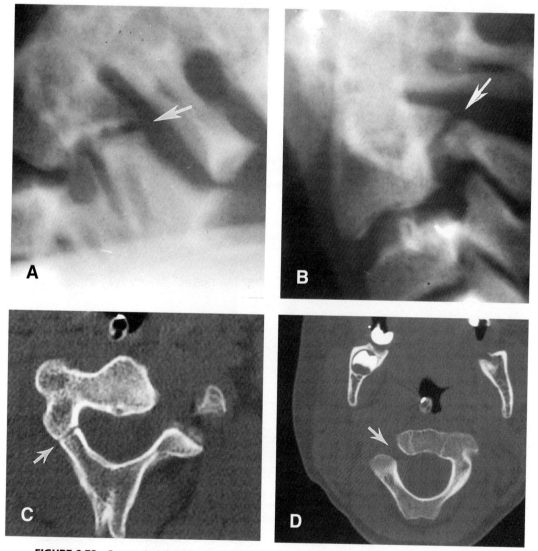

FIGURE 6.72. *Congenital defects, posterior arch of C2.* **(A)** Note the defect with smooth sclerotic edges (*arrow*). **(B)** With flexion there is no change in the configuration of the defect (*arrow*). (Courtesy John Dorst, M.D.) **(C)** Axial computed tomographic scan demonstrates a smooth-edged defect (*arrow*). **(D)** Another patient with a large defect (*arrow*).

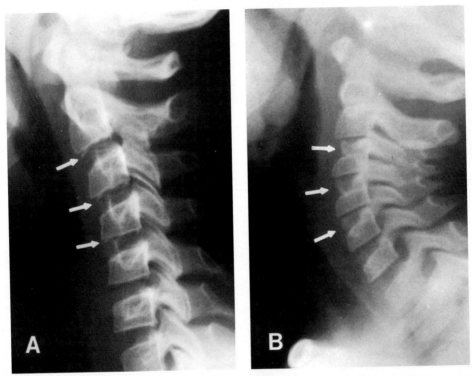

FIGURE 6.73. (A) *Ring epiphyses.* Note normal ring epiphyses (*arrows*). The one off C3 appears tilted and avulsed. This, however, is a normal appearance. (B) Transverse processes projected through intervertebral discs. Note the transverse processes of the cervical vertebrae (*arrows*) projected through the intervertebral discs. They should not be confused with intervertebral disc calcifications.

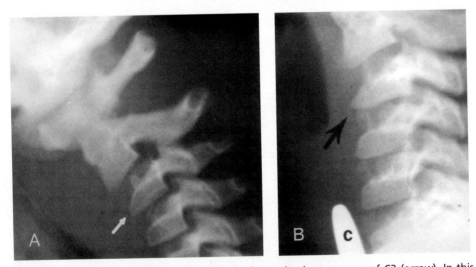

FIGURE 6.74. *Normal wedging of C3.* (A) Note the wedged appearance of C3 (*arrow*). In this patient, also note other normal findings often misinterpreted as pathology. The C1-to-dens distance is wide but normal. The interspinous distance between C1 and C2 also is wide but is normal. The apophyseal joint at the C2-3 level shows considerable anterior displacement, but this is also normal. (B) Note the wedged appearance of C3 (*arrow*). A compression fracture might be suggested; however, this patient was examined for a coin (C) in the esophagus. (From Swischuk LE, Swischuk PN, John SD: Wedging of C3 in infants and children: Usually a normal finding and not a fracture. *Radiology* 1993;188:523–526, with permission.)

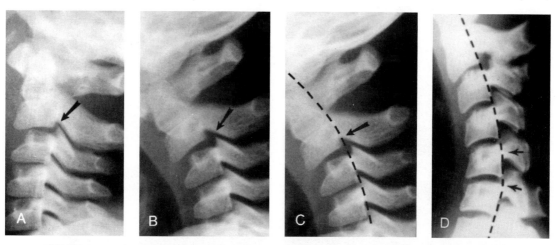

FIGURE 6.75. *Physiologic motion through C2-3.* (**A**) In the neutral position note the alignment of the apophyseal joints of the various vertebrae. Specifically, note the configuration of the joints at the C2-3 level (*arrow*). Also note that C3 is slightly wedged. (**B**) With flexion, most motion occurs through the C2-3 level (*arrow*). (**C**) The apex of the curve during flexion is at the C2-3 level. (**D**) In older children and adults it is located in the midcervical spine (*arrows*).

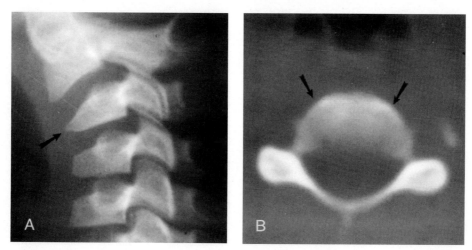

FIGURE 6.76. *Wedging of C3.* (**A**) Note marked wedging of C3 (*arrow*). Is a fracture present? Angulation of C2 on C3 is normal. (**B**) Computed tomographic scan through C3 demonstrates no fracture (*arrows*). (From Swischuk LE, Swischuk PN, John SD: Wedging of C3 in infants and children: Usually a normal finding and not a fracture. *Radiology* 1993;188:523–526, with permission.)

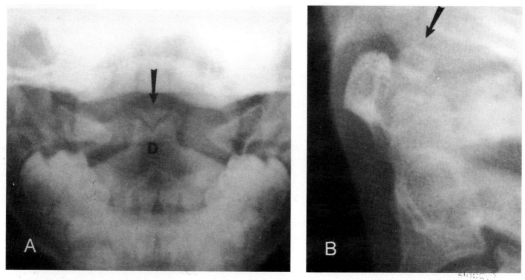

FIGURE 6.77. *Normal os terminale.* (**A**) Frontal, open-mouth odontoid view demonstrates the typical normal os terminale (*arrow*) seated in the wedge at the top of the dens (**D**). (**B**) On lateral view, the os terminale usually is not visible, but in some cases it is located high, above the wedge of the dens, and becomes visible (*arrow*).

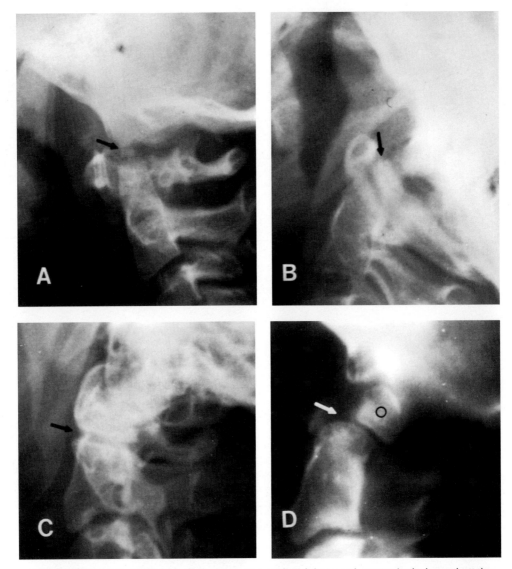

FIGURE 6.78. *Os terminale–os odontoideum anomalies.* **(A)** Normal os terminale (*arrow*) at the tip of the dens. **(B)** Large os odontoideum (*arrow*). This actually is an overgrown os terminale associated with a hypoplastic dens. (Courtesy of D. Binstadt, M.D.) **(C)** This 15-year-old boy was in an automobile accident, and at first the defect through the base of the dens (*arrow*) was thought to represent a dens fracture. Note how smooth it appears, however, and note that considerable anomalous development of the upper cervical spine is present. More specifically, C1 is markedly hypoplastic and deformed. **(D)** Subsequent laminography demonstrates that the defect is not a fracture, but rather a persistent congenital defect between the hypoplastic dens and overgrown os terminale or os odontoideum (*O*). The os odontoideum shows marked posterior displacement, attesting to the instability of this lesion.

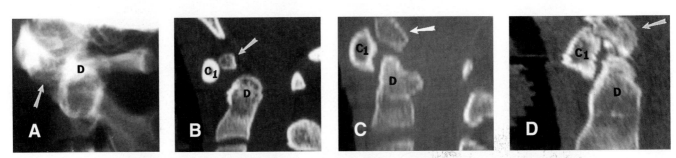

FIGURE 6.79. *Os odontoideum–os terminale anomalies.* **(A)** In this patient note the wide C1-to-dens distance (*arrow*). The dens (*D*) is hypoplastic. **(B)** Sagittal reconstructed computed tomographic scan demonstrates the anteriorly displaced os odontoideum (*arrow*). The anterior arch of C1 (*C1*) also is displaced anteriorly. The dens (*D*) is hypoplastic. **(C)** Another patient with a hypoplastic dens (*D*). An osteophyte is present posteriorly os odontoideum. **(D)** The anterior arch of C1 (*C1*) is enlarged, and there is a large irregular os odontoideum (*arrow*) (D) hypoplastic dens. **(C** and **D** are from Swischuk, LE: The os terminale-os odontoideum complex. *Emerg Radiol* 1997;4:7–81, with permission.)

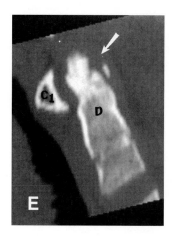 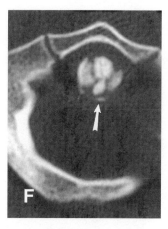

FIGURE 6.79. *(continued)* (E) Another patient with a fragmented-appearing dens and os terminale. *D*, dens. *C1*, Anterior arch of C1. **(F)** Axial view demonstrates similar fragmentation *(arrow)*. This patient was normal. (**E** and **F** are from Swischuk, LE: The os terminale-os odontoideum complex. *Emerg Radiol*, 1997;4:72–81, with permission.)

dens. Ordinarily it is not seen on lateral view, because it is seated deeply in the notch. In some cases, however, it is located higher and then becomes visible (Fig. 6.77B).

If the os terminale becomes the os odontoideum, it is associated with dens hypoplasia and usually some degree of hypermobility at the C1-2 area (Fig. 6.78). Indeed, in advanced cases, the entire lesion is quite unstable and frequently requires surgical stabilization. Occasionally an os odontoideum can be acquired (3,5), resulting from pronounced dens resorption (interrupted blood supply) after dens injuries in infancy. Most are congenital in origin, however, and a variety of configurations of the os odontoideum are presented in Fig. 6.79.

REFERENCES

1. Currarino G. Primary spondylolysis of the axis vertebra (C2) in three children, including one with pylenocysostosis. *Pediatr Radiol* 1989;19:535–538.
2. Fardon DF, Fielding JW. Defects of the pedicle and spondylolisthesis of the second cervical vertebra. *J Bone Joint Surg* 1981;63B:526–528.
3. Hawkins RJ, Fielding JW, Thompson WJ. Os odontoideum-congenital or acquired: A case report. *J Bone Joint Surg* 1978;58A:413–414.
4. Nordstrom REA, Lahdenranta TV, Kaitila II, Laasonen EMI. Familial spondylolisthesis of the axis vertebra. *J Bone Joint Surg Br* 1086;68:704–706.
5. Ricciardi JE, Kaufer H, Louis DS. Acquired os odontoideum following acute ligament injury: Report of a case. *J Bone Joint Surg* 1976;58A:410–412.
6. Smith JT, Skoinner SR, Shonnard NH. Persistent synchondrosis of the second cervical vertebra simulating a hangman's fracture in a child. *J Bone Joint Surg* 1993;75A:1228–1230.
7. Swischuk LE, Hayden CK Jr, Sarwar M. The dens-arch synchondrosis versus the hangman's fracture. *Pediatr Radiol* 1979;8:100–102.
8. Swischuk LE, John SD, Moorthy C. The os terminale-os odontoideum complex. *Emerg Radiol* 1997;4:72–81.
9. Swischuk LE, Swischuk PN, John SD. Wedging of C3 in infants and children: Usually a normal finding and not a fracture. *Radiology* 1993;188:523–526.
10. von Torklus D, Gehle W. The upper cervical spine: Regional morphology, pathology and traumatology. *An X-ray atlas.* New York: Grune and Stratton, 1972.
11. Watanabe M, Toyama Y, Fujimura Y. Atlanto-axial instability in os odontoideum with myelopathy. *Spine* 1996;21:1435.

THORACOLUMBAR SPINE TRAUMA

In the thoracolumbar spine, much as in the cervical spine, injuries can result from flexion, extension, lateral flexion, rotation, or axial compression forces.

Flexion Injuries

Most often flexion injuries of the thoracolumbar spine result in anterior compression of the vertebral bodies (Figs. 6.80

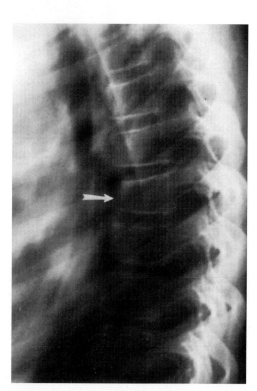

FIGURE 6.80. *Compression fracture: thoracic vertebra.* Note the typical appearance of the anteriorly compressed vertebra *(arrow)*.

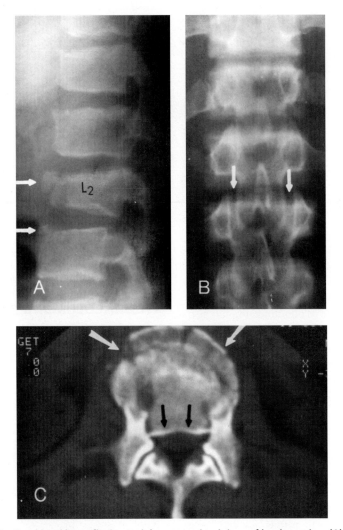

FIGURE 6.81. *Combined hyperflexion–axial compression injury of lumbar spine.* **(A)** Lateral view demonstrating marked anterior compression of L2, anterior teardrop fractures of L2 and L3 (*arrows*), and minimal anterior compression of T12. Also note that the posterior portion of L2 is minimally displaced posteriorly into the spinal canal. **(B)** Frontal view demonstrating widening of the apophyseal joints of L2 (*arrows*) and some widening of the corresponding interpedicular distance. These findings result from the compression-induced bursting of the vertebra. This patient fell directly on his buttocks and sustained an axial compression–hyperflexion injury of the thoracolumbar spine. **(C)** Computed tomographic scan demonstrating the compression fracture of the lumbar vertebra (*white arrows*) and protrusion of the posterior fragment (*black arrows*) into the spinal canal.

and 6.81). The more severe the injury, however, the greater is the likelihood that there is posterior ligament injury, widening of the interspinous distance, and associated spinous-tip or neural-arch avulsion fracturing. Actually, the mechanics of injury are exactly the same as those encountered in flexion injuries of the cervical spine, and in addition to the preceding fractures, teardrop fractures also can be seen (Fig. 6.81). In the lumbar spine, teardrop fractures often are referred to as *limbus fractures.* If the injury is severe enough, patients with these fractures also demonstrate anterior subluxation through the apophyseal joints, and once this finding, or widening of the interspinous distance, is present, the fracture is considered unstable.

Extension Injuries

Extension injuries of the thoracolumbar spine are not as common as flexion injuries. In some cases, nothing more than nondisplaced neural-arch and spinous-process fractures result, but in other cases a hangman's fracture–type mechanism is at play.

Another fracture that might be sustained if excessive extension forces are applied to the thoracolumbar spine is the so-called corner fracture of the vertebral body. Actually, this is the same fracture as the extension teardrop fracture seen in the cervical spine and should indicate underlying ligamentous injury with instability. In addition, there may be associated disc space widening and actual posterior displacement of the involved vertebral body.

Lateral Flexion Injuries

As in the cervical spine, lateral flexion injuries can result in ipsilateral compression fractures of the vertebral bodies or contralateral transverse process fractures. Most often, these injuries are not particularly serious if lateral flexion is the sole force involved. If other forces are involved, more serious injuries can occur. Transverse process fractures must be differentiated from rudimentary lumbar ribs or bipartite transverse processes (see Fig. 6.87).

Rotation Injuries

These are either rotation–flexion or rotation–extension injuries. The upper thoracic spine is especially prone to severe wrenching injuries, and considerable spinal damage can result (Fig. 6.82).

Axial Compression Injuries

Axial compression results in a "burst" vertebra, and often this type of injury is associated with some degree of hyperflexion injury (Fig. 6.81). If axial compression is a promi-

nent component of such an injury, the vertebral body bursts and spreads outward in all directions. Once again, the mechanics are the same as those seen in the cervical spine. On frontal view, one may note widening of the interpedicular distance or widening of the apophyseal joints. On lateral view, the compressed vertebra is squashed, and the posterior portion of it protrudes into the spinal canal. If significant associated interspinous ligament laxity or tearing occurs, the lesion becomes unstable.

Other Injuries of the Thoracolumbar Spine

The transverse fracture of the vertebral body with anterior or lateral dislocation of the upper half of the fractured vertebra is a well-known injury occurring in patients wearing lap seat belts (1,3,7,8,14,15,17,20). These are termed "chance" fractures (3) and can be detected on frontal views (Fig. 6.83). It is not uncommon, however, for the fracture to remain undetected for some time, for often in these patients supine roentgenograms for abdominal pain are obtained, and not enough attention is paid to the lumbar spine. In addition, these fractures often are ignored in cases of multiple body injuries, especially if CT studies are obtained first (20). It is important to examine the topogram of these CT studies, because it often provides the clue to the underlying fracture (Fig. 6.83B).

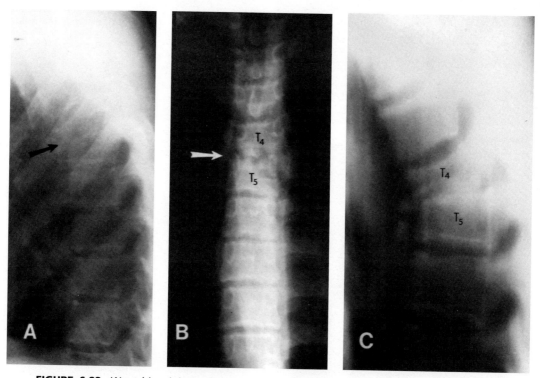

FIGURE 6.82. *Wrenching injury of thoracic spine.* **(A)** Note acute kyphosis at the T4-5 level *(arrow)*. The vertebral bodies and intervening disc space are difficult to identify. **(B)** Frontal view demonstrating obliteration of the disc space between T4 and T5 *(arrow)* and lateral displacement of T4 on T5. **(C)** Subsequent laminagraphy demonstrates the extensive nature of the rotation–flexion injury of T4 and T5.

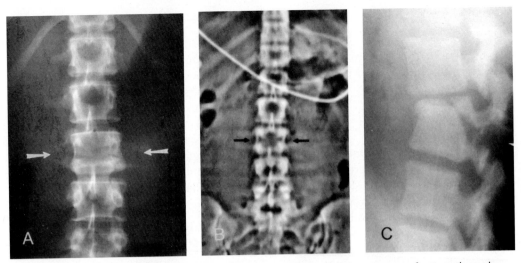

FIGURE 6.83. *Chance fracture of lumbar vertebral body.* **(A)** Note the transverse fracture through the third lumbar vertebra (*arrows*) in this teenager who was in a car accident. The film was obtained because of abdominal pain. Note, however, that the vertebra and its transverse processes are completely fractured. Also note that the pedicles of the involved vertebra are distorted because of the fracture. **(B)** Topogram in another patient demonstrating suspicious findings involving L3 (*arrows*). **(C)** Lateral view demonstrates a classic Chance fracture through the pedicles and vertebral body (*arrows*). There is some associated compression of the anterior aspect of the third lumbar vertebra.

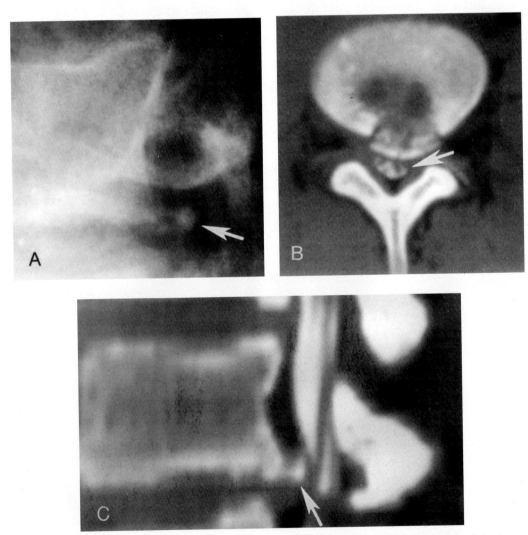

FIGURE 6.84. *Ring epiphysis fracture.* **(A)** Note the avulsed, posteriorly displaced ring epiphysis (*arrow*). **(B)** Computed tomographic scan demonstrates the posteriorly displaced fracture fragment and avulsed ring epiphysis (*arrow*). **(C)** Sagittal reconstruction demonstrates the displaced ring epiphyseal fragment (*arrow*) causing spinal canal compression.

Concomitant abdominal injuries, especially compressive injuries to the intestine, are not uncommon (9), and the so-called lap belt echimosis, a bruise along the line of the seat belt, is a valuable clinical tipoff to the problem (18). In addition to the lumbar seat belt fracture complex, it recently has been noted that diagonal seat belts can lead to serious cervical spine injuries in infants and young children.

Another unusual fracture of the vertebral body is the fracture of the ring epiphysis (2,11). With flexion injuries the superior ring is involved; with extension injuries the inferior ring is involved (11). In addition, these fractures can be associated with disc herniation. The fracture fragment can be seen

to be displaced into the spinal canal, and this can be demonstrated both with CT scanning and MR imaging (Fig. 6.84).

Still another relatively uncommon injury of the thoracolumbar spine is the anterior chronic compression injury or anterior Schmorl's node (6,8,19,21). In these cases, chronic trauma leads to disc damage and herniation of nuclear material into the anteriosuperior corner of the vertebral body, with a resultant triangular teardrop-like fracture fragment (Fig. 6.85). In some cases, considerable sclerosis is seen at the site, indicating a chronic problem with attempt at healing. The condition is a source of chronic back pain and usually is seen in the lower thoracic and upper lumbar regions. The fact that

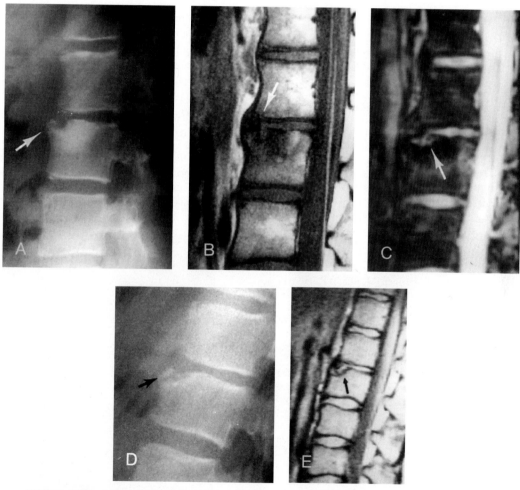

FIGURE 6.85. *Anterior Schmorl's nodes.* **(A)** Note the classic appearance of a chronic anterior Schmorl's node *(arrow)* of the involved lumbar vertebra. The adjacent disc space shows narrowing, and there is reactive sclerosis in the vertebral body. **(B)** T1-weighted sagittal magnetic resonance image demonstrates loss of signal in the disc anteriorly, narrowing of the disc, and loss of signal in the vertebral body because of the sclerosis. **(C)** T2-weighted image demonstrates how the nuclear material has extruded into the upper anterior corner of the vertebral body *(arrow)*. **(D)** Another patient with similar findings *(arrow)*. **(E)** T1-weighted sagittal magnetic resonance scan demonstrates extrusion of disc material into the upper anterior corner of the vertebral body *(arrow)*. The involved disc space is narrower than normal. This also has been called a *limbus vertebra.*

disc material herniates into the vertebral body now is clearly demonstrable with MR scanning (Fig. 6.85).

Spinal injuries in the battered child syndrome also can be encountered. Although they are not particularly common, one can see simple compression fractures, compression fractures with notched vertebrae, actual fracture dislocations, and spinous-tip avulsions (2,4,5,12,19). In addition, as might be expected, hangman's fractures also can occur in child abuse (12,15,17). Interestingly, this fracture, and other cervical spine fractures, may be relatively silent and unsuspected (12,17). This is an important point to appreciate, because hangman's fractures in infants often are misinterpreted as physiologic defects.

REFERENCES

1. Ashton CJ, Yu JS, Chung CB. The chance fracture: Anteroposterior radiographic signs. *Emerg Radiol* 1997;4:320–325.
2. Carrion WV, Dormans JP, Drukmond DS, Christofersen MR. Circumferential growth plate fracture of the thoracolumbar spine from child abuse. *J Pediatr Orthop* 1996;16:210–214.
3. Chance GQ. Note on type of flexion fracture of spine. *Br J Radiol* 1948;21:452–453.
4. Diamond P, Hansen CM, Christofersen MR. Child abuse presenting as a thoracolumbar spinal fracture dislocation: A case report. *Pediatr Emerg Care* 1994;10:83–86.
5. Gabos PG, Tuten HR, Leet A, Stanton RP. Fracture-dislocation of the lumbar spine in an abused child. *Pediatrics* 1998;101:473–477.
6. Greene TL, Hensinger RN, Hunter LY. Back pain and vertebral changes simulating Scheuermann's disease. *J Pediatr Orthop* 1985;5:1–7.
7. Hayes CW, Conway WF, Walsh JW, Coppage L, Gervin AS. Seat belt injuries: Radiologic findings and clinical correlation. *RadioGraphics* 1991;11:23–36.
8. Henales V, Hervas JA, Lopez P, Martinez JM, Ramos R, Herrera M. Intervertebral disc herniations (limbus vertebrae) in pediatric patients: Report of 15 cases. *Pediatr Radiol* 1993;23:608–610.
9. Hoy GA, Cole WG. Concurrent paediatric seat belt injuries of the abdomen and spine. *Pediatr Surg Int* 1992;7:376–379.
10. Hoy GA, Cole WG. The paediatric cervical seat belt syndrome. *Injury* 1993;24:297–299.
11. Keller RH. Traumatic displacement of the cartilaginous vertebral rim: A sign of intervertebral disc prolapse. *Radiology* 1974;110:21–24.
12. Kleinman PK, Shelton YA. Hangman's fracture in an abused infant: Imaging features. *Pediatr Radiol* 1997;27:776–777.
13. Kleinman PK, Zito JL. Avulsion of the spinous processes caused by infant abuse. *Radiology* 1984;151:389–392.
14. Lynch JM, Meza MP, Pollach IF, Adelson PD. Direct injury to the cervical spine of a child by a lap-shoulder belt resulting in quadriplegia: case report. *J Trauma* 1996;41:747–749.
15. McGrory BE, Fenichel GM. Hangman's fracture subsequent to shaking an infant. *Ann Neurol* 1977;2:82.
16. Rogers LF. The roentgenographic appearance of transverse or chance fractures of the spine: The seat belt fracture. *AJR* 1971;111:844–849.
17. Rooks VJ, Sisler C, Burton B. Cervical spine injury in child abuse: Report of two cases. *Pediatr Radiol* 1998;28:193–195.
18. Sivit CJ, Taylor GA, Newman KD, Bulas DI, Gotschall CS, Wright CJ, Eichelberger MR. Safety belt injuries in children with lap-belt ecchymosis: CT findings in 61 patients. *AJR* 1991;157:111–114.
19. Sovio OM, Bell HM, Beauchamp RD, Tredwell SJ. Fracture of the lumbar vertebral apophysis. *J Pediatr Orthop* 1985;5:550–552.
20. Sturn PF, Glass RBJ, Sivit CJ, Eichelberger MR. Lumbar compression fractures secondary to lap-belt use in children. *J Pediatr Orthop* 1995;15:521–523.
21. Swischuk LE. Spine and spinal cord trauma in battered child syndrome. *Radiology* 1969;92:733–738.
22. Swischuk LE, John SD, Allbery S. Disk degenerative disease in childhood: Scheuermann's disease, Schmorl's nodes, and the limbus vertebra. MRI findings in 12 patients. *Pediatr Radiol* 1998;28:334–338.
23. Taylor GA, Eggli KD. Lap-belt injuries of the lumbar spine in children: A pitfall of CT diagnosis. *AJR* 1988;150:1355–1358.
24. Walters G, Coumas JM, Akins CM, Ragland RL. Magnetic resonance imaging of acute symptomatic Schmorls' node formation. *Pediatr Emerg Care* 1991;7:294–296.

SACROCOCCYGEAL SPINE TRAUMA

Injuries of the coccyx are quite uncommon except in older children, who can fall on their buttocks; if the injury is severe enough, the lateral view demonstrates tilting of the fractured coccyx. Sacral fractures are dealt with in the section of this chapter covering pelvic injuries.

Normal Variations Causing Problems in the Thoracolumbar Spine

One of the most common normal variations causing problems is the normal ring epiphysis of the vertebral body (Fig.

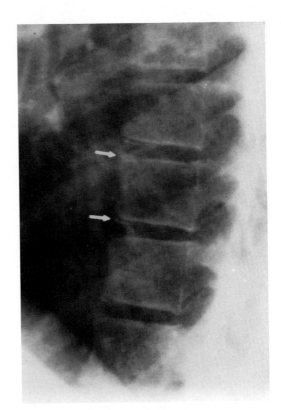

FIGURE 6.86. *Ring epiphyses.* Note the sliver-like appearance of the normal ring epiphyses of the vertebral bodies (*arrows*). These should not be misinterpreted as teardrop fractures.

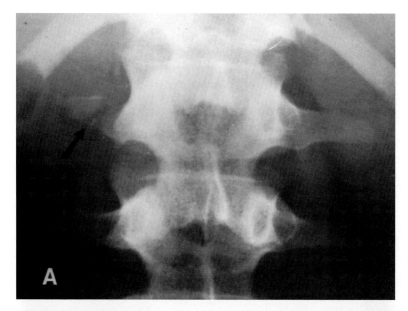

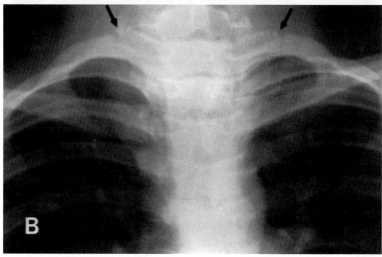

FIGURE 6.87. (A) *Rudimentary lumbar rib or bipartite transverse process (arrow). This finding should not be misinterpreted as a fracture.* (B) *Normal secondary ossification centers of the upper thoracic transverse processes (arrows).*

6.86). These ring-like growth plates of the vertebral bodies occur throughout the entire spine in childhood and to the uninitiated can suggest a corner, avulsion, teardrop, or limbus fracture. This, however, is not to say that the ring epiphysis is never involved in this type of fracture, however, because in children a portion of the ring epiphysis can be avulsed with certain flexion or extension injuries. In these cases, the ring-epiphysis fragment constitutes a true teardrop fracture (Fig. 6.84). If this occurs, however, it is not located in its normal place.

The ***apparent bipartite transverse process of a lumbar vertebra, which is really a rudimentary rib,*** can be misinterpreted as a fracture (Fig. 6.87A), and a similar problem can arise in the upper thoracic spine, in which ***accessory ossicles of the transverse processes*** also are prone to misinterpretation (Fig. 6.87B).

REFERENCES

1. Azouz EM, Kozlowski K, Marton D, Sprague P, Zerhouni A, Asselah F: Osteoid osteoma and osteoblastoma of the spine in children. *Pediatr Radiol* 1986;16:25–31.
2. Kricun R, Shoemaker EI, Chovanes GI, Stephens HW: Epidural abscess of the cervical spine: MR findings in five cases. *AJR* 1992; 158:1145–1149.
3. Schweich PJ, Hurt TL: Spinal epidural abscess in children: Two illustrative cases. *Pediatr Emerg Care* 1992;8:84–87.

MISCELLANEOUS PROBLEMS OF THE SPINE

Infections of the Spine

Generally speaking, infections of the spine consist of osteomyelitis and so-called "spondyloarthritis" or "discitis" of childhood (1,6). In all of these conditions, the hallmark of radiographic diagnosis is disc-space narrowing, with destruction of the two adjacent vertebral-body surfaces (Fig. 6.88). Most often these patients present with back pain, hip pain, or a limp, but abdominal pain also has been noted (3). The degree of systemic reaction is variable, and the underlying organism usually is *Staphylococcus aureus*. In some of

these cases, however, an infectious agent is not demonstrable, and this has prompted some to consider such cases traumatic rather than infectious in origin. Bone scanning is worthwhile for the detection of these infections (6), especially because the roentgenographic changes are somewhat late in onset (Fig. 6.88). CT and MR imaging (2,4, 5) also are excellent in demonstrating the disc and bony

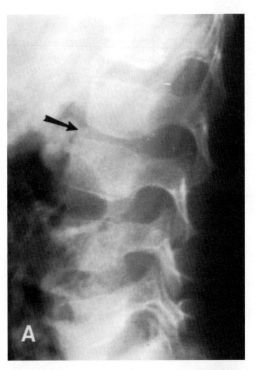

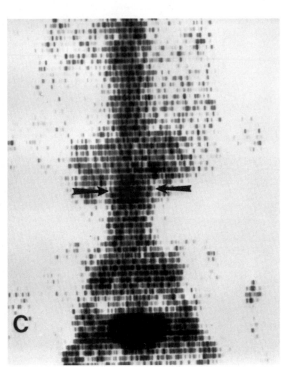

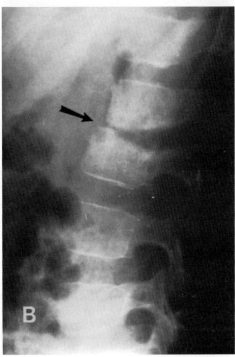

FIGURE 6.88. *Discitis or spondyloarthritis.* **(A)** Typical early changes consisting of disc-space narrowing only (*arrow*). **(B)** Two weeks later, note how much destruction has occurred at the site of infection (*arrow*). In addition, there has been some posterior displacement of the upper vertebral body. **(C)** Bone scan obtained after the first roentgenogram demonstrates increased activity over the lesion (*arrows*).

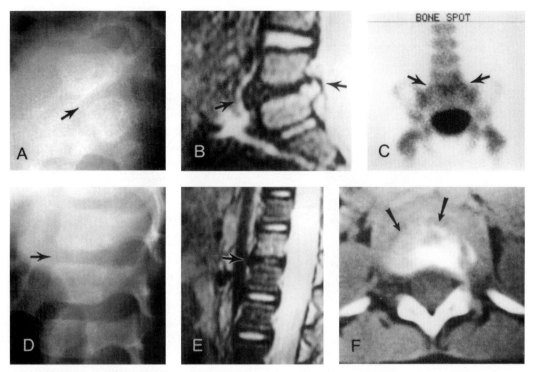

FIGURE 6.89. *Discitis: Magnetic resonance image and computed tomographic findings.* **(A)** Note subtle suggestion of narrowing of the disc space between L5 and S1 (*arrow*). **(B)** Sagittal T1-weighted magnetic resonance image demonstrates loss of signal in the disc, bulging of the ligament anteriorly (*anterior arrow*), and bulging of the posterior ligament with a portion of the disc protruding (*posterior arrow*) into the spinal canal. **(C)** Nuclear scintigraphy demonstrates increased activity at the L5-S1 level (*arrows*). **(D)** Another patient with virtually normal findings at the involved disc space (*arrow*). **(E)** Sagittal T2-weighted magnetic resonance study demonstrates loss of signal in the involved disc (*arrow*) and increased signal in the vertebral body above it. **(F)** Computed tomographic scan in another patient demonstrates vertebral body destruction (*arrows*).

changes, but MR imaging is probably the more informative of the two (Fig. 6.89). On MR imaging, the disc loses its normal signal, either in its entirety or in part. In addition, on T1-weighted images, signal loss often is seen in the vertebral bodies (Fig. 6.89). On T2-weighted images, there is increased signal in the involved areas of the vertebral bodies (Fig. 6.89). In some cases, disc material may herniate beyond the confines of the normal disc space. These herniations may be anterior or posterior (Fig. 6.89).

REFERENCES

1. Alexander CJ: The aetiology of juvenile spondyloarthritis (discitis). *Clin Radiol* 1970;21:178–187.
2. Forster A, Pothmann R, Winter K, Baumann-Rath CA: Magnetic resonance imaging in non-specific discitis. *Pediatr. Radiol* 1987;17: 162–163.
3. Leahy AL, Fogarty EE, Fitzgerald RJ, Regan BF: Diskitis as a cause of abdominal pain in children. *Surgery* 1984;95:412–414.
4. Sartoris DJ, Moskowitz PS, Kaufman RA, Ziprkowski MN, Berger PE: Childhood diskitis: Computed tomographic findings. *Radiology* 1983;149:701–708.
5. Szala, EA, Green NE, Heller RM, Horev G, Kirchner SG: Magnetic resonance imaging in the diagnosis of childhood discitis. *J Pediatr Orthop* 1987;7:164–167.
6. Wenger DR, Bobechko WP, Gilday DL: The spectrum of intervertebral disc-space infection in children. *J Bone Joint Surg* 1978; 60A:100–108.

Pathologic Fractures

Pathologic fractures of the spine are an occasional cause of acute back pain. The most commonly encountered condition is eosinophilic granuloma or histiocytosis X. Metastatic neuroblastoma, other metastatic disease, or underlying solitary primary bone lesions such as aneurysmal bone cysts or interosseous hemangiomas, however, also can lead to pathologic compression. Histiocytosis X and eosinophilic granuloma differ a little from the last conditions, in that they produce a very flat vertebra, the so-called vertebra plana (Fig. 6.90). Patients with leukemia or lymphoma also can present with compression fractures of the vertebrae, but most often these patients also are receiving steroid therapy. Compression fracture secondary to poorly mineralized bone such as might be seen with hyperparathyroidism, rickets,

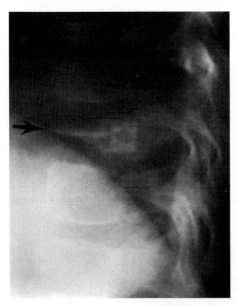

FIGURE 6.90. *Pathologic fracture of vertebral body.* Note typical flat vertebra (vertebra plana) associated with pathologic compression secondary to histiocytosis X (*arrow*).

and osteogenesis imperfecta also can be encountered, especially if the children with these conditions are active and ambulant.

The roentgenographic hallmark of all these fractures is loss of vertebral body height resulting from compression. The adjacent intervertebral discs, however, remain normal. This is a very important point, for the configuration is completely opposite to that which is seen with osteomyelitis or discitis. The only exception to this rule is coccidioidomycosis or other fungal disease, which can be associated with retention of the integrity of the disc space.

Calcified Intervertebral Discs

Commonly this condition occurs in the cervical spine (Fig. 6.91), but it also can be seen in the thoracic spine. Usually, it is associated with neck pain and stiffness, but the cause is unknown (1,2,5). There is debate as to whether the calcification results from trauma or inflammation, but even though no conclusive data to support either cause are currently available, inflammation seems more plausible. Systemic response in these patients is variable, and although some show signs of marked inflammation and muscle spasm, others are less symptomatic. Continuing observa-

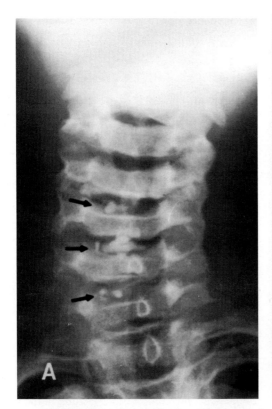
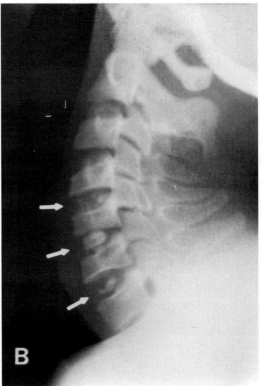

FIGURE 6.91. *Disc calcifications.* **(A)** Frontal view demonstrating acute scoliosis and multiple disc calcifications (*arrows*). This boy presented with acute neck pain and torticollis. **(B)** Lateral view demonstrating characteristic appearance of the calcified intervertebral discs (*arrows*). Note that the spine is normal in other respects.

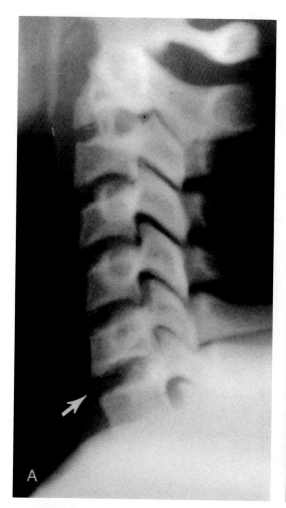
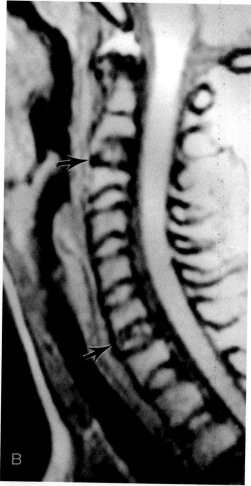

FIGURE 6.92. *Discitis: magnetic resonance findings.* **(A)** In this patient there is subtle widening of the disc space between C6 and C7 (*arrow*). In addition, there is some suggestion of widening of the disc space between C2 and C3. These findings are subtle. There is no evidence of calcification. **(B)** Proton-density magnetic resonance image demonstrates loss of signal in the disc space between C2 and C3 (*upper arrow*) and the disc space between C6 and C7 (*lower arrow*). The discs also are expanded. (From Swischuk LE, Stansberry SD: Calcific discitis: MRI changes in discs without visible calcification. *Pediatr Radiol* 1991;21:365–366, with permission.)

tion shows that these calcifications eventually disappear, and little in the way of residual vertebral bony change remains (7). In the interval, however, some of these discs have been noted to herniate and protrude either anteriorly or posteriorly (3,6). Of course, those protruding posteriorly do so into the spinal canal, but they do not seem to cause cord injury (3,6). MR imaging is useful in delineating this generally benign entity (4) and can show changes even before calcification occurs (7) (Fig. 6.92).

REFERENCES

1. Girodias J-B, Azouz EM, Marton D: Intervertebral disk space calcification: A report of 51 children with a review of the literature. *Pediatr Radiol* 1991;21:541–546.

2. Heinrich SD, Zembo MM, King AG, Zerkle AJ, MacEwen GD: Calcific cervical intervertebral disc herniation in children. *Spine* 1991;16:228–231.

3. Mainzer F: Herniation of the nucleus pulposus: A rare complication of intervertebral disk calcification in children. *Radiology* 1973; 107:167–170.

4. McGregor JC, Butler P: Disc calcification in childhood: Computed tomographic and magnetic resonance imaging appearances. *Br J Radiol* 1986;59:180.

5. Sonnabend DH, Taylor TKF, Chapman GK: Intervertebral disc calcification syndromes in children. *J Bone Joint Surg* 1982;64B: 25–31.

6. Sutton TJ, Turcotte B: Posterior herniation of calcified intervertebral discs in children. *Can J Assoc Radiol* 1973;24:131–136.

7. Swischuk LE, Stansberry SD: Calcific discitis: MRI changes in discs without visible calcification. *Pediatr Radiol* 1991;21: 365–366.

8. Urso S, Colajacomo M, Migliorini A, Fassari FM: Calcifying dis-

copathy in infancy in the cervical spine: Evaluation of vertebral alterations over a period of time. *Pediatr Radiol* 1987;17:387–391.

Spondylolysis and Spondylolisthesis

Generally not a cause of acute pain, spondylolysis occasionally can result from acute trauma. Nonetheless, most cases are chronic in nature, and generally accepted opinion is that most are acquired (1,4,6–8). In this regard, there is considerable feeling that the initial problem may be a fatigue fracture (8). Some familial tendency toward the problem has been documented (1), but most cases are sporadic. In support of a traumatic cause is the prevalence of the problem in adolescent athletes (2,5). In some cases the findings have been shown to be progressive (5).

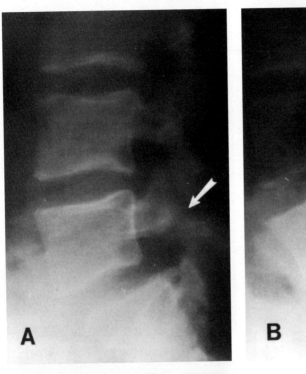

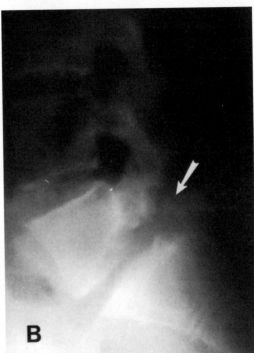

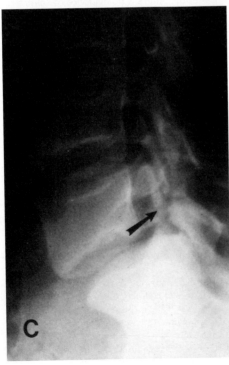

FIGURE 6.93. *Spondylolisthesis.* **(A)** Note typical spondylolysis (*arrow*) with minimal spondylolisthesis. **(B)** More extensive lytic changes producing a dysplastic appearance through the pedicle (*arrow*). Also note bone resorption along the posterior aspect of the vertebral bodies, some disc-space narrowing, and a spondylolisthesis of at least grade II (i.e., 50% or ½ of the vertebral body). **(C)** Acute spondylolysis in a patient with acute back pain who had been in a car accident. Note defect in the pedicle (*arrow*). On this oblique view, spondylolisthesis is suggested, but on true lateral view, none was present.

In early cases, the defect is rather straight and subtle (Fig. 6.93A), but later on, bony resorption occurs and a more dysplastic appearance results (Fig. 6.93B). This has prompted dividing the condition into those cases with a small defect and those with a dysplastic-appearing pedicle, but probably both represent different stages of abnormality in the same problem (1). Oblique views are very helpful in detecting this injury (3).

Spondylolysis usually is associated with spondylolisthesis (anterior displacement of the upper vertebral body) and spondylolisthesis generally is graded on the basis of degree of anterior slippage of the vertebral body. The grades usually run from I through IV and reflect anterior slippage as related to quarters of the underlying vertebral body (Fig. 6.93).

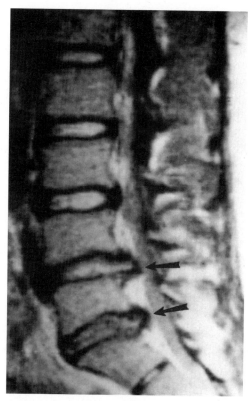

FIGURE 6.94. *Disc herniation: magnetic resonance findings.* Note posteriorly herniated discs at two levels (*arrows*). The disc spaces are irregular and the discs themselves have lost some signal.

REFERENCES

1. Abanese M, Pizzutillo PD: Family study of spondylolysis and spondylolisthesis. *J Pediatr Orthop* 1982;2:496–499.
2. Letts M, Smallman T, Afanasiev R, Gouw G: Fracture of the pars interarticularis in adolescent athletes: A clinical biomechanical analysis. *J Pediatr Orthop* 1986;6:40–46.
3. Libson E, Bloom RA, Dinari G, Robin GC: Oblique lumbar spine radiographs: Importance in young patients. *Radiology* 1984;151:89–90.
4. McKee BW, Alexander WJ, Dunbar JS: Spondylosis and spondylolisthesis in children. *Can J Assoc Radiol* 1971;22:100–109.
5. Muschik M, Hahnel H, Robinson PN, Perka C, Muxchik C: Competitive sports and the progression of spondylolisthesis. *J Pediatr Orthop* 1996;16:364–369.
6. Oakley RH, Carty H: Review of spondylolisthesis and spondylolysis in paediatric practice. *Br J Radiol* 1984;57:877–885.
7. Wertzberger J, Peterson H: Acquired spondylolysis and spondylolisthesis in the young child. *Spine* 1980;5:437.
8. White LL, Widell EH, Jackson DW: Fatigue fracture: The basic lesion in isthmic spondylolisthesis. *J Bone Joint Surg* 1975;57A:17–22.

Intervertebral Disc Herniation

Disc herniations are extremely uncommon in infants and young children but are not so uncommon in the active adolescent (1–6). Clinically, often the same problem arises as in adults: If a disk protrusion is present, it may or may not be symptomatic or even responsible for the symptoms in the patients (3).

Roentgenographically, there is little to see except for muscle spasm causing straightening or curvature of the spine. For the most part, these patients require CT scanning or MR imaging for final diagnosis (Fig. 6.94). In some cases disc herniation is associated with fractures of the ring epiphysis (1).

REFERENCES

1. Banerian KG, Wang A.-MF, Samberg LC, Kerr HH, Wesolowski DP: Association of vertebral end plate fracture with pediatric lumbar intervertebral disk herniation: Value of CT and MR imaging. *Radiology* 1990;177:763–765.
2. Clarke NMP, Cleak DK: Intervertebral lumbar disc prolapse in children and adolescents. *J Pediatr Orthop* 1983;3:202–206.
3. Erkintalo MO, Salminen JJ, Alanen AM, Paajanen HEK, Kormano MJ: Development of degenerative changes in the lumbaar intervertebral disk: Results of a prospective MR imaging study in adolescents with and without low-back pain. *Radiology* 1995;196:529–533.
4. Hashimoto K, Fujita K, Kojimoto H, Shimomura Y: Lumbar disc herniation in children. *J Pediatr Orthop* 1990;10:394–396.
5. Kurihara A, Kataoka O: Lumbar disk herniation in children and adolescents. *Spine* 1980;5:443.
6. Zamani MH, MacEwen GD: Herniation of the lumbar disc in children and adolescents. *J Pediatr Orthop* 1982;2:528–533.

Miscellaneous Thoracolumbar Spine Problems

Occasionally patients present to the trauma center with intraspinal or bony tumors. These are relatively rare, however, and a complete discussion of them is beyond the scope of this book. Similarly, patients may present with spinal epidural abscesses. Metastatic disease leading to vertebral compression has been discussed elsewhere. Almost invariably, spine and spinal cord lesions such as those just mentioned are best evaluated with MR imaging. Plain-film findings usually are absent with epidural abscesses; with bony tumors they usually are present. With intraspinal tumors, the plain films may be normal or may show evidence of intracannulicular expansion consisting of scalloping of the posterior vertebral bodies and erosion of the medial aspects of the pedicles.

SUBJECT INDEX

Note: Page number followed by f refer to figures; page numbers followed by t refer to tables.

A

Abdomen, 146–289. *See also specific organs and disorders*
  abscess of, 169–173, 170f, 171f, 172f, 173f
    CT of, 172, 172f
    vs. normal findings, 287, 287f
    ultrasound of, 172, 172f
  acute, 149
    pneumonia and, 173–174, 173f, 174f
    systemic disease and, 217
  airless, 149, 150f
    in appendicitis, 177, 178f
    in gastroenteritis, 175, 176f
  calcifications of, 279–280, 280f
  distension of, 165, 166f
  extraluminal gas in, abnormal patterns of, 155–162. *See also specific disorders*
  fluid collections in, 165–169, 166f, 167f, 168f
  inflammatory disorders of, 173–217. *See also Appendicitis*
  intraluminal gas in, abnormal patterns of, 149–155, 151f, 152f, 153f, 154f
  masses of, 276–278, 277f
  normal, 146–149, 287–289, 287f, 288f
    CT of, 146, 148f
    plain film of, 146, 146f
    ultrasound of, 146, 147f
  in systemic disease, 217
  trauma to, 243–263. *See also specific organs*
    in battered child syndrome, 262–263, 262f, 263f
    CT in, 243–244, 244f
    hemoperitoneum with, 169
    periportal fluid tracking in, 244, 244f
    shock in, 244, 244f
    vascular, 262
Abscess
  abdominal, 169–173, 170f, 171f, 172f, 173f
    CT of, 172, 172f
    vs. normal findings, 287, 287f
    ultrasound of, 172, 172f
  amebic, 169, 172–173, 173f
  in appendicitis, 185, 185f, 186f, 187f, 189, 192, 192f
  of brain, 526, 527f–528f
  epidural, 526, 528f
  hepatic, 169, 170f–171f, 172–173, 173f
  intestinal, in battered child syndrome, 262, 263f
  pancreatic, 203, 203f
  perinephric, 171, 209f
  psoas, 171–172, 172f, 278, 279f
  pulmonary, 70f, 71
  pyogenic, 169

renal, 210, 210f
retropharyngeal, 134–137, 135f, 136f, 137f
  CT in, 135, 136f, 137t
  ultrasound in, 135, 136f
soft tissue, 473, 474f–475f
subphrenic, 171, 171f
testicular, 282, 284f
tuboovarian, 212, 213f, 214f
Acetabulum
  fracture of, 374–377, 375f, 376f–377f, 388–389
  normal, 385, 385f, 399f
Achilles tendonitis, 445, 446f
Acid ingestion, 263–264
Acidosis, chest film in, 111f, 112
Acromioclavicular separation, 309, 309f
Acromium, fracture of, in battered child syndrome, 315f, 466–467, 467f
Actinomycosis, 39, 39f
Acute chest syndrome, 110, 111f
Adenitis
  epitrochlear, 344, 344f
  mesenteric, 195–200. *See also Mesenteric adenitis*
Adenoids, 536, 537f
Adrenal gland
  calcification in, 280, 280f
  trauma to, 261, 261f
Adult respiratory distress syndrome, pulmonary edema and, 80f, 81
Airless abdomen, 149, 150f
  in appendicitis, 177, 178f
  in gastroenteritis, 175, 176f
Airway (upper). *See also Lungs; Respiratory tract*
  displacement of, prevertebral soft-tissue swelling and, 536, 537f
  normal, 119–121, 119f, 120f
  obstruction of, 121–129
    angioneurotic edema and, 132, 133f
    chest film in, 130
    in croup, 124–129, 125f, 126f, 127f, 128f
    in epiglottitis, 122–123, 122f, 123f, 124f
    foreign bodies in, 130–132, 130f, 131f, 132f
    laryngeal trauma and, 132, 133f
    pulmonary edema and, 130
    stridor with, 121–122, 121f
    in uvulitis, 129, 129f
    vascular rings in, 132, 134f
  poor film of, 119, 120f
Alkaline disk battery, ingestion of, 264
Allergic pneumonitis, 109–110, 110f
Aluminum foil, in trachea, 131f
Amebic abscess, 169, 172–173, 173f
Ammonium hydroxide, ingestion of, 263
Angiofibroma, nasopharyngeal, 143f–144f
Angioneurotic edema, stridor with, 132, 133f

Ankle, 436–453. *See also* Fibula, distal; Tarsal bones; Tibia, distal
  accessory ossicles of, 448, 450f–451f
  buckle fracture of, 436, 437f
  edema of, 448, 449f
  epiphyseal–metaphyseal fracture of, 436–440, 438f, 439f, 440f
  eversion injury to, 440, 440f, 441f
  fat pads of, 436, 436f
  fluid in, 292t, 436, 436f, 437f
  inversion-rotation injury to, 439–440, 439f–440f
  normal, 448, 450f–451f, 451–453, 452f
  osteomyelitis of, 448, 449f–450f
  septic arthritis of, 448, 448f
  sprain of, 445
  teardrop sign in, 436, 437f
  tendonitis of, 445, 446f
Antacid, bismuth-containing, in gastroenteritis, 271, 272f
Anterior cruciate ligament, avulsions of, 405–406, 405f–406f, 407f
Anterior humeral line, in elbow fracture, 324, 324f
Aorta, trauma to, 97, 101–102, 102f
Apnea, cervical spine injury and, 578
Apophyseal joints
  abnormal configurations of, 543, 543f–544f
  dislocation of, 549, 550f
  fanned, 544f
Appendices epiploicae
  idiopathic infarction of, 202
  torsion of, 202
Appendicitis, 177–194
  air in, 180, 181f
  airless abdomen in, 177, 178f
  clinical findings in, 177
  color flow Doppler in, 188, 189f
  compression in, 185
  vs. Crohn's disease, 201, 201f
  CT in, 192–192, 192f, 193f
  gangrenous, 188, 188f
  vs. gastroenteritis, 175f, 177, 179f
  lymphadenopathy in, 180, 189, 190f, 196
  vs. Meckel's diverticulitis, 201
  vs. mesenteric adenitis, 195–200. *See also Mesenteric adenitis*
  perforation in, 177, 179f, 181–185
    abscess with, 185, 185f, 186f, 187f, 189, 192, 192f
    colon cutoff sign with, 181–182, 182f, 183f
    fecalith with, 179f, 180–181, 182f, 183f, 185f, 186f, 188, 189f
    flank-stripe sign in, 186f
    free peritoneal fluid with, 189, 191f
    functional obstruction with, 182, 184f